INTERNAL MEDICINE ON CALL

INTERNAL MEDICINE ON CALL

Second Edition

Edited by

Steven A. Haist, MD, MS
Associate Professor of Medicine
Division of General Internal Medicine and Geriatrics
Department of Internal Medicine
University of Kentucky Medical Center
Lexington, Kentucky

John B. Robbins, MD
General Internist
Private Practice
Gallatin Internal Medicine Clinic
Bozeman, Montana

Series Editor

Leonard G. Gomella, MD
The Bernard W. Godwin, Jr. Associate Professor of
    Prostate Cancer
Department of Urology
Jefferson Medical College
Thomas Jefferson University Medical Center
Philadelphia, Pennsylvania

APPLETON & LANGE
Stamford, Connecticut

Notice: The authors and the publisher of this volume have taken care to make certain that the doses of drugs and schedules of treatment are correct and compatible with the standards generally accepted at the time of publication. Nevertheless, as new information becomes available, changes in treatment and in the use of drugs become necessary. The reader is advised to carefully consult the instruction and information material included in the package insert of each drug or therapeutic agent before administration. This advice is especially important when using, administering, or recommending new or infrequently used drugs. The authors and publisher disclaim all responsibility for any liability, loss, injury, or damage incurred as a consequence, directly or indirectly, of the use and application of any of the contents of this volume.

Prentice Hall International (UK) Limited, *London*
Prentice Hall of Australia Pty. Limited, *Sydney*
Prentice Hall Canada, Inc., *Toronto*
Prentice Hall Hispanoamericana, S.A., *Mexico*
Prentice Hall of India Private Limited, *New Delhi*
Prentice Hall of Japan, Inc., *Tokyo*
Simon & Schuster Asia Pte. Ltd., *Singapore*
Editora Prentice Hall do Brasil Ltda., *Rio de Janeiro*
Prentice Hall, *Upper Saddle River, New Jersey*

ISBN: 0-8385-4056-2
ISSN: 1052-6854

Acquisitions Editor: Shelley Reinhardt
Managing Editor, Development: Gregory R. Huth
Production Editor: Chris Langan
Designer: Mary Skudlarek
Senior Art Manager: Eve Siegel

Dedicated to our patients, students, and mentors, who through the years have taught us the art of medicine.

Contents

Contributors

Jerri L. Alley, MD
Intern
Department of Dermatology
University of Arkansas for Medical Sciences
Little Rock, Arkansas
(Coma, Acute Mental Status Changes; Dysuria; Headache)

James A. Barker, MD
Scott & White Clinic
Assistant Professor
Pulmonary & Critical Care Medicine
Texas A & M College of Medicine
Temple, Texas
(Cough; Hemoptysis; Wheezing; Ventilator Management)

David J. Bensema, MD
General Internist
Private Practice
Creekside Internal Medicine
Lexington, Kentucky
(Hematuria; Insomnia; Syncope)

Karen M. Blumenschein, PharmD
Assistant Professor
College of Pharmacy
University of Kentucky Medical Center
Lexington, Kentucky
(Section V, Multiple Problems)

Marianne Billeter, PharmD
Assistant Professor of Clinical Pharmacy
College of Pharmacy
Xavier University of Louisiana
New Orleans, Louisiana
(Commonly Used Medications)

Larry T. Breeding, MD
Fellow
Division of Cardiology
Department of Internal Medicine
University of Kentucky Medical Center
Lexington, Kentucky
(Pacemaker Problems)

John S. Bruner, MD
Intern
Department of Obstetrics and Gynecology
Greenville Memorial Hospital
Greenville, South Carolina
(Dyspnea; Hypernatremia; Hyponatremia)

David W. Dozer, MD
Gastroenterologist
Private Practice
Milwaukee Digestive Diseases Consultants, S.P.
Milwaukee, Wisconsin
(Diarrhea; Nausea and Vomiting)

Rita M. Egan, MD, PhD
Assistant Professor of Medicine
Division of Rheumatology
Department of Internal Medicine
University of Kentucky Medical Center
Lexington, Kentucky
(Joint Swelling; Arthrocentesis)

Kim R. Emmett, MD
Assistant Professor
Division of General Internal Medicine and Geriatrics
Department of Internal Medicine
University of Kentucky Medical Center
Lexington, Kentucky
(Falls)

G. Paul Eleazer, MD
Associate Professor of Medicine
Department of Internal Medicine
University of South Carolina
Columbia, South Carolina
(Hyperglycemia; Hypoglycemia; Hypomagnesemia)

Douglas L. Fraker, MD
Associate Professor of Surgery
Head, Division of Surgical Oncology
University of Pennsylvania School of Medicine
Philadelphia, Pennsylvania

Amiee Gelhot, PharmD
Ambulatory Care Specialist
Assistant Professor
College of Pharmacy
University of Kentucky
Lexington, Kentucky
(Commonly Used Medications)

David K. Goebel, MD
Hematologist/Oncologist
Private Practice
Tri-State Regional Cancer Center
Ashland, Kentucky
(Leukopenia)

John J. Gohmann, MD
Medical Oncologist
Private Practice
Central Baptist Hospital
Lexington, Kentucky
(Leukocytosis)

Tricia L. Gomella, MD
Neonatal Consultant
Division of Neonatology
Department of Pediatrics
Francis Scott Key Medical Center
Baltimore, Maryland

C. Gary Grigsby, Jr., MD
Cardiologist
Private Practice
Lexington, Kentucky
(Arterial Line Placement; Arterial Puncture)

Steven A. Haist, MD, MS
Associate Professor of Medicine
Division of General Internal Medicine and Geriatrics
Department of Internal Medicine
University of Kentucky Medical Center
Lexington, Kentucky
(Acidosis; Alkalosis; Delirium Tremens; Hypercalcemia; Oliguria and Anuria; Seizures; Laboratory Diagnosis; Paracentesis; Commonly Used Medications)

David P. Haynie, MD
Cardiovascular Specialist PA
Private Practice
Lewisville, Texas
(Bradycardia; Irregular Pulse; Tachycardia)

William J. John, MD
Assistant Professor of Medicine
Division of Hematology and Oncology
Department of Internal Medicine
University of Kentucky Medical Center
Lexington, Kentucky
(Hematemesis and Melena; Jaundice; Hematochezia; Gastrointestinal Tubes)

Ross E. Kerns, MD
Hematologist-Oncologist
Private Practice
Knoxville, Tennessee
(Coagulopathy)

Alan T. Lefor, MD
Associate Professor of Surgery and Oncology
Department of Surgery and the University of Maryland Cancer Center
University of Maryland School of Medicine
Baltimore, Maryland

Jerry J. Lierl, MD
Cardiologist
Private Practice
Cardiology Associates
Crestview Hill, Kentucky
(Central Venous Line Problems; Central Venous Catheterization)

Shantae L. Lucas, MD
Fellow
Division of Hematology and Oncology
Department of Internal Medicine
University of Kentucky Medical Center
Lexington, Kentucky
(Fever in the HIV Patient)

Ralph A. Manchester, MD
Medical Chief
University Health Service
Associate Professor of Medicine
General Medicine Unit
Department of Medicine
University of Rochester School of Medicine and Dentistry
Rochester, New York
(Hypocalcemia; Hypophosphatemia)

Rick R. McClure, MD, FACC
Cardiologist
Cardiovascular Consultants, PSC
Private Practice
Lexington, Kentucky
(Hypotension)

Thomas B. Montgomery, MD
Section of General Internal Medicine
Department of Medicine
Tulane University Medical Center
New Orleans, Louisiana
(Fever; Hypertension; Hypothermia)

Rita K. Munn, MD
Assistant Professor
Division of Hematology and Oncology
Department of Internal Medicine
University of Kentucky Medical Center
Lexington, Kentucky
*(Anemia; Polycythemia; Transfusion Reaction; Bone Marrow
Aspiration and Biopsy; Blood Component Therapy)*

Carol B. Peddicord, MD
General Internist
Private Practice
Albany, Kentucky
(Chest Pain)

John B. Robbins, MD
General Internist
Private Practice
Gallatin Internal Medicine Clinic
Bozeman, Montana
*(Abdominal Pain; Anaphylactic Reaction; Aspiration; Arterial Line
Problems; Cardiopulmonary Arrest; Foley Catheter Problems;
Heart Murmur; Pain Management; Pulmonary Artery Catheter
Problems; Thrombocytopenia; Bladder Catheterization; Endo-
trachial Intubation; Intravenous Techniques; Lumbar Puncture;
Pulmonary Artery Catheterization; Skin Biopsy; Thoracentesis;
Fluid and Electrolytes)*

Steven I. Shedlofsky, MD
Professor of Medicine
Division of Digestive Diseases and Nutrition
Department of Internal Medicine
University of Kentucky Medical Center
and Veteran's Administration Hospital
Lexington, Kentucky
(Laboratory Diagnosis; Hepatitis)

Benjamin J. Stahr, MD, FCAP
Pathologist
Greensboro Pathology Associates
Moses H. Cone Memorial Hospital
Greensboro, North Carolina
(Laboratory Diagnosis)

R. Douglas Strickland, MD
Gastroenterologist
Private Practice
Holston Valley Hospital
Gastroenterology Associates
Kingsport, Tennessee
(Constipation)

Eric C. Westman, MD, MHS
Assistant Professor
Division of General Internal Medicine
Department of Medicine
Duke University Medical Center
Durham, North Carolina
(Phlebitis)

Eric A. Wiebke, MD
Assistant Professor
Department of Surgery
Indiana University College of Medicine
Indianapolis, Indiana

Timothy A. Winchester, MD
General Internist
Private Practice
Creekside Internal Medicine
Lexington, Kentucky
(Hyperkalemia; Hypokalemia)

Preface

The second edition of *Internal Medicine on Call* is a user-friendly reference that will assist in the initial evaluation and treatment of the most frequently encountered problems in internal medicine. It will serve as an aid to house officers and medical students when they are called about medical problems, whether common or potentially life-threatening. *Internal Medicine on Call* provides a concise and practical approach to these problems and serves to bridge the gap between textbooks and patient care. Unlike many books or manuals, *Internal Medicine on Call* is organized by the presenting problem or complaint rather than the diagnosis. We have not attempted to provide a comprehensive discussion, but rather the essential elements in the initial assessment and management of each problem. This will aid the house officer or student when called to evaluate a patient with a specific problem.

Each on-call problem is introduced with a case scenario. This is followed by the questions the clinician should initally ask. A differential diagnosis is given with key points to help one arrive at the final diagnosis. A database section includes key points on the physical examination and laboratory and other tests that are important in making the diagnosis. A plan for the treatment of specific diagnoses is also included. Recommendations for treatment are specific with regard to dosage and dosing intervals, but it is emphasized that hepatic and renal disease as well as other factors (eg, age) can greatly affect the metabolism of drugs. In addition, variations in institutional practices exist. For these reasons, treatment may need to be individualized from patient to patient or from institution to institution.

House officers and medical students often have questions regarding frequently used medications, laboratory tests, procedures including step-by-step instruction, as well as indications and contraindications. These areas, as well as ventilator management and transfusion therapy, have been included to provide house officers and medical students a manual to answer many of the questions that arise in the day-to-day care of their patient.

We are grateful to Tricia Gomella, MD, for providing the "on-call" concept originally used in her book *Neonatology: Basic Management, On Call Problems, Diseases, and Drugs*, published by Appleton & Lange in 1988. We thank Appleton & Lange for providing us the forum to present a unique approach for medical student and house officer education. In particular, we want to thank Rebecca J. Frey, M Div, our copy editor, whose diligence and eye for detail has helped us improve the quality of the second edition of *Internal Medicine on Call*.

Finally, we want to thank Susan Brodie, Robin Lavy, and Nancy Brigham, PhD, for their efforts in the completion of this book. Without their assistance and support, the completion of this manual would not have been possible.

We sincerely hope that this manual will enhance your training and help you to provide the best care for your patients.

Steven A. Haist, MD
Lexington, Kentucky
John B. Robbins, MD
Bozeman, Montana

October, 1996

I. On Call Problems

1. ABDOMINAL PAIN

I. Problem. A 34-year-old woman admitted for control of her diabetes develops acute abdominal pain that increases in severity over several hours.

II. Immediate Questions

A. What are the patient's vital signs? Acute abdominal pain may signify a condition as benign as gastroenteritis or as catastrophic as an infarcted bowel or perforated viscus. The significant morbidity and mortality of the acute surgical abdomen can be obviated by early diagnosis. *Tachycardia* and *hypotension* would suggest circulatory or septic shock from perforation, hemorrhage, or fluid loss into the intestinal lumen or peritoneal cavity. Orthostatic blood pressure and pulse changes would also be helpful in ascertaining the presence of volume loss. *Fever* occurs in inflammatory conditions such as cholecystitis and appendicitis. When the temperature exceeds 102°F, gangrene or perforation of a viscus should be suspected. Fever may not be present in elderly patients, patients on corticosteroids, or patients who are immunocompromised.

B. Where is the pain located? Abdominal pain is produced by three mechanisms: (1) *tension* within the walls of the alimentary tract (biliary or intestinal obstruction); (2) *ischemia* (strangulated bowel, mesenteric vascular occlusion); and (3) *peritoneal irritation*. The first two causes result in visceral pain, a dull pain perceived in the midline and *poorly localized*. Generally, *midepigastric pain* is caused by disorders of the stomach, duodenum, pancreas, liver, and biliary tract. Disease of the small intestine, appendix, upper ureters, testes, and ovaries results in *periumbilical pain*. *Lower abdominal pain* is caused by processes in the colon, bladder, lower ureters, and uterus. Inflammation of the parietal peritoneum results in more severe pain that is *well localized* to the area of inflammation.

C. Does the pain radiate? Pain that becomes rapidly generalized implies perforation and leakage of fluid into the peritoneal cavity. Biliary pain can radiate from the right upper quadrant to the right inferior scapula. Pancreatic and abdominal aneurysmal pain may radiate to the back. Ureteral colic may be referred to the groin and thigh.

D. When did the pain begin? Sudden onset suggests perforated ulcer, mesenteric occlusion, ruptured aneurysm, or ruptured ectopic pregnancy. A more gradual onset (>1 hour) implies an inflammatory condition such as appendicitis or cholecystitis or an obstructed viscus such as bowel obstruction.

E. What is the quality of the pain? Intestinal colic occurs as cramping abdominal pain interspersed with pain-free intervals. Biliary colic is not a true colicky pain in that it usually presents as sustained, persistent pain. Unfortunately, the terms *sharp, dull, burning,* and *tearing,* although used by patients to describe pain, seldom assist in determining the etiology.

F. What relieves the pain or makes it worse? Pain with deep inspiration is associated with diaphragmatic irritation, such as with pleurisy or upper abdominal inflammation. Patients with intestinal or ureteral colic tend to be restless and active, whereas patients with peritonitis attempt to avoid all motion. Coughing frequently exacerbates abdominal pain from peritonitis.

G. Are there any associated symptoms? *Vomiting* may result from intestinal obstruction or may result from a visceral reflex caused by pain. In conditions causing an acute surgical abdomen, the vomiting usually follows rather than precedes the onset of pain. *Hematemesis* suggests gastritis or peptic ulcer disease. *Diarrhea* may result from gastroenteritis, but may also result from ischemic colitis or inflammatory bowel disease. *Obstipation* (absence of passage of stool or flatus) suggests mechanical bowel obstruction. *Hematuria* would suggest genitourinary disease such as nephrolithiasis. *Cough* and *sputum* production might occur if lower lobe pneumonia is present.

H. If female, what is the patient's menstrual history? A missed period in a sexually active woman would suggest ectopic pregnancy. A foul vaginal discharge might indicate pelvic inflammatory disease.

I. What is the patient's past medical history? Does the patient have a history of peptic ulcer disease, gallstones, alcohol abuse, abdominal operations suggesting adhesions, or an abdominal aortic aneurysm? Is there any known history of cardiac arrhythmias or other cardiac disease that could result in embolization to a mesenteric artery?

III. Differential Diagnosis. There are several potential causes of acute abdominal pain, some of which are listed in Table 1–1. Many of these diseases can be managed medically; others require urgent surgery. Abdominal pain can result from extra-abdominal processes as well as intra-abdominal disease.

A. Intra-abdominal disease

1. Hollow viscera. Perforation of a hollow viscus represents a surgical emergency.

a. Upper abdomen: Esophagitis, gastritis, peptic ulcer disease, cholecystitis.

b. Midgut: Small bowel obstruction or infarction.

TABLE 1–1. COMMON CAUSES OF ACUTE ABDOMEN: CONDITIONS IN ITALIC TYPE OFTEN REQUIRE SURGERY

■ **Gastrointestinal tract disorders**
  Appendicitis
  Small and large bowel obstruction
  Strangulated hernia
  Perforated peptic ulcer
  Bowel perforation
  Meckel's diverticulitis
  Boerhaave's syndrome
  Diverticulitis
  Inflammatory bowel disorders
  Mallory-Weiss syndrome
  Gastroenteritis
  Acute gastritis
  Mesenteric adenitis

■ **Liver, spleen, and biliary tract disorders**
  Acute cholecystitis
  Acute cholangitis
  Hepatic abscess
  Ruptured hepatic tumor
  Spontaneous rupture of the spleen
  Splenic infarct
  Biliary colic
  Acute hepatitis

■ **Pancreatic disorders**
  Acute pancreatitis

■ **Urinary tract disorders**
  Ureteral or renal colic
  Acute pyelonephritis
  Acute cystitis
  Renal infarct

■ **Gynecologic disorders**
  Ruptured ectopic pregnancy
  Twisted ovarian tumor
  Ruptured ovarian follicle cyst
  Acute salpingitis
  Dysmenorrhea
  Endometriosis

■ **Vascular disorders**
  Ruptured aortic and visceral aneurysms
  Acute ischemic colitis
  Mesenteric thrombosis

■ **Peritoneal disorders**
  Intra-abdominal abscesses
  Primary peritonitis
  Tuberculous peritonitis

■ **Retroperitoneal disorders**
  Retroperitoneal hemorrhage

Boey JH: Acute abdomen, In Way LW, Ed. Current Surgical Diagnosis and Treatment. 1988.

    c. Lower abdomen: Inflammatory bowel disease, appendicitis, large bowel obstruction, diverticulitis.
  2. Solid organ
    a. Hepatitis
    b. Pancreatitis
    c. Splenic infarction
    d. Pyelonephritis/Urolithiasis
  3. Pelvis
    a. Pelvic inflammatory disease
    b. Ruptured ectopic pregnancy
  4. Vascular system
    a. Ruptured aneurysm
    b. Dissecting aneurysm
    c. Mesenteric thrombosis or embolism
 B. Extra-abdominal disease. These causes of acute abdominal pain should be considered to spare the patient unnecessary surgery.
  1. Diabetic ketoacidosis
  2. Acute adrenal insufficiency
  3. Acute porphyria

4. **Pneumonia involving lower lobes**
5. **Pulmonary embolism involving lower lobes**
6. **Pneumothorax**
7. **Sickle cell crisis**

IV. Database

A. Physical examination key points (See Table 1–2.)

1. **Vital signs** (See Section II.A.)
2. **Lungs.** Percuss for dullness at the bases which would suggest a pleural effusion or consolidation. In addition to dullness, the presence of crackles or bronchial breath sounds suggests a pneumonia, infarction, or atelectasis associated with decreased inspiratory effort because of pain.
3. **Heart.** Look for jugular venous distension, S_3 gallop, or a displaced point of maximal impulse indicative of congestive heart failure that might predispose to passive congestion of the liver or mesenteric ischemia. An irregular pulse could indicate atrial fibrillation which might result in mesenteric artery embolism.
4. **Abdomen**
   a. **Inspection.** Examine for the presence of distension (obstruction, ileus, ascites), ecchymoses (hemorrhagic pancreatitis), caput medusae (portal hypertension), and surgical scars.

TABLE 1–2. PHYSICAL FINDINGS WITH VARIOUS CAUSES OF ACUTE ABDOMEN.[1]

Condition	Signs
Perforated viscus	Scaphoid, tense abdomen; diminished bowel sounds (late); loss of liver dullness; guarding or rigidity
Peritonitis	Motionless, absent bowel sounds (late); rebound tenderness; guarding or rigidity
Inflamed mass or abscess	Tender mass (abdominal, rectal, or pelvic); punch tenderness; special signs (Murphy's, psoas, or obturator)
Intestinal obstruction	Distension; visible peristalsis (late); hyperperistalsis (early) or quiet abdomen (late); diffuse pain without rebound tenderness; hernia or rectal mass (some)
Paralytic ileus	Distension; minimal bowel sounds; no localized tenderness
Ischemic or strangulated bowel	Not distended (until late); bowel sounds variable; severe pain but little tenderness; rectal bleeding (some)
Bleeding	Pallor, shock; distension; pulsatile (aneurysm) or tender (eg, ectopic pregnancy) mass; rectal bleeding (some)

[1] Reproduced with permission from Boey, JH: Acute abdomen, In Way LW, ed. *Current Surgical Diagnosis and Treatment.* 10th ed. Appleton & Lange; 1994.

b. **Auscultation.** Listen for bowel sounds (absent or occasional tinkle with ileus, hyperperistaltic with gastroenteritis, high-pitched rushes with small bowel obstruction).

c. **Percussion.** Tympany is associated with distended loops of bowel. Shifting dullness and a fluid wave suggest the presence of ascites. Loss of liver dullness may occur if a viscus has ruptured and free air has entered the abdominal cavity.

d. **Palpation.** Involuntary guarding, rigidity, and rebound tenderness are hallmarks of peritonitis. Localized tenderness and guarding suggest perforation with spillage of gastrointestinal contents into the peritoneal cavity. Costovertebral angle tenderness is common with pyelonephritis. **Murphy's sign** is inspiratory arrest on palpation of the gall bladder and is seen with acute cholecystitis. Pain with active hip flexion or with extension of the patient's right thigh while lying on the left side (**psoas sign**) could result from an inflamed appendix. The **obturator sign** (pain on internal rotation of the flexed thigh) can occur with appendicitis.

5. **Rectum.** Evaluation of acute abdominal pain is not complete until a rectal exam has been performed. A mass could suggest the presence of rectal carcinoma. Lateral rectal tenderness occurs with appendicitis, a condition in which examination of the abdomen may not reveal localized findings. If stool is present, evaluate for occult blood.

6. **Female genitalia.** Examine for pain with cervical motion and cervical discharge that may suggest pelvic inflammatory disease. Also palpate for adnexal masses that would indicate an ectopic pregnancy, ovarian abscess, cyst, or neoplasm.

B. **Laboratory data.** The decision to operate on a patient with acute abdominal pain is seldom made solely on the basis of laboratory data. This information serves mainly as an adjunct in those cases in which the etiology of the pain is not clear, or to assist preoperative assessment in those individuals for whom the diagnosis is certain and the decision to perform surgery has already been made.

1. **Hematology.** An increased hematocrit suggests hemoconcentration from volume loss. A low hematocrit may suggest a process that has resulted in chronic blood loss, or possibly acute intra-abdominal hemorrhage or an acute gastrointestinal hemorrhage. With acute blood loss, however, the hematocrit may not decrease for several hours. An elevated white blood cell count (WBC) suggests an inflammatory process such as appendicitis or cholecystitis.

2. **Electrolytes, blood urea nitrogen (BUN), creatinine.** Bowel obstruction with vomiting can result in hypokalemia, azotemia, and volume contraction alkalosis. A strangulated bowel or sepsis may result in a metabolic gap acidosis.

3. **Liver function tests including bilirubin, transaminases, and alkaline phosphatase.** These may be elevated in acute hepatitis, cholecystitis, and other liver diseases.
4. **Amylase.** Markedly elevated levels are associated with pancreatitis. However, in up to 30% of patients with acute pancreatitis, amylase may be initially normal, especially in patients with lipemic serum. Conversely, amylase can also be elevated in conditions other than pancreatitis; such as acute cholecystitis, perforated ulcer, small bowel obstruction with strangulation, and ruptured ectopic pregnancy.
5. **Arterial blood gases (ABG).** Hypoxemia is often an early sign of sepsis and may occur with pancreatitis. As mentioned, metabolic acidosis may result from ischemic bowel or sepsis.
6. **Pregnancy test.** All premenopausal women with acute right or left lower abdominal pain should be tested for human chorionic gonadotropin (HCG) to rule out ectopic pregnancy whether or not they missed their last period.
7. **Urinalysis.** Hematuria may indicate nephrolithiasis; pyuria and hematuria can be present in urinary tract infections. In addition, pyuria is occasionally present with appendicitis.
8. **Cervical culture.** Obtain a cervical culture for chlamydia and gonorrhea when pelvic inflammatory disease (PID) is suspected.

C. **Radiology and other studies**
1. **Flat & upright abdominal films.** These films can be readily obtained and may provide important information. Watch for the following indicators: gas pattern; evidence of bowel dilation; air-fluid levels; presence or absence of air in the rectum; pancreatic calcifications; biliary and renal calcifications; aortic calcifications; loss of psoas margin (suggesting retroperitoneal bleeding); and presence or absence of air in the biliary tract.
2. **Chest film.** A CXR may reveal lower lobe pneumonia, pleural effusion, or elevation of a hemidiaphragm indicating a subdiaphragmatic inflammatory process. Free air under the diaphragm suggests a perforated viscus and is most often seen on the upright chest film. As many as 15% to 20% of cases of perforation do not manifest this sign.
3. **Ultrasound.** This readily obtainable and noninvasive test may reveal the presence or absence of gallstones, biliary tract dilation, or ectopic pregnancy.
4. **Electrocardiogram (ECG).** An ECG is needed to rule out an acute myocardial infarction (MI) or pericarditis which may present with acute upper abdominal pain.
5. **Paracentesis.** (See Section III, Chapter X, Paracentesis, p 369) In a patient with known ascites presenting with acute abdominal pain, this test is required to rule out the possibility of spontaneous bacterial peritonitis. If ascites is suspected but has not

been documented, then an ultrasound should be performed prior to an attempted paracentesis.

6. **Other studies** may be obtained in a more leisurely fashion to determine the nature of the pain, provided the patient does not appear to have a case of acute abdominal pain requiring surgery. These tests can include the following:

   a. **Intravenous pyelogram (IVP)**

   b. **Abdominal CT scan**

   c. **Hepato-iminodiacetic acid (HIDA) scan,** to rule out acute cholecystitis

   d. **Contrast bowel study,** such as an upper GI and small bowel series, to look for evidence of occult perforation or mechanical obstruction. A barium enema may be helpful in evaluation for sigmoid or cecal volvulus.

   e. **Endoscopic studies,** such as esophagogastroduodenoscopy (EGD), colonoscopy, or endoscopic retrograde cholangiopancreatography (ERCP).

   f. **Arteriography.** This may be necessary in those patients in whom mesenteric artery ischemia is suspected.

V. Plan. As mentioned previously, the initial goal in evaluating a patient with acute abdominal pain is to determine whether or not surgical treatment is indicated to prevent further morbidity. When pain has been present 6 or more hours and has not improved, there is an increased likelihood that the patient will require surgical exploration to determine the cause of pain. Often the specific etiology of the patient's abdominal pain is not determined until laparotomy. The use of analgesics remains controversial, but many surgeons now favor the use of moderate doses of pain medication to make the patient more comfortable and facilitate further examination.

A. Observation. With the exception of those conditions that require urgent surgical exploration (Table 1–3), most cases of abdominal pain can be initially managed with close observation, correction of any fluid or electrolyte disturbances, and judicious use of analgesics.

1. Any patient on a medical service developing acute abdominal pain should be evaluated by a general surgeon.

2. In those cases in which mechanical obstruction is suspected or vomiting is present, nasogastric decompression should be initiated. (See Section III, Chapter X, Gastrointestinal Tubes, p 360)

3. Patients who present with septic or circulatory shock should receive vigorous intravenous volume replacement. If hypotension persists, they may require a vasopressor such as dopamine. (See Section I, Chapter 41, Hypotension, p 207)

4. Meperidine (Demerol) 50–75 mg IM Q 3–4 hours may be used to provide patient comfort; however, avoid oversedation which could obscure patient evaluation.

5. Serial physical examinations by the same examiner are very helpful in determining the patient's symptoms and establishing the diagnosis or need for surgery.

B. Surgery. Indications that mandate urgent operation without a period of observation or establishment of a specific preoperative diagnosis are outlined in Table 1–3.

TABLE 1–3. INDICATIONS FOR URGENT OPERATION IN PATIENTS WITH ACUTE ABDOMEN.[1]

■ **Physical findings**
Involuntary guarding or rigidity, especially if spreading
Increasing or severe localized tenderness
Tense or progressive distention
Tender abdominal or rectal mass with high fever or hypotension
Rectal bleeding with shock or acidosis
Equivocal abdominal findings along with
  Septicemia (high fever, marked or rising leukocytosis, mental changes, or increasing glucose intolerance in a diabetic patient)
  Bleeding (unexplained shock or acidosis, falling hematocrit)
  Suspected ischemia (acidosis, fever, tachycardia)
  Deterioration on conservative treatment

■ **Radiologic findings**
Pneumoperitoneum
Gross or progressive bowel distension
Free extravasation of contrast material
Space-occupying lesion on CT scan, with fever
Mesenteric occlusion on angiography

■ **Endoscopic findings**
Perforated or uncontrollably bleeding lesion

■ **Paracentesis findings**
Blood, bile, pus, bowel contents, or urine

[1] Reproduced with permission from Boey JH: Acute abdomen. In Way LW, ed. *Current Surgical Diagnosis and Treatment,* 10th ed. Appleton & Lange; 1994.

REFERENCES

Hendrix TR, Bulkley GB, Schuster MM: Abdominal Pain. In: Harvey AM, Johns RJ, McKusick VA et al, eds. *The Principles and Practice of Medicine.* 22nd ed. Appleton & Lange;1988:787.

Jung PJ, Merrell PC: Acute abdomen. Gastroenterol Clin North Am 1988;17:227.

Ridge JA, Way LW: Abdominal pain. In: Sleisenger MH, Fordtran JS, eds. *Gastrointestinal Disease: Pathophysiology, Diagnosis, Management.* 5th ed. WB Saunders;1993:150.

Silen W: *Cope's Early Diagnosis of the Acute Abdomen.* 18th ed. Oxford University Press;1991.

2. ACIDOSIS

I. **Problem.** A 30-year-old male is brought into the emergency room unconscious. He was found at home by a friend. No other history is available. Physical examination is unremarkable except for rapid, shallow breathing. An arterial blood gas reveals a pH of 7.10.

II. **Immediate Questions**
  A. **Is the acidemia from a metabolic, respiratory, or mixed acidosis?** A quick look at the pCO_2 on the arterial blood gas slip will reveal whether the disturbance is a primary metabolic or respiratory acidosis. If the pCO_2 is less than 40 mm Hg, then the primary disturbance is a metabolic acidosis. If the pCO_2 is greater than 40 mm Hg, the disturbance may be a primary respiratory acidosis or may be a mixed disturbance. Many arterial blood gas slips list the base excess (BE). The BE may help determine the etiology of the acidosis. If the BE is positive, the acidosis is respiratory; if the BE is negative, the acidosis is at least partially metabolic. Remember, the BE is calculated from the pH; the calculation assumes that both the pH and pCO_2 are correct.
  B. **What are the patient's vital signs?** A common cause of metabolic acidosis is lactic acidosis from hypoperfusion. If there is hypotension or if the patient is orthostatic, immediate fluid resuscitation is indicated. Vasopressor agents may also be needed. (See Section X, Chapter 41, Hypotension, p 203). Bradypnea may suggest a narcotics overdose. Tachypnea may arise from hyperventilation as respiratory compensation for a metabolic acidosis; or from increased respiratory effort but hypoventilation, resulting in a respiratory acidosis.
  C. **Are there any arrhythmias or ectopy?** With a profound acidemia from any cause, there may be disturbances of cardiac rhythm or ventricular ectopy. Obtain an ECG and monitor the patient.
  D. **What is the serum bicarbonate?** To fully understand an acid-base problem, it is imperative to obtain the serum bicarbonate from an electrolyte panel. A high serum bicarbonate is evidence for a primary respiratory acidosis. A low serum bicarbonate is evidence for either a primary metabolic acidosis, or a mixed metabolic and respiratory acidosis.
  E. **Do the values for serum bicarbonate, pH, and pCO_2 fit?** Once you have the serum bicarbonate, you should make sure the pH, pCO_2 and HCO_3^- fit:

$$pH = pK_a + \log \frac{HCO_3^-}{H_2CO_3}$$

which can be simplified to:

$$H^+ = 24 \times \frac{pCO_2}{HCO_3^-}$$

In this patient with a pH of 7.10, if the pCO_2 is 20 mm Hg and the serum bicarbonate is 6 mmol/L, then:

$$H^+ = 24 \times \frac{20}{6}$$

$$H^+ = 80$$

Does a pH of 7.10 equal a $[H^+]$ of 80 nmol/L? There are some simple rules to help convert pH to $[H^+]$. At a pH of 7.40, the $[H^+] = 40$ nmol/L. pH is a log scale, and for every 0.3 change in pH, the $[H^+]$ doubles or is halved. For instance, if pH = 7.70, $[H^+]$ = 20 nmol/L, and at pH = 8.00, $[H^+]$ = 10 nmol/L. In this patient, if pH = 7.10, then $[H^+]$ = 80 nmol/L. Also, around a pH of 7.40 (7.25–7.48), the $[H^+]$ changes 1 nmol/L for every 0.01 change in pH. Lastly, on the back of many arterial blood gas slips, there may be a scale showing the relationship between pH and $[H^+]$. If the numbers do not fit reasonably well into the equation

$$[H^+] = 24 \times \frac{pCO_2}{HCO_3^-}$$

then it is difficult to determine the acid–base disturbance, and the blood gas and serum bicarbonate should be repeated. For instance, if pH = 7.30, pCO_2 = 45 mm Hg, and HCO_3^- = 30 mmol/L, a superficial interpretation might be respiratory acidosis; however, closer scrutiny is necessary.

a pH of 7.30 corresponds to a H^+ of 50 mmol/L

$$50 = 24 \times \frac{45}{30}$$

Either the pH, the pCO_2, or the HCO_3^- is in error. For instance, if there had been too much heparin in the syringe, the pH would be falsely low.

F. Is the compensation appropriate? Checking to see whether the compensation is appropriate may unmask mixed disturbances.

1. For respiratory acidosis, immediate compensation is through buffers. In the short term, one expects the HCO_3^- to increase by 1 mmol/L for every 10 mm Hg increase in pCO_2 over normal (40 mm Hg). Renal compensation is not present for up to 24 hours. For chronic respiratory acidosis, expect an increase in the HCO_3^- of 3.5 to 4.0 mmol/L for every 10 mm Hg increase in pCO_2. For instance, in a 25-year-old with an acute episode of asthma, the ABG revealed a pCO_2 of 90. One would expect the

bicarbonate to increase by 5 mmol/L from the calculation 1 mmol/L × (90 mm Hg − 40 mm Hg)/10 mm Hg. One would also expect the HCO_3^- to be 31 mmol/L from the calculation 26 mmol/L (normal bicarbonate range 23–29) + 5 mmol/L. If the bicarbonate were 25 mmol/L, then a relative metabolic acidosis would be present along with the primary respiratory acidosis. If the bicarbonate were 36 mmol/L, then a metabolic alkalosis would also be present along with the primary respiratory acidosis.

2. For metabolic acidosis, compensation begins immediately through buffers and hyperventilation; however, steady state may not be reached for up to 24 hours. The expected change in pCO_2 is 1–1.5 times the change in HCO_3^-. For instance, in a 40-year-old with renal failure, the serum bicarbonate was found to be 15 mmol/L. The change in bicarbonate from normal should be 11 mmol/L or 26 mmol/L − 15 mmol/L. The expected change in pCO_2 would be between 11 and 16 mm Hg (11 × 1 and 11 × 1.5). One would expect the pCO_2 to be between 24 and 29 mm Hg (40 − 16 and 40 − 11). If the actual pCO_2 were 19 mm Hg, then a respiratory alkalosis would also be present along with the primary metabolic acidosis. If the actual pCO_2 were 36 mm Hg, then a relative respiratory acidosis would be present along with the primary metabolic acidosis.

III. **Differential Diagnosis.** An acidemia is either from a metabolic or respiratory acidosis. There are many causes for both, and sometimes a patient may have more than one cause.
   A. **Respiratory acidosis.** By definition, respiratory acidosis occurs secondary to hypoventilation. Hypoventilation can be caused by lung, chest, or central nervous system (CNS) disorders.
      1. **Lungs**
         a. **Asthma.** May progress from a respiratory alkalosis to respiratory acidosis. A normal or elevated pCO_2 indicates impending respiratory failure, and may require prompt intubation.
         b. **Pulmonary edema.** Mild pulmonary edema usually causes a respiratory alkalosis. Severe pulmonary edema may cause a respiratory acidosis, and intubation will probably be required.
         c. **Pneumonia.** Again, pneumonia usually causes respiratory alkalosis. But if more than one lobe is involved, or if there is underlying chronic obstructive disease, pneumonia may cause a respiratory acidosis.
         d. **Upper airway obstruction.** Causes of obstruction may include foreign bodies, tumors, or a laryngospasm.
         e. **Pneumothorax.** Usually causes respiratory alkalosis; can cause a respiratory acidosis.

      f. Large pleural effusion. Usually causes a respiratory alkalosis; can cause a respiratory acidosis.
  2. Chest abnormalities
    a. Kyphoscoliosis. Resulting in a restrictive defect.
    b. Scleroderma. Resulting in a restrictive defect.
    c. Marked obesity (Pickwickian syndrome).
    d. Muscular disorders. These include muscular dystrophy, severe hypophosphatemia, or myasthenia gravis.
    e. Peripheral neurologic disorders, such as Guillain-Barré syndrome.
  3. CNS disorders
    a. Drugs or toxins causing depression of respiratory drive.
      i. Ethanol intoxication at levels of 400–500 mg%
      ii. Barbiturates, especially overdoses
      iii. Narcotics
      iv. Benzodiazepines, especially when taken with alcohol
    b. Cerebrovascular accident
    c. Brain stem bleed or cervical spinal cord injuries
B. Metabolic acidosis. This can be divided into gap and nongap acidosis. The anion gap can be calculated as follows:

$$\text{Anion gap} = [Na^+] - ([Cl^-] + [HCO_3^-])$$

The normal anion gap is 8–12 mmol/L. An increase in anion gap may result from an increase in an unmeasured anion. Other causes of an elevated anion gap include dehydration; alkalosis; use of penicillin antibiotics that contain large amounts of sodium such as carbenicillin; and therapy with sodium salts or organic acids such as sodium lactate, acetate, and citrate. Sodium citrate is used in whole blood and packed red cells as an anticoagulant. However, only a metabolic acidosis will cause an appreciable increase in the anion gap.
  1. Normal anion gap (metabolic nongap acidosis)
    a. Loss of bicarbonate through the GI tract
      i. Diarrhea
      ii. Small bowel fistula
      iii. Pancreatocutaneous fistula
      iv. Ureterosigmoidostomy
      v. Chloride-containing exchange resins, such as cholestyramine; or with calcium chloride or magnesium chloride.
    b. Loss of bicarbonate through the kidneys
      i. Renal tubular acidosis. Distal and proximal.
      ii. Carbonic anhydrase inhibitors
    c. Other causes not from gastrointestinal or renal loss of HCO_3^-
      i. Early renal failure

        ii. Hydrochloric acid
        iii. Hyperalimentation
        iv. Dilutional

2. **Elevated anion gap (metabolic gap acidosis)**

    a. **Lactic acidosis.** Results from overproduction or impairment of lactate utilization by the liver, often from tissue hypoperfusion.

        i. Shock. Cardiogenic, hypovolemic, septic.
        ii. Severe anemia
        iii. Hypoxia
        iv. Malignancy
        v. Seizures
        vi. Ethanol
        vii. Crush injury

    b. **Renal failure.** Loss of acid secretion, and failure to filter anions.

    c. **Ketoacidosis**

        i. Diabetic ketoacidosis
        ii. Alcoholic ketoacidosis
        iii. Starvation ketoacidosis

    d. **Toxins**

        i. Salicylates. These compounds cause an isolated metabolic gap acidosis (10%), an isolated respiratory alkalosis (30%), but most commonly a mixed metabolic gap acidosis and respiratory alkalosis (57%).

        ii. Methanol. Metabolized to formic acid and formaldehyde. May cause blindness, abdominal pain, and headache.

        iii. Ethylene glycol. Metabolized to oxalate, glycolaldehyde, and hippurate. Renal failure, neurologic disturbances, hypertension, and cardiovascular collapse may occur.

        Caution: Isopropyl alcohol ingestion does not cause an acidosis, because isopropyl alcohol is metabolized to acetone. It may therefore cause a positive nitroprusside test for ketones.

    e. The anion gap is also helpful in differentiating a pure metabolic acidosis, a mixed metabolic gap acidosis and metabolic nongap acidosis, and a mixed metabolic gap acidosis and metabolic alkalosis. For instance, if the HCO_3^- were 14 with a gap of 23, this would most likely represent a **pure metabolic gap acidosis** as calculated by:

          23 mmol/L   Actual gap
   − <u>10</u> mmol/L   Normal gap
          13 mmol/L   Expected change in HCO_3^- from normal

26 mmol/L   Normal HCO_3^- (range 23–29)
− 13 mmol/L   Expected change
13 mmol/L   Expected HCO_3^-

Actual HCO_3^- 14 mmol/L ≈ expected gap of 13 mmol/L

An HCO_3^- of 19 with a gap of 25 would most likely represent a **mixed metabolic acidosis and metabolic alkalosis** as calculated by:

25 mmol/L   Actual gap
− 10 mmol/L   Normal gap
15 mmol/L   Expected change in HCO_3^- from normal

26 mmol/L   Normal HCO_3^- (range 23–29)
− 15 mmol/L   Expected change in HCO_3^-
11 mmol/L   Expected HCO_3^-

The actual HCO_3^-, however, is 19 mmol/L, 8 mmol/L higher than expected. Thus, there must also be a metabolic alkalosis in addition to the metabolic gap acidosis.
An HCO_3^- of 8 mmol/L with a gap of 22 mmol/L would most likely represent a **mixed metabolic gap acidosis and metabolic nongap acidosis** as calculated by:

22 mmol/L   Actual gap
− 10 mmol/L   Normal gap
12 mmol/L   Expected change in HCO_3^-

26 mmol/L   Normal HCO_3^- (range 23–29)
− 12 mmol/L   Expected change in HCO_3^-
14 mmol/L   Expected HCO_3^-

The actual HCO_3^-, however, is 8 mmol/L or 6 mmol/L lower than expected. Thus, there must also be a metabolic nongap acidosis in addition to the metabolic gap acidosis.

IV. Database
A. Physical examination key points
1. **Vital signs.** A low respiratory rate suggests hypoventilation; a high rate points toward respiratory failure or compensation for a metabolic acidosis. Hypotension suggests hypoperfusion.
2. **Skin.** Changes which characterize scleroderma indicate a restrictive defect. Cool, clammy, and mottled skin on the extremities suggests shock.
3. **HEENT.** Ketosis or fruity odor on breath suggests diabetic ketoacidosis. Look for tracheal shift from a space-occupying lesion or venous distension (congestive heart failure or tension pneumothorax). Pinpoint pupils are consistent with drug overdose.

4. **Lungs.** Evaluate for absent or decreased breath sounds, stridor in upper airway obstruction, wheezes, and rales.
5. **Abdomen.** Peritoneal signs indicate an acute abdomen; marked distension may inhibit respiration.
6. **Neuromuscular examination.** Generalized weakness or focal neurologic signs, depressed level of consciousness, obtundation, and coma should be noted.

B. **Laboratory data**
1. **Hemograms.** Anemia may be associated with renal failure. Anemia may cause ischemia resulting in lactic acidosis. Leukocytosis may suggest sepsis.
2. **Electrolytes.** Serum chloride is usually elevated in metabolic nongap acidosis. Serum potassium is usually increased with acidosis, but may be low in diabetic ketoacidosis, or renal tubular acidosis. The serum potassium may be especially helpful in determining the acid-base status given the serum bicarbonate prior to the arterial blood gas analysis. For instance, a serum bicarbonate of 34 mmol/L could indicate a primary metabolic alkalosis, or compensation for a chronic respiratory acidosis. If the potassium were 5.6 mmol/L, this would argue that the bicarbonate of 34 mmol/L was from compensation for a chronic respiratory acidosis. If the potassium were 3.1 mmol/L, this would argue that the bicarbonate of 34 mmol/L was from a metabolic alkalosis. The potassium, BUN, and creatinine may be elevated with renal failure. The creatinine may be falsely elevated with ketoacidosis.
3. **Metabolic gap acidosis.** The following tests *must* be ordered:
   a. **Glucose.** If elevated, may indicate diabetic ketoacidosis.
   b. **Ketone levels.** May indicate alcoholic, starvation, or diabetic ketoacidosis.
   c. **Lactate.** Lactic acidosis may be seen with alcohol use, severe anemia, sepsis, hypoperfusion (either generalized or local), hypoxemia, end-stage liver disease, and postictally.
   d. **Salicylate level**
   e. **Ethanol**
   f. **Methanol**
   g. **Ethylene glycol**
   h. **Paraldehyde.** Very rare cause of metabolic acidosis.
   i. **BUN and creatinine**
4. **Metabolic nongap acidosis.** If the history does not reveal an obvious cause such as diarrhea, then you need to consider renal tubular acidosis.
   a. **Distal renal tubular acidosis.** Inability to lower urine pH below 5.5 with NH_4Cl (ammonium chloride).
   b. **Proximal renal tubular acidosis.** Urine pH will decrease to <5.5; however, the excretion of HCO_3^- is increased to >15% when serum HCO_3^- is raised to the normal range.

5. **Respiratory acidosis.** Order a serum and urine drug screen. If there is hypoventilation with decreased respirations, you need to rule out a drug overdose. Also, with an intentional salicylate overdose, ingestion of other substances must be ruled out, as intentional overdoses often involve multiple substances.

C. **Radiologic and other studies**
   1. If there is respiratory acidosis:
      a. **Chest x-ray (CXR).** Rule out pneumothorax, pulmonary edema, infiltrative processes.
      b. **CT scan of head.** Consider with hypoventilation and altered mental status or with focal neurologic exam.
      c. **Electromyography (EMG).** May be helpful in assessment of neuromuscular disorders.

V. **Plan.** In general, for both respiratory and metabolic acidosis, treatment of the underlying cause of the acidemia is the primary goal. In emergent situations, the two methods for short-term reversal of metabolic and respiratory acidosis are: 1) to administer IV sodium bicarbonate; and 2) to hyperventilate the patient. Be sure to check serial pH values to monitor the progress of therapy.

A. **Severe acidosis (pH < 7.20).** Use continuous cardiac monitoring for potential arrhythmia.

B. **Metabolic acidosis**
   1. **Bicarbonate therapy.** Although controversial, the present recommendation is to administer IV bicarbonate if the pH < 7.10. The goal is to raise the HCO_3^- to 10–15 mmol.
      a. Calculate the amount of sodium bicarbonate needed to raise the HCO_3^- to a given level.

      $$NaHCO_3 \text{ needed} = wt \text{ (in Kg)} \times {}^*0.50 \times (desired\ HCO_3^- - measured\ HCO_3^-).$$

      *(If pH is < 7.10, 0.80 should be used to estimate HCO_3^- volume of distribution instead of 0.50).

      b. Give 50% of this amount over the first 12 hours as a mixture of bicarbonate with D5W. A normal bicarbonate drip is made by adding 3 ampoules of $NaHCO_3$ (50 mmol/ampoule) to 1 L of D5W.
      c. Complications of bicarbonate therapy include:
         i. **Hypernatremia**
         ii. **Volume overload**
         iii. **Hypokalemia.** Caused by intracellular shifts of potassium as the pH increases.
   2. **Treatment of underlying causes**
      a. Volume resuscitation with normal saline is indicated for sepsis and hemorrhagic shock. Vasopressors may be needed. See Section 1, Chapter 41, Hypotension, Section V, p 207.
      b. Dialysis as needed for renal failure.

    c. Normal saline and insulin for diabetic ketoacidosis. See Section 1, Chapter 31, Hyperglycemia, Section V.

    d. Normal saline and dextrose for alcoholic ketoacidosis along with replacement of other electrolytes and vitamins such as thiamine and folate as needed.

    e. Starvation ketosis is treated with normal saline and dextrose.

    f. Salicylate intoxication is treated with alkalinization of urine. Intravenous fluids containing $NaHCO_3$ (3 ampoules 50 mEq in 1 L of D5W or 2 ampoules in 1 L D5 1/4NS) are administered at 100–250 mL/h. Check urine pH every 1–2 hours. Urine pH should be maintained at or above 7.5–8.0. ABG and serum bicarbonate should be followed closely, and severe alkalemia (pH > 7.55) avoided. Hemodialysis may be required.

    g. Methanol and ethylene glycol ingestion is treated with ethanol infusion, which decreases the accumulation of toxic metabolites. Hemodialysis may be required.

C. Respiratory acidosis. The main goal is to treat the underlying cause.

    1. If indicated, intubate the patient and treat with mechanical ventilation. If a patient is already intubated and has a significant respiratory acidosis, then increase alveolar ventilation either by increasing tidal volume (up to 8–10 mL/kg), while following peak inspiratory pressures, or by increasing the respiratory rate. See Section 1, Chapter 18; Dyspnea, p 99; and Section VI, Ventilator Management, p 387.

    2. In an emergent situation, disconnect the patient from the ventilator and hyperventilate by hand. The importance of good pulmonary toilet (ie, suctioning of secretions) cannot be overemphasized. Sedation is often a necessary adjunct to mechanical ventilation. See Section VI, Ventilator Management, p 387.

REFERENCES

Kaehny WD: Pathogenesis and management of respiratory and mixed acid-base disorders. In: Schrier RW ed.: *Renal and Electrolyte Disorders.* 4th ed. Little, Brown;1992:211.

Narins RG, Emmett A: Simple and mixed acid-base disorders: A practical approach. Medicine. 1980;59:161.

Shapiro JI, Kaehny WD: Pathogenesis and management of metabolic acidosis and alkalosis. In: Schrier RW ed.: *Renal and Electrolyte Disorders.* 4th ed. Little, Brown;1992:161.

3. ALKALOSIS

I. Problem. You are consulted to see a 60-year-old male with a pH of 7.65, who is 3 days' status post cholecystectomy.

II. Immediate Questions

A. Is the alkalemia from a metabolic, respiratory, or mixed alkalosis? A quick look at the pCO_2 on the ABG slip will reveal whether the disturbance is a primary metabolic or respiratory alkalosis. If the pCO_2 is >40 mm Hg, the primary disturbance is a metabolic alkalosis with at least partial respiratory compensation. If the pCO_2 is <40 mm Hg, the disturbance may be a primary respiratory alkalosis or a mixed disturbance. Many arterial blood gas slips list the base excess (BE), which may help determine the etiology of the alkalosis. If the BE is negative, the alkalosis is respiratory; if the BE is positive, the alkalosis is at least partially metabolic. Remember, the BE is calculated from the pH, and assumes that both the pH and pCO_2 are correct.

B. What are the patient's vital signs? An elevated respiratory rate, fever, hypotension, or all three may indicate sepsis. Respiratory alkalosis is associated with sepsis. Tachypnea may also indicate anxiety, CNS disease, or pulmonary disease.

C. What medications is the patient taking? Thiazide diuretics can cause a contraction alkalosis. Acetate in hyperalimentation solutions, antacids, exogenous steroids, or large doses of penicillin or carbenicillin may cause an alkalosis. Salicylate overdose and progesterone can cause a respiratory alkalosis.

D. Is a nasogastric tube in place? Is the patient vomiting? Loss of HCl from the stomach is a common cause of metabolic alkalosis.

E. Is there any history of mental status changes, seizures, paresthesias, or tetany? Alkalemia may cause the above; and if so, prompt action is indicated.

F. Is there any ventricular ectopy? Severe alkalemia may cause ventricular arrhythmias unresponsive to the usual pharmacologic treatments.

Caution: Mortality in critically ill surgical patients is associated with a high serum pH. One study indicated that mortality was 69% in patients with a pH >7.60, but fell to 44% in patients with a pH between 7.55 and 7.59.

G. What is the serum bicarbonate? To fully understand an acid-base problem, you must obtain the serum bicarbonate from an electrolyte panel. A low serum bicarbonate is evidence of a primary respiratory alkalosis with at least partial metabolic compensation. A high serum bicarbonate is evidence for either a primary metabolic alkalosis or a mixed metabolic and respiratory alkalosis.

H. Does the serum bicarbonate fit the pH and pCO_2? See Section 1, Chapter 2, Acidosis, Section II E, p 9.

I. Is the compensation appropriate? Checking to see if the compensation is appropriate may unmask mixed disturbances.

1. In a respiratory alkalosis, immediate compensation takes place through buffers. The compensation for acute respiratory alkalosis is a decrease of 2 mmol of HCO_3^- (range 1–3 mmol) for each

10 mm Hg decrease in pCO_2. Renal compensation is complete between 24 and 48 hours. The compensation for chronic respiratory alkalosis is a decrease of about 5 mmol of HCO_3^- for each 10 mm Hg decrease in pCO_2. For instance, in a 35-year-old woman who is 36 weeks pregnant, the ABG revealed a pCO_2 of 25. One would expect the HCO_3^- to decrease by 7.5 mmol from the calculation 5 mmol/L × (40 mm Hg − 25 mm mg)/10 mm Hg. One would expect the HCO_3^- to be 18.5 or 26 mmol/L (normal HCO_3^-) − 7.5 mmol (expected change in HCO_3^-). If the HCO_3^- were 25 mmol, a relative metabolic alkalosis would be present along with the primary respiratory alkalosis, since the serum bicarbonate is higher than expected. If the HCO_3^- were 12 mmol, there would be a metabolic acidosis along with the primary respiratory alkalosis, since the serum bicarbonate is lower than expected.

2. For metabolic alkalosis, compensation begins immediately through buffers and hypoventilation. Hypoventilation as a means of compensation is limited by resulting hypoxemia. Seldom will the pCO_2 be >55 mm Hg secondary to compensation. The expected increase in pCO_2 is 0.6 mm Hg (range 0.25–1.0 mm Hg) for each 1-mmol increase in HCO_3^-. For instance, in a 60-year-old status post cholecystectomy, the HCO_3^- was 36 mmol/L. The expected pCO_2 is 46 mm Hg (36 mmol/L − 26 mmol/L) × 0.6 mm Hg per 1 mmol/L change in HCO_3^-. If the pCO_2 were 40 mm Hg, there would be a relative respiratory alkalosis along with the primary metabolic alkalosis. If the pCO_2 were 55 mm Hg, there would be a respiratory acidosis along with a primary metabolic alkalosis.

III. **Differential Diagnosis.** Alkalemia results either from a metabolic or respiratory alkalosis. There may be many causes for both; and sometimes a patient may have more than one cause.
  A. **Respiratory alkalosis.** By definition, respiratory alkalosis occurs secondary to hyperventilation. Hyperventilation can result from either central or peripheral stimulation of respiration. Common causes include medications, CNS disease, pulmonary disease, anxiety, and systemic disorders.
    1. **Medications**
      a. **Salicylate overdose.** Causes an isolated respiratory alkalosis (30%), isolated metabolic gap acidosis (10%), and most commonly a mixed metabolic gap acidosis and respiratory alkalosis (57%).
      b. **Progesterone**
    2. **CNS disease.** See Section 1, Chapter 13, Coma, Acute Mental Status Changes, p 70.
      a. **Cerebrovascular accident**

        b. Infection
        c. Tumor. Primary or metastatic.
        d. Trauma
    3. Pulmonary disease. See Section 1, Chapter 18, Dyspnea, p 99.
        a. Interstitial lung disease
        b. Pneumonia. If multiple lobes, may cause respiratory acidosis.
        c. Asthma. If mild to moderate, will cause a respiratory alkalosis; if severe, respiratory acidosis may result.
        d. Pulmonary emboli
        e. Pneumothorax
    4. Anxiety
    5. Pulmonary edema. If mild, causes a respiratory alkalosis; if severe, may cause a respiratory acidosis.
    6. Pain
    7. Pregnancy. Secondary to progesterone.
    8. Liver disease. Cirrhosis.
    9. Fever
   10. Early sepsis
   11. Hyperthyroidism
   12. Iatrogenic
   13. Hypoxemia
B. Metabolic alkalosis. Can be divided into chloride-responsive and chloride-unresponsive. The urine Cl^- is $< 10–20$ mmol/L with the chloride-responsive causes, and $>20–30$ mmol/L with the chloride-unresponsive causes. Provided no diuretic has been given.
    1. Chloride-responsive causes
        a. Gastric losses. Vomiting or nasogastric tube.
        b. Diarrhea. Chloride wasting.
        c. Diuretics
        d. Correction of chronic hypercapnia
        e. Sulfates, phosphates, or high-dose penicillins
        f. Massive blood transfusion. Citrate is used as an anticoagulant and is metabolized to HCO_3^-. One unit of whole blood and one unit of packed red cells contain 17 and 5 mEq of citrate, respectively.
    2. Chloride-unresponsive causes
        a. Cushing's syndrome. Elevated glucocorticoids from a variety of causes including pituitary adenoma, adrenal adenoma, and ectopic production. Also results in hypertension, glucose intolerance, fluid retention, and osteoporosis.
        b. Hyperaldosteronism. Rare cause of hypertension. Also associated with hypokalemia and hypernatremia.
        c. Exogenous steroid ingestion
        d. Bartter's syndrome. Also hypokalemia. Hyperreninemia and hyperaldosteronemia secondary to hyperplasia of the juxtaglomerular apparatus. Patients are normotensive.

      e. Potassium or magnesium deficiency
      f. Calcium carbonate-containing antacids
      g. Milk-alkali syndrome
      h. Refeeding with glucose after starvation

IV. Database
A. Physical examination key points
1. **Vital signs.** Tachypnea may indicate pulmonary disease, pulmonary edema, or CNS respiratory stimulation. An elevated temperature may indicate an infection or sepsis.
2. **Chest.** Examination must be thorough; look for evidence of pneumothorax, pleural effusion, bronchospastic disease, and pulmonary edema.
3. **Abdomen.** Look for evidence of chronic liver disease such as ascites and caput medusae.
4. **Skin.** Check for evidence of chronic liver disease such as palmar erythema, Dupuytren's contractures, and spider angiomas. Also look for changes associated with Cushing's syndrome, such as buffalo hump, purple striae, and easy bruisability.
5. **Neurologic exam.** Check for focal abnormalities as evidence for tumor, cerebrovascular accident, and infection. Tremor and hyperreflexia may suggest hyperthyroidism.

B. Laboratory data
1. **Anion gap.** May unmask a mixed metabolic gap acidosis and metabolic alkalosis. See Section 1, Chapter 2, Acidosis, III B 2e, p 19.
2. **Serum electrolytes.** Hypokalemia and hypomagnesemia may cause a metabolic alkalosis. Hypokalemia may also result from alkalosis as potassium ions shift intracellularly in exchange for hydrogen ions.
3. **Respiratory alkalosis**
   a. **Salicylate level.** If elevated, check serum and urine drug screen for other ingested substances.
   b. **Liver function tests**
   c. **Thyroid function studies**
   d. **Blood cultures**
4. **Metabolic alkalosis.** You will need a spot urine for chloride. A urine chloride below 10–20 mmol/L represents a **chloride-responsive** alkalosis. A urine chloride above 20 mmol/L represents a **chloride-unresponsive** alkalosis.
5. **Chloride-unresponsive metabolic alkalosis.** You may need to rule out Cushing's syndrome and primary aldosteronism.

C. Radiologic and other studies. If respiratory alkalosis, consider the following:
1. **Chest x-ray.** To look for pulmonary disease and pulmonary edema.
2. **CT scan of head.** Rule out CNS disease.

V. Plan. It is essential to identify the cause of the alkalemia and treat it.

A. Respiratory alkalosis

1. If hypoxic, give supplemental oxygen.
2. If anxious, give sedative such as diazepam 1–5 mg PO or 1–2 mg IV; or lorazepam 1–2 mg PO or 0.5 mg IV.
3. If nonintubated, increase $FiCO_2$ (fraction of inspired carbon dioxide) by use of a rebreathing mask. Would consider for pH >7.55.
4. If the patient is intubated, you will need to decrease minute ventilation by decreasing the rate or tidal volume. Be sure the tidal volume is set for 8–10 mL/kg. The respirator may need to be changed from assist control to intermittent ventilation.
5. If salicylate overdose, consider alkalinization of urine. Alkalinization of urine should be done cautiously in a patient who is already alkalotic. Follow serum pH and serum bicarbonate closely. See Section 1, Chapter 2, Acidosis, Section V, p 17, for instructions on alkalinization of urine. Hemodialysis may be required.

B. Metabolic alkalosis

1. In the presence of severe alkalemia with seizures or ventricular arrhythmias, prompt, immediate action is needed. Treatment includes increasing the pCO_2, or administering an acid such as hydrochloric acid. Hydrochloric acid must be given slowly through a central line.
2. Bicarbonate precursors such as acetate salts (amino acids) found in hyperalimentation solutions or solutions containing lactate should be eliminated if possible.
3. If chloride-responsive, give normal saline.
4. If chloride-unresponsive, treat underlying disorder.
   a. If potassium or magnesium deficient, will often need massive replacement.
   b. Evaluation and specific treatment of endogenous mineralocorticoid disorders.

REFERENCES

Kaehny WD: Pathogenesis and management of respiratory and mixed acid-base disorders. In: Schrier RW ed.: *Renal and Electrolyte Disorders.* 4th ed. Little, Brown;1992:211.

Narins RG, Emmett M: Simple and mixed acid–base disorders: A practical approach. Medicine 1980;59:161.

Shapiro JI, Kaehny WD, Gabow PA: Pathogenesis and management of metabolic acidosis and alkalosis. In: Schrier RW ed.: *Renal and Electrolyte Disorders.* 4th ed. Little, Brown;1992:161.

Wilson RF, Gibson D, Percinel AK et al: Severe alkalosis in critically ill surgical patients. Arch Surg 1972;105:197.

4. ANAPHYLACTIC REACTION

I. **Problem.** Within 10 minutes of receiving an intramuscular injection, a patient develops respiratory distress and diffuse pruritus.

II. **Immediate Questions.** Anaphylaxis can be a life-threatening situation and requires immediate evaluation and treatment.
   A. **What are the patient's vital signs?** Tachycardia is a common finding and could result from an arrhythmia or as a response to hypoxia, fear, or hypotension. Hypotensive shock, which can occur with or without other symptoms, poses the greatest danger from anaphylaxis and must be recognized and treated promptly.
   B. **Can the patient still communicate?** The ability to provide appropriate answers to simple questions implies adequate cerebral oxygenation. Inability to speak, or stridor, could indicate upper airway obstruction from laryngospasm or laryngeal edema.
   C. **What medication(s) did the patient receive?** Anaphylaxis can result from a variety of agents, including medications, foods, venoms, pollens, and serum. The most common medications causing anaphylaxis are penicillins, cephalosporins, sulfonamides, and local anesthetics. Anaphylactoid reactions nonimmunologically mediated result from opiates, nonsteroidal anti-inflammatory drugs, and radio contrast material.

III. **Differential Diagnosis.** Signs and symptoms of anaphylaxis are produced by the release of biologically active mediators such as histamine from basophils and mast cells. This release can either be mediated immunologically through the interaction of antigen with IgE residing on the basophils and mast cells, or can occur as the result of a nonimmunologic release of mediators. These mediators affect several organ systems, including the skin, upper and lower airways, vascular system, and gastrointestinal tract. Anaphylaxis may involve only one or all of the preceding organ systems, and thus must be distinguished from other disease processes occurring at these sites.
   A. **Upper airway obstruction.** This could result from epiglottitis, aspiration of a foreign body, or may occur with other causes of laryngeal edema such as hereditary angioneurotic edema.
   B. **Acute asthmatic attack.**
   C. **Wheezing, from other causes.** See Section 1, Chapter 61, Wheezing, p 297.
   D. **Pulmonary embolus.** This diagnosis must be considered in any patient developing acute shortness of breath.
   E. **Other causes of dyspnea.** See Section 1, Chapter 18, Dyspnea, p 99.

    F. Vasovagal reaction. This can also cause acute cardiovascular collapse, but is usually associated with bradycardia and resolves quickly with recumbency.

    G. Urticaria. This condition can be produced by a wide variety of causes other than anaphylaxis.

IV. Database. Knowledge of the patient's prior history of allergies and current medications is essential. The temporal relationship between administration of medication and the onset of symptoms is also important, since anaphylaxis usually occurs within one hour of administration.

    A. Physical examination key points

        1. Vital signs. Hypotension must be recognized immediately.

        2. Lungs. Listen for wheezing (suggests bronchospasm) and stridor (suggests upper airway obstruction).

        3. Skin. Generalized flushing, urticaria, and angioedema may occur.

        4. Extremities. Look for cyanosis.

        5. Mental status. Impaired mentation may indicate significant respiratory compromise or hypotension, and would suggest the need for immediate respiratory and/or blood pressure support.

    B. Laboratory data—Arterial blood gases. Hypoxia and hypercapnia occur with respiratory compromise; however, most often the problem must be addressed before results of this test are available.

    C. Radiologic and other studies

        1. Chest x-ray. Can be obtained after the patient is stabilized to exclude other causes of respiratory distress, such as pneumonia and congestive heart failure.

        2. Electrocardiogram. Acute myocardial infarction can present with severe dyspnea. Anaphylaxis can also cause myocardial ischemia and arrhythmias.

V. Plan. Treatment should be initiated quickly without waiting for the results of laboratory testing. If the patient is pulseless, external cardiac compression should be initiated. Initial therapy consists of epinephrine, oxygen, and a nebulized beta$_2$-agonist.

    A. Epinephrine. Epinephrine 0.3–0.5 mL of 1:1000 dilution (0.3–0.5 mg) subcutaneously should be given immediately for laryngeal edema, bronchospasm, angioedema, or urticaria, and then every 10–20 minutes if needed. The goal is to maintain airway patency, reduce fluid extravasation, and pruritus. Patients with hypotension and poor tissue perfusion will require intravenous epinephrine: 1 mL of 1:1000 dilution in 500 mL D5W at a rate of 0.5–5 µg (0.25–2.5 mL) per minute.

    B. Oxygen. Oxygen by face mask should be instituted if the patient appears dyspneic. Intubation may be required if the patient is severely somnolent or hypoxemic. Tracheostomy may be necessary if upper airway edema precludes intubation. The goal is to maintain a pO2 > 60 mm Hg.

C. Bronchodilators. Metaproterenol (0.3 ml of 5% solution in 2.5 mL of saline) or albuterol (0.5 mL of 0.5% solution in 2.5 mL of saline) can be administered by nebulizer for persistent bronchospasm.

Secondary therapy is utilized to prevent recurrent or prolonged reactions. These agents have little or no efficacy during the acute anaphylactic reaction.

D. Diphenhydramine (Benadryl). Diphenhydramine (25–50 mg) IM or PO Q 6 hr should follow epinephrine to reduce the effects of histamine release. This may alleviate hypotension as well as lessen the symptoms associated with mild urticaria.

E. High-dose glucocorticosteroids. These have questionable benefit in anaphylactic shock, but hydrocortisone 250 mg IV Q 6 hr should be given for episodes of anaphylactic bronchospasm. This may also help the late phase response that sometimes occurs several hours after the initial presentation.

F. Aminophylline. For patients whose bronchospasm does not respond to epinephrine and beta$_2$-agonists, aminophylline 6 mg/kg over 20–30 minutes should be given, followed by a maintenance dose of 0.4–0.9 mg/kg per hour.

G. Blood pressure support. Hypotension usually responds to the administration of epinephrine; however, normal saline may be necessary for those patients failing to respond. Patients taking beta-adrenergic blockers may be refractory to epinephrine; in these cases hypotension may respond to intravenous glucagon.

H. Monitoring. Relapse of anaphylaxis can occur hours after the initial presentation. Close monitoring through the first 24 hours is essential. Even with rapid and appropriate treatment, patients may not respond. Always be prepared for the possible need of emergent intubation or tracheostomy.

REFERENCE

Bochner BS, Lichtenstein LM. Anaphylaxis. N Engl J Med 1991;324:1785.

5. ANEMIA

I. Problem. A patient is admitted for pneumonia. The hematocrit (HCT) is noted to be 25%.

II. Immediate Questions

A. What are the patient's vital signs? If the patient is not hypotensive or severely tachycardic, transfusion therapy is probably not emergently indicated.

B. Is the patient symptomatic? In the absence of angina or hemodynamic compromise, transfusion therapy is not emergently indicated.

C. Is there evidence of acute or recent blood loss such as hematemesis, melena, hematochezia, or menorrhagia? Gastrointestinal (GI) blood loss can be divided into acute or chronic, upper GI (See Section I, Chapter 26, Hematemesis, Melena, p 140) and lower GI (See Section I, Chapter 27, Hematochezia, p 143). Patients more frequently succumb from acute upper GI blood loss; however, lower GI blood loss, though not seen as frequently by internists, can still be fatal.

D. What medications does the patient take? Aspirin and nonsteroidal anti-inflammatory drugs (NSAIDs) may lead to GI blood loss. Alkylating agents (melphalan, *cis*-platinum), folate antagonists (Bactrim, pentamidine), anticonvulsants (Dilantin), and anti-inflammatory drugs (phenylbutazone) may cause marrow suppression or aplasia. Penicillin, sulfonamides, and methyldopa (Aldomet) may cause hemolysis. Alcohol, isoniazid, and trimethoprim may cause maturation defects.

E. Is there significant organ dysfunction or a current inflammatory disease? Severe liver, kidney, adrenal, and thyroid dysfunction may lead to anemia. Rheumatoid arthritis, systemic lupus erythematosus (SLE), and vasculitides are associated with anemia of chronic disease.

F. Does the patient have other medical problems associated with excess total body water that may lead to a pseudoanemia, such as congestive heart failure, cirrhosis, and pregnancy? In settings with increased plasma volume relative to the red cell mass, an apparent anemia may be manifest or an existing anemia may be made more apparent.

G. Does the patient have a personal or family history of anemia, thalassemia, sickle cell anemia, or glucose 6-phosphatase deficiency? Hereditary disorders of hemoglobin usually present nonacutely and a family history may be suggestive of an inherited cause of the anemia.

III. Differential Diagnosis. There are well over 100 causes of anemia. A look at the peripheral smear with careful attention to the red cell indices is of particular importance when evaluating a patient with anemia. Anemia may result from decreased production of red blood cells (RBCs), blood loss, or increased destruction of RBCs.

A. Pancytopenia. The platelet and white blood cell (WBC) counts are decreased along with the hemoglobin (HGB) and HCT. Pancytopenia is usually caused by either marrow invasion, failure, or suppression; most commonly caused by drugs, solid tumors, hematologic malignancies, and inflammatory diseases. It may be idiopathic.

B. **Anemia with a low mean corpuscular volume (MCV).** Associated with microcytic red cells on the peripheral smear. Iron deficiency is the most common etiology and is seen in approximately 20% of menstruating females. Thalassemias also fall in this category. Hypochromic, microcytic red blood cells (RBCs), target cells, basophilic stippling, marked anisocytosis, and poikilocytosis are noted. Sideroblastic anemia and anemia of chronic disease may also be associated with low MCV. The MCV should never be <70 if it is due to chronic disease. Microcytic anemias can easily be differentiated by looking at the peripheral smear and various laboratory studies. Serum iron, total iron-binding capacity or transferrin, ferritin, and hemoglobin electrophoresis may be helpful (Table 1–4).

C. **Normal-MCV anemias.** Many anemias are associated with a normal MCV. Anemia of chronic disease is probably the most common normocytic anemia. Chronic infections (tuberculosis, osteomyelitis), collagen vascular diseases, and malignancies may produce an anemia with a normal MCV. Kidney, liver, thyroid, and adrenal dysfunction may also lead to a normal-MCV anemia. Correction of the underlying disorder should correct the anemia.

D. **High-MCV anemias.** Many anemias are macrocytic, but only a few are megaloblastic. Folate and vitamin B_{12} deficiencies are the most common megaloblastic anemias. Vitamin B_{12} deficiency can be secondary to pernicious anemia (lack of intrinsic factor), bacterial overgrowth, ileal disease, and rarely, dietary deficiency. Vitamin B_{12} stores last 3–4 years. Folate deficiency is often caused by dietary deficiency but may be secondary to increased needs such as with pregnancy or hyperthyroidism. If there is no obvious cause of folate deficiency, then the possibility of malabsorption must be considered. Along with macrocytic RBCs, the peripheral smear of folate or vitamin B_{12} deficiency may demonstrate hypersegmented neutrophils and nucleated RBCs. Other anemias that may be associated with macrocytes are myelodysplasias, aplastic anemias, acquired sideroblastic anemias, anemias induced by chemotherapy (antimetabolites), and anemia associated with hypothyroidism and chronic liver disease. An increased MCV may be seen in the

TABLE 1–4. CAUSES OF MICROCYTIC ANEMIA.

	Iron Deficiency	β-Thalassemia	Chronic Disease	Sideroblastic Anemia
Iron	Low	Normal/increased	Low	Increased
TIBC	Increased	Normal	Low	Normal
Ferritin	Low	Normal/increased	Normal/increased	Increased
Hemoglobin A_2[1]	Normal	Increased	Normal	Normal

[1] A type of hemoglobin detected by hemoglobin electrophoresis.

presence of a markedly increased reticulocyte count, as reticulo-cytes are large cells that increase the mean RBC size.

E. Anemias with increased reticulocytosis. Many anemias listed above are associated with an increased reticulocyte count. A reticulocyte is a very young red cell ~1 day old. As the RBC life span is ~100 days (actually 120), the normal reticulocyte count is ~1/100 or 1%. An increased reticulocyte count indicates that the bone marrow is producing red cells faster than normal. This is usually due to red cells having a shortened life span or to blood loss. The peripheral smear may reveal large polychromatophilic RBCs which are reticulocytes; however, a reticulocyte stain is needed to perform a definitive reticulocyte count. Examples of anemias with an increased reticulocyte count include acquired or autoimmune hemolytic anemias and congenital hemolytic anemias (sickle cell anemia, thalassemias). Correction of a particular deficit such as B_{12} deficiency by the administration of vitamin B_{12} will also lead to a reticulocytosis.

IV. Database
A. Physical examination key points
1. **Vital signs.** Make sure the patient is not hypotensive. The patient may be **orthostatic.** Look for a decrease in systolic blood pressure of 10 mm Hg and/or an increase in heart rate of 20 bpm on movement from a supine to a standing position after 1 minute.
2. **Skin.** Telangiectasia, palmar erythema, and jaundice may indicate liver disease. Isolated jaundice may point toward hemolysis.
3. **Oropharynx.** Glossitis is commonly seen in iron and B_{12} deficiency.
4. **Heart.** Murmurs may be either indicative of hemolysis from valvular disease or merely a flow murmur resulting from anemia.
5. **Abdomen.** Check for splenomegaly, which is associated with hemolysis, thalassemias, chronic leukemias, lymphomas, and occasionally acute leukemias. Could also indicate portal hypertension secondary to cirrhosis. Also look for ascites and hepatomegaly.
6. **Rectum.** Test for stool hemoccult to look for GI blood loss.
7. **Neurologic examination.** Loss of vibration and position sense as well as dementia are associated with B_{12} deficiency but may also represent effects of alcohol and hypothyroidism.

B. Laboratory data
1. **Peripheral smear.** Review on all patients with anemia. Note the size and shape of the RBCs and the presence or absence of platelets. Nucleated RBCs, reticulocytes, schistocytes, sickle cells, and target cells may aid in the diagnosis. Examine WBC morphology for hypersegmented neutrophils.

2. **Reticulocyte count.** The most important laboratory test after reviewing the peripheral smear. An increased count indicates either an appropriate response to anemia or shortened RBC survival through blood loss or hemolysis. A low reticulocyte count indicates that the marrow is responding inappropriately to the anemia.

3. **Iron and total iron binding capacity (TIBC) or transferrin.** Occasionally a ferritin should also be obtained if the anemia is microcytic. Will aid in the diagnosis of iron deficiency anemia. Iron deficiency anemia results in a low iron and a normal or elevated TIBC or transferrin; the ferritin is also low. If the patient has a very low MCV (<70) and a normal iron and TIBC, the likelihood of thalassemia is high. It is important to realize that many acute and chronic illnesses can dramatically affect the iron and TIBC, making their utility in the diagnosis of anemia low. If the question of iron deficiency requires a definite answer, a bone marrow exam with iron stains is indicated.

4. **B$_{12}$ and folate.** Order these tests for any patient suspected of having B$_{12}$ and folate deficiency prior to transfusion. If folate deficiency is secondary to malnutrition, a serum folate may be normal after one or two well-balanced meals. If folate deficiency is suspected and the patient has recently eaten, then consider checking a red blood cell folate.

5. **Haptoglobin and urine hemosiderin.** A low haptoglobin and a positive urine hemosiderin are indicative of hemolysis.

6. **Direct and indirect Coombs' test.** These tests may indicate that the hemolysis is immunologic. A direct Coombs' measures the presence of antibody and/or complement on the RBC; an indirect Coombs' detects antibody in the plasma that has dissociated from the RBC but is directed at the RBC. The direct Coombs' is the more valuable test in evaluating the possibility of immunohemolytic disease, whereas the indirect Coombs' is primarily of value as a blood banking procedure. Detection of an antibody in the plasma but not on the RBC indicates it is an alloantibody rather than an autoantibody. Most immunohemolytic anemias are due to warm–reacting antibodies, usually IgG. These are manifest by a direct Coombs' that is positive for IgG with or without complement.

7. **Platelet count.** May be elevated in early iron deficiency. Decreased in folate and vitamin B$_{12}$ deficiency as well as with marrow replacement.

C. **Radiologic and other studies.** Not usually needed unless GI blood loss is suspected; then order as clinically indicated.

V. Plan

A. **Anemia with hemodynamic compromise or complications**

1. If the patient is hemodynamically unstable or having angina, a transfusion is urgently indicated. In such cases, the source of

blood loss is usually obvious. For specific information on transfusion, consult Chapter 5.

2. Be sure the patient has adequate intravenous access if there is evidence of acute bleeding.

B. Anemia without hemodynamic compromise or complications. If the patient is not hemodynamically compromised, proceed with the workup in an orderly fashion. In many cases, the cause of the anemia is not obvious. Furthermore, laboratory testing is not always diagnostic. If the patient has an unremarkable history and physical, ambivalent laboratory testing, and no obvious underlying infectious, malignant, or inflammatory disease, a bone marrow biopsy is indicated.

C. Iron deficiency anemia. In this condition a source of blood loss must be found. This usually entails a flexible sigmoidoscopy and air-contrast barium enema, or a colonoscopy and either an upper endoscopy or a barium study of the upper GI tract. Keep in mind that heavy menstrual losses are the most common cause of iron deficiency anemia in young women. Once the source of blood loss is determined, the iron stores need to be repleted. Most patients tolerate oral iron as ferrous sulfate 325 mg PO TID between meals. Treatment must be continued for 3–6 months after normalization of the CBC to ensure adequate repletion of iron stores. Gradually increasing the dose over several days from Q day to BID to TID will improve tolerance to oral iron. Vitamin C 500–1000 units with each dose of iron may improve absorption.

D. Folate deficiency. This condition is usually due to dietary insufficiency (pregnancy, chronic alcoholism). In this setting, daily folate supplementation at 1 mg PO is indicated.

E. Vitamin B_{12} deficiency. Inadequate dietary intake is a rare cause of B_{12} deficiency. True pernicious anemia can be diagnosed by the use of Schilling's test, which involves giving a loading dose of 1000 μg vitamin B_{12} to saturate receptor sites. This dose is followed by the administration of radiolabeled B_{12} and measurement of the radioactivity in a 24-hour urine sample. If the amount of radioactive B_{12} in the urine is small, oral intrinsic factor can be given along with a second dose of radioactive B_{12} and a 24-hour urine recollected. An abnormal first step and a normal second step help differentiate between pernicious anemia and other causes of vitamin B_{12} deficiency (eg, bacterial overgrowth and ileal diseases). The history may also give an obvious etiology for B_{12} deficiency (status post gastrectomy or ileal resection). Vitamin B_{12} is replaced by administration of 30–100 μg IM daily for 2–3 weeks, then 100–200 μg IM every 2–4 weeks for life.

F. Hemolytic anemia. In the face of an elevated reticulocyte count with no obvious source of blood loss, a destructive process must be considered. Immune-mediated processes can be diagnosed by use of the Coombs' test. In the setting of Coombs' negative hemolytic anemia, other processes must be considered such as disseminated intravascular coagulation or microangiopathic hemolytic anemia. A review of the peripheral smear will be helpful. A concomitant low platelet count, low fibrinogen, and elevated prothrombin time, partial thromboplastin time, and fibrin degradation products point toward disseminated intravascular coagulation (see Coagulopathy, p 64). The possibility of an inherited disorder such as thalassemia, sickle cell anemia, or an enzymopathy must be ruled out. Hemoglobin electrophoresis and review of the peripheral smear are indicated. If an enzymopathy is considered, specific assays are indicated (glucose-6-phosphate dehydrogenase, pyruvate kinase, and so on). The possibility of paroxysmal nocturnal hemoglobinuria must be considered in cases where the etiology is unclear. Ham's test is indicated in this instance. Discussion of specific treatments for hemolytic anemia is beyond the scope of this book.

G. **Anemia of chronic disease.** This is usually a diagnosis of exclusion. The etiology may be obvious as in a patient with advanced malignancy. There is no specific diagnostic test for this disorder; treatment is of the underlying disease. It is generally manifest by a low reticulocyte count, a low iron and TIBC or transferrin, and normal bone marrow morphology. These are not specific findings, however.

REFERENCES

Bolinger A: Anemias. In: Koda-Kimbal MA, Young LY eds. *Applied Therapeutics: The Clinical Use of Drugs*, 5th ed. Applied Therapeutics, Inc., 1992.

Lux SE: Introduction to anemia. In: Handin RI, Lux SE, Stossel TP, eds.: *Blood: Principles and Practice of Hematology*. Lippincott;1995:1383.

6. ARTERIAL LINE PROBLEMS

(See also Section 3, Arterial Line Placement, p 341)

I. **Problem.** You are called to the intensive care unit to see a patient in whom a low, dampened arterial line pressure is being obtained.

II. **Immediate Questions**
   A. **Does the pressure accurately reflect the patient's status?** Mental status changes (See Section I, Chapter 13, Coma, Acute Mental Status Changes, p 69), tachycardia, and a decreased urine output would be expected with hypotension.
   B. **Is the problem with the catheter itself or with the monitoring apparatus (tubing, transducer, electronic equipment)?** If the

patient's clinical status does not reflect the low blood pressure obtained by the arterial line, the problem may lie in the equipment.
C. Is an extremity at risk? Thrombosis secondary to the arterial line can cause ischemia and tissue loss.
D. Has the quality of the tracing changed recently? Find out if the tracing was satisfactory earlier. A good tracing followed by a poor one suggests either deterioration in clinical status or a new problem with the catheter.

III. Differential Diagnosis. A low or dampened blood pressure may result from problems with the monitoring equipment, problems with the arterial line catheter, or actual hemodynamic deterioration of the patient.
A. Patient status. If the patient's hemodynamic status has deteriorated, the decrease in blood pressure or dampening of the waveform is actually indicative of the patient's status. Often, other clinical indicators of the patient's status such as mental status changes, tachycardia, decreased urine output, and electrocardiographic changes suggest that the patient is genuinely hypotensive.
B. Monitoring apparatus problems
   1. Air is present in the tubing/transducer.
   2. The tubing is kinked.
   3. Electrical equipment is faulty.
C. Catheter problems
   1. There are kinks in the catheter.
   2. A thrombus is present in the catheter or in the vessel.
   3. The catheter tip is resting against the wall of the artery because of the way the catheter was anchored (by suture or taping).
   4. The catheter has punctured the arterial wall, causing bleeding and compression of the catheter.

IV. Database
A. Physical examination key points
   1. Blood pressure. If the arterial line pressure is low, perform a brachial artery cuff pressure. If the reading confirms hypotension, prompt action is indicated. The manual blood pressure is usually within 10–20 mm Hg of the arterial line pressure, unless severe vasoconstriction is present; in which case indirect measurement may underestimate direct measurement by 20–30 mm Hg.
   2. Pulses. Check at once for distal pulses and for swelling or tenderness in the area of the catheter insertion. Failure to find a pulse or the presence of a decrease in pulse, with significant swelling at the catheter site, represents a potentially serious vascular compromise.
   3. Inspection of the equipment

a. Check for air in the lines or the transducer. The search must be thorough and will almost certainly require the assistance of the nursing staff.
b. Have nursing staff confirm that the electrical equipment is working properly.
c. Attempt to withdraw blood through the catheter. Inability to do so suggests either that the catheter tip is poorly positioned, or that there is a kink or a thrombus in the catheter, at the catheter tip, or in the artery. *Caution:* Do not attempt to flush a catheter through which blood cannot be drawn!

V. Plan

A. Maintaining perfusion to the extremity.
A limb may be susceptible to ischemic injury as the result of systemic hypotension, a large catheter-to-vessel ratio, bleeding into surrounding tissues, inadequate flushing techniques, or prolonged catheter indwelling time.

1. Failure of the pulse to return will probably necessitate a surgical attempt at thrombus removal or repair of the artery. Consult a vascular surgeon immediately.
2. If bleeding from the artery into the surrounding tissue seems likely, watch carefully for compartmental syndrome (pain, pain with extension of the digits, pallor, hypesthesia, and loss of motor function). Surgical evacuation of the blood may be necessary. Consult a vascular surgeon at once if compartmental syndrome is suspected.
3. Search for evidence of infection. If infection is present, culture and treat appropriately, and remove the catheter.

B. Monitoring apparatus problems
1. Flush the transducer and tubing thoroughly.
2. Retape the tubing to eliminate kinks.
3. Replace faulty electrical equipment.
4. An armboard may prevent the catheter or tubing from extra-arterial kinking.

C. Catheter problems
1. Loosen sutures or tape to reposition catheter tip away from the wall.
2. If a thrombus or kink in the intra-arterial catheter is suspected, the line will probably have to be removed and relocated.
3. In general, do not attempt to place a new arterial line over a guide wire. Remove the old catheter and replace it with a new one, preferably at a different site. Perforation of the catheter with the guide wire may cause a foreign body embolus, damage to the arterial wall, or dislodgement of a thrombus in or at the tip of the catheter. All these potentially serious complications make the risk of using a catheter guide wire to assess a dampened waveform unwise.

7. ASPIRATION

I. **Problem.** After a generalized seizure, a patient is observed to vomit and subsequently develops acute respiratory distress.

II. **Immediate Questions**
   A. **What are the vital signs?** On the basis of the history, it must be assumed that the patient has aspirated gastric contents. This can result in acute respiratory compromise, either through lodging of particulate matter in the larynx or trachea, by induction of laryngospasm, or through the rapid onset of pulmonary edema. In any of these cases, both **tachycardia** and **tachypnea** are often present. In severe episodes of respiratory compromise, **apnea, respiratory arrest,** or **shock** may also occur.
   B. **Is the patient able to communicate?** Aphonia may result from lodging of particulate matter in the larynx or trachea, and requires immediate endotracheal suctioning.
   C. **Is the patient cyanotic?** Cyanosis would indicate severe respiratory compromise and probable need for emergent intubation.
   D. **Does the patient need to be repositioned?** If the patient continues to vomit, to prevent further aspiration of gastric contents, the patient should be placed in a lateral decubitus position with the head down.

III. **Differential Diagnosis.** Three distinct aspiration syndromes are recognized, depending on the nature of the aspirated contents: (1) acidic gastric contents; (2) nonacid and/or particulate material; and (3) oropharyngeal bacterial pathogens. These syndromes should be distinguished from one another as well as from other causes of acute respiratory distress, because the complications and treatment differ for each.
   A. **Acid aspiration.** Aspiration of gastric contents with a pH < 2.5 results in immediate alveolar injury and chemical pneumonitis. Noncardiogenic pulmonary edema and shock may occur. Clinically, there is abrupt onset of dyspnea, fever, wheezing, rales, and hypoxemia.
   B. **Particulate aspiration.** This can result in mechanical obstruction and bronchospasm. Pneumonia can ensue if particulate material remains lodged in peripheral airways.
   C. **Oropharyngeal bacteria.** Saliva contains 10^8 organisms per milliliter. Aspiration of saliva into the lower airway can cause an early pneumonitis followed by necrotizing pneumonia or abscess in 3–14 days.
   D. **Asthma.** See Section 1, Chapter 61, Wheezing, p 297.

E. **Pneumonia.** Pneumonia can be very difficult to distinguish from acute aspiration of gastric contents, as both can result in sputum production, tachycardia, tachypnea, fever, rales, and radiographic infiltrates.

F. **Pulmonary embolism.** This diagnosis must be considered in the differential of any patient developing acute respiratory distress.

G. **Foreign body aspiration.** This occurs mainly in younger children and occasionally in debilitated elderly people who aspirate a food bolus.

H. **Upper airway obstruction.** Acute edema of the vocal cords or glottis may follow aspiration. A high-pitched wheeze is heard over the larynx (stridor) with the stethoscope.

IV. **Database.** Attempt to identify those conditions that predispose to aspiration, including impairment of consciousness, swallowing, and esophageal dysfunction. Disorders resulting in **impairment of consciousness** include anesthesia, alcohol abuse, seizure disorder, cerebrovascular accident, cardiopulmonary arrest, and drug overdose. **Esophageal dysfunction** predisposes to aspiration, and includes esophageal stricture, hiatal hernia, and nasogastric intubation. **Impaired swallowing** may result from a cerebrovascular accident, polymyositis, myasthenia gravis, Parkinson's disease, a tracheostomy, or cancer involving the head and neck.

A. **Physical examination key points**

1. **Vital signs.** See Section II.A.

2. **HEENT.** Check dentition for loose or missing teeth and evidence of gingivitis.

3. **Neck.** Examine for evidence of tumor involving the oropharynx. Also look for any evidence of prior surgical procedures or radiation of the head and neck.

4. **Lungs.** Wheezing and crackles can occur after aspiration of gastric contents. Wheezing and diminished breath sounds may result from aspiration of particulate material. Listen for stridor (laryngeal wheeze).

5. **Skin.** Examine for presence of cyanosis.

6. **Neurologic examination.** Determine the degree of consciousness and the presence or absence of a gag reflex.

B. **Laboratory data**

1. **Arterial blood gases.** Hypoxemia and hypercapnia may occur and, if present, intubation may be required.

2. **Hemogram.** Aspiration of acid contents and pneumonia can cause a leukocytosis and left shift.

3. **Sputum Gram's stain and culture.** If the patient manifests fever, leukocytosis, and sputum production 2–3 days after aspiration, a sputum Gram's stain and culture may be helpful in con-

firming pneumonia and directing subsequent antibiotic therapy. However, aspiration pneumonia is often anaerobic and may be polymicrobial.

C. Radiologic and other studies

  1. Chest x-ray may show:

   a. Hyperaeration from air trapping on the side of foreign body aspiration.

   b. Infiltrate in dependent segments of the lungs. Infiltrates may not be seen immediately after aspiration; therefore, if the initial CXR is normal but there is a strong clinical suspicion of aspiration, repeat the CXR in 4–5 hours.

   c. A wedge-shaped pleural-based density suggests pulmonary infarction from pulmonary embolism.

   d. Clear fields and hyperinflation are common in uncomplicated asthma.

   e. Lung abscess formation does not generally occur until 7–14 days following aspiration, and will not be observed on initial films.

  2. Other studies. Ventilation/perfusion ($\dot{V}/\dot{Q}$) scan if a pulmonary embolism is suspected.

V. Plan. Aspiration should be suspected in any patient with a predisposing factor who develops sudden respiratory distress. Early treatment is important, as death from respiratory failure can occur if the condition is not recognized early. Ideally, the best treatment is prevention.

A. Prevention

  1. For patients being administered tube feedings, gastric emptying should be confirmed and the head of the bed elevated. Small silastic feeding tubes are preferable to large-bore Salem sump tubes. Placement of the feeding tube into the duodenum or jejunum markedly decreases the risk of aspiration.

  2. Unconscious patients should be placed in a lateral, slightly head-down position whenever possible.

  3. When not being used for enteral feedings, nasogastric tubes should be placed only when continuous suction is required.

  4. Patients with recent strokes should not be fed by mouth until they have demonstrated an intact gag reflex.

  5. Patients on tube feedings should be elevated 30–45 degrees at all times.

B. Oxygenation. Supplemental oxygen should be given in an amount sufficient to ensure oxygen saturation greater than 90%.

C. Intubation and positive pressure breathing. Will be required in the patient for whom supplemental oxygen therapy is not sufficient to maintain adequate oxygenation; or in the patient who is obtunded and unable to protect her or his airway.

D. Endotracheal suction. Should be attempted in any patient who is observed to aspirate.

E. Medications
1. Bronchodilators such as albuterol 0.5 mL with 3 mL normal saline may relieve bronchospasm.
2. Prophylactic corticosteroids have not been shown to decrease subsequent morbidity and mortality from aspiration, and are not indicated.
3. Prophylactic antibiotics likewise have not been shown to diminish morbidity and mortality. Antibiotics should be administered only if the patient continues to manifest fever, leukocytosis, purulent sputum, and infiltrates 2–3 days after the initial aspiration. For those patients with in-hospital aspiration, a regimen that provides coverage for gram-negative aerobes, anaerobes, and possibly *Staphylococcus aureus* should be used.
F. Fiberoptic bronchoscopy. Is indicated only when lobar or segmental collapse is present, or when foreign body aspiration is suspected.

REFERENCES

Ibanez J et al: Gastroesophageal reflux in intubated patients receiving enteral nutrition: Effect of supine and semi-recumbent positions. JPEN 1992;16:419.
Russin SJ, Adler AG: Pulmonary aspiration. Postgrad Med 1989;85:155.
Tietjen PA, Kaner RD, Quin CE: Aspiration emergencies. Clin Chest Med 1994;15:117.

8. BRADYCARDIA

I. **Problem.** A nurse on the telemetry unit calls to notify you that a 66-year-old woman has a heart rate of 40 beats per minute (bpm) on the telemetry monitor. She was admitted earlier in the day with atypical chest pain and dizziness.

II. **Immediate Questions**
A. **What are the patient's other vital signs?** Any given heart rate must always be considered in the context of its relationship with the blood pressure (BP) and other signs of the patient's condition. A patient with a BP below 90 mm Hg and bradycardia requires more thought and action than a patient with bradycardia, a normal BP, and no adverse symptoms.
B. **What has the patient's heart rate been since admission?** The range of normal heart rates is wide and is influenced by many factors, such as activity, age of the patient, medications, presence of pain, type of illness that caused the patient to be hospitalized, and presence of fever. The resting heart rate can be expected to rise approximately 10 bpm for each degree of temperature above normal in a febrile patient.

C. Does the patient have any symptoms possibly related to the bradycardia? Such as profound fatigue, dizziness, nausea, dyspnea, chest pain, decreased urinary output, or mental status changes.

III. Differential Diagnosis

A. Sinus bradycardia. Defined as a sinus node rhythm below 60 bpm. Changes in sinus rate are modulated by changes in sympathetic and parasympathetic tone. Causes of sinus bradycardia include the following:

1. **Increased parasympathetic tone.** Sinus bradycardia can be precipitated many times by sudden stressful or painful events. An example is a vasovagal syncopal episode related to nervousness, or to fear experienced by a patient having a peripheral blood sample taken.

2. **Sinus node dysfunction.** Characterized by the presence of bradycardia at times that are inappropriate for the patient's current state. Sinus node dysfunction can also be manifested by periods of sinoatrial arrest, or sinoatrial exit block, or by alternating sinus bradycardia and atrial tachyarrhythmias, commonly referred to as sick sinus syndrome.

3. **Myocardial infarction.** Sinus bradycardia is seen most frequently with inferior wall infarctions, involving the proximal portion of the right coronary artery and its branch to the sinoatrial node. The presence of sinus bradycardia during the early phases of an acute myocardial infarction is a good prognostic sign. It does not require therapy, as long as left ventricular cardiac output is adequate and CHF is absent. In fact, raising the heart rate in this instance may raise cardiac demand and precipitate recurrent angina pectoris.

4. **Cushing's reflex.** Sinus bradycardia is associated with an increase in intracranial pressure secondary to a variety of causes, such as hemorrhagic stroke, meningitis, intracranial tumor, or trauma. Hypertension is seen in addition to the bradycardia.

5. **Other medical disorders.** Sinus bradycardia can occur in patients with hypothyroidism, hypothermia, and certain infiltrating diseases of the myocardium.

6. **Drug effect.** Sinus bradycardia is a common secondary effect of several classes of medications, including beta-blockers, and calcium channel blockers, as well as clonidine (Catapres), lithium carbonate, and certain antiarrhythmic drugs such as amiodarone (Cordarone).

B. Atrioventricular (AV) node blocks

1. **Mobitz type I second-degree AV Block (Wenckebach).** Characterized by progressive, cyclical prolongation of the PR interval with each cardiac cycle until a ventricular beat is dropped. This results in intermittent AV block in a repeated cycle.

      a. Acute myocardial infarction. Most commonly seen early in inferior wall infarctions related to ischemia affecting the atrioventricular nodal branch of the right coronary artery.

      b. Drug effect. Excessive serum levels of certain cardiac medications can result in the development of Wenckebach-type second-degree AV block. Examples would include: digitalis (Lanoxin), beta-blockers, calcium channel blockers, and amiodarone.

      c. Infections. A Wenckebach rhythm is occasionally seen during the acute phases of rheumatic fever and Lyme disease, when the inflammatory process affects the cardiac conduction system.

      d. Other. Wenckebach rhythms can occasionally be seen in asymptomatic, otherwise normal adults; they are related to the level of parasympathetic nervous system tone, such as in highly-trained aerobic athletes, particularly during sleep.

2. Mobitz type II second-degree AV block. Cyclical AV block without the progressive prolongation of the PR interval. The QRS complex of conducted beats is often wide because of involvement of the bundle of His.

      a. Acute myocardial infarction. Large anterior wall infarctions are a more common cause than inferior infarctions.

      b. Degenerative diseases. Involving the bundle of His.

      c. Infectious diseases. Such as viral myocarditis, acute rheumatic fever, and Lyme disease.

3. Third-degree AV block. This ominous rhythm is associated with the same conditions as Mobitz type II second-degree heart block. Third-degree AV block occurs when there is no conduction of the P waves from the sinoatrial node through the atrioventricular node to the ventricle. This results in the P waves and QRS complexes being independent of one another. Usually the ventricular rate and rhythm are controlled by a secondary intraventricular pacemaker which is normally suppressed when AV conduction is intact.

IV. Database

A. Physical examination key points

1. Vital signs. Obtain the patient's blood pressure during the bradycardic rhythm, and assess the patient's level of consciousness.

2. Neck veins. Intermittent cannon "A" waves in the jugular venous pulsations are observed in the presence of complete AV dissociation. A cannon "A" wave is an exaggerated A wave in the jugular venous pulse that results from right atrial contraction on an already closed tricuspid valve, caused by simultaneous atrial and ventricular contraction. This results in backward ejec-

tion of right atrial blood into the superior vena cava and jugular
veins.

   3. **Lungs.** Rales on lung exam, during periods of bradycardia, sug-
      gest inadequate left ventricular cardiac output or congestive
      heart failure. This is referred to as a chronotropic incompetence.
   4. **Heart.** Listen for murmurs and gallops. An S_4 may be present
      during an acute myocardial infarction. A new cardiac murmur may
      be seen in myocardial infarction, acute rheumatic fever, and
      myocarditis. See Section 1, Chapter 25, Heart Murmur, p 133.
   5. **Skin.** Cool, pale extremities suggest an inadequate cardiac out-
      put, possibly as a result of the bradycardic rhythm.
   6. **Mental status.** Inadequate cerebral perfusion may result in al-
      tered level of consciousness.
  B. **Laboratory data**
   1. **Electrolytes.** Exclude hypokalemia if the patient is on digoxin.
   2. **Digoxin level.** A must if the patient is on digoxin. Bradycardia
      can be a sign of digitalis intoxication.
   3. **Thyroid hormone levels.** Rule out hypothyroidism as a cause.
  C. **Electrocardiogram and rhythm strip**
   1. Identify P waves and their timing and relationship to the QRS
      complexes. Leads I, aVR, V_1, and the inferior leads demonstrate
      the morphology of the P waves best. The absence of P waves
      suggests an AV nodal rhythm, or atrial fibrillation with a slow
      ventricular response, as the cause of the bradycardia.
   2. An increasing PR interval with a dropped QRS complex, recur-
      ring in a cyclical pattern, indicates Mobitz type I second-degree
      heart block.
   3. P waves that occur intermittently without an associated QRS
      complex, but with an otherwise constant PR interval, suggest
      Mobitz type II second-degree heart block. The QRS duration is
      usually prolonged.
   4. Third-degree heart block is present when the P waves and QRS
      complexes demonstrate no relationship to each other.
   5. Look for evidence of myocardial ischemia or infarction. ST seg-
      ment elevation or depression, T wave inversion, and the pres-
      ence of new Q waves are common findings.
   6. Look for the presence and timing of pacemaker spikes, if
      appropriate.

V. Plan. Therapy is dictated by the most likely causes and the presence
   of symptoms related to the bradycardia. Some bradycardic rhythms do
   not require any treatment. React appropriately.
  A. **Drugs**
   1. Consider stopping or holding doses of medications associated
      with bradycardic rhythms. If the patient is asymptomatic, and

otherwise fine, discontinuing a medication such as propranolol is all that needs to be done.

2. Atropine. 0.5–1.0 mg IV push, up to a total dose of 2.0 mg, is the initial treatment of **symptomatic** sinus bradycardia, second-degree AV block, or third-degree AV block. Remember, be careful in raising the heart rate of a patient with a recent myocardial infarction, because myocardial demand could increase the likelihood of precipitating angina pectoris.

3. Since atropine is only a temporary measure, its effects are not likely to last beyond an hour or so. Temporary cardiac pacing (TCP) if available, dopamine 5–20 µg/kg/min or epinephrine 2–10 µg/min can be used following atropine if the heart rate is not maintained adequately to maintain hemodynamic stability.

4. If digitalis overdose or intoxication is responsible for a potentially life-threatening, hemodynamically unstable arrhythmia, and rapid treatment is necessary, consider giving the patient intravenous digoxin immune Fab fragments, or **Digibind**. Refer to the *Physician's Desk Reference* (PDR) for dosing information.

B. Treatment of bradycardia secondary to a CNS event. Decrease the intracranial pressure in patients with CNS disturbances. Initial steps would include: hyperventilation, furosemide, and dexamethasone if there is an increase in intracranial pressure resulting in bradycardia. See Section 1, Chapter 13, Coma, Acute Mental Status Changes, p 69.

C. Temporary artificial pacemakers. Temporary pacemakers include: external and transvenous devices. External pacemakers can be applied quickly in an emergent situation such as cardiac arrest. A transvenous pacemaker can be placed at the bedside using central venous cannulation when the patient is more hemodynamically stable.

1. Indications for temporary pacing.

    a. Mobitz type II second-degree or third-degree AV block associated with an acute myocardial infarction.

    b. Symptomatic AV block associated with drug toxicity that is likely to be recurrent, such as may occur occasionally with amiodarone toxicity.

    c. Sinus bradycardia with severe congestive heart failure.

    d. Prolonged sinus pauses (>3.5 seconds) associated with syncope. This may be the clue to sick sinus syndrome.

2. Indications for permanent pacing.

    a. Sick sinus syndrome **with** symptoms as a result of bradycardia or sinus pauses.

    b. Mobitz type II second-degree or third-degree AV block.

    c. Occasionally, patients with cardiomyopathies and class III congestive heart failure may benefit from placement of a dual-chambered permanent pacemaker in order to raise heart rate and cardiac output.

REFERENCES

Fisch C: *Electrocardiography of Arrhythmias*. Lea & Febiger 1990.
Marriott H: *Practical Electrocardiography*. 7th ed. Williams and Wilkins;1983.
Reiffel JA: Bradyarrhythmias. In: Horowitz LN, ed. *Current Management of Arrhythmias*. Decker;1991:225.
Zipes DP: Management of cardiac arrhythmias: Pharmacological, electrical, and surgical techniques. In: Braunwald E ed. *Heart Disease: A Textbook of Cardiovascular Medicine*. 4th ed. Saunders;1992:628.

9. CARDIOPULMONARY ARREST

I. **Problem.** You are the first member of a code team to arrive at the bedside of a patient found unresponsive by the nurse.

II. **Immediate Questions**
   A. **Is the patient unresponsive?** Cardiopulmonary resuscitation (CPR) begins with an attempt to arouse the patient. Call the patient by name and gently shake him or her by the shoulders. If the patient is unresponsive, begin CPR.
   B. **Is the patient in optimal position for CPR?** The patient must be supine and lying on a firm, flat surface to provide effective external chest compression. The head must be at the same level as the thorax for optimal cerebral perfusion.
   C. **Is the airway obstructed?** In an unconscious patient, the tongue and epiglottis may fall backward and occlude the airway. A head tilt/chin lift maneuver will lift these structures and open the airway. Vomitus or foreign material should be removed from the mouth by either a finger sweep or suction.
   D. **After establishment of airway patency, is the patient breathing?** Respiration can be assessed within 3–5 seconds by looking for chest movement, listening for air movement, and feeling for breath on the rescuer's face (rescuer's face is turned to face the patient's chest; rescuer's cheek is above the patient's mouth). If breathing is not present, then institute rescue breathing with two full breaths, preferably via either a pocket mask or Ambu bag if available.
   E. **Is there evidence of adequate circulation?** Establish the presence of a carotid pulse. If no pulse is felt after 10 seconds of palpation, begin external chest compressions. After basic and then advanced cardiac life support has been instituted, other questions may help elucidate the cause of the patient's arrest.

F. **What medications has the patient been taking?** Cardiac medications are particularly important. Drugs that prolong the QT interval, such as quinidine and procainamide, may predispose to torsades de pointes, characterized by recurrent ventricular tachycardia and ventricular fibrillation. Phenothiazines and tricyclic antidepressants may also cause this condition. Digoxin (Lanoxin) is a frequent cause of a variety of cardiac arrhythmias.

G. **Has the patient received any administered medications that could have resulted in an anaphylactic reaction?** See Section 1, Chapter 4, Anaphylactic Reaction, p 23.

H. **Is there any history of electrolyte disturbance or conditions that could predispose to electrolyte disturbance?** Hypokalemia and hypomagnesemia can predispose to arrhythmias. Hyperkalemia can cause complete heart block and cardiac arrest.

I. **What are the patient's medical problems?** Inquire specifically regarding a prior history of coronary artery disease or other cardiac disease. Is there any recent history to suggest an acute stroke or any conditions that predispose to acute pulmonary embolism such as recent surgery? The aggressiveness of CPR can be determined by knowing if the patient has any terminal medical problems such as advanced cancer.

III. **Differential Diagnosis.** Cardiopulmonary arrest can result from either a primary cardiac disturbance or from primary respiratory arrest. There are a wide variety of causes of cardiopulmonary arrest; some of the more common are listed here:

A. **Cardiac**
   1. **Acute myocardial infarction**
   2. **Acute pulmonary edema**
   3. **Ventricular arrhythmias**
   4. **Cardiac tamponade**

B. **Pulmonary**
   1. **Pulmonary embolism (usually massive)**
   2. **Acute respiratory failure**
   3. **Aspiration**
   4. **Tension pneumothorax (large)**

C. **Hemorrhagic.** Acute severe hemorrhage such as from a ruptured aortic aneurysm or rapid gastrointestinal bleeding.

D. **Metabolic**
   1. **Electrolyte disturbances.** Hypokalemia, hyperkalemia, and hypomagnesemia can induce arrhythmias.
   2. **Acidosis and alkalosis**
   3. **Hypothermia and rewarming.** During the treatment of acute hypothermia, rewarming may induce ventricular fibrillation or other arrhythmias.

  E. Drug overdoses. Especially tricyclic antidepressants, digitalis, and beta-blockers.

IV. Database
  A. Physical examination key points. The initial assessment of airway, breathing, and circulation is described in Section II, p 42. Resuscitation should obviously be initiated before a detailed physical examination is performed. Other signs to watch for:
  1. **Tracheal deviation.** This would indicate the possibility of tension pneumothorax.
  2. **Distended neck veins.** May also indicate a tension pneumothorax or pericardial tamponade.
  B. Laboratory data. These should be obtained early in resuscitation efforts but should not delay initiation of therapy.
  1. **Arterial blood gases.** Acidosis could be the cause of an arrhythmia or result from prolonged hypoperfusion. A low pO$_2$ can result from a variety of causes, including pulmonary edema and pulmonary embolus, or again it may result from prolonged hypoperfusion.
  2. **Serum electrolytes.** Particularly potassium and magnesium.
  3. **Complete blood count.** Keep in mind that with massive hemorrhage the hematocrit may not have had sufficient time to equilibrate and therefore may not be an accurate indicator of the severity of blood loss.
  C. Radiologic and other studies
  1. **Continuous cardiac monitoring.** Preferably with a 12-lead electrocardiogram. Should be obtained as early as possible. 3-lead monitoring is acceptable.
  2. **Chest x-ray.** A CXR should be obtained to determine the position of the endotracheal tube or any central venous line. This should obviously be performed after the patient is stabilized.

V. Plan. A full description of definitive therapy for each of the causes of cardiopulmonary arrest is beyond the scope of this text. The reader is referred to the excellent references at the end of this section. In general, the best success in performing CPR has been achieved in those patients in whom basic life support has been initiated *within 4 minutes* of the time of arrest and advanced cardiac life support *within 8 minutes.* Fairly early recognition of unresponsiveness and initiation of CPR is crucial. Once basic life support has been instituted, the next goal should be to determine the cardiac rhythm. Ventricular fibrillation is treated with immediate defibrillation. The next priority is endotracheal intubation followed by establishment of venous access via an antecubital vein or other large, visible superficial vein. Once a 12-lead ECG has been obtained, the physician may be able to establish a specific cause of the arrest and direct treatment accordingly. Listed here are brief summaries of the management of the major cardiac causes of arrest.

A. Ventricular fibrillation (See Figure 1–1.) Immediate defibrillation is the most important step in the treatment of ventricular fibrillation. In fact, defibrillation should be attempted prior to attempts to intubate the patient or establish intravenous access. Defibrillation is facilitated by the use of quick-look paddles now available on most defibrillators.

1. The first attempt should be with 200 joules. If the patient remains in ventricular fibrillation, the second attempt should use 300 joules, administered immediately. If fibrillation still persists, a third countershock with 360 joules should be delivered.

2. If the patient remains in ventricular fibrillation after three countershocks, CPR should be resumed. The patient should be intubated, intravenous access should be established, and the patient should be connected to a 12-lead ECG. Epinephrine (1 mg of a 1:10,000 solution) should be administered every 3–5 minutes. This drug is probably the most important pharmacologic agent used during CPR.

3. After 30–60 seconds, defibrillation should be attempted again with 360 joules. If the patient remains in ventricular fibrillation, a 1.5 mg/kg IV bolus of lidocaine should be administered.

4. After administration of lidocaine, defibrillation should again be attempted. If fibrillation persists, a second 1.5 mg/kg bolus of lidocaine can be administered, followed by another attempt at defibrillation.

5. Upon return to spontaneous circulation after either step 3 or 4, a constant infusion of 2–4 mg/min (15–50 mg/kg/min) of lidocaine should be started.

6. If ventricular fibrillation still persists, bretylium 5 mg/kg IV push can be given followed by defibrillation. A second dose of 10 mg/kg can be given after 5 minutes.

B. Sustained ventricular tachycardia with no palpable pulse. This arrhythmia should be managed like ventricular fibrillation.

C. Ventricular tachycardia with a palpable pulse

  1. Stable ventricular tachycardia

    a. Lidocaine is the drug of choice, an initial loading dose of 1.0 to 1.5 mg/kg IV push followed by an IV infusion of 2 mg/min should be administered. An additional 0.5 to 0.75 mg/kg IV bolus of lidocaine can be administered every 5–10 minutes as necessary until a total loading dose of 3 mg/kg has been given.

    b. If lidocaine fails, procainamide can be administered IV in 100-mg increments Q 5 min until either the arrhythmia is suppressed, the QRS complex widens more than 50%, or a loading dose of 17 mg/kg has been given.

   c. Finally, if both lidocaine and procainamide have been unsuccessful, bretylium 5–10 mg/kg infused over 10 min can be administered, followed by continuous infusion of 2 mg/min.

   d. If none of the preceding agents has succeeded in converting the patient, *synchronized* cardioversion with an initial energy level of 100 joules may be attempted, followed by 200 joules,

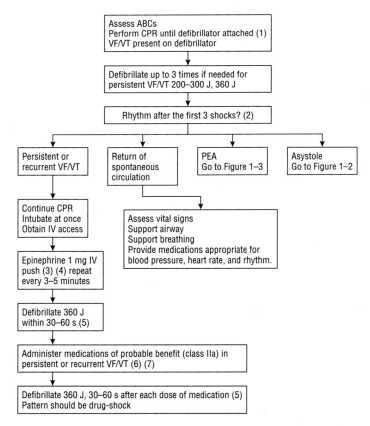

Figure 1–1. Algorithm for ventricular fibrillation and pulseless ventricular tachycardia (VF/VT). (Modified and reproduced, with permission, from JAMA 1992;268:2217.)

300 joules, and 360 joules if necessary. Premedicate the patient with a sedative and analgesic whenever possible.

   2. **Unstable ventricular tachycardia**
      a. If the patient has a pulse but is hemodynamically unstable (hypotension, unconsciousness, pulmonary edema), antiarrhythmic therapy should be deferred; instead, immediate *synchronized* cardioversion with 100 joules should be administered.
      b. If an unstable ventricular tachycardia does not convert with 100 joules, administer 200–300 joules; if still unsuccessful, 360 joules.

Footnotes to Figure 1–1
Class I: Definitely helpful.
Class IIa: Acceptable, probably helpful.
Class IIb: Acceptable, possibly helpful.
Class III: Not indicated, may be harmful.

(1) Precordial thump is a class IIb action in witnessed arrest, no pulse, and no defibrillator available.
(2) Hypothermic cardiac arrest is treated differently after this point. See Section I, Chapter 42, Hypothermia p. 208.
(3) The recommended dose of epinephrine is 1 mg IV push every 3–5 min. If this approach fails, several class IIb dosing regimens can be considered:
   Intermediate: epinephrine 2–5 mg IV push, every 3–5 min.
   Escalating: epinephrine 1 mg–3 mg–5 mg IV push (3 min apart).
   High: epinephrine 0.1 mg/kg IV push, every 3–5 min.
(4) Sodium bicarbonate (1 mEq/kg) is class I if patient has known preexisting hyperkalemia.
(5) Multiple sequenced shocks (200 J, 200–300 J, 360 J) are acceptable here (class I), especially when medications are delayed.
(6) Lidocaine 1.5 mg/kg IV push. Repeat in 3–5 min to total loading dose of 3 mg/kg; then use:
   Bretylium 5 mg/kg IV push. Repeat in 5 min at 10 mg/kg.
   Magnesium sulfate 1–2 g IV in torsades de pointes or suspected hypomagnesemic state or severe refractory VF.
   Procainamide 30 mg/min in refractory VF (maximum total 17 mg/kg).
(7) Sodium bicarbonate (1 mEq/kg IV):
   Class IIa
   If known preexisting bicarbonate-responsive acidosis.
   If overdose with tricyclic antidepressants.
   To alkalinize the urine in drug overdoses.
   Class IIb
   If intubated and continued long arrest interval.
   Upon return of spontaneous circulation after long arrest interval.
   Class III
   Hypoxic lactic acidosis.

Figure 1–1. (*continued*)

      c. Following cardioversion, a continuous infusion of lido-
      caine should be administered to prevent recurrence of the
      arrhythmia.

D. Asystole (See Figure 1–2.) This rhythm has an extremely poor
prognosis.

  1. Epinephrine 1 mg should be administered IV and repeated Q
3–5 min.

  2. Because massive parasympathetic discharge can occasionally
result in asystole, an initial dose of atropine 1 mg may be administered if there is no response to the epinephrine. This dose
may be repeated after 3–5 min if there is no response.

  3. Sodium bicarbonate and calcium chloride are no longer recommended for management of asystole.

  4. In general, pacemaker therapy will not be successful if the heart
fails to respond to either of the preceding measures.

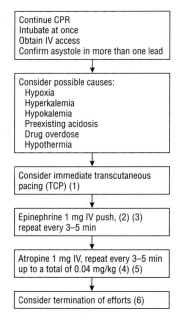

Figure 1–2. Asystole treatment algorithm. (Modified and reproduced, with permission, from
JAMA 1992;268:2220.)

5. Keep in mind that occasionally fine ventricular fibrillation may be mistaken as asystole. This problem can be avoided by evaluating the ECG in several leads.

E. Pulseless electrical activity (PEA) (See Figure 1–3.) This condition is characterized by the presence of electrical activity on the ECG but no detectable pulse. It is important to recall that some causes of this condition can be reversed if they are recognized and treated appropriately.

1. PEA is caused by a variety of conditions including hypoxemia, severe acidosis, pericardial tamponade, tension pneumothorax, hypovolemia, and pulmonary embolus. It is therefore important to evaluate for potentially reversible causes such as pericardial tamponade and pneumothorax.

2. If tamponade is suspected, pericardiocentesis should be performed.

Footnotes to Figure 1–2
Class I: Definitely helpful.
Class IIa: Acceptable, probably helpful.
Class IIb: Acceptable, possibly helpful.
Class III: Not indicated, may be harmful.

(1) TCP is a class IIb intervention. Lack of success may be due to delays in pacing. To be effective TCP must be performed early, simultaneously with drugs. Evidence does not support routine use of TCP for asystole.
(2) The recommended dose of epinephrine is 1 mg IV push every 3–5 min. If this approach fails, several class IIb dosing regimens can be considered:
    Intermediate: epinephrine 2–5 mg IV push, every 3–5 min.
    Escalating: epinephrine 1 mg–3 mg–5 mg IV push (3 min apart).
    High: epinephrine 0.1 mg/kg IV push, every 3–5 min.
(3) Sodium bicarbonate 1 mEq/kg is class I if patient has known preexisting hyperkalemia.
(4) Shorter atropine dosing intervals are class IIb in asystolic arrest.
(5) Sodium bicarbonate 1 mEq/kg IV:
    Class IIa
    If known preexisting bicarbonate-responsive acidosis.
    If overdose with tricyclic antidepressants.
    To alkalinize the urine in drug overdoses.
    Class IIb
    If intubated and continued long arrest interval.
    Upon return of spontaneous circulation after long arrest interval.
    Class III
    Hypoxic lactic acidosis.
(6) If patient remains in asystole or other agonal rhythms after successful intubation and initial medications and no reversible causes are identified, consider termination of resuscitative efforts by a physician.
    Consider interval since arrest.

Figure 1–2. (*continued*)

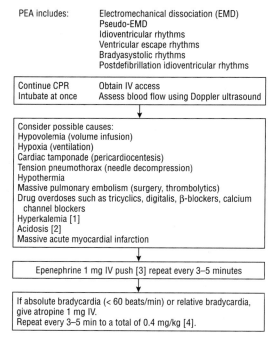

PEA includes: Electromechanical dissociation (EMD)
                       Pseudo-EMD
                       Idioventricular rhythms
                       Ventricular escape rhythms
                       Bradyasystolic rhythms
                       Postdefibrillation idioventricular rhythms

Continue CPR	Obtain IV access
Intubate at once	Assess blood flow using Doppler ultrasound

Consider possible causes:
Hypovolemia (volume infusion)
Hypoxia (ventilation)
Cardiac tamponade (pericardiocentesis)
Tension pneumothorax (needle decompression)
Hypothermia
Massive pulmonary embolism (surgery, thrombolytics)
Drug overdoses such as tricyclics, digitalis, β-blockers, calcium
    channel blockers
Hyperkalemia [1]
Acidosis [2]
Massive acute myocardial infarction

Epenephrine 1 mg IV push [3] repeat every 3–5 minutes

If absolute bradycardia (< 60 beats/min) or relative bradycardia,
give atropine 1 mg IV.
Repeat every 3–5 min to a total of 0.4 mg/kg [4].

Figure 1–3. Algorithm for pulseless electrical activity (PEA) (electromechanical dissociation [EMD]). (Modified and reproduced, with permission, from JAMA 1992;268:2219.)

3. If tension pneumothorax is suspected, insertion of a catheter-over-needle device in the second intercostal space in the mid-clavicular line should be attempted.
4. Otherwise, treatment consists of epinephrine 1 mg IV Q 3–5 minutes along with CPR.
5. A fluid challenge should also be administered. Give 500 mL of normal saline over 15 min.
6. The administration of calcium chloride for this condition is no longer recommended.

REFERENCES

Cummins RO, ed.: *Textbook of Advanced Cardiac Life Support.* 3rd ed. American Heart Association;1994.
Graver K, Cavallaro D, eds.: An approach to the key algorithms for cardiopulmonary resuscitation. In: *ACLS Certification and Preparation.* 3rd ed. Mosby;1993.

Footnotes to Figure 1–3
Class I: Definitely helpful.
Class IIa: Acceptable, probably helpful.
Class IIb: Acceptable, possibly helpful.
Class III: Not indicated, may be harmful.

[1] Sodium bicarbonate 1 mEq/kg is class I if patient has known preexisting hyperkalemia.
[2] Sodium bicarbonate 1 mEq/kg:
   Class IIa
   If known preexisting bicarbonate-responsive acidosis.
   If overdose with tricyclic antidepressants.
   To alkalinize the urine in drug overdoses.
   Class IIb
   If intubated and continued long arrest interval.
   Upon return of spontaneous circulation after long arrest interval.
   Class III
   Hypoxic lactic acidosis.
[3] The recommended dose of epinephrine is 1 mg IV push every 3–5 min. If this approach fails, several class IIb dosing regimens can be considered:
   Intermediate: epinephrine 2–5 mg IV push, every 3–5 min.
   Escalating: epinephrine 1 mg–3 mg–5 mg IV push (3 min apart).
   High: epinephrine 0.1 mg/kg IV push, every 3–5 min.
[4] Shorter atropine dosing intervals are possibly helpful in cardiac arrest (class IIb).

Figure 1–3. (*continued*)

10. CENTRAL VENOUS LINE PROBLEMS

(See also Section 1, Chapter 55, Pulmonary Artery Catheter Problems)

 I. Problem. The nursing staff calls to report a subclavian line has stopped functioning.

 II. Immediate Questions
   A. If the central line is used for central venous pressure (CVP) monitoring, what does the waveform look like? The CVP waveform drops on inspiration, rises with expiration, and should show monophasic to triphasic fluctuations with each cardiac cycle. If there is no waveform, the catheter may not be patent, or there may be a thrombus in the vein or catheter.
   B. Do intravenous fluids flow easily into the catheter or does fluid leak from the insertion site? Again, these developments might indicate a thrombosed central vein or a kinked catheter.
   C. Is the patient febrile? A fever in conjunction with a malfunctioning catheter suggests either a central line infection, deep vein thrombosis, or both. If any suspicion of associated infection or thrombosis exists, malfunctioning lines should be removed immediately and cultured.

D. **Are there any arrhythmias?** A central line catheter that extends into the right atrium or right ventricle can cause atrial or ventricular ectopy and arrhythmias.

E. **What is the line's purpose? What is its relative necessity?** If drugs are being administered centrally that should not be given peripherally (vincristine or adriamycin as a continuous infusion), the situation is different from one in which the central line could be replaced by a peripheral line.

III. Differential Diagnosis

A. **Clotted catheter.** This can occur when central lines are allowed to run dry or are running very slowly. Blood backs up into the catheter lumen and thrombosis occurs.

B. **Misdirected catheter.** Subclavian catheters from either the right or the left side may be inadvertently placed retrograde into the ipsilateral internal jugular vein. This results in a line that cannot be used to measure central venous pressure. Much more rarely, subclavian or internal jugular attempts end up in the long thoracic vein and fail to function properly. The catheter may also extend into the right atrium or right ventricle rather than the proximal venous circulation.

C. **Kinked catheter.** Catheters can kink at the skin or more deeply. From the right subclavian insertion site, it is not uncommon for catheters within relatively stiff sheaths to kink at the turn from the subclavian vein to the brachiocephalic vein as it joins the superior vena cava. Kinking at this bend is uncommon for single-lumen catheters or triple-lumen catheters not inside a sheath. Internal jugular lines and left subclavian lines are not generally subject to this problem. It should be stressed that any line can be misdirected and kink. The catheters are easily seen fluoroscopically and radiographically; a chest x-ray will usually diagnose the problem.

D. **Infected catheter.** Central line sepsis will usually not result in any apparent malfunction of the catheter. Fever, sepsis, and positive blood cultures may all result from the spread of skin flora to the intravascular segment of the catheter.

E. **Thrombosis of the vein of insertion.** Any deep vein accessed for central line insertion can thrombose as a result of the trauma associated with the procedure, as well as the presence of a foreign body within the vein. Clinically, these events resemble natural deep vein thrombosis, and can result in associated bland or septic pulmonary emboli.

IV. Database

A. **Physical examination key points**

1. **Vital signs.** An elevated temperature suggests an infection. If the catheter has been in place more than 3 days, you must consider the central venous catheter as the source of the fever.

2. **Extremities.** Look for evidence of deep vein thrombosis. Unilateral edema and venous engorgement suggest deep vein thrombosis.
3. **Skin.** Examine the insertion site for evidence of tissue infiltration, bleeding, catheter kinking, or leakage. Also, erythema around the insertion site may result from a localized infection.

B. **Laboratory data**
   1. **Complete blood count with differential.** An elevated white count with an increase in banded neutrophils is often present with catheter-related sepsis.
   2. **Prothrombin time (PT), partial thromboplastin time (PTT), platelet count.** Should be obtained if a central line needs to be changed and a coagulopathy is suspected, such as in patients with severe liver disease or malnutrition.
   3. **Blood cultures.** Should be obtained as part of routine evaluation of a fever. Remember, if a central venous catheter has been in place more than 3 days, there is a significant risk of catheter-related sepsis.

C. **Radiologic and other studies**
   1. **Chest x-ray.** Useful in determining whether a catheter is in the correct position or kinked.
   2. **Culture of catheter tip.** If catheter-related sepsis or infection is suspected, the catheter must be removed and the tip sent for culture.
   3. **Impedance plethysmography and Doppler ultrasound.** Noninvasive tests for suspected extremity venous thrombosis.
   4. **Venography.** The gold standard for diagnosing venous thrombosis. If there is a history of allergy to contrast, venography should be preceded by treatment with corticosteroids and diphenhydramine.
   5. **Nuclear venogram.** Can diagnose venous thrombosis and pulmonary embolism simultaneously with lower extremity injection.

V. **Plan.** (For replacement of central venous catheters, see Section III, Central Venous Catheterization, p 350)
   A. **Clotted catheter.** A line can sometimes be salvaged by aspirating the catheter while it is slowly pulled out. Sterile technique and a small syringe are necessary. Use of a guide wire, manual flushing, or injection of urokinase 5000 U (5000 U/mL) may result in embolization. However, these measures seldom cause any significant problem, probably because of the small volume of the embolus. The only completely safe approach, however, is aspiration. The risk of replacement of the line has to be weighed against the risk of using any of the other techniques besides aspiration. Other factors must be considered, such as the length of time the catheter has been in place, the necessity of central rather than peripheral placement, and the presence of fever or local evidence of infection.

B. **Misdirected catheter.** This situation usually requires removal and replacement. Sometimes you can use a guide wire with fluoroscopic assistance to manipulate the catheter to the superior vena cava, but most often you will need to do a new puncture. If the catheter is in the right atrium or right ventricle and does not have to be removed for other reasons, it can be partially withdrawn, using sterile technique, so that it is in the inferior or superior vena cava.

C. **Kinked catheter.** A new line that is kinked at the site of insertion can sometimes be salvaged by repositioning the line with new skin sutures. More proximal kinks can sometimes be fixed by replacing the catheter over a guide wire. If the kink is within a sheath or directly after the catheter emerges from the sheath, the sheath can sometimes be withdrawn leaving the catheter in the same place, provided there is enough catheter left onto which the sheath can be withdrawn. The best way to deal with this problem is to prevent it, by avoiding the right subclavian approach in patients who have shallow chests in the lateral dimension. In these patients, the lines must negotiate a sharp angle from the subclavian to the superior vena cava.

D. **Infected catheter.** An infected or possibly infected central line *must be removed.* This virtually always requires replacement elsewhere if central venous access is still desired. Intravenous line-associated sepsis is caused in large part by skin contamination. The practice of removing the line over a guide wire and traversing the same insertion site with the replacement line is not recommended. A new site is a better idea. It is important to draw two sets of blood cultures from the suspect line as well as two sets from the peripheral veins before the line is removed, and to culture the tip of the catheter after it is removed.

E. **Thrombosis of the vein of insertion.** This also requires line removal and replacement at a site distant from the thrombosed vein. Heparin 80 U/kg IV bolus followed by 18 U/kg continuous infusion is recommended unless contraindicated for other reasons. The PTT should be checked 6 hours after the infusion is begun; the heparin dose should be adjusted so that the PTT is one and one-half to two times the control. If sepsis is also suspected, antibiotics are necessary, as is a surgical consultation for possible removal of the infected vein. Vancomycin 1000 mg every 12 hours is the preferred antibiotic if normal renal function is present. Vancomycin covers *Staphylococcus epidermidis* as well as *Staphylococcus aureus.* Be sure to decrease the dose if renal insufficiency is present.

REFERENCES

Fares LG, Block PH, Feldman SD: Improved house staff results with subclavian cannulation. Am Surg 1986;52:108.

Gil RT, Kruse JA, Thill-Baharozian MC et al: Triple- vs. single-lumen central venous catheters. Arch Intern Med 1989;149:1139.
Mansfield PF, Hohn DC, Fornage BD et al: Complications and failures of subclavian-vein catheterization. N Engl J Med 1994;331:1735.

11. CHEST PAIN

I. **Problem.** A 48-year-old man with a history of tobacco abuse is admitted for elective bronchoscopy. On the evening of his admission, he develops substernal chest pain that persists approximately 15 minutes.

II. **Immediate Questions.** Because potentially serious conditions may cause chest pain, patients with this complaint should be evaluated on an urgent basis. By far, the most important tool in identifying the cause of chest pain is a meticulous history.

   A. **Does the patient have a prior history of coronary artery disease, and if so, does the current pain resemble previous episodes of angina pectoris?** If the patient has a documented history of coronary artery disease, particularly if the current episode resembles previously known anginal attacks, assume the pain represents myocardial ischemia and treat accordingly.

   B. **What are the locations, quality, and severity of the pain?** Location (substernal, epigastric); radiation (jaw, arms, back); quality (burning, crushing, tearing, stabbing, sharp); and severity of pain are features that may suggest a particular diagnosis. Because several intrathoracic and extrathoracic structures are innervated by the same spinal cord segments, the location and quality of different causes of chest pain may overlap.

   C. **Are there any factors that are known to precipitate or relieve the pain?** Sharp pain that is worsened by coughing or deep inspiration suggests pleuritis, pericarditis, or pneumothorax. Although classical angina is brought on by exertion, acute myocardial infarction (MI) may produce chest pain at rest, especially in the early morning. Movement of the arms or trunk that reproduces pain would indicate a musculoskeletal origin; however, pericarditis can also cause chest pain that is worsened by movement of the trunk. The pain of esophagitis is frequently exacerbated by recumbency. The relief of chest pain with sublingual nitroglycerin implies myocardial ischemia, although chest pain resulting from esophageal spasm and gallbladder colic may also be relieved. Myocardial ischemia is relieved in 3–5 minutes, whereas esophageal spasm is relieved in 10 minutes by sublingual nitroglycerin.

   D. **Has there been any recent trauma, fall, or thoracic procedure?** Fractured ribs, chest wall contusions, or other musculoskeletal conditions such as recent excessive physical activity can result in chest pain.

III. **Differential Diagnosis.** The differential diagnosis of chest pain includes a variety of conditions, ranging from musculoskeletal chest wall pain to life-threatening conditions such as acute MI and dissecting aneurysm. The clinician's initial goal is to exclude potentially catastrophic conditions, and if such conditions are identified, institute immediate therapy.

   A. **Cardiac causes of chest pain**

      1. **Acute myocardial infarction**

         a. Pain is characterized as a severe, crushing, retrosternal pain that may radiate into the arms and neck. This pain is generally described as the worst ever experienced, and generally persists 30 minutes or longer. It is seldom relieved by one or two nitroglycerin tablets, and frequently requires morphine sulfate for relief. The pain of MI may begin at rest or even during sleep, and is only infrequently preceded by strenuous physical activity.

         b. Associated symptoms include nausea, diaphoresis, dyspnea, and palpitations.

         c. Because more than 50% of the deaths caused by acute MI occur within the initial 2 hours, the physician must maintain a high index of suspicion for MI when evaluating any patient with acute chest pain.

      2. **Angina pectoris**

         a. The pain of angina is similar to that of MI, although it generally lasts less than 20 minutes and is not nearly as severe. Relief can generally be obtained with sublingual nitroglycerin. The pain is generally exacerbated by exertion, but can also occur at rest, or with emotional stress.

         b. Any recent change in a stable pattern of angina, such as occurrence with rest or increased frequency or severity, should imply an unstable pattern that mandates close monitoring and aggressive medical therapy.

         c. Although coronary artery disease is the most common cause of angina pectoris, other potential causes include coronary artery spasm, aortic stenosis, and angina precipitated by thyrotoxicosis, anemia, and low diastolic blood pressure.

      3. **Acute pericarditis**

         a. Pain is usually described as sharp, but may be dull, and is frequently pleuritic. The pain may be worsened by recumbency and relieved by sitting and leaning forward. Rotation of the trunk may precipitate pain.

         b. Possible causes include the following:

            i. Infection. Most commonly viral, but may also be bacterial, fungal, or tuberculous.

  ii. Myocardial infarction. Pericarditis may occur in the first 2–3 days after infarction, or may not occur until 1–4 weeks after MI (Dressler's syndrome).

  iii. Uremia

  iv. Malignancy. Most often breast cancer, bronchogenic carcinoma, or lymphoma.

  v. Connective tissue diseases. These include rheumatoid arthritis, scleroderma, systemic lupus erythematosus, or acute rheumatic fever.

B. Vascular causes of chest pain

 1. Acute aortic dissection

  a. This is usually described as an excruciatingly severe pain that is tearing in nature and may radiate to the back (especially if the descending aorta is involved). The pain is most severe at its onset.

  b. The condition most frequently occurs in patients with a prior history of hypertension or connective tissue disorders such as Marfan's syndrome. On presentation, however, the blood pressure may be normal or even low.

  c. Aortic dissection is a potentially life-threatening condition that must be recognized and treated early.

 2. Primary pulmonary hypertension. The pain in this condition is frequently similar to that of angina. It is usually mild, may be associated with syncope or dyspnea, and may occur with exertion.

C. Pulmonary causes of chest pain

 1. Pulmonary embolism (PE) with infarction

  a. Infarction results in inflammation of the overlying pleura and thus causes pleuritic chest pain. Embolism without infarction may cause a more vague, nondescript, substernal chest pain. Dyspnea is often present. Hemoptysis may be present if there is underlying pulmonary infarction.

  b. A number of conditions predispose to deep venous thrombosis or PE, and include the following: pregnancy, postoperative state, prolonged immobilization, malignancy (especially adenocarcinoma), obesity, exogenous estrogen use, paraplegia, cerebral vascular accident with resultant hemiplegia, congestive heart failure, and hypercoagulable states such as protein C, protein S, or antithrombin III deficiency, or the presence of a lupus anticoagulant or anticardiolipin antibody.

  c. Pulmonary embolism (PE) is a potentially fatal condition that is too often underdiagnosed. It should be suspected in any hospitalized patient who develops acute shortness of breath or chest pain, especially with any of the above risk factors.

 2. Pneumothorax

  a. This is characterized by the acute onset of pleuritic chest pain associated with dyspnea.

    b. Tension pneumothorax is a potentially life-threatening condition that is characterized by hypotension, tracheal deviation, venous distension, and severe respiratory distress.

    c. There are three broad categories of causes of pneumothorax:

        i. Spontaneous causes. This most often occurs in 20- to 30-year-old males and in older patients with bullous emphysema.

        ii. Iatrogenic causes. Pneumothorax may be a complication of subclavian vein catheterization or thoracentesis. Barotrauma from mechanical ventilation, especially in patients requiring high inspiratory pressures, may also result in pneumothorax.

        iii. Traumatic causes. Any patient with a penetrating chest injury, as well as patients with rib fractures, may sustain a pneumothorax.

3. Pleurodynia. This is frequently associated with Coxsackie virus.

4. Pneumonia/pleuritis. The pain is typically pleuritic and associated with fever, productive cough, and rigors.

D. Gastrointestinal causes of chest pain

  1. Gastroesophageal reflux. This condition is usually described as a burning pain that is made worse with recumbency and relieved by antacids.

  2. Esophageal spasm. This condition is easily confused with angina pectoris. It may cause substernal chest pain or tightness that is relieved by nitrates. Intermittent dysphagia, if it occurs, suggests esophageal disease; however, it may be difficult by history alone to distinguish esophageal spasm from angina. Remember that both conditions may occur together.

  3. Gastritis. Alcoholism, stress that is associated with severe burns, trauma, major surgery, or intensive care unit admission, and use of NSAIDs may all induce inflammation of the gastric mucosa, resulting in epigastric and lower chest pain.

  4. Peptic ulcer disease (PUD). This is typically described as an epigastric discomfort that may be burning or gnawing and frequently radiates to the back. Pain may be either relieved or exacerbated by eating. It is frequently relieved by antacids.

  5. Biliary colic. This condition is characterized by postprandial pain that occurs 1–2 hours after eating, and may last several hours. In contrast to the term colic, the pain is actually constant, intense, and may last several hours. The pain is usually located in the right upper quadrant and radiates to the right scapula; however, the pain may also be perceived largely in the epigastrium and lower chest, and therefore may be confused with angina.

  6. Pancreatitis. There is usually a prior history of gallstones or alcohol ingestion. Pain is usually midepigastric with radiation to the back. Similar to pericarditis, it may be exacerbated by recumbency and relieved by sitting upright and leaning forward. There are often associated nausea and vomiting.

- E. **Musculoskeletal chest pain.** Pain is usually reproduced by palpation over the costochondral or sternochondral junctions. Pain is fairly well localized.
    1. **Costochondritis.** Point tenderness is elicited over the costochondral junction.
    2. **Muscle strain/spasm.** Most typically, there is a preceding history of exercise or overexertion.
    3. **Rib fractures after trauma**

IV. Database
A. Physical examination key points
1. **Vital signs**
    a. Hypotension is an ominous sign that may result from any one of several potentially catastrophic causes, including massive MI, cardiac tamponade from pericarditis, tension pneumothorax, acute massive PE, rupture of a dissecting aneurysm, or gastritis or peptic ulcer disease with hemorrhage.
    b. Hypertension may result from any painful condition, but must be particularly looked for in the setting of acute MI or aortic dissection where emergent therapy to reduce the pressure is mandated.
    c. Fever may result from PE, MI, pneumonia, or pericarditis.
    d. Tachycardia may result from sinus tachycardia associated with pain, but could also indicate ventricular tachycardia that has developed because of myocardial ischemia. If untreated, ventricular tachycardia may progress into ventricular fibrillation. (See Section I, Problem 58, Tachycardia, p 279). PE frequently causes sinus tachycardia or acute atrial fibrillation.
    e. Bradycardia is a frequent occurrence with inferior MI and may result from either sinus node dysfunction or atrioventricular heart block (second- or third-degree). (See Section I, Problem 8, Bradycardia, p 37).
2. **HEENT.** Evidence of thrush, especially in an immunosuppressed patient, could indicate *Candida* esophagitis.
3. **Neck.** Significant venous distension may occur with either an acute tension pneumothorax or cardiac tamponade. Pain with hyperextension of the neck may indicate a cervical nerve or disk problem as a cause of referred shoulder and chest pain. Tracheal deviation suggests tension pneumothorax.
4. **Chest.** Localized chest wall tenderness may result from a contusion, costochondritis, or rib fracture.
5. **Lungs**
    a. Absent breath sounds and hyperresonance to percussion indicate a pneumothorax.
    b. Crackles and signs of pneumonic consolidation such as increased tactile fremitus or egophony may occur with pneumonia or a pulmonary infarction.

     c. A pleural friction rub may result from pneumonia, pulmonary infarction, or any process resulting in pleuritis.

     d. Bibasilar crackles and/or wheezes may occur with decompensated congestive heart failure resulting from myocardial ischemia or infarction.

     e. Lung examination may be normal in a patient with acute PE.

  6. Heart

     a. The point of maximal impulse (PMI) may not be palpable in a patient with a pericardial effusion. The heart sounds may be likewise distant. In a patient with acute pericarditis, a friction rub may be present, but this is an evanescent finding and therefore the patient must be reexamined periodically.

     b. Most often, the cardiac exam is normal in a patient with acute MI or angina pectoris. If there is significant associated left ventricular dysfunction, an S_3 gallop may be heard. An S_4 gallop may also be present. A harsh systolic ejection murmur over the aortic outflow area may indicate aortic stenosis, which can cause angina pectoris even in the presence of normal coronary arteries. In the setting of a recent MI, a new holosystolic murmur at the apex suggests papillary muscle dysfunction or rupture. If dissection is suspected, listen for a decrescendo diastolic murmur of aortic regurgitation at the left lower sternal border, which may develop if the dissection spreads to involve the aortic ring.

  7. Abdomen. For a discussion of the various abdominal conditions that can also produce epigastric and lower chest pain, see Section I, Problem 1, Abdominal Pain, p 1.

  8. Neurologic examination. A careful and detailed exam is important in any patient in whom aortic dissection is suspected. The dissection may occlude cerebral or spinal arteries, and thereby cause a variety of neurologic deficits.

  9. Extremities

     a. In a patient with suspected PE, examine for evidence of deep venous thrombosis; however, the physical exam is notoriously inaccurate in this condition and may be entirely normal despite the presence of significant venous thrombosis. Be sure to examine the upper extremities.

     b. In patients with suspected dissection, it is important to examine the pulses bilaterally in both upper and lower extremities for symmetry.

B. Laboratory data

  1. Hemogram. Leukocytosis may result from any form of inflammation such as pulmonary infarction or MI. If there is an increase in banded neutrophils, suspect a bacterial infection such as pneumonia.

  2. Arterial blood gases. This should be obtained if a pulmonary process is suspected, such as embolism, pneumothorax, and pneumonia. It should also be ordered for any patient with de-compensated cardiac function resulting in pulmonary edema.

3. **Cardiac isoenzymes.** Serial measurements of creatine phos-phokinase (CK) with isoenzymes every 8–12 hours over the first 24–48 hours may help to confirm or exclude an MI. Note that CK may not become elevated until several hours after the beginning of infarction. Therefore, a single measurement of CK cannot be used to exclude the diagnosis of MI.

C. **Radiologic and other studies**

1. **Electrocardiogram.** An ECG should be obtained in any patient with a new complaint of chest pain. If available for comparison, an old ECG is helpful. New T wave changes, ST segment de-pression or elevation, or the presence of new Q waves will be helpful in identifying the cause of the chest pain as myocardial ischemia/infarction. Note again that patients presenting with my-ocardial infarction may initially have an entirely normal ECG, and that the diagnosis of MI cannot be excluded on the basis of a normal ECG.

2. **Chest x-ray.** Request a CXR in any patient in whom the etiol-ogy of the chest pain is unclear. It may be helpful in diagnosing pneumothorax, pneumonia, and pleural and pericardial effu-sions. A widened mediastinum suggests dissection of the tho-racic aorta.

3. **Echocardiogram.** This can be performed on a nonemergent basis if pericarditis is suspected and if the patient does not ap-pear to be in tamponade. Also helpful in diagnosis of thoracic aortic dissection and assessing regional wall abnormalities in acute MI.

4. **Contrast CT scan.** This should be obtained in any patient in whom aortic dissection is suspected.

5. **Ventilation/perfusion ($\dot{V}/\dot{Q}$) lung scan.** A lung scan may be helpful if pulmonary emboli are suspected. Impedance plethys-mography and Doppler ultrasound of the lower extremities may also be obtained if there is a strong suspicion for acute deep ve-nous thrombosis.

V. **Plan.** In assessing any patient with acute chest pain, the physician's overriding goal is to exclude the presence of the previously mentioned life-threatening conditions. In the acute setting, it is better to maintain a high index of suspicion for these conditions and to overtreat rather than undertreat.

A. **Emergency management** (for all patients with chest pain)

1. Treat with oxygen. Administer oxygen therapy with 2–4 L/min by nasal cannula. If the patient has a history of chronic obstructive airway disease, it is preferable to administer 24% O_2 by Venturi face mask initially.

   2. Establish an intravenous line for administration of medications
   should the patient deteriorate.
   3. If chest pain is still present and the systolic blood pressure is
   above 90, administer 0.4 mg nitroglycerin sublingually.
   4. Obtain a 12-lead ECG.
   5. If your initial assessment suggests any evidence of a pneumothorax, pneumonia, or heart failure, obtain a stat portable
   CXR and ABG.
   B. Myocardial ischemia. If your initial assessment suggests the possibility of acute MI, the following are brief guidelines offered for the
   initial treatment. A full discussion of acute MI is beyond the scope
   of this section.
   1. Aspirin. Administer two chewable aspirin (consider ticlopidine
   [Ticlid] if there is a history of aspirin hypersensitivity).
   2. Nitrates
   a. Nitroglycerin in a dose of 0.4–0.6 mg may be administered
   sublingually every 5 minutes, provided that the systolic blood
   pressure remains above 90. It is preferable to administer the
   nitroglycerin while the patient is recumbent. This may provide relief for angina pectoris and possibly unstable angina
   pectoris.
   b. The pain of acute MI is seldom relieved by the administration
   of nitroglycerin sublingually, and requires treatment with either intravenous nitroglycerin or morphine. If the nitroglycerin
   is effective but pain recurs, begin a nitroglycerin infusion initially at 10 μg/min and increase by 10 μg/min every 10 minutes until relief of pain. The systolic blood pressure must be
   maintained above 90 during the administration of nitroglycerin. Hemodynamic monitoring with a pulmonary artery
   catheter (see Section 3, Pulmonary Artery Catheterization)
   is advised.
   3. Morphine sulfate
   a. If pain is not relieved by nitroglycerin sublingually or intravenously, 3–5 mg of morphine IV every 5–10 minutes can be
   administered for relief. Close monitoring of the patient's
   blood pressure and respirations is necessary, because hypotension and respiratory suppression may occur. These effects may be reversed with naloxone (Narcan) 0.4 mg IV.
   4. Beta-blockers should be considered. Metoprolol 5 mg every
   2–5 min for 3 doses intravenously; or atenolol 5 mg every 5 min
   for 2 doses intravenously.
   5. Arrangements for transfer to a coronary care unit or intensive
   care unit should be made. This is especially important in the first
   24 hours of myocardial infarction, when arrhythmia monitoring
   and ready access to a defibrillator are essential.
   6. Discussion of thrombolytic therapy is beyond the scope of this
   section, but *should always be considered* in any patient pre-

senting with chest pain that is consistent with a MI; at least 1 mm ST-segment elevation in two contiguous leads and no contra-indication to thrombolytics. See the discussions of alteplase, anistreplase, and streptokinase in Section 7, Commonly Used Medications.

C. Aortic dissection. The initial treatment goal is to reduce pain and, if the patient is hypertensive, to reduce blood pressure. Surgical correction is indicated for all ascending thoracic aneurysms.

1. Make arrangements for immediate transfer to an intensive care unit where hemodynamic monitoring can be instituted.
2. Obtain immediate vascular surgical consult.
3. A continuous infusion of nitroprusside (Nipride) 0.5–1.0 mg/kg/min or labetalol (Trandate, Normodyne) 20–80 mg bolus, then 2 mg/min should be initiated and titrated upward to control systolic blood pressure in the range of approximately 100–120 mm Hg systolic. Labetalol may be the preferred agent because of associated increases in contractility and shearing force with nitroprusside.
4. Administration of nitroprusside with the resultant short-term decrease in systolic blood pressure may result in a rebound increase in contractility and shearing force, which might worsen the dissection. Propranolol (Inderal) 0.5 mg IV should therefore be administered prior to beginning nitroprusside. The initial bolus of propranolol should be followed by 1 mg IV every 5 minutes until the pulse pressure has been reduced to 60 mm Hg. Once this dose of propranolol has been established, it can be administered every 4–6 hours IV. Other intravenous beta-blockers such as metoprolol (Lopressor), esmolol (Brevibloc), atenolol (Tenormin), and labetalol (Trandate, Normodyne) can be used.
5. To relieve pain, morphine sulfate 3–5 mg may be administered IV every 10 minutes. Again, close monitoring of the blood pressure and respirations is necessary.

D. Pulmonary embolism

1. Ensure adequate oxygenation.
2. After checking a baseline prothrombin time and partial thromboplastin time, administer a bolus of heparin 80 units/kg IV and follow it with a continuous IV infusion of 18 units/kg/hr. Repeat the PTT in approximately 4–6 hours and adjust the heparin to maintain a PTT approximately 1.5–2 times the control value (50–70 sec).
3. If systemic anticoagulation is contraindicated, surgical consultation will be necessary to place a venocaval filter.
4. **Massive PE with hypotension.** Thrombolytic therapy or surgical consultation for embolectomy should be considered.

E. Acute pneumothorax

1. An acute tension pneumothorax should be treated by immediate placement of a 16-gauge needle into the second intercostal

space in the midclavicular line. This potentially life-saving measure can be instituted while awaiting placement of a chest tube.
2. A spontaneous pneumothorax occurring in an otherwise healthy person and involving 20% or less of the lung can usually be treated with oxygen and observation. All other pneumothoraces should be treated by chest tube insertion.

F. Pericarditis
1. Indomethacin (Indocin) 50 mg TID is generally effective for pain relief in most cases of pericarditis.
2. If tamponade is suspected, an emergent echocardiogram should be performed. If tamponade is confirmed, consultation with cardiology for pericardiocentesis should be requested.

G. Gastritis/esophagitis
1. Antacids such as Mylanta-II 30 mL every 4–6 hours may provide immediate relief.
2. H_2 antagonists such as cimetidine (Tagamet), ranitidine (Zantac), famotidine (Pepcid), or nizatidine (Axid) may also relieve symptoms. Prokinetic agents such as metoclopramide (Reglan) and cisapride (Propulsid); and hydrogen proton pump inhibitors such as omeprazole (Prilosec) are also effective.
3. Elevating the head of the bed on 6-in. blocks may help to reduce the reflux that occurs with recumbency.

H. Costochondritis.
Treat with nonsteroidal anti-inflammatory drugs such as ibuprofen (Motrin) 800 mg every 8 hours.

REFERENCES

Fortuin NJ, Walford GD: Thoracic pain and angina pectoris. In: Harvey AM, Johns RJ, McKusick VA et al, eds. *The Principles and Practice of Medicine.* 22nd ed. Appleton & Lange;1988:88.

Raschke RA, Reilly BM, Guidry JR et al: The weight-based heparin dosing nomogram compared with a "standard care" nomogram. Ann Intern Med 1993;119:874.

Silverman ME: *Examination of the Heart—The Clinical History.* 3rd ed. American Heart Association;1990.

12. COAGULOPATHY

I. **Problem.** After emergent exploratory laparotomy, a patient has bleeding from the incision site and blood oozing from an intravenous site.

II. **Immediate Questions**
A. **What is the patient's blood pressure?** Determine immediately if the bleeding is extensive enough to cause hypovolemia and shock. Assess volume status by blood pressure, urine output, and central pressures if available. If the patient has tachycardia (pulse > 100) or hypotension (blood pressure ≤ 90), establish intravenous ac-

cess and begin fluid resuscitation at once. If central lines need to be placed, determine extent of the coagulopathy before inserting needles into major noncompressible vessels.

B. How much external bleeding is there? Look at wounds or needle puncture sites to see if there is active bleeding.

C. Do factors exist that increase the likelihood of generalized bleeding? In the example given, disseminated intravascular coagulation (DIC) could be suspected. In general, when confronted with a bleeding patient, inquire about liver disease, nutritional status, family history of bleeding disorders, any bleeding with prior surgical procedures (including dental extractions), and use of medications such as aspirin, nonsteroidal anti-inflammatory drugs (NSAIDs), or anticoagulants.

III. Differential Diagnosis

A. Inadequate hemostasis. This is the most common cause of localized bleeding in the postoperative patient. The bleeding is usually minimal.

B. Platelet disorders

1. **Thrombocytopenia** (See Section I, Problem 59, Thrombocytopenia, p 289.)

   a. **Decreased production.** Often secondary to chemotherapy fibrosis or neoplasia involving the bone marrow. Tuberculosis and histoplasmosis are two granulomatous diseases that can invade the bone marrow. Vitamin B_{12}, folic acid, or iron deficiencies may result in decreased production.

   b. **Sequestration.** Caused by splenic enlargement resulting from portal hypertension, neoplasia, infection or storage diseases.

   c. **Destruction.** Idiopathic thrombocytopenic purpura (ITP), thrombotic thrombocytopenic purpura (TTP), collagen vascular diseases, and reactions to drugs (penicillins, sulfa drugs, thiazides, and heparin) can cause platelet destruction.

   d. **Dilution.** May occur in patients who have been transfused with large volumes of blood over a short interval.

2. **Qualitative platelet disorders**

   a. **von Willebrand's disease.** This is an autosomal dominant disease characterized by decreased platelet adhesion; it has many different variants.

   b. **Acquired disorder.** Results from interference with cyclooxygenase metabolism by aspirin and NSAIDs. Aspirin will affect platelet function for the life of the platelet (7–10 days after aspirin is discontinued); NSAIDs affect platelet function only in the presence of the drug.

   c. **Glanzmann's thrombasthenia.** Inherited abnormality in which platelets do not aggregate.

    d. Bernard-Soulier syndrome. Inherited abnormality characterized by giant platelets with abnormal platelet adhesion.

    e. Uremia. Abnormal platelet aggregation caused by an unknown mechanism.

C. Coagulation defects

  1. Congenital

    a. Hemophilia A. Factor VIII deficiency, X-linked recessive. Incidence of 1/10,000 male births.

    b. Hemophilia B. Factor IX deficiency, X-linked recessive. Incidence of 1/100,000 male births.

    c. Congenital deficiencies of other coagulation factors. These are much less common than factor VIII and IX deficiencies.

  2. Acquired

    a. Disseminated intravascular coagulation (DIC). DIC is associated with sepsis, trauma, burns, and malignancy; it may be a complication of pregnancy and delivery, liver disease, and heat stroke.

    b. Vitamin K deficiency. Vitamin K is required for synthesis of factors II, VII, IX, and X. Most frequent setting for deficiency is the malnourished patient receiving antibiotics.

    c. Severe liver disease. Cirrhosis, hepatitis, hemochromatosis, biliary cirrhosis, or cancer. Coagulopathy is caused by decreased production of coagulation factors, production of abnormal coagulation factors, or a failure to clear activated coagulation factors.

IV. Database. The most important factor in diagnosing a coagulopathy is understanding and utilizing appropriate laboratory tests. It is imperative to draw blood for needed tests prior to instituting therapy or transfusions.

  A. Physical examination key points

    1. Vital signs. Orthostatic hypotension signifies a major loss of blood. By definition it is a decrease of 10 mm Hg in the systolic blood pressure and/or an increase in the heart rate of 20 bpm on movement from a supine to a standing position after one minute. Also look for tachycardia or hypotension.

    2. Skin. Petechiae, purpura, easy bruising, and oozing from intravenous sites suggest a systemic rather than a local cause.

    3. Incisions. Examine any incision for hematoma or for active bleeding.

    4. Abdomen. Splenomegaly, hepatomegaly, or ascites suggest cirrhosis.

    5. Extremities. Hemarthrosis may be seen with hemophilia or other causes of coagulopathy.

    6. Neurologic examination. To assess for CNS bleeding.

B. Laboratory data
1. **Hemogram.** Follow serial hematocrits with ongoing bleeding.
2. **Platelet count.** An adequate platelet count does not imply adequate function of platelets. Generally, platelet counts of 50,000–100,000 are adequate to maintain hemostasis if function is normal.
3. **Prothrombin time (PT) and partial thromboplastin time (PTT).** The PTT assesses all coagulation proteins except factors VII and XIII. The PT will be elevated if there is a deficiency of factor I, II, V, VII, or X. Factor VII has the shortest half-life; a deficiency in factor VII is the usual cause in generalized problems such as liver disease. In systemic lupus erythematosus, there may be a circulating anticoagulant, which usually prolongs the PTT and less frequently the PT. This condition generally does not cause a bleeding diathesis but may predispose to thrombosis.
4. **Thrombin time.** The TT assays functional fibrinogen; it can also assay for heparin effect and presence of fibrinogen degradation products.
5. **Fibrinogen, fibrin split products and D-dimer assay.** In DIC, fibrinogen may be decreased and fibrin split products are increased. The absolute fibrinogen level may be normal but a downward trend is helpful. D-dimer increase may suggest ongoing DIC.
6. **Bleeding time.** This test evaluates platelet function. Uremia, liver disease, and aspirin therapy within the last week may adversely affect function. Bleeding time is also prolonged by rare disorders of collagen that may impair integrity of the vessel wall. Thrombocytopenia by itself will also increase the bleeding time.
7. **Peripheral blood smear.** May reveal fragments and helmet cells in DIC and TTP. May suggest other causes of thrombocytopenia such as vitamin B_{12} or folate deficiency. The presence of nucleated red blood cells suggests the presence of marrow infiltrative disorders (eg, prostate cancer) as the cause.
8. **Blood replacement.** Type and cross-match if needed.
9. **Future studies.** Save one or two tubes of blood prior to transfusion therapy to assay for any coagulation factors or other studies that may be ordered later.

C. Radiologic and other studies
1. **Chest x-ray.** Obtain a CXR if there is indication of intrathoracic bleeding.
2. **Bone marrow aspiration and biopsy.** Might be performed to assess platelet production in the presence of unexplained thrombocytopenia or if leukemia or another infiltrative marrow disorder is suspected.

V. Plan. Assess the rate of bleeding and differentiate between mechanical bleeding and true coagulopathy. Almost all external bleeding that is mechanical can be controlled by applying direct pressure and elevation. Treatment of coagulopathy requires appropriate laboratory tests to make the diagnosis and then institution of the correct treatment. In any case, in the acute setting assess the amount of blood loss and the volume status, and treat with IV fluids if hypovolemia is present. For further information regarding transfusion of blood products, refer to Section V—Blood Component Therapy, p 383.

  A. Thrombocytopenia

    1. Use random donor platelet transfusion, usually 5–10 U at a time, for a platelet count below 20,000 or with higher platelet counts if there is ongoing bleeding. Platelet transfusions are generally not indicated in immune thrombocytopenias unless there is active bleeding. Patients receiving multiple platelet transfusions may develop HLA antibodies and have better incremental increases in the platelet count with HLA-matched single donor platelets. Immunocompromised patients should receive irradiated platelets to avoid a graft-versus-host reaction (bone marrow transplant patients, possibly patients with acute leukemia or aggressive lymphoma undergoing aggressive therapy).

    2. For a drug reaction, discontinue the drug and transfuse platelets if necessary.

    3. In the presence of ITP, no treatment is usually needed until the platelet count is below 10,000 unless there is bleeding. Chronic ITP is treated with prednisone, cyclophosphamide (Cytoxan), azathioprine (Imuran), or danazol (Danocrine). The best long-term results are obtained with splenectomy. Platelet transfusions prior to splenectomy are very short-lived in ITP.

    4. Document functional defect with bleeding time and treat the underlying condition such as uremia. Discontinue drugs adversely affecting function.

  B. von Willebrand's disease (VWD)

    1. Cryoprecipitate or fresh-frozen plasma are plasma products of choice. (See Section V, Blood Component Therapy, p 385.)

    2. Deamino-8-d-arginine vasopressin (DDAVP), a vasopressin analog, increases von Willebrand factor (vWF) levels by releasing stores from endothelium. DDAVP can be effective for certain types of VWD for mild bleeding, but is contraindicated in type IIb since it may exacerbate thrombocytopenia.

  C. Hemophilia A. Specific recommendations for factor replacement depend on site of bleeding and severity of factor deficiency and are beyond the scope of this book. The reader is referred to a standard hematology text for this information. The half-life of factor VIII is about 8–12 hours. As many factor VIII concentrates are now available, treatment of choice should be with genetically engineered products which minimize risk of transmission of viral hepatitis and human immunodeficiency virus (HIV).

D. Hemophilia B. As with hemophilia A, the reader is referred to a standard hematology text for specific recommendations for factor replacement. Factor IX concentrate has a half-life of approximately 24 hours. Several factor IX preparations are available. There is concern about some preparations containing activated coagulation factors which may induce thrombosis or DIC. New preparations probably avoid this risk. Newly diagnosed patients should receive only heat-treated products to avoid transmission of viral hepatitis or HIV virus.

E. DIC. Treat the underlying cause. Support the bleeding patient with fresh-frozen plasma, platelet transfusions, and blood transfusions.

F. Vitamin K deficiency/liver disease. If immediate treatment is needed, transfuse with 2–4 units of fresh-frozen plasma and follow the PT/PTT. As factor VII, which has a half-life of 6 hours, is metabolized quickly, repeated infusions may be needed in 6–12 hours. In all cases, begin treatment with vitamin K 10 mg SC every day for 3 consecutive days. Vitamin K may be given intravenously, but because of rare anaphylactic reactions, it must be given slowly over several minutes. IV vitamin K has a faster onset and shorter time to maximal effect than SC vitamin K. If the coagulopathy is secondary to vitamin K deficiency, a response to vitamin K should be evident after 24 hours. If there is no response to vitamin K, the coagulopathy is not due to vitamin K deficiency.

REFERENCES

Bithell TC: Disorders of hemostasis and coagulation. In: Lee GR, Bithell TC, Foerster J et al, eds.: *Wintrobe's Clinical Hematology.* 9th ed. Lea & Febiger;1993:1299.
Schrier SL: Disorders of hemostasis and coagulation. In: Dale DC, editor-in-chief, Federman DD ed.: *Scientific American Medicine*, vol.1, sect. 5, part VI, 1. Scientific American, Inc.;1993.

13. COMA, ACUTE MENTAL STATUS CHANGES

I. **Problem.** You are called to evaluate a 63-year-old man in the emergency room because of confusion and lethargy.

II. **Immediate Questions**

A. **What are the patient's vital signs?** Shock of any etiology can cause poor cerebral perfusion and altered mental status. Fever could result from an infectious process which frequently in the elderly can cause an acute confusional state. Meningitis should be suspected in any patient presenting with acute mental status changes and fever. A normal breathing pattern suggests the absence of brain stem damage. Cheyne-Stokes respirations, characterized by periods of waxing and waning hyperpnea alternating with shorter periods of apnea, require an intact brain stem. Hyperventilation can be compensation for metabolic acidosis. Apneustic or ataxic breathing strongly suggests brain stem damage.

B. What is the time course of the mental status changes? It is important to question other sources such as the patient's family or friends, if possible, when obtaining the history. If the disorientation is long-standing, then the patient may have Alzheimer's disease or some other cause of dementia.

C. What medications is the patient taking? Medications, especially in the elderly, may alter mental status. The following are but a few of the drugs or medications that may cause mental status changes: narcotics (morphine, codeine, meperidine); street drugs (phencyclidine [PCP] and cocaine); barbiturates; amphetamines; atropine; scopolamine; and commonly prescribed medications such as H_2 blockers (cimetidine, ranitidine, famotidine, nizatidine); digitalis; sedatives (benzodiazepines); tricyclic antidepressants; and steroids. If the patient is hospitalized, check the medication records to see how much pain medication and sedatives the patient has actually received, not just how much was ordered.

D. Is there a history of trauma? This information is especially important in a patient receiving anticoagulant therapy. Recent head trauma may result in a subdural or epidural hematoma, often resulting in increasing lethargy and coma. The elderly, and alcoholic patients, are particularly susceptible.

E. Is there evidence of central nervous system pathology such as headache, hemiparesis, ataxia, or vomiting? A cause of increased intracranial pressure such as tumor, subdural hematoma, or cerebral hemorrhage may lead to delirium, lethargy, or coma as well as the previously mentioned symptoms.

F. Does the patient drink or use any recreational medications? Exposure to drugs or toxins is the most common cause of coma. Intoxication with ethanol or other substances, as well as alcohol withdrawal or delirium tremens (see Section 1, Chapter 16, Delirium Tremens, p 85), can cause disorientation.

G. Is the patient a diabetic? Either hypoglycemia (see Section 1, Chapter 36, Hypoglycemia, p 36) or hyperglycemia (see Section 1, Chapter 31, p 161, Hyperglycemia) may cause altered mental status.

H. Does the patient have any known systemic illnesses? Severe liver disease, renal failure, hypothyroidism. and respiratory failure can cause mental status changes and lethargy.

I. Is there a history of psychiatric illness? Patients with depression may present with confusion and disorientation. Patients with catatonic schizophrenia may not be responsive to verbal and other cues.

  J. **In the perioperative patient, did the patient receive any anticholinergic medications? Was there any prolonged hypotension during surgery?** Postoperative delirium is common; there are many potential causes including hypotension; anoxia; myocardial ischemia/infarction; and medications including anticholinergics, sedatives, and narcotics.

  K. **Does the patient have a prior history of pulmonary problems?** Hypoxemia can cause acute confusion but patients are initially agitated rather than lethargic.

III. Differential Diagnosis

A. Trauma

1. **Subdural hematoma.** The most common intracranial mass lesion resulting from head injury.

2. **Epidural hematoma.** Usually associated with a skull fracture and a lacerated meningeal vessel, particularly the middle meningeal artery.

3. **Concussion.** A clinical diagnosis of cerebral dysfunction that clears within 24 hours.

4. **Contusion.** Usually associated with neurological deficits that persist longer than 24 hours after injury. Small hemorrhages are present in the cerebral parenchyma on CT scan.

B. Metabolic causes

1. **Exogenous.** Intoxication with ethanol or alcohol withdrawal (either minor withdrawal or delirium tremens, see Section 1, Chapter 16, Delirium Tremens (DTs): Major Alcohol Withdrawal, p 85); drugs (see Section 1, Chapter 16, II D, p 86) including drug withdrawal, anesthetic agents with delayed clearance postoperatively, carbon monoxide poisoning, and poisoning from plants such as *Psilocybe* or *Panaeolus* mushrooms that often cause hallucinations and inability to concentrate.

2. **Endogenous**

   a. **Endocrine**

      i. **Pancreas.** Hypoglycemia (most often secondary to treatment of diabetes) or marked hyperglycemia resulting in a hyperosmolar state.

      ii. **Pituitary.** Hypopituitarism leading to adrenal insufficiency and hypothyroidism.

      iii. **Thyroid.** Hyperthyroidism and hypothyroidism. Both may have associated mental status changes. Hyperthyroidism is associated with agitation and nervousness, whereas hypothyroidism is associated with lethargy. Must have a high index of suspicion in elderly because mental status changes may be the only sign.

        iv. **Parathyroid.** Either hyperparathyroidism resulting in hypercalcemia or hypoparathyroidism resulting in hypocalcemia can cause mental status changes.

  b. Fluids/electrolytes

        i. **Sodium.** Hyponatremia (see Section 1, Chapter 39, Hyponatremia, p 193) and hypernatremia (see Section 1, Chapter 33, Hypernatremia, p170) may cause confusion. With hyponatremia, the severity of the mental status changes is related to the level and the rate of sodium decrease.

        ii. **Potassium.** Hypokalemia (see Section 1, Chapter 37, Hypokalemia, p 185) or hyperkalemia (see Section 1, Chapter 32, Hyperkalemia, p 166). Potassium abnormalities infrequently cause mental status changes. Hypokalemia may precipitate hepatic encephalopathy in cirrhotics.

        iii. **Calcium.** Hypocalcemia (see Section 1, Chapter 35, Hypocalcemia, p 178) or hypercalcemia (see Section 1, Chapter 30, Hypercalcemia, p 156).

        iv. **Magnesium.** Hypomagnesemia (see Section 1, Chapter 38, Hypomagnesemia, p 190). Often there is associated hypokalemia and hypocalcemia. In addition to being delirious, the patient may be anxious or psychotic.

        v. **Acidemia or alkalemia.** Mental status changes often result from underlying acidemia or alkalemia. Acute, and to a lesser extent, chronic hypercapnia, can cause confusion, hallucinations, and coma.

        vi. **Hypoxia.**

        vii. **Osmolarity disturbances; hyperosmolar coma.** Common causes are hypernatremia and marked hyperglycemia as well as foreign substances such as mannitol.

        viii. **Thiamine deficiency (Wernicke's encephalopathy).** This condition is often seen in alcoholics but is also observed in other conditions such as hyperemesis gravidarum, AIDS, peritoneal dialysis, and eating disorders. Mental status changes range from mild confusion to coma. Patients presenting in coma with Wernicke's encephalopathy are often not diagnosed until autopsy. Ataxia and ophthalmoplegia (usually bilateral horizontal nystagmus) are also frequently present.

  c. Organ failure

        i. **Renal failure.** Usually with markedly elevated blood urea nitrogen.

        ii. **Hepatic encephalopathy.** Seen in fulminant hepatitis and cirrhosis. Often precipitated by worsening hepatic function, gastrointestinal bleeding, dehydration, azotemia, hypokalemic alkalosis, constipation, and medications such as sedatives.

        iii. **Respiratory failure.** Hypoxia and/or hypercapnia.

C. Infection
    1. Central nervous system infections (meningitis, encephalitis)
    2. Sepsis

D. Tumors
    1. Primary or metastatic to CNS
    2. Hypercalcemia from metastatic disease
    3. Paraneoplastic syndromes. Hypercalcemia from parathyroid-like substance (squamous cell carcinoma) or hyponatremia from syndrome of inappropriate antidiuretic hormone (SIADH) release.

E. Psychiatric causes
    1. Psychogenic coma. The neurologic and laboratory profile is completely normal.
    2. Depression. May cause dementia or vegetative state, especially in the elderly.
    3. ICU psychosis

F. Miscellaneous
    1. Seizures. Including postictal confusion.
    2. Cerebrovascular disease
        a. Infarction or hemorrhage. Will often have focal neurologic findings.
        b. Arteriovenous malformation
        c. Hypertensive encephalopathy. Blood pressure is markedly elevated; fundoscopic exam is notable for exudates, hemorrhages, and often papilledema.
        d. Ruptured aneurysm
    3. Syncope See Section 1, Chapter 57, Syncope, p 274.
    4. Decreased cardiac output (shock) See Section 1, Chapter 41, Hypotension, p 207.
    5. Other CNS diseases
        a. Alzheimer's dementia
        b. Normal pressure hydrocephalus. Triad of ataxia, incontinence, and dementia.
        c. Korsakoff's psychosis (thiamine deficiency). This condition results from untreated, unrecognized Wernicke's encephalopathy; characterized by anterograde amnesia, impaired ability to learn, and confabulation. Recovery can be expected in only 50% of cases.
    6. Hypothermia See Section 1, Chapter 42, Hypothermia, p 208. Results most commonly from exposure; frequently observed in patients with alcoholic or barbiturate intoxication, extracellular fluid deficit, peripheral circulatory failure, and myxedema.
    7. Hyperthermia. See Section 1, Chapter 21, Fever, p 112. Most commonly from heat stroke. Also seen in patients taking phenothiazines.

IV. Database

A. Physical examination key points

1. **Vital signs.** Hypotension can cause decreased cerebral perfusion. It is a common finding in acute mental status changes due to diabetes, ethanol or barbiturate intoxication, internal hemorrhage, myocardial infarction, dissecting aortic aneurysm, and gram negative septicemia. Bradyarrhythmias or tachyarrhythmias can cause hypotension. Tachycardia may be associated with other causes of mental status changes such as sepsis, pulmonary embolus, hypoglycemia, and myocardial infarction. Severe hypertension may indicate hypertensive encephalopathy or cerebral hemorrhage, and is sometimes seen in patients with increased intracranial pressure. Bradycardia in association with hypertension may indicate CNS pathology (Cushing's reflex). Bradypnea may indicate ethanol intoxication or barbiturate overdose. Tachypnea may indicate significant hypoxia or sepsis. A fever suggests infection or possibly loss of thermoregulation associated with thyroid storm; a markedly elevated temperature from heat stroke or malignant hyperthermia can cause mental status changes. The elderly may not have a fever in response to an infection/sepsis. Hypothermia may suggest hypothyroidism (myxedema coma), sepsis, or exposure.

2. **HEENT**

   a. **Head.** Look for evidence of trauma that may point to a subdural or epidural bleed, or a cerebral contusion.

   b. **Eyes.** Pinpoint pupils may indicate narcotic use. Unilateral, fixed, and dilated pupils suggest ipsilateral temporal lobe herniation. Bilateral, fixed, and dilated pupils suggest anoxia and brain death. Pupils may be dilated or sluggish to direct and indirect light in hypothermia or hyperthermia. Assessment of unprovoked eye movements can be valuable. Smooth, fully conjugate, spontaneous eye movements in a comatose patient suggest an intact brain stem with a bihemispheric cause of coma. Nystagmus is seen with Wernicke's encephalopathy. Conjunctival or fundal petechiae suggest fat embolism or endocarditis. Papilledema suggests a mass, an intracranial bleed, or hypertensive encephalopathy. Subhyaloid hemorrhages may be seen trapped behind the vitreous humor at the edge of the optic disc, suggesting a sudden rise in intracranial pressure.

   c. **Ears.** Blood behind the tympanic membranes suggests head trauma with a basilar skull fracture. An otitis media could be a source of meningitis.

   d. **Nasopharynx.** A fruity odor suggests diabetic ketoacidosis. A uriniferous odor suggests uremia.

   e. **Neck.** Resistance to passive flexion of the neck without resistance to other neck movements is evidence for meningitis or subarachnoid bleed. Tests for Kernig's and Brudzinski's signs should be performed as well to rule out meningeal irritation. Bruits suggest a stroke; however, many patients have incidental bruits. Thyroid enlargement points to hypothyroidism or hyperthyroidism. A bruit over an enlarged thyroid gland is pathognomonic of Graves' disease.

3. **Chest.** Thorough exam to rule out significant pulmonary disease resulting in hypoxia or hypercapnia.
4. **Heart.** An irregularly irregular apical pulse (atrial fibrillation) points to embolization from a mural thrombus. A new murmur with fever and/or leukocytosis suggests endocarditis. A right-to-left shunt may also cause hypoxia.
5. **Abdomen.** Splenomegaly, ascites, and other evidence of chronic liver disease suggest hepatic encephalopathy.
6. **Skin.** Jaundice, spider angiomata, and palmar erythema point to hepatic encephalopathy. A maculohemorrhagic rash suggests meningococcal infection, staphylococcal endocarditis, or other infection. In carbon monoxide poisoning, the skin is usually cherry–red. Needle marks on extremities indicate possible drug abuse.
7. **Neurologic examination**
   a. A thorough neurologic exam including mental status examination is essential in any patient with coma or mental status changes, acute or chronic. Focal findings suggest an intracranial process. Hyperreflexia may be seen with upper motor neuron lesions or hyperthyroidism. Clonus is absent with hyperthyroidism and present in upper motor neuron lesions. Absent or sluggish reflexes are seen in hypothyroidism and hypothermia. The relaxation phase of the reflexes is delayed in hypothyroidism and increased in hyperthyroidism.
   b. In evaluating the comatose patient, the Glasgow Coma Scale is helpful; it assesses spontaneous movement and response to pain. (See Appendix, Table A–3, p 539). Testing the oculocephalic reflex is also helpful: Hold the eyes open and turn the patient's head quickly to one side. The eyes should move toward the midline as if staring at a fixed point (intact doll's eyes). Movement of the eyes in the direction the head is turned (absent doll's eyes) suggests a brain stem lesion. Doll's eyes' movements are not present in a normal, alert person.

B. **Laboratory data**
   1. **Complete blood count with differential, platelet count.** To evaluate for infection and anemia.
   2. **Complete blood chemistry.** Includes electrolytes, glucose, blood urea nitrogen, creatinine, bilirubin, alkaline phosphatase, and transaminases (ALT and AST [SGOT and SGPT]), calcium,

magnesium, and osmolality. Will rule out many organ-failure or metabolic causes. A serum glucose can be rapidly checked with a glucometer via a "finger stick."

3. **Arterial blood gases.** Along with serum bicarbonate, these measurements will uncover a metabolic or respiratory acid-base disturbance, which may point to the underlying cause. Also necessary to rule out hypoxemia.

4. **Serum ammonia.** Elevation indicative of hepatic failure; however, not all patients with hepatic encephalopathy have an elevated ammonia.

5. **Thyroid-stimulating hormone (TSH) and thyroxine (T_4) levels.** To rule out suspected hypothyroidism or hyperthyroidism; must have high index of suspicion. Occasionally the T_4 will be normal with hyperthyroidism and only the triiodothyronine (T_3) will be elevated along with a low TSH.

6. **Urine and serum toxicology screening.** If there is an unexplained metabolic gap acidosis, salicylate, ethanol, methanol, and ethylene glycol ingestion/overdose must be ruled out.

7. **Blood and urine cultures.** If sepsis is suspected.

C. **Radiologic and other studies**

1. **Chest x-ray.** Especially if an infectious or pulmonary source is possible.

2. **CT scan of the head.** If there are any indications of a CNS etiology, especially in the presence of headache, vomiting, focal neurologic signs, or papilledema.

3. **Lumbar puncture.** See Section III, Chapter 10, p 364. Should be performed in any patient with unexplained fever and mental status changes.

4. **Electrocardiogram.** Look for myocardial infarction or atrial fibrillation. Myocardial infarction, especially in the elderly, may present with acute mental status changes.

5. **Electroencephalogram.** Diffuse theta and delta changes may be present with most metabolic causes. Often not diagnostic except for herpes encephalitis.

V. **Plan.** Although the therapy of changing neurological status must be directed at the underlying cause, certain steps should be taken immediately: ensure adequate airway, breathing, and circulation (the ABCs of basic life support). Intubation may be necessary to protect the airway. If possible, the patient should be placed in a lateral position to prevent aspiration.

A. **Metabolic causes.** Treat the underlying defect. Refer to specific abnormality in the index. Any patient in coma should receive thiamine 100 mg slow IV push. Hypoglycemia should be considered in anyone in a coma. Some experts recommend doing a finger-stick glucose to rule out hypoglycemia rather than empirically giving an ampoule of D50 because the administration of D50 has been associated with a poorer outcome in patients with cerebral hemorrhage.

B. **Exogenous causes.** Any suspicion of narcotic-induced somnolence can be safely treated with naloxone 0.4–0.8 mg IV push. A repeat dose may be necessary (up to 4–5 ampoules are commonly given in this situation).

C. **Tumor.** Somnolence in the presence of metastatic or primary CNS tumors is an emergency usually treated by radiotherapy; however, the intracranial pressure must be acutely decreased. This can be done with steroids, hyperventilation, and osmotic diuresis. Give dexamethasone IV bolus 0.1–0.2 mg/kg. The patient should be intubated to protect the airway and can be hyperventilated by increasing the rate of the respirator and following the pCO_2. You should attempt to decrease the pCO_2 to 20–25 mm Hg. Osmotic diuresis with mannitol 50 g in a 20% solution over 20 minutes is also beneficial if there is associated cerebral edema.

D. **Infection.** Treat with appropriate antibiotics. Gram's stain may help direct initial antibiotic therapy prior to culture results.

E. **Cardiac syncope or low cardiac output.** Treat the underlying cardiac problem.

F. **Vascular problems.** Intracranial bleeding is usually treated like other causes of increased intracranial pressure. Contact a neurosurgical consultant immediately. Increased intracranial pressure should be emergently treated to circumvent herniation. Intubation with hyperventilation, osmotic diuresis with mannitol 50 g in a 20% solution over 20 minutes, and dexamethasone 0.1–0.2 mg/kg may acutely decrease intracranial pressure.

REFERENCES

Adams RD, Victor M: Coma and related disorders of consciousness. In: *Principles of Neurology*. 4th ed. McGraw-Hill Information Services Co;1993:300.

Adams RD, Victor M: Delirium and other acute confusional states. In: *Principles of Neurology*. 4th ed. McGraw-Hill Information Services Co;1993:353.

Browning RG, Olsen DW, Steven HA: 50% Dextrose: Antidote or toxin? Ann Emerg Med 1990;19:113.

Samuels MA: The evaluation of comatose patients. Hosp Pract 1993;165.

14. CONSTIPATION

I. **Problem.** A 75-year-old bedridden woman from a nursing home admitted with dehydration and a urinary tract infection has not had a bowel movement in 7 days.

II. **Immediate Questions**

A. **What are the patient's normal bowel habits?** Normal bowel habits vary from three stools per day to three stools per week.

Some individuals develop a dependence on bowel stimulants and other laxatives.

B. What medications is the patient taking? Constipation is a side effect of many drugs, including narcotics, antidepressants (tricyclics), nonabsorbable antacids (aluminum hydroxide), diuretics, and calcium channel blockers (especially verapamil [Calan, Isoptin]).

C. Is the abdomen distended, tender, or tense? Is the patient passing flatus or vomiting? Mechanical obstruction from sigmoid volvulus, intussusception, and hernia can lead to constipation. Mechanical obstruction often has other symptoms. Flatus signifies an intact, functioning gastrointestinal tract.

D. Does the patient have a history of hemorrhoids or rectal bleeding? Rectal lesions, including hemorrhoids, proctitis, and fissures, may induce constipation.

E. Has the patient undergone any recent radiographic or surgical procedures? Barium from x-ray studies can cause constipation. Many postoperative patients will have an ileus resulting in constipation.

III. Differential Diagnosis

A. Systemic disorders

1. **Drugs.** Constipation is a side effect of many medications including analgesics (inhibitors of prostaglandin synthesis, opiates); anticholinergics (antihistamines, antiparkinsonism agents, phenothiazines, tricyclic antidepressants); antacids containing aluminum hydroxide or calcium carbonate; barium sulfate; clonidine; diuretics (non-potassium sparing); calcium channel blockers (especially verapamil); ganglionic blockers; iron preparations; muscle blockers, and polystyrene sodium sulfonate.

2. **Endocrine disorders.** Hypothyroidism, diabetes, and hyperparathyroidism.

3. **Metabolic disorders.** Hypercalcemia and hypokalemia.

4. **Volume status.** Dehydrated patients, especially the elderly, can become constipated.

B. Gastrointestinal disorders

1. **Tumors.** Benign or malignant tumors can lead to constipation through obstruction by mass effect.

2. **Inflammatory lesions.** With induction of pain, the patient suppresses the urge to defecate, resulting in constipation. Common inflammatory disorders include diverticulitis, proctitis, hemorrhoids, fistula-in-ano, and inflammatory bowel diseases (IBD), such as ulcerative colitis and Crohn's disease.

3. **Mechanical obstruction.** Constipation can be secondary to physical blockage from adhesions, incarcerated hernias, volvulus, or intussusception.
C. **Neurologic conditions**
   1. **Spinal or pelvic trauma.** Results in colonic dysmotility or anal sphincter dysfunction.
   2. **Autonomic neuropathy.** Results in colonic dysmotility and can even cause pseudo-obstruction.
   3. **Cerebral vascular accident.** Constipation may develop via an associated decrease in activity level.

IV. **Database**
   A. **Physical examination key points**
      1. **Vital signs.** Fever suggests an inflammatory source such as diverticulitis or IBD. Orthostasis suggests dehydration.
      2. **Abdomen.** Distension may result from obstruction. Evidence of prior surgery suggests adhesions. Listen for bowel sounds and quality to assess for ileus or obstruction. Absence of bowel sounds is consistent with any cause of complete obstruction. On palpation, assess for tenderness or rebound. Rebound suggests peritoneal inflammation. Feel for stool-filled colon.
      3. **Rectum.** Rule out external lesions (hemorrhoids or fissures) as the cause. Be sure the anal sphincter is not stenotic. Check the quality of sphincter tone. Absence of sphincter tone suggests a spinal cord lesion. Presence of blood suggests an inflammatory cause or a benign or malignant tumor.
      4. **Neurologic examination.** Look for evidence of prior cerebrovascular accident or spinal injury, such as decreased motor function or asymmetric reflexes. A delay in the relaxation phase of the reflexes suggests hypothyroidism.
   B. **Laboratory data**
      1. **Electrolytes and calcium.** Hypokalemia or uremia is a rare cause of constipation. Check calcium level to rule out hypercalcemia.
      2. **Complete blood count.** Elevated white blood cell count may indicate an inflammatory disorder. A low hemoglobin accompanies blood loss and can result from a variety of causes, such as benign or malignant tumors, diverticulitis, or IBD.
      3. **Sedimentation rate.** With active IBD, the sedimentation rate is elevated, but it can be elevated with any inflammatory process.
      4. **Stool for occult blood.** Inflammatory disorders and tumors result in blood loss.
      5. **Thyroid function studies.** If history and physical examination are consistent with hypothyroidism, thyroid function studies (TSH, T_4) should be obtained.

C. Radiologic and other studies
   1. **Acute abdominal series.** If acute obstruction is considered likely.
   2. **Proctosigmoidoscopy.** To further assess the presence of obstructing or inflammatory lesions.
   3. **Barium enema.** For demonstrating partial obstruction or mass lesion. Colonoscopy is the procedure of choice if colon carcinoma or colonic polyps are suspected.
   4. **CT scan of abdomen.** To further evaluate for partial obstruction.

V. Plan. Once the etiology is demonstrated, the underlying cause should be corrected. Medicines inducing constipation should be discontinued whenever possible. Electrolyte abnormalities should be corrected or obstruction relieved.
   A. Prevention. Patients taking narcotics should be started on stool softeners and bowel stimulants. Bedridden patients should also be given stool softeners. Place patients on high-fiber diets; encourage activity and adequate fluid intake.
   B. Laxatives and enemas. There are several modalities from which to choose, depending on preference and etiology (Table 1–5). Use bulk laxatives (psyllium) and high-fiber diets for control and prevention of constipation. Surfactants or wetting agents, osmotic lax-

TABLE 1–5. LAXATIVES.

Type	Name	Dosage
Bulk—daily use	Effer-syllium	1 teaspoon (6–7 g) in fluid 1 or 2 times daily
	Metamucil	1 teaspoon (6–7 g) in fluid 1 or 2 times daily
Softeners/wetting agents—daily use	Docusate sodium (Colace)	50–200 mg 1 or 2 times daily Available: Capsules 50–100 mg Solution 10 mg/mL Syrup 25 mg/mL
	Docusate calcium (Surfak)	240 mg 1 or 2 times daily
	Lactulose (Chronuluc)	15–30 mL 1 or 2 times daily
	Mineral oil	14–45 mL; one-time dose
Stimulants—prn	Bisacodyl (Dulcolax)	Oral 5–15 mg, 5-mg tablets Rectal 10 mg, 10-mg suppository
	Senna (Senokot)	1 tablet 1 or 2 times daily
	Glycerine suppository	3 g; 1 rectally
Osmotic—prn	Milk of Magnesia	15–30 mL 1 or 2 times daily
	Magnesium citrate	200 mL; one-time dose
Enema—prn	Fleet enema	120 mL rectally
	Oil retention enema	

atives, and colonic stimulants for rapid action can also be used to relieve constipation. Suppositories or enemas such as gentle tap-water enemas, oil retention enemas, and glycerin suppositories are useful for rapid action.

C. Disimpaction. Digital disimpaction is occasionally required when hard stool will not pass through the rectum. This is more common in the elderly. After disimpaction, the patient should receive laxatives or preferably enemas to relieve the constipation. Use stool softeners or bulk laxatives to prevent recurrence.

D. Other. If obstructing or inflammatory lesions are demonstrated, they should be treated with surgery, anti-inflammatory medicines, or antibiotics.

REFERENCES

Camilleri M, Thompson WG, Fleshman JW et al: Clinical management of intractable constipation. Ann Intern Med 1994;121:520.

Floch MH, Wald A: Clinical evaluation and treatment of constipation. Gastroenterologist 1994;2:50.

Harari D, Gurwitz JH, Minaker KL: Constipation in the elderly. J Am Geriatr Soc 1993;41:1130.

Lange RL, DiPiro JT: Diarrhea and constipation. In: DiPiro JT, Talbert RL, Hayes PE, et al, eds.: *Pharmacotherapy: A Pathophysiologic Approach.* 2nd ed. Appleton & Lange;1993:566.

Rousseau P: Treatment of constipation in the elderly. Postgrad Med 1988:83;339.

Wald A: Constipation in elderly patients. Drugs & Aging 1993;3:220.

15. COUGH

I. **Problem.** A nurse notifies you that one of your patients is unable to sleep because of a persistent cough.

II. **Immediate Questions**

A. Is the cough acute or chronic? Acute onset of cough most often results from infections such as the common cold, but can result from urgent conditions such as acute bronchospasm (see Section I, Chapter 61, Wheezing, p 297), pulmonary embolus (see Section I, Chapter 11, Chest Pain, p 55), aspiration (see Section I, Chapter 7, Aspiration, p 34), or decompensated congestive heart failure. A chronic cough is unlikely to represent a condition that could pose immediate danger to the patient.

B. Is the cough productive of sputum? If so, what does the sputum look like? A productive cough implies an inflammatory condition such as infection. Blood in the sputum leads to consideration of several other causes. (See Section I, Chapter 29, Hemoptysis, p 51).

    C. Is the patient tachypneic or dyspneic? Either of these could suggest a significant underlying respiratory disease such as pulmonary embolus or pneumonia.

    D. Is the patient on an angiotensin-converting enzyme (ACE) inhibitor? Cough has been reported as a side effect in 1–19% of patients on ACE inhibitors. The cough is nonproductive and persistent. It can begin 3–12 months after initiation of therapy and remits 1–7 days after the drug is discontinued. There is a female predominance.

III. Differential Diagnosis. Cough reflex receptors are present in the ear, pharynx, sinuses, nose, larynx, trachea, bronchi, and pleural surfaces. Thus, disorders stimulating receptors in these locations can result in cough.

    A. Ear. Impacted cerumen, foreign body, or hair in the ear can produce cough.

    B. Oropharynx/nasopharynx. Postnasal drip from allergic and nonallergic rhinitis or sinusitis is a common cause of cough.

    C. Larynx. Acute viral laryngitis can produce cough.

    D. Tracheobronchial tree. Any process irritating the mucosal receptors or preventing clearance of secretions can result in cough.

        1. Bronchospasm. Asthma is a frequent cause of nonproductive cough, especially nocturnal cough. Wheezing may be absent.

        2. Bronchitis. Both acute and chronic bronchitis can cause irritation of mucosal receptors and result in cough.

        3. Pneumonia. Viral, bacterial, tuberculous, and fungal causes should all be considered, especially in any immunocompromised patient. Such patients include persons with acquired immunodeficiency syndrome, persons receiving immunosuppressive treatment, or persons with an underlying lymphoproliferative or hematologic malignancy.

        4. Gastroesophageal reflux. Aspiration of oropharyngeal and gastric contents can produce cough. Symptoms typically worsen at night or during meals.

        5. Inhaled irritants. The most common cause of a chronic cough is inhaled tobacco smoke.

        6. Bronchogenic carcinoma. This condition produces mechanical irritation of mucosal receptors. The majority of patients with bronchogenic carcinoma develop chronic cough at some point.

    E. Others. There are many other causes of cough; a few are listed here.

        1. Congestive heart failure. A nocturnal cough may be the only manifestation of early congestive heart failure.

        2. Interstitial lung disease. This includes interstitial fibrosis and granulomatous disease such as tuberculosis and sarcoidosis.

3. **Thoracic aneurysm.** This can cause cough by producing bronchial or tracheal compression.

IV. Database
A. Physical examination key points
1. **Vital signs.** Fever occurs with infection and pulmonary infarction. Tachypnea and use of accessory respiratory muscles suggest significant underlying pulmonary disease.
2. **HEENT**
   a. Examine the ears for impacted cerumen, foreign body, or hair in the external auditory canal.
   b. Examine the posterior pharynx for evidence of sinusitis or rhinitis, such as a postnasal drip or cobblestoning resulting from lymphoid hyperplasia.
   c. Check for evidence of sinus tenderness or opacification.
3. **Lungs**
   a. **Stridor.** This is a manifestation of upper airway obstruction resulting from laryngeal edema or epiglottitis.
   b. **Rhonchi.** Occur with bronchitis and inhalation injuries.
   c. **Signs of consolidation.** Peripheral bronchial breath sounds, egophony, and increased tactile fremitus occur with pneumonia.
   d. **Crackles.** Occur in congestive heart failure, pneumonia, and interstitial lung disease.
   e. **Wheezing.** Occurs in asthma. If localized, may signify a foreign body or obstructing neoplasm.
4. **Heart.** Jugular venous distension, displaced point of maximal impulse, and third heart sound (S_3) gallop indicate congestive heart failure.
5. **Lymph nodes.** Lymphadenopathy suggests metastatic carcinoma, a lymphoproliferative disorder, or a granulomatous disease such as sarcoidosis.
6. **Extremities.** Clubbing occurs in patients with bronchiectasis, bronchogenic carcinoma, or idiopathic pulmonary fibrosis.

B. Laboratory data
1. **Hemogram.** Leukocytosis with left shift occur with infectious diseases. Thrombocytosis may result from underlying malignancy.
2. **Arterial blood gases.** These results should be obtained only if the patient appears dyspneic or cyanotic.

C. Radiologic and other studies
1. **Chest x-ray.** Evidence of congestive heart failure, neoplasm, pneumonia, interstitial lung disease, hilar adenopathy and thoracic aortic aneurysm may appear on CXR.
2. **Ventilation/perfusion ($\dot{V}/\dot{Q}$) scan.** Should be obtained if there is a high suspicion of pulmonary embolism.

3. **Sputum.** Examine for color, viscosity, odor, and amount. Perform Gram's stain.
4. **Purified protein derivative (PPD) skin test.** Should be performed if tuberculosis is a possibility.
5. **Pulmonary function tests.** A restrictive pattern occurs in interstitial lung disease. A restrictive pattern is a decrease in all lung volumes: forced expiratory volume at 1 second (FEV_1), forced vital capacity (FVC), total lung capacity (TLC), and other lung volumes. The FEV_1/FVC ratio is maintained near normal or may be high. A reversible obstructive defect (a decrease in the FEV_1 and FEV_1/FVC ratio) would suggest underlying emphysema or asthma. Bronchial provocation with methacholine may be necessary to diagnose occult asthma if baseline pulmonary function tests are normal.
6. **Bronchoscopy.** This is of value only if there is an abnormality noted on CXR, or a localized wheeze.

V. Plan. The treatment of cough is dependent on identifying the etiology, and then directing treatment toward that cause.
   A. Infectious conditions (See Section III for drug dosages.)
      1. **Community-acquired pneumonia.** Penicillin is recommended for pneumococcal infections; however, erythromycin should be used in those situations in which mycoplasma or Legionnaires' pneumonia is a diagnostic possibility.
      2. **Acute bronchitis.** Most often, acute bronchitis has a viral etiology; however, in those instances in which mycoplasma or bacteria is suspected, erythromycin or ampicillin can be given.
      3. **Chronic bronchitis.** Most often occurs in smokers; cough resolves with cessation of smoking.
   B. Rhinitis/sinusitis. In these instances, cough is best managed by treatment with an antihistamine and decongestant. Antibiotics are indicated if bacterial sinusitis is suspected.
   C. Asthma. Inhaled bronchodilators such as metaproterenol (Alupent) and albuterol (Ventolin) represent the best treatment for those whose cough is due to asthma. Oral bronchodilators may be necessary for patients in whom inhalation therapy provokes cough; however, a trial with a spacer is warranted prior to changing to oral therapy. Spacers have been useful in eliminating the cough provoked by inhalation therapy in some patients. Initially, steroids (oral or inhaled) may be required to eliminate the cough.
   D. Gastroesophageal reflux. These patients should have the head of their beds elevated and should not eat before retiring for bed. Antacids, histamine H_2 antagonists such as cimetidine (Tagamet) or proton pump blockers such as omeprazole (Prilosec) may also be required.

E. **General measures.** In patients with a nonproductive cough in whom infection is not a concern, cough suppression can provide much-needed symptomatic relief.
   1. **Cough suppression**
      a. Codeine phosphate is the most effective cough suppressant. The usual dose is 10–30 mg Q 4–6 hr (maximum dose is 120 mg/d).
      b. Dextromethorphan, a codeine derivative, acts centrally and is the best non-narcotic for cough suppression. This dose is 30 mg Q 6–8 hr.
      c. Diphenhydramine HCl acts centrally to suppress cough; the dose is 25 mg Q 4 hr.
   2. **Expectorants.** Have been shown to be of no value and should not be used.

REFERENCES

Bryant BG, Lombardi TP: Cold, cough, and allergy products. In: Covington TR, Lawson LC, Young LL et al eds. *The Handbook of Non-Prescription Drugs.* 10th ed. American Pharmaceutical Association;1993:89.

Irwin RS et al: Persistent cough in the adult: Spectrum and frequency of causes and successful outcome of specific therapy. Am Rev Respir Dis 1981;123:413.

Poe RH et al: Chronic persistent cough: Experience in diagnosis and outcome using an anatomic diagnostic protocol. Chest 1989;95:723.

16. DELIRIUM TREMENS (DTs): MAJOR ALCOHOL WITHDRAWAL

I. **Problem.** A 55-year-old intoxicated man is admitted with abdominal pain and an elevated amylase. Narcotic analgesia is initiated. On the third day post admission, he is found talking to the walls and shaking violently.

II. **Immediate Questions**
   A. **What are the patient's vital signs?** Hypertension, tachycardia, and fever may represent signs of autonomic overactivity, common in DTs. A fever may also point to an infectious etiology as the cause of the delirium.
   B. **What is the patient's mental status?** Altered levels of consciousness and impaired cognitive function define delirium. Hallucinations and confusion are important observations. These, coupled with autonomic hyperactivity, are typical of DTs. Delirium tremens can also present as unresponsiveness. Visual hallucinations (eg, "pink elephants") are more commonly associated with

toxic psychosis (eg, ethanol). Auditory hallucinations are more commonly associated with psychiatric illness (eg, schizophrenia).

C. What is the patient's airway status? Any patient with an altered level of consciousness is at increased risk of aspiration.

D. What medications or illicit drugs is the patient taking? Medications may cause disorientation. Likely offenders include: narcotics (morphine, codeine, meperidine), phencyclidine (PCP), cocaine, barbiturates, amphetamines, atropine, scopolamine, and commonly prescribed medications such as H_2 blockers (cimetidine, ranitidine, famotidine, nizatidine) or aspirin; and especially in the elderly, digitalis, sedatives (benzodiazepines), tricyclic antidepressants, and steroids. Individuals who abuse one substance are more likely to abuse others. A thorough drug history, including illicit drugs, is essential. Ask specifically regarding the use of narcotics, sedatives, barbiturates, and atropine-like substances.

E. Is there a history of alcohol abuse? This is central to an accurate diagnosis. Historical information may need to be obtained from family or friends because of the delirium.

F. Is there a previous history of DTs? Many times there is a past history of DTs. The absence of such a history does not exclude DTs as the cause of the delirium.

G. Is there a history of alcohol withdrawal seizures? One-third of patients with a history of alcohol withdrawal seizures develop DTs, whereas only 5% of patients with minor alcohol withdrawal develop DTs.

H. When was the patient's last drink? The length of time since the last drink will assist in the diagnosis of DTs. Minor alcohol withdrawal usually begins 6–8 hours after cessation of drinking, peaks at about 24 hours and usually resolves within 48 hours. The onset of DTs is between day 2 and days 10–14 from cessation of ethanol intake.

III. Differential Diagnosis. DTs is a manifestation of diffuse cerebral dysfunction. Focal neurologic deficits point to a structural abnormality (stroke or brain tumor). The differential diagnosis of delirium is more extensive than given here and includes any source of diffuse cerebral dysfunction. (See Section I, Chapter 13, Coma, Acute Mental Status Changes, p 69). Patients presenting with DTs may have a wide range of concomitant problems. The patient described in this case may be delirious because of any of the following diagnoses:

A. Withdrawal syndromes

   1. Minor alcohol withdrawal. A less severe form of alcohol withdrawal, which occurs between 8 and 48 hours after the last drink. Disorientation is usually mild. Tachycardia, diaphoresis, and tremor are often present. Seizures and hallucinations may occur.

   2. Barbiturate withdrawal. Indistinguishable from DTs clinically.

3. **Opioid withdrawal.** Occurs up to 48 hours after cessation of agent (most rapid with heroin). Symptoms include restlessness, rhinorrhea, lacrimation, nausea, diarrhea, and hypertension.

B. **Metabolic abnormalities.** There are multiple metabolic abnormalities that can cause altered levels of consciousness and impaired cognitive function similar to DTs.

   1. **Fever** (See Section I, Chapter 21, Fever, p 112).
   2. **Hepatic encephalopathy**
   3. **Hypercalcemia** (See Section I, Chapter 30, Hypercalcemia, p 156).
   4. **Hyperkalemia** (See Section I, Chapter 32, Hyperkalemia, p 166).
   5. **Hyperosmolar states.** Can result in delirium. Most common causes are hypernatremia (see Section I, Chapter 33, Hypernatremia, p 170), and hyperglycemia (see Section I, Chapter 31, Hyperglycemia, p 161); but can also include hyperproteinemia and foreign substances such as mannitol.
   6. **Hypocalcemia** (See Section I, Chapter 35, Hypocalcemia, p 178).
   7. **Hyponatremia** (See Section I, Chapter 39, Hyponatremia, p 72).
   8. **Hypothermia** (See Section I, Chapter 42, Hypothermia, p 208).
   9. **Hypoxia.** Congestive heart failure can produce hypoxia and delirium in an indolent fashion.
   10. **Uremia**
   11. **Wernicke's encephalopathy.** Results from nutritional deficiency of thiamine. Characterized by a triad of symptoms: (1) mental status changes (confusion to coma); (2) ataxia; and (3) ophthalmoplegia (most commonly lateral-gaze nystagmus from bilateral lateral rectus palsies).

C. **Endocrine abnormalities**

   1. **Hypoglycemia** (See Section I, Chapter 36, Hypoglycemia, p 181). Either from an insulin-secreting tumor or from intentional or accidental insulin overdose.
   2. **Hyperglycemia** (See Section 1, Chapter 31, Hyperglycemia, p 161. Extreme hyperglycemia, especially in the elderly, can result in delirium.
   3. **Hyperthyroidism.** The signs/symptoms of hyperthyroidism may mimic alcohol withdrawal syndrome; there may be mental status changes, diaphoresis, tachycardia, tremor, and agitation. There is often a history of weight loss, hot weather intolerance, and hyperdefecation. The thyroid gland is often enlarged. The T_3 or T_4 will be elevated and the TSH level suppressed. The signs and symptoms of hyperthyroidism are usually more subacute or chronic; however, thyroid storm can develop acutely if there is a precipitating event such as an operation or infection. Thyroid storm is characterized by thermoderegulation (hyperthermia), mental status changes, and an identifiable precipitating event.

D. **Hypertensive encephalopathy.** Encephalopathy induced by poorly controlled hypertension. Headache is common. Exudates and hemorrhages are present on fundoscopic examination. Papilledema may be present.

E. Central nervous system (CNS) infections. In anyone with disorientation, consider CNS infection, including meningitis, brain abscess, and encephalitis. With bacterial causes, fever and leukocytosis with an increase in banded neutrophils are often present, as well as other signs (meningismus or papilledema). If there are focal findings or papilledema, a CT scan should be performed initially.

F. Psychiatric disturbances
   1. **ICU psychosis**. Secondary to unfamiliar setting; often seen in elderly patients. May be secondary to or aggravated by medications such as lidocaine and digoxin.
   2. **"Sundowning."** Nighttime agitation and confusion are common problems, especially in the elderly. The agitation and confusion resolve in the morning.

G. Sepsis. Sepsis can cause mental status changes. A fever and elevated white blood cell count with an increase in banded neutrophils are common. A source for sepsis is often evident, such as pyuria or an infiltrate on chest x-ray.

H. Low cardiac output states. Either from ischemia or cardiomyopathy. Can cause confusion secondary to decreased cerebral perfusion and may result in agitation. A history of chest pain or myocardial infarction may be helpful. Previous symptoms of congestive heart failure (orthopnea, paroxysmal nocturnal dyspnea, and dyspnea on exertion) may also be present. On physical examination, hypotension or relative hypotension is seen, as are increased jugular vein distension and bibasilar wet inspiratory crackles.

IV. Database
   A. Physical examination key points
      1. **Vital signs.** Tachycardia, hypertension, and fever are common manifestations of DTs. Fever from DTs may be as high as 104°F (40°C). With severe hypertension and delirium, consider hypertensive encephalopathy. Fever may also be a manifestation of a localized infection or sepsis. Hypothermia could be associated with sepsis or could be the cause of the delirium. Carpal spasm with inflation of the blood pressure cuff between the diastolic and systolic blood pressure for 3 minutes (Trousseau's sign) is seen with hypocalcemia.
      2. **Eyes.** Nystagmus suggests Wernicke's encephalopathy. Lid lag or proptosis suggests hyperthyroidism. Papilledema may be seen in meningitis or hypertensive encephalopathy, or with a space-occupying lesion.
      3. **Neck.** Thyromegaly suggests hyperthyroidism as a cause of the delirium. Jugular venous distension points toward congestive heart failure.
      4. **Chest.** Signs of congestive heart failure and other causes of pulmonary edema and hypoxia should be sought.

5. **Abdomen.** Check for bladder distension, a common cause of agitation in the elderly.
6. **Skin.** Profuse sweating is typical of DTs. Telangiectasias and gynecomastia are associated with chronic ethanol use and chronic liver disease.
7. **Neurologic examination.** Mental status changes define delirium. Hallucinations, confusion, and disorientation are typical. Reflexes will be exaggerated but symmetrical. Hyperreflexia is also seen in hyperthyroidism. Twitching at the corner of the mouth with tapping over the facial nerve (Chvostek's sign) is seen in hypocalcemia. Any focal findings on motor, sensory, deep tendon, or cranial nerve examination point to a structural abnormality, either spinal or intracranial.

B. **Laboratory data.** There are multiple electrolyte abnormalities that may cause delirium, or that may be associated with heavy ethanol use.
1. **Sodium.** Hyponatremia could be the etiology of the delirium.
2. **Glucose.** Eliminate hypoglycemia or hyperglycemia as a cause of delirium; both may be associated with heavy ethanol ingestion.
3. **Calcium.** May reveal hypocalcemia or hypercalcemia as the cause.
4. **Potassium.** Hypokalemia often complicates heavy ethanol ingestion. Hyperkalemia may also cause delirium.
5. **Blood urea nitrogen and creatinine.** May point to uremia/renal failure as etiology of the delirium.
6. **Liver function tests.** Transaminases (AST and ALT), total bilirubin, and alkaline phosphatase to rule out hepatic failure as a cause of the delirium. Liver dysfunction is common in patients who chronically use alcohol.
7. **Arterial blood gases.** To eliminate hypoxemia as a cause.
8. **Complete blood count with differential.** An elevated white blood cell count with an increase in banded neutrophils suggests a bacterial etiology. An elevated mean corpuscular volume may be from associated folate or vitamin B_{12} deficiency. Vitamin B_{12} deficiency can cause mental status changes. Anemia from a variety of causes is commonly seen in heavy ethanol use.
9. **Thyroid function tests.** Thyroid-stimulating hormone (TSH) is suppressed and thyroxine is usually elevated with hyperthyroidism. Hypothyroidism may cause changes in mental status and result in an elevated TSH and a decrease in the thyroxine.
10. **Phosphorus.** Hypophosphatemia is associated with heavy ethanol use as a result of either poor nutritional intake, diarrhea, vomiting, or refeeding after prolonged starvation.
11. **Magnesium.** Hypomagnesemia is often seen with heavy ethanol use. Hypomagnesemia may result from poor intake, diarrhea, renal losses, and excessive sweating.

C. **Radiologic and other studies**
   1. **Chest x-ray.** May reveal cardiomegaly, pulmonary edema, or pneumonia.
   2. **Electrocardiogram.** To rule out myocardial ischemia as an etiology of delirium. Also tachyarrhythmias are associated with alcohol withdrawal (major or minor).
   3. **CT scan of head.** May be indicated if there are focal findings on examination, or seizures associated with DTs. Alcohol withdrawal seizures should occur before the onset of DTs.
   4. **Lumbar puncture.** Indicated in any patient with mental status changes and fever. May be difficult to rule out meningitis in a patient with DTs without lumbar puncture.
   5. **Electroencephalogram.** May help diagnose encephalitis. Usually increased nonfocal activity with DTs. Rarely is an electroencephalogram needed.

V. **Plan**
   A. **Strategies.** There are four types of treatment strategies for alcohol withdrawal (minor or moderate):
      1. **Supportive care.** A calm environment with frequent assessment and nursing care is all that is required for many patients with *mild* alcohol withdrawal. Individuals with a history of alcohol withdrawal seizures or delirium tremens, or a co-existing acute illness will require medical management in addition to supportive care.
      2. **Scheduled dosing.** The gold standard is a treatment regimen in which a fixed dose of a benzodiazepine is given on a regular schedule and tapered over several days, eg diazepam (Valium) 20 mg every 6 hours for 1 day decreasing the dose by 1/2 every day, with an additional 10–20 mg every 2–4 hours as needed. Chlordiazepoxide (Librium) 100 mg every 6 hours for 1 day, decreasing the dose by 1/2 every day with an additional 25–50 mg every 2–4 hours as needed. Lorazepam (Ativan) or oxazepam (Serax) PO or IM should be considered with moderate to severe hepatic dysfunction.
      3. **Front-load dosing.** A long-acting benzodiazepine is given every 1–2 hours until symptoms abate; eg, diazepam (Valium) 20 mg PO every 2 hours until symptoms subside; or lorazepam (Ativan) 2 mg IM every 2 hours can be used.
      4. **Symptom-triggered dosing.** The benzodiazepines are administered according to the patient's symptoms. This method requires frequent assessment and has been shown to require a lower amount of benzodiazepine than the scheduled dosing regimen; moreover, the duration of treatment is shorter. Initially diazepam (Valium) 20 mg PO or chlordiazepoxide (Librium) 50 mg PO is given; or lorazepam (Ativan) 2 mg IM initially with ad-

ditional doses every 1–2 hours if assessment indicates a need for more medication. The assessment should include the use of a scale such as the Clinical Institute Withdrawal Assessment for Alcohol, to determine need for additional medication.

B. Delirium tremens
1. **ICU setting**
2. **Intravenous fluids.** May require 3 to 6 liters per day; use D5 NS.
3. **Correction of electrolyte disorders**
   a. **Hypokalemia.** Replacement with potassium supplements either PO or IV. A total replacement dose of 100 mEq of potassium is required to raise a potassium of 3.0 mEq/L to 4.0 mEq/L. Intravenous replacement is generally 10–15 mEq per hour. Oral replacement is 20–60 mEq per dose, and can be repeated in 2–4 hours.
   b. **Hypophosphatemia.** IV replacement is reserved for severe, life-threatening hypophosphatemia (levels < 1.5 mg/dL). IV replacement is with 5–10 mmol over 4–6 hours. PO replacement can be with Neutra-Phos capsules (250 mg per capsule) or skim milk (1 quart contains 1 g of phosphorus or about 30 mmol).
   c. **Hypomagnesemia.** Replacement is generally either IV or IM. The oral route often causes diarrhea. Magnesium sulfate can be given 1 g IM in each hip or 1 g IV per hour for 4 hours. The magnesium level should be checked 1–2 hours after the fourth gram has been infused. This regimen may need to be repeated. Magnesium is mostly an intracellular cation. With extremely low levels of magnesium, often 10–15 g will be required.
4. **Thiamine replacement.** Thiamine 100 mg IV or IM should be given prior to the administration of any intravenous fluids containing glucose. Glucose can precipitate Wernicke's encephalopathy in a patient with marginal thiamine stores. Thiamine should be given for 3 days.
5. **Other vitamins.** Multivitamins and folate should be given daily either orally or intravenously.
6. **Restraints.** Are often needed to prevent injury.
7. **Benzodiazepines.** Diazepam (Valium) 5–10 mg intravenously every 5–10 minutes until sedated, or lorazepam (Ativan) 1–2 mg intravenously every 5–10 minutes. The dose of diazepam should not exceed 100 mg/hr or 250 mg over 8 hours.
8. **Other treatments.** Phenobarbital 100–200 mg IM or IV every 1–2 hours can be used if benzodiazepines cannot be used. Carbamazepine (800 mg/d, taper over 7 days) has been used for mild and moderate withdrawal as a single agent. Advantages are that it is non-addictive, non-sedating, and metabolism is not affected by liver dysfunction.

9. **Adjunct therapy.** A beta-blocker, atenolol (Tenormin 50–100 mg/d) has been shown to be beneficial for mild to moderate withdrawal, both in an outpatient and inpatient setting. Clonidine (Catapres) 0.1–0.2 mg PO BID or clonidine transdermal (Catapres TTS-1 or TTS-2) can also be used.
10. **Haloperidol (Haldol).** 2–10 mg PO, IV or IM can be used for hallucinations or for agitation not responding to benzodiazepines. Neuroleptics decrease the seizure threshold, however, and may precipitate alcohol withdrawal seizures. Butyrophenones are a better choice than phenothiazines.
11. **Antipyretics.** Acetaminophen 650–1000 mg or aspirin 650 mg and a cooling blanket may be required because of fever associated with DTs.

REFERENCES

Kraus ML, Gottlieb LD, Horwitz RI et al: Randomized clinical trial of atenolol in patient with alcohol withdrawal. N Engl J Med 1985;313:905.

Lerner WD, Fallon HJ eds.: The alcohol withdrawal syndrome. N Engl J Med 1985;313:951.

Lohr RH: Treatment of alcohol withdrawal in hospitalized patients. Mayo Clin Proc 1995;70:777.

Saitz R: Recognition and management of occult alcohol withdrawal. Hosp Pract 1995;June 15:49.

Saitz R, Mayo-Smith MF, Roberts MS et al: Individualized treatment for alcohol withdrawal. JAMA 1994;272:519.

Turner RC, Lichstein PR, Peden JG, et al: Alcohol withdrawal symptoms: A review of pathophysiology, clinical presentations, and treatment. J Gen Intern Med 1989;4:432.

17. DIARRHEA

I. **Problem.** A 50-year-old woman is admitted with a history of diarrhea for 36 hours.

II. **Immediate Questions**
   A. **What are the patient's vital signs?** Hypotension suggests volume depletion or possible septic shock. Fever implies an infectious etiology. Diarrhea with associated hypotension or fever should be evaluated immediately.
   B. **Is the diarrhea grossly bloody?** This usually is seen with ischemic bowel or infarction, invasive infections, neoplasms, or inflammatory bowel disease. Bloody diarrhea requires more active and immediate intervention.
   C. **Is this an acute or chronic problem?** *Acute diarrhea* is usually a self-limited disease and can often be treated symptomatically. The

most common cause of acute diarrhea in the outpatient setting is infection, and in the inpatient setting, drugs. *Chronic diarrhea* is diarrhea that has been present 4–6 weeks or longer. Common causes include lactose intolerance, irritable bowel syndrome, inflammatory bowel disease (IBD), postsurgical procedures, malabsorptive syndromes, drugs, and various infections. Some causes of chronic diarrhea can present with an acute phase.

D. Are there risk factors that suggest a specific cause? Risk factors include drug-induced diarrhea, travel, homosexual relationships, abdominal surgery, vascular disease, and various endocrine disorders such as diabetes and Addison's disease.

E. Is there associated abdominal pain? Absence of pain makes inflammatory causes such as ischemic bowel disease or ulcerative colitis less likely.

F. What is the volume of the stool? Large volumes suggest small bowel or right colon; small volumes suggest left colon.

III. Differential Diagnosis
A. Infection
1. **Viruses.** Viral syndromes usually resolve in a few days and can be treated symptomatically. Rotavirus and Norwalk virus are the most common viruses causing diarrhea.
2. **Bacteria.** *Shigella dysenteriae, Salmonella typhimurium, Campylobacter jejuni, Yersinia species, Staphylococcus aureus, Vibrio cholerae, Vibrio parahaemolyticus, Escherichia coli, Bacillus cereus, Clostridium perfringens,* and *Clostridium difficile* all cause diarrhea by producing enterotoxins or by enteroinvasion. The spectrum of illness may range from asymptomatic to a life-threatening illness with diarrhea and abdominal pain. *S aureus, B cereus,* and *C perfringens* are often associated with food poisoning. *C jejuni* and enterohemorrhagic *E coli* often cause a bloody diarrhea. *V cholerae* can cause severe, life-threatening diarrhea and is commonly associated with consumption of raw shellfish.
3. **Parasites.** *Giardia lamblia, Entamoeba histolytica,* and *Cryptosporidium. G lamblia* is often contracted by drinking contaminated water. *E histolytica* is seen in travelers to developing countries and in institutionalized patients. *Cryptosporidium* can cause a self-limited diarrhea in individuals who work with animals, especially livestock. *G lamblia, E histolytica,* and *Cryptosporidium* are common etiologic agents causing diarrhea in homosexual men. *Cryptosporidium* results in a severe, unremitting diarrhea in patients infected with human immunodeficiency virus.

B. Inflammatory diseases
1. **Ischemic bowel** secondary to thrombosis, embolism, or vasculitis such as polyarteritis nodosa and systemic lupus erythe-

matosus can result in bloody or guaiac-positive diarrhea. Atrial fibrillation is a common source of embolism.

2. **Inflammatory bowel disease (IBD).** Ulcerative colitis (UC) begins in the rectum and spreads proximally in a continuous manner. Presenting complaints begin abruptly and usually include rectal bleeding and diarrhea. Patients with Crohn's disease may also present with diarrhea; however, the onset of symptoms is more insidious than with UC, and the diarrhea is less often bloody.

C. **Tumor**
   1. **Malignant carcinoid syndrome.** Flushing is also common.
   2. **Colon carcinoma.** Bright red blood per rectum as well as occult blood loss or anemia is common.
   3. **Medullary thyroid carcinoma**
   4. **Lymphoma involving the bowel**
   5. **Villous adenomas**
   6. **Gastrinomas**

D. **Endocrinopathies**
   1. **Hyperthyroidism.** Hyperdefecation (loose, frequent stools) rather than diarrhea. Diarrhea may be present with thyroid storm.
   2. **Diabetes.** Associated with long-standing diabetes with neuropathy.
   3. **Hypoparathyroidism**
   4. **Addison's disease.** Nausea, vomiting, abdominal pain, weight loss, and lethargy along with diarrhea.

E. **Drugs**
   1. **Laxatives.** Chronic laxative abuse causes chronic diarrhea.
   2. **Antacids.** Magnesium-containing antacids can cause osmotic diarrhea.
   3. **Lactulose.** Used to treat hepatic encephalopathy; should be titrated to two to three loose stools per day but can result in severe, life-threatening hypernatremia secondary to an osmotic diarrhea if not dosed properly.
   4. **Cardiac agents.** Diarrhea is a common reason for discontinuation of quinidine. Digoxin and digitalis may also cause diarrhea.
   5. **Colchicine.** In treatment of acute gout, diarrhea can occur with increasing doses.
   6. **Antibiotics.** Antibiotics can produce diarrhea by altering gut flora. This leads to malabsorption or induction of *C difficile* overgrowth and toxin production, which can result in pseudomembranous colitis. Pseudomembranous colitis is most often secondary to antibiotics, especially broad-spectrum antibiotics such as clindamycin and the cephalosporins.
   7. **Selected antihypertensives.** Reserpine, guanethidine, methyldopa, guanabenz, and guanadrel can all cause diarrhea.

8. **Cholinergic agents.** Bethanechol, metaclopromide, and neostigmine all cause diarrhea.

F. **Abdominal surgery.** Can cause chronic diarrhea.
 1. **Gastric surgery.** Either vagotomy, resection, or bypass procedures.
 2. **Cholecystectomy**
 3. **Bowel resection**

G. **Malabsorption.** A common cause of chronic diarrhea that may result in deficiencies of fat-soluble vitamins A, D, E, and K, weight loss, and hypoalbuminemia.
 1. **Chronic pancreatitis**
 2. **Bowel resection**
 3. **Bacterial overgrowth**
 4. **Celiac or tropical sprue**
 5. **Whipple's disease**
 6. **Eosinophilic gastroenteritis**

H. **Lactose intolerance.** A common cause of chronic diarrhea resulting from lactose enzyme deficiency. Often associated flatulence.

I. **Irritable bowel syndrome.** Intermittent diarrhea may alternate with constipation. Symptoms are aggravated by stress. Abdominal pain may be present. Physical examination and routine laboratory tests are normal.

J. **Fecal impaction.** Can present with diarrhea. Often occurs in older age group.

K. **Human immunodeficiency virus (HIV) infection.** Diarrhea is common in patients positive for HIV or with acquired immunodeficiency syndrome (AIDS). Parasitic infections mentioned in Section III.A.3 are common in homosexual men with or without HIV infection. *Isospora belli* and *Microsporidia* are two other parasites that can cause diarrhea in HIV patients. Other nonparasitic etiologies associated with HIV infection include *Salmonella typhimurium,* which often results in bacteremia, *Campylobacter jejuni, Mycobacterium avium-intracellulare,* and cytomegalovirus. Often the diarrhea is idiopathic, associated with fever and weight loss, and may precede other manifestations of AIDS by months.

IV. **Database**
 A. **Physical examination key points**
 1. **General.** Cachexia suggests a chronic process such as carcinoma, AIDS, IBD, or malabsorption.
 2. **Vital signs.** Hypotension or postural changes suggest significant sepsis or volume depletion. Tachycardia implies volume depletion or infection, or could be secondary to pain. Tachypnea may indicate fever, anxiety, pain, or sepsis or may represent compensation for a metabolic acidosis from a variety of causes including sepsis and bowel infarction.

3. **HEENT.** Aphthous ulcers are associated with IBD. An enlarged thyroid suggests hyperthyroidism or medullary carcinoma.
4. **Abdomen.** Look for surgical scars. Distension may be from carbohydrate malabsorption. Absent bowel sounds suggest bowel infarction or associated peritoneal inflammation. Metastatic cancer can result in hepatomegaly.
5. **Rectum.** Rule out rectal carcinoma. Look for fissures suggesting UC. Fecal impaction can present with diarrhea.
6. **Musculoskeletal exam.** Arthritis is associated with IBD, Whipple's disease, and infection by *Yersinia enterocolitica.*
7. **Skin.** Hyperpigmentation can be seen with Addison's disease or celiac sprue. Erythema nodosum and pyoderma gangrenosum point to IBD. Dermatitis herpetiformis suggests celiac sprue, a rare cause of diarrhea.

B. **Laboratory data**
1. **Electrolytes.** With severe diarrhea various electrolyte abnormalities can occur, including hypokalemia, metabolic acidosis, hypernatremia, and hyponatremia.
2. **Complete blood count with differential.** An elevated hematocrit suggests volume depletion. An anemia (See Section I, Problem 5, Anemia, p 25) may be associated with IBD, carcinoma, or HIV infection. A microcytic anemia suggests chronic gastrointestinal blood loss or malabsorption of iron. Macrocytic anemia may be secondary to vitamin B_{12} deficiency after gastric surgery, or folate or vitamin B_{12} malabsorption.
3. **Sedimentation rate.** Expect to be increased in IBD, metastatic carcinoma, and systemic infections.
4. **Prothrombin time and partial thromboplastin time.** An elevated PT and PTT could be secondary to vitamin K deficiency from malabsorption or associated liver disease.
5. **Albumin.** Expect a low albumin in diarrhea secondary to malabsorption, IBD, and metastatic carcinoma.
6. **Calcium.** To rule out hypoparathyroidism as a cause. Hypocalcemia associated with vitamin D deficiency secondary to steatorrhea may also be seen.
7. **Endocrine tests.** Helpful as clinically indicated; include thyroid tests (thyroxine, thyroid-stimulating hormone), parathyroid hormone, cortrosyn stimulation test, and gastrin.
8. **24- to 72-hour collection of stool for fecal fat.** Essential for workup of malabsorption.
9. **Stool for occult blood.** Follow with serial exams to increase sensitivity. Occult blood suggests UC, neoplasm, ischemic bowel, or various infections such as *C jejuni.*
10. **Stool for leukocytes.** Presence of fecal leukocytes suggests an inflammatory etiology such as infection, ischemia, or IBD. In the absence of fecal leukocytes, viruses, enterotoxic food poisoning, or parasites can be suspected as can drugs, causes of malabsorption or endocrinopathies, cancer, irritable bowel, lactose intolerance, and abdominal surgery.

11. **Stool cultures.** Indicated for clinical dysentery (fever, abdominal cramps, fecal leukocytes), inflammatory causes, prolonged diarrhea (longer than 7–14 days), symptoms suggestive of acute proctitis, or a prolonged illness. Contact lab regarding special procedures to identify *Yersinia, Vibrio,* or *E coli* 0157:H7 if clinically indicated.

12. **Stool for ova and parasites (O&P)**
    a. Parasitic infections often require a "fresh" specimen within several hours of collection.
    b. Amebic dysentery diagnosed with presence of trophozoites. Cysts suggest the carrier state in the absence of trophozoites. Serology may help in the diagnosis.
    c. Identification of *Giardia* cysts is diagnostic of active infection. A small bowel aspirate may be required to recover *Giardia*.

13. *Clostridium difficile* **toxin**. If antibiotics have been given in the last 2–4 weeks. The presence of *C difficile* without the toxin should not cause diarrhea. Toxin-negative pseudomembranous colitis must also be considered.

C. **Radiologic and other studies**
1. **Proctosigmoidoscopy.** Indicated if pseudomembranous colitis is a possible etiology, if patient remains ill with negative stool cultures, or if diarrhea is bloody. An unprepped study is useful in determining the presence of mucosal inflammation suggesting IBD, obtaining cultures and biopsies, and examining for masses or stool impaction. Enemas or suppositories may obscure the presence of disease.
2. **Colonoscopy.** May be indicated if bleeding is seen on sigmoidoscopy.
3. **Barium enema.** May reveal carcinoma or IBD.
4. **Upper GI series** with small bowel follow-through. May suggest Crohn's disease, celiac sprue, Whipple's disease, or lymphoma.
5. **D-Xylose test.** Abnormal in diseases involving the small bowel mucosa such as Crohn's disease, celiac sprue, Whipple's disease, and lymphoma.

V. **Plan.** Symptomatic treatment with fluids, electrolytes and antidiarrheal agents is usually all that is required. The initial use of antibiotic therapy should be avoided; and implemented only in specific situations guided by stool culture results. Many causes of diarrhea resolve with treatment or removal of the underlying cause (eg, discontinuation of a drug like quinidine). For further recommendations regarding treatment other than those listed, please refer to any general medicine text.
A. **Fluid replacement.** This is the most important early intervention in diarrhea.
1. **Oral.** Helpful if given as hyposmolar solution and with glucose to facilitate uptake of sodium and water.

      2. Intravenous. Necessary if patient is markedly volume-depleted or has accompanying nausea and vomiting. Patient may need potassium replacement as well.

B. Diet. Place patient on a lactose-free diet to prevent the development of diarrhea secondary to lactose deficiency which may be transient as a result of acute gastroenteritis. Diarrhea could also be secondary to lactose intolerance. Administer clear liquid diet for 24–48 hours, and then advance diet slowly.

C. Antidiarrheal agents. Often helpful but should not be used if invasive diarrhea is clinically suspected. Antimotility drugs are contraindicated in patients with pseudomembranous colitis or IBD because of the risk for precipitating toxic megacolon. Commonly used agents include kaolin and pectin (Kaopectate) 30–120 mL after each loose stool; bismuth subsalicylate (Pepto-Bismol) 30 mL Q 30 min as needed up to 8 doses Q day; diphenoxylate with atropine (Lomotil 5 mg) 1–2 tablets QID, not to exceed 20 mg/day; and loperamide (Imodium) 4 mg initially, then 2 mg after each loose stool, not to exceed 16 mg Q day.

D. Antibiotics. Antibiotic treatment usually does not shorten the duration of illness. It may select out resistant strains of organisms and often lead to pseudomembranous colitis.

      1. *Salmonella.* Does not usually require antibiotics unless the patient remains ill or is predisposed to osteomyelitis from sickle cell disease or endocarditis. Treatment is chloramphenicol, ampicillin, trimethoprim-sulfamethoxazole (Bactrim or Septra), or ciprofloxacin.

      2. Shigellosis. Antibiotics recommended to decrease duration of illness and fecal shedding. Antibiotic sensitivity is crucial because resistance is common. Treatment is ciprofloxacin, norfloxacin, trimethoprim-sulfamethoxazole, or ampicillin for 7 days.

      3. Pseudomembranous colitis. Recommended treatment with vancomycin 125 mg PO Q 6 hr or metronidazole (Flagyl) 250 mg PO Q 6 hr for 7–10 days. Metronidazole is less expensive and is equally effective. Addition of cholestyramine (Questran) QID may help control diarrhea if given with antibiotics.

      4. *Campylobacter* infection. Often self-limiting illness. With severe or persistent diarrhea, erythromycin or ciprofloxacin for 5–7 days is effective.

REFERENCES

Ahnen DJ: Nutrient assimilation. In: Kelly WN (editor-in-chief). *Textbook of Internal Medicine.* 2nd ed. Lippincott;1992:404.

Lange RL, DiPiro JT: Diarrhea and constipation. In: *Pharmacotherapy: A Pathophysiologic Approach.* 2nd ed. Appleton & Lange;1993:566.

Levine MM: Antimicrobial therapy for infectious diarrhea. Rev Infect Dis 1986;8:5207.

Powell DW: Approach to the patient with diarrhea. In: Kelly WN (editor-in-chief). *Textbook of Internal Medicine.* 2nd ed. Lippincott;1992:618.

18. DYSPNEA

I. **Problem.** A patient admitted to the coronary care unit to rule out a myocardial infarction complains of difficulty breathing.

II. **Immediate Questions**
   A. **Was the onset of dyspnea acute or gradual?** The differential diagnosis for acute dyspnea differs from subacute or chronic dyspnea. Causes of acute dyspnea include bronchospasm, pulmonary embolism (PE), pneumothorax, acute pulmonary edema, and anxiety. Chronic dyspnea can present with an acute exacerbation.
   B. **Are there other associated symptoms such as chest pain?** The patient may focus on the shortness of breath and fail to disclose chest pain or discomfort unless specifically asked. Dyspnea rather than angina may be the primary or the only symptom of acute myocardial ischemia.
   C. **Is the patient cyanotic?** Hypoxemia is a potentially lethal condition. If cyanosis is noted, immediate oxygen therapy is indicated.
   D. **What is causing the dyspnea?** Precipitating activities, including exposure to chemicals and other irritants, and the degree of dyspnea are important in its evaluation.

III. **Differential diagnosis.** Dyspnea is the subjective sensation of difficult, labored, uncomfortable breathing. It may occur through increased respiratory muscle work, stimulation of neuroreceptors throughout the respiratory tract, or stimulation of peripheral and central chemoreceptors. Although many diseases produce dyspnea, two-thirds of the cases are caused by pulmonary or cardiac disorders.
   A. **Pulmonary**
      1. **Pulmonary embolism.** This diagnosis must be considered in any patient presenting with acute dyspnea. Also, recurrent pulmonary emboli can cause intermittent dyspnea at rest. This diagnosis should be especially considered in any patient with risk factors such as prolonged immobilization, recent surgery, obesity, malignancy (especially adenocarcinomas), venous trauma, or high-dose estrogen therapy.
      2. **Pneumothorax.** This can occur after trauma, or spontaneously in patients with bullous emphysema, or in young males with a tall, thin body habitus. Patients on ventilators receiving positive end-expiratory pressure (PEEP) ventilation are at increased risk of pneumothorax. Iatrogenic pneumothoraces may occur after subclavian or internal jugular line placement or after thoracentesis.

3. **Asthma/chronic obstructive airway disease.** These patients usually have a prior history of dyspnea; however, anaphylaxis can also produce acute asthma. (See Section I, Chapter 4, Anaphylactic Reaction, p 23). In addition to bronchospasm, these patients often demonstrate other evidence of anaphylaxis, such as stridor and urticaria.
4. **Aspiration** (See Section I, Chapter 7, Aspiration, p 34).
5. **Pneumonia.** Characterized by fever, productive cough, radiographic infiltrates, and leukocytosis.
6. **Interstitial lung disease.** This usually produces progressive dyspnea, and is caused by a large number of diseases.
7. **Pleural effusion.** More likely to cause chronic or subchronic dyspnea rather than acute dyspnea.

B. **Cardiac**
1. **Acute myocardial infarction.** As mentioned earlier, patients experiencing acute myocardial ischemia can present complaining of dyspnea rather than chest pain. In addition, patients with acute myocardial infarction (MI) can develop acute PE.
2. **Congestive heart failure.** Accumulation of fluid in the interstitial spaces of the lung stimulates neuroreceptors, which produce a sensation of dyspnea. These patients frequently experience orthopnea and paroxysmal nocturnal dyspnea. Orthopnea also occurs in patients with chronic obstructive pulmonary disease (COPD).
3. **Pericardial tamponade.** Dyspnea is frequently a significant complaint.
4. **Arrhythmias.** Dyspnea is a common complaint.
5. **Valvular diseases.** Aortic stenosis, aortic insufficiency, mitral stenosis, and mitral insufficiency can cause dyspnea.

C. **Psychogenic breathlessness.** Dyspnea associated with hyperventilation can be difficult to separate from organic causes. Typically, these patients are anxious and develop acral paresthesias and lightheadedness. Their dyspnea is often worse at rest and improve during exercise. In patients with this history, the clinician should strongly suspect a psychogenic origin. Nevertheless, this diagnosis should not be made until organic causes have been excluded.

D. **Neuromuscular.** Dyspnea can be caused by CNS disorders, myopathies, neuropathies, phrenic nerve and diaphragmatic disorders, spinal cord disorders, or systemic neuromuscular disorders.

E. **Other organic causes.** Anemia, gastroesophageal reflux, hyperthyroidism, and hypothyroidism can all cause dyspnea.

IV. **Database**
A. **Physical examination key points**
1. **Vital signs.** Fever may signify infection, but also occurs with pulmonary and myocardial infarction. Tachypnea oc-

curs in most cases of dyspnea; however, dyspnea can occur in patients with a normal respiratory rate. Hypotension may result from a tension pneumothorax, anaphylaxis, pericardial tamponade, or acute MI. Pulsus paradoxus may occur with acute exacerbation of asthma, COPD, or pericardial tamponade.

2. **Lungs.** Observe the patient for accessory muscle use. Listen for wheezes, stridor, crackles, and absent breath sounds. Paradoxical abdominal movement during respiration suggests diaphragmatic and respiratory muscle fatigue.

3. **Heart.** Elevated jugular venous pressure, a displaced point of maximal impulse, or an S_3 gallop suggest decompensated heart failure. Irregular heart beat and murmurs are also important signs.

4. **Extremities.** Examine for swelling or other evidence of deep venous thrombosis which predisposes to pulmonary embolus. Also evaluate for peripheral cyanosis and clubbing.

5. **Neurologic exam.** Confusion and impaired mentation may signify severe hypoxemia.

B. **Laboratory data**
1. **Hemogram.** Leukocytosis with an increase in banded neutrophils occurs with pneumonia. Anemia can cause dyspnea on exertion.

2. **Arterial blood gases.** Should be obtained in any patient with significant dyspnea, or if hypoxemia is suspected.

3. **Sputum Gram's stain and culture.** Obtain these tests in patients with suspected pneumonia.

4. **Thyroid function test.** If thyroid disease is considered.

C. **Radiologic and other studies**
1. **Chest x-ray.** Obtain a stat portable upright CXR if there is obvious distress. If the patient is unable to sit for an adequate film, obtain lateral decubitus films to rule out the possibility of a basilar pneumothorax.

2. **Electrocardiogram.** Should always be obtained in any patient with acute dyspnea to rule out the possibility of pericarditis (PR depression; ST elevation—diffuse and concave upward; T wave inversion); myocardial ischemia or infarction (ST depression; ST elevation—convex upward; T wave inversion; new Q waves); arrhythmia; or pulmonary embolism ($S_1Q_3T_3$; right-axis deviation; right bundle branch block; T wave inversion).

3. **Pulmonary function tests.** These are not applicable to the acute situation, but can assist in the evaluation of patients with obstructive or restrictive lung disease. Bronchoprovocation testing may help increase yield of pulmonary function testing. (See Section I, Chapter 15, Cough, Section IV.C.5., Pulmonary Function Tests, p 84)

4. **Ventilation perfusion ($\dot{V}/\dot{Q}$) scan.** To evaluate for PE.

5. **Pulmonary angiogram.** In patients with a low or moderate probability V̇/Q̇ scan in whom there still exists a suspicion for PE, this test is the gold standard to diagnose PE. A venogram or impedance plethysmography, and Doppler ultrasound of lower extremities may be helpful.
6. **Echocardiogram.** Should be obtained emergently if there is a strong clinical suspicion for cardiac tamponade. Otherwise, an echocardiogram can be useful for assessing left ventricular function, valvular function, and whether or not cardiac disease is responsible for the dyspnea.
7. **Cardiopulmonary exercise testing.** It can be useful if the diagnosis is unclear, by helping to determine whether a cardiac or pulmonary abnormality exists.

V. Plan
A. Emergent therapy
1. **Oxygen supplementation.** The initial goal of treatment in patients with acute dyspnea should be to ensure adequate oxygenation; thus, the majority of patients should be treated with 100% oxygen therapy. In those patients with a history of chronic obstructive airway disease in whom one is concerned about the possibility of suppression of their hypoxic ventilatory drive, therapy should be initiated with 24–28% oxygen by Venturi mask. In either case, an ABG should be obtained to direct subsequent adjustments of the oxygen. Continuous oxygen saturation monitoring can also be helpful.
2. **Stat portable CXR, ECG, and ABG.** Indicated in any patient who complains of acute dyspnea.

B. Asthma
1. Request a stat nebulizer treatment with albuterol (Proventil, Ventolin) 0.5 mL in 2–3 mL normal saline.
2. In patients with anaphylaxis or in young patients with acute asthma, epinephrine 0.25–0.4 mL of a 1:1000 concentration can be given SC.
3. Methylprednisolone (Solu-Medrol) 125 mg stat IV will provide relief of bronchospasm in 3–6 hours as the effectiveness of the albuterol dissipates.

C. Anaphylaxis (See Section I, Chapter 4, Anaphylactic Reaction, Section V, p 24)

D. Myocardial ischemia. If initial assessment suggests myocardial ischemia, administer sublingual nitroglycerin, provided the systolic blood pressure is > 100. (See Section I, Chapter 11, Chest Pain, Section V, p 61)

E. Acute congestive heart failure. Furosemide (Lasix) 40–80 mg IV may be given, provided the patient is not hypotensive. Morphine sulfate 2–5 mg IV may also be helpful initially if acute pulmonary edema is present.

   F. Pneumonia. Treat with pulmonary toilet and antibiotics as directed by results of the sputum Gram's stain.

   G. Pleural effusion. Removal of pleural fluid by thoracentesis can often produce a significant improvement in a patient's dyspnea. (See Section III, Chapter 14, Thoracentesis, p 377)

   H. Aspiration (See Section I, Chapter 7, Aspiration, Section V, p 36)

REFERENCES

Gillespie DJ, Staats BA: Concise review for primary-care physicians: Unexplained dyspnea. Mayo Clin Proc 1994;69:657.

Mahler DA: Acute dyspnea. In: Mahler DA ed. *Dyspnea*. Futura;1990:127.

Manning HL, Schwartzstein RM: Pathophysiology of dyspnea. N Engl J Med 1995;327:1547.

Robertson HT II: Approach to the patient with dyspnea. In: Kelly WN, ed-in-chief: *Textbook of Internal Medicine*. 2nd ed. Lippincott;1992:1877.

19. DYSURIA

  I. Problem. A 38-year-old sexually active woman complains of pain with urination.

  II. Immediate Questions

    A. How long has this symptom been present? A gradual onset of several days' duration suggests a chlamydial or gonorrheal infection. Prostatitis and subclinical pyelonephritis may also present with several days of symptoms.

    B. Does the patient have a prior history of urinary tract infection (UTI) or urologic abnormality? Females and any patient with urinary tract abnormalities are more prone to recurrent UTIs.

    C. Are there any other associated symptoms? Fever, chills, nausea and vomiting, and back pain are often signs of upper UTIs such as pyelonephritis. Frequency, urgency, and dysuria are lower UTI signs and occur in cystitis, prostatitis, and urethritis. A vaginal discharge would suggest a vaginitis, such as caused by *C albicans* or *T vaginalis*, as a cause of dysuria. In men, ask about a history of recent penile discharge.

    D. Has the patient recently had a Foley catheter removed? Catheter placement may result in an infection or transient urethral irritation.

    E. What type of contraception or sexual protection is used by the patient? Use of diaphragm and spermicide enhance UTI susceptibility in females. In males, unprotected anal intercourse or intercourse with an infected partner are risk factors for UTIs.

III. Differential Diagnosis. The principal causes of dysuria differ for men and women.

   A. Female. Women presenting with acute dysuria are likely to have one of seven conditions, each of which may require different management.

   1. **Acute pyelonephritis.** Suggested by fever, flank pain, rigors, nausea, and vomiting.

   2. **Subclinical pyelonephritis.** As many as 30% to 80% of patients presenting with signs of only lower UTI (dysuria, frequency, urgency) have in fact an upper UTI as well. This condition should be especially suspected in patients with urinary tract abnormalities, diabetes, immunocompromising conditions, long-term cystitis symptoms, or history of relapsing infection.

   3. **Lower UTI.** These patients have either cystitis or urethritis, with bacteria confined to either the bladder or the urethra.

   4. **Chlamydial urethritis.** This is characterized by a prolonged onset over several days. The patient often reports intercourse with a partner having similar symptoms. An associated mucopurulent endocervical secretion may be noted on pelvic exam.

   5. **Other urethral infections.** Urethritis may also be caused by *N gonorrhoeae* and *T vaginalis*.

   6. **Vaginitis.** In contrast to internal sensations of dull pain associated with dysuria caused by cystitis, vaginitis causes external burning pain as the urine stream flows over inflamed labia.

   7. **No recognized pathogen.** These patients have no pyuria and no evidence of infection. The most common cause is atrophic vaginitis. Consider bladder or urethral carcinoma. "Urethral syndrome" is seen in some women who may be exquisitely sensitive to pH changes in the urine.

   B. Male

   1. **Cystitis/pyelonephritis**

   2. **Urethritis**
      a. **Nongonococcal.** Discharge occurs 8–21 days after exposure and is typically thin and clear.
      b. **Gonococcal.** In contrast, the discharge associated with this condition is heavy and purulent. Symptoms occur 2–6 days after exposure.
      c. **Nongonococcal/gonococcal.** Keep in mind that both conditions frequently coexist.

   3. **Prostatitis.** Symptoms include complaints of vague groin or back pain. Associated fever and chills suggest acute prostatitis. Chronic bacterial prostatitis is less common. Chronic abacterial prostatitis is more common and is sometimes called "prostatosis" or "prostatodynia."

   4. **Cancer (bladder, prostate, urethral)**

   5. **Benign condition (urethral stricture, meatal stenosis, benign prostatic hypertrophy)**

IV. Database

A. Physical examination key points

1. **Vital signs.** Check for fever, tachycardia, or hypotension which suggest urosepsis.
2. **Abdomen.** Examine for evidence of suprapubic tenderness or costovertebral angle tenderness.
3. **Genitalia.** In women who present with acute dysuria and also report a vaginal discharge, pelvic examination is mandatory to rule out vaginitis or cervicitis. In men with a history of urethral discharge, penile stripping may be necessary to produce a discharge. Examine for evidence of epididymitis or orchitis.
4. **Prostate.** In acute prostatitis, the gland is swollen, tender, and boggy. In patients presenting with acute prostatitis, digital exam of the prostate could result in bacteremia; therefore, examination of the prostate is best deferred until the patient has been treated with several days of antibiotics. In patients with chronic prostatitis, examination of the prostate may be unremarkable.

B. Laboratory data

1. **Urinalysis.** Pyuria, which can be quickly detected by testing urine for the presence of leukocyte esterase, is present in almost all cases of UTI. Bacteriuria, which can be detected using the nitrite test, confirms a bacterial cause. It is important to remember that false negative nitrite results may occur in patients who consume a low nitrate diet or who take diuretics. Also examine for white blood cell casts, which occur with pyelonephritis. Hematuria frequently occurs with cystitis/pyelonephritis but is seldom seen with urethritis. A Gram's stain of uncentrifuged urine is also helpful in assessing the presence of bacteria.
2. **Urine culture.** Although useful in determining a bacterial cause of dysuria, a urine culture is usually indicated in women only if acute pyelonephritis or subclinical pyelonephritis is suspected; or if the patient is presenting with a relapse from a UTI. In men, a urine culture should always be obtained to confirm and direct subsequent treatment.
3. **Blood cultures.** Should be ordered in all patients who appear septic and are admitted for presumed acute pyelonephritis.
4. **CBC with differential.** Leukocytosis and a left shift are seen with acute pyelonephritis and sometimes with acute prostatitis. They are seldom seen in urethritis, chronic prostatitis, or cystitis.
5. **Urethral discharges.** In both men and women, the discharge should be gram-stained and cultured on Thayer-Martin medium. The presence of intracellular gram-negative diplococci on Gram's stain is sufficient presumptive evidence of gonorrhea in men and warrants therapy. In women with endocervical discharge, cultures for gonorrhea should be obtained.

6. **Vaginal discharge.** Wet mount to look for *T vaginalis*, which have flagella and, when viewed on wet mount, move rapidly and erratically. Clue cells, or activated squamous cells coated with bacteria, indicate infection with *Gardnerella vaginalis*. The presence of hyphae, indicating infection with *C albicans*, should be assessed on a slide of vaginal discharge treated with 2–3 drops of 10% potassium hydroxide.

C. **Radiologic and other studies.** Full urologic evaluation is indicated in men with pyelonephritis, recurrent infections, or other complicating factors. Women who have had more than two recurrences of pyelonephritis, as well as women in whom complicating factors such as anatomic abnormalities are suspected, should also undergo full urologic evaluation. An ultrasound or intravenous pyelography should be obtained in patients admitted for acute pyelonephritis if they remain febrile after 2–3 days of treatment with an appropriate antibiotic.

V. Plan

A. **Acute pyelonephritis**

1. In patients who appear septic or are unable to tolerate oral medications, administer gentamicin 1.5–2.0 mg/kg IV loading dose; then give about 1.5 mg/kg Q 8–24 hr depending on renal function (see Aminoglycoside Dosing, Table 7–15) plus ampicillin 1.5–2.0 gm Q 4–6 hr. A third-generation cephalosporin such as ceftriaxone 1 g IV/24 hr is an alternative. After the patient is afebrile and clinically improved, and results of urine culture and sensitivity testing are known, the patient can be switched to oral medications. Duration of therapy should be at least 10–14 days. Patients with diabetes mellitus should receive the same treatment.

2. Indications for hospitalization include dehydration; inability to tolerate oral medications; concern about compliance; uncertainty about diagnosis; and severe illness with high fever, severe pain, and marked debility.

3. In patients with acute uncomplicated pyelonephritis, a 14-day outpatient course of trimethoprim-sulfamethoxazole (Bactrim DS), 1 tablet BID can be administered. If the patient is allergic to sulfa, give a quinolone antibiotic such as ciprofloxacin 500 mg BID for 14 days.

4. Patients should have urine cultures checked 2–3 weeks after completion of therapy.

B. **Subclinical pyelonephritis.** These patients should be treated with a 14-day course of the same oral agents as described above for uncomplicated pyelonephritis.

C. **Uncomplicated lower UTI.** In patients presenting with acute dysuria who are noted to have pyuria and bacteriuria on urinalysis, but do not have the clinical picture of acute pyelonephritis, an uncomplicated lower UTI can be presumed and treated. A urine culture is not mandatory in these patients. Studies indicate that trimethoprim-sulfamethoxazole (Bactrim) is the most efficacious treatment. A 3-day regimen of Bactrim DS, 1 tablet PO BID, is sufficient for uncomplicated lower UTIs. A 7-day regimen should be considered in patients with diabetes mellitus; > 7 days of symptoms; a recent UTI; or an UTI associated with the use of a diaphragm. Alternative antibiotics in patients with a history of intolerance to sulfa are trimethoprim 100 mg BID for 3 days or nitrofurantoin 100 mg QID for 3 days. The patient should be instructed to return for follow-up if symptoms persist or recur after therapy. Follow-up culture is not necessary.

D. Vaginitis. Therapy is directed to the specific cause of the vaginitis. For patients with candidal vaginitis, miconazole (Monistat) cream topically for 7 days is effective. An alternative is a single 150-mg dose of fluconazole (Diflucan) PO. For bacterial vaginosis metronidazole (Flagyl) 500 mg BID for 7 days, or 2 grams as a single dose are effective. For trichomonal vaginitis, metronidazole 2 g PO in a single dose is recommended for the sex partner as well as the patient. Topical Premarin cream is effective for atrophic vaginitis. The cream should be applied nightly for 1 week and 2–3 times weekly thereafter.

E. Chlamydial urethritis. This should be suspected in patients who have dysuria and pyuria but no bacteriuria, and who have a partner with symptoms. Doxycycline 100 mg BID for 7 days is effective. An alternative therapy is tetracycline 500 mg QID for 7 days or ofloxacin (Floxin) 300 mg PO BID for 7 days. These patients should have their partner evaluated and treated as well. Verify that females are not pregnant before prescribing tetracycline or doxycycline.

F. Gonococcal urethritis. With the emergence of penicillin resistance, ceftriaxone 250 mg IM is now recommended. Because of the frequent coexistence of chlamydial urethritis, a course of doxycycline is suggested as well.

G. Acute prostatitis. Patients who are septic should be admitted and a regimen of either ampicillin and gentamicin or a third-generation cephalosporin instituted, followed by 3 weeks of an oral fluoroquinolone (ciprofloxacin) or trimethoprim-sulfamethoxazole.

H. Chronic prostatitis. Patients with chronic bacterial prostatitis may respond to a 3-week course of an oral agent such as fluoroquinolone (ciprofloxacin). Many patients have nonbacterial prostatitis and should be referred for urologic evaluation if symptoms do not resolve on a course of antibiotics.

I. Urethral syndrome. Identify foods or medications that cause symptoms. Alkalinization of urine may help some patients.

REFERENCES

Hooton TM: A simplified approach to urinary tract infection. Hosp Pract 1995;30:23.
Hooton TM, Stamm WE: Management of acute uncomplicated urinary tract infection in adults. Med Clin North Am 1991;75:339.
Pappas PG: Laboratory in the diagnosis and management of urinary tract infections. Med Clin North Am 1991;75:313.
Ronald AR, Nicolle LE, Harding GKM: Standards of therapy for urinary tract infections in adults. Infection 1992;20:S164.
Stamm WE, Hooton TM: Management of urinary tract infection in adults. N Engl J Med 1993;329:1328.

20. FALLS

I. **Problem:** You are called to evaluate an 84-year-old female patient with pneumonia who has fallen on her way to the bathroom.

II. **Immediate Questions**

A. **What were the circumstances of the fall?** Determine, if possible, exactly how the fall occurred; what activity the patient was involved in; how the patient felt at the time of the fall. Causes of falls can be characterized as intrinsic (ie, due to some disease state or characteristic of the patient, such as orthostatic hypotension) or extrinsic (ie, due to some environmental cause, such as a slippery floor). In many cases, the causes are intermingled. Certain premonitory symptoms, such as dizziness or chest pain, may be helpful to determine a cause for the fall.

B. **What complaints (if any) does the patient have?** Determine whether premonitory symptoms such as dizziness, palpitations, dyspnea, chest pain, weakness, confusion, incontinence, loss of consciousness or tongue biting occurred. In addition, inquire about pain involving the neck, ribs, arms, back, or hips.

C. **What are the patient's vital signs?** Hypotension and tachycardia may be associated with many conditions such as an acute infection, dehydration or acute myocardial infarction (MI). Tachypnea may also be noted with the above conditions or a pulmonary embolus. A fever, a decreased temp or a temperature elevated a few degrees above baseline (especially in elderly patients) may be indicative of an infection.

D. **What medical conditions does the patient have?** Many conditions predispose to dizziness. A history of diabetes mellitus (DM) may be associated with autonomic dysfunction leading to orthostatic hypotension or poorly controlled DM can cause an osmotic diuresis and lead to volume depletion.

E. **What medications is the patient taking?** Medication side effects such as dizziness, hypotension, or confusion may predispose to falls. Vasodilators and diuretics are medications that commonly cause hypotension and dizziness.

III. **Differential Diagnosis.** With younger patients, the cause of the fall may be readily apparent. However, the differential diagnosis with an older patient may be quite extensive.
   A. **Extrinsic causes:** Are environmental.
      1. **Slippery floors/sidewalks.** Floor wax, water or urine; in the case of sidewalks, snow or ice.
      2. **Inadequate or excessive lighting**
      3. **Transfers.** A weakened patient attempting to make a transfer from the bed to a wheelchair may fall.
      4. **Bed side-rails.** If side rails are up, a delirious patient attempting to climb over them can fall.
      5. **Unavailability of walking aids.** Often a hospitalized patient will not have his/her cane or walker immediately available and may attempt to walk to the bathroom unaided.
   B. **Intrinsic**
      1. **"Normal" aging.** Physical changes such as visual impairment (ie, presbyopia or cataracts). Patients with visual or hearing loss may be unable to move well in a new environment.
      2. **Neurologic**
         a. **CVA with hemiparesis.** The patient may have decreased mobility.
         b. **Parkinson's disease.** The patient may have decreased mobility.
         c. **Dementia.** From any number of causes such as multi-infarct dementia, Alzheimer's disease or hypothyroidism. The demented patient may use poor judgment about his/her ability to move in a new environment.
         d. **Seizures**
         e. **Carotid sinus hypersensitivity.**
         f. **Peripheral neuropathy.** Vitamin B_{12} deficiency is more common among the elderly, also consider peripheral neuropathy with a history of diabetes mellitus or alcohol abuse.
         g. **Vestibular dysfunction**
      3. **Cardiovascular** (See Section I, Chapter 57, Syncope, p 274)
         a. **Orthostatic hypotension.** Should be considered in patients who are dehydrated, infected, have a GI bleed or who may have autonomic dysfunction, such as patients with diabetes mellitus.
         b. **Arrhythmias.** Tachy- or bradyarrhythmias should be considered especially in the elderly or if there is a history of heart disease. (See Section I, Chapter 58, Tachycardia, p 279; and Section I, Chapter 8, Bradycardia, p 37)
         c. **Angina or myocardial infarction (MI).** Syncope or hypotension can be a sign of ischemic heart disease.

d. **Vagal response disorders.** Valsalva (defecation, micturition or other) maneuvers may cause an increase in vagal tone resulting in a decrease in heart rate and blood pressure resulting in a fall.

4. **Fluid/volume loss.** From any cause, including diuretics, diarrhea, vomiting or nasogastric suction, GI hemorrhage, high fever, or decreased oral intake.

5. **Musculoskeletal disorders.** Degenerative joint disease or osteoarthritis is very common in the elderly. Deconditioning can be a problem especially during hospitalization. In addition, a patient who fell earlier may now have a hip fracture, predisposing him/her to fall again.

6. **Metabolic disorders**
   a. **Hypothyroidism**
   b. **Hypoglycemia.** There may be associated diaphoresis, tachycardia, or syncope.
   c. **Electrolyte imbalance.** Hypokalemia or hypomagnesemia can lead to arrhythmias. Hypercalcemia can cause confusion.
   d. **Diabetes mellitus (DM).** Uncontrolled DM can lead to an osmotic diuresis leading to volume depletion. A peripheral neuropathy can result from long standing DM.
   e. **Metabolic encephalopathy.** Uremia and hepatic failure can cause confusion.

7. **Psychological factors**
   a. **Refusal of assistance or ancillary devices.** Patients may think that they do not need a walker or assistance with transfer.
   b. **Disorientation.** From any number of causes, including dementia, acute bacterial infection, "sundowning," and ICU psychosis, as well as others. (See Section I, Chapter 13, Coma and Acute Mental Status Changes, p 69)
   c. **Depression.** In the elderly, depression may present as dementia. These patients may become increasingly immobile, or less likely to notice obstacles or changes in their environment.

8. **Medications.** Including diuretics, antihypertensives (especially vasodilators such as calcium channel blockers) nonsteroidal anti-inflammatory agents (NSAIDs), analgesics, anticonvulsants, antiarrhythmics, sedatives, and antipsychotics. Also, medications that may affect the vestibular system at either normal or toxic doses, such as aminoglycosides (gentamicin, tobramycin); aspirin; furosemide (Lasix); quinine; quinidine; and alcohol.

9. **Congestive heart failure**

10. **Infection.** Any infection can be associated with a change in mental status, particularly in the elderly. In addition, patients

admitted because of an infection (ie, pneumonia) may become weakened during the hospitalization, and may be unable to move about safely unassisted.

IV. Database
A. Physical examination key points
1. **Vital signs.** Look for hypotension, tachycardia or bradycardia, tachypnea or a change in the temperature from baseline (increase or decrease). Check for orthostatic changes, a decrease in systolic blood pressure of 10 mm Hg, and/or an increase in heart rate of 20 bpm, (16 bpm in the elderly) 1 minute after moving from a supine to a standing position.
2. **HEENT.** Look for evidence of trauma from the fall, such as soft tissue swelling and tenderness.
3. **Extremities.** Look for evidence of fractures, such as an externally rotated and flexed hip.
4. **Neurologic examination.** This should include a mini-mental status examination.

B. Laboratory data.
If there are obvious clues from the history and/or physical examination, an extensive laboratory evaluation may not be indicated.
1. **Complete blood count (CBC)**
2. **Electrolytes.** Hypokalemia or hypomagnesemia can cause arrhythmias, hypercalcemia can cause confusion.
3. **BUN, creatinine and glucose**
4. **Liver function tests.** Aspartate aminotransaminase (AST), alanine aminotransaminase (ALT), total bilirubin, alkaline phosphatase or γ-glutamyltransferase (GGT) to rule out hepatic dysfunction.

C. Radiologic and other studies
1. **Skeletal x-rays.** As indicated.
2. **CT scan of head**
3. **Electrocardiogram.** Look for evidence of ischemia/infarction, tachy- or bradyarrhythmia, or electrolyte abnormalities such as hypokalemia. Check the QT interval, especially if the patient is taking any medication which prolongs the QT interval (eg, quinidine or procainamide).

V. Plan
A. Prevention.
Preventive measures can greatly reduce the number of falls and are essential for good patient care. The primary preventive measure is environmental modification. Avoid use of restraints if possible; obstacles which interfere with patient movement should be removed. Assistive devices that the patient routinely uses, such as a walker, cane, or hearing aid, should be made available if possible.

   B. **Medication modification**
   C. **Further studies**. Such as CT scans as indicated.
   D. **Observation.** The patient who has suffered a head injury should
      be fully evaluated and monitored by neurologic checks by the nurs-
      ing staff.

21. FEVER

   I. **Problem.** You are called to see a 57-year-old man who has been hos-
      pitalized for 3 days and now has a fever of 39.5°C (103.1°F).

  II. **Immediate Questions**
   A. **How long has the patient been febrile and how high is the tem-
      perature?** It is important to know if this elevation in temperature
      signals the abrupt onset of fever or represents the gradual
      worsening of a prior fever. Fever above 40.0°C (104.0°F) requires
      immediate action.
   B. **What is the fever pattern?** Is the fever intermittent (it falls to nor-
      mal at some time during the day), sustained (it remains elevated),
      or relapsing (febrile periods are followed by one to several days of
      normal temperatures)? Drug fever is often sustained but can be
      intermittent. Examples of relapsing fever include malaria and the
      Pel-Ebstein fever of Hodgkin's disease.
   C. **Does the patient have any other pertinent medical illnesses,
      or is he or she immunocompromised?** Such information is vital
      before you can properly assess the patient. Also see Section I,
      Chapter 22, Fever in the HIV-Positive Patient, p 119.
   D. **Are any intravenous lines in place?** Indwelling Foley catheters,
      intravenous access sites, nasogastric tubes (which can predispose
      to sinusitis), and central venous catheter sites are frequent sources
      of nosocomial fever.
   E. **Are there any associated symptoms?** The symptoms to ascer-
      tain include chills, rigors, rash, myalgias, arthralgias, cough, spu-
      tum production, post-nasal drainage, chest pain, headache, dys-
      uria, abdominal pain, nausea, vomiting, pain at an intravenous site,
      night sweats, and change in mental status. Such questions may
      point toward a specific cause.
   F. **What medications is the patient taking?** Ask if the patient is tak-
      ing any antipyretics or current antibiotics. Also consider a drug-in-
      duced fever and review all medications.
   G. **Have any recent procedures such as bronchoscopy been
      done, or has the patient recently received blood?** A fever to
      38.3°C (101°F) is common after bronchoscopy; also following
      transfusions.

H. **Are there any factors relating to the patient's psychosocial history that need to be assessed?** The clinician should inquire about recent travel, especially in countries with poor sanitation; HIV risk factors (intravenous drug use; homosexual or bisexual male; promiscuous sexual activity; or sexual intercourse with a person with AIDS or who is HIV positive); exposure to dogs, cats, birds, ticks, and cattle; and health of family members.

III. **Differential Diagnosis.** An exhaustive list is extraordinarily long; only the major categories are presented here:
   A. **Infections**
      1. **Bacterial**
      2. **Viral**
      3. **Mycobacterial**
      4. **Fungal**
      5. **Parasitic**
   B. **Neoplasms.** Solid tumors, lymphoma, Hodgkin's disease, leukemia. Fever with leukemia is often due to infection but may be caused by the primary disease, especially in chronic myelogenous leukemia. Solid tumors causing fever include renal cell and hepatocellular carcinoma, osteogenic sarcoma, and atrial myxoma.
   C. **Connective tissue disease**
      1. **Acute rheumatic fever**
      2. **Rheumatoid arthritis**
      3. **Adult Still's disease**
      4. **Systemic lupus erythematosus (SLE)**
      5. **Vasculitis.** Including hypersensitivity vasculitis, polymyalgia rheumatica, temporal arteritis, and polyarteritis nodosa.
   D. **Thermoregulatory disorders.** Heat stroke, malignant hyperthermia, thyroid storm, and malignant neuroleptic syndrome. Thyroid storm may be a postoperative complication in a hyperthyroid patient. Features of malignant neuroleptic syndrome include hyperthermia, hypertonicity of skeletal muscle, mental status changes, and autonomic nervous system instability in patients on neuroleptics.
   E. **Drug-induced fever.** Potential culprits include antibiotics (penicillins, cephalosporins, sulfonamides); methyldopa (Aldomet); quinidine; hydralazine (Apresoline); procainamide; phenytoin (Dilantin); chlorpromazine (Thorazine); carbamazepine (Tegretol); anti-inflammatory agents such as ibuprofen (Motrin); antineoplastic agents; and allopurinol (Zyloprim). Other agents that may cause fever include: steroids, antidopaminergic neuroleptic agents, sympathetic agents, cocaine, LSD, hallucinogens, phencyclidine, and tricyclic antidepressants (increase thermoset point via action at the anterior hypothalamus). Withdrawal from ethanol, barbiturates, benzodiazepines, and sedative hypnotics also increases ther-

moset point via action at the anterior hypothalamus, as well as producing excessive muscular activity with consequent increased heat production. Dystonic reactions due to butyrophenones, phenothiazines, and metoclopramide can stimulate excess muscular activity as well. Salicylate toxicity can cause increased heat production. Parasympatholytic agents (anticholinergics, antihistamines, antiparkinsonism agents, phenothiazines and tricyclic antidepressants) decrease sweating, with consequent decreased heat dissipation.

  F. **Miscellaneous disorders.** Including pulmonary embolus with infarction, myocardial infarction, inflammatory bowel disease, and Addisonian crisis.
  G. **Fever of unknown origin (FUO).** Manifested by fever > 38.3°C (101.0°F) on several occasions for a duration of at least 3 weeks, with no definite etiology.
  H. **Unknown source.** 18% in one series of inpatients.
  I. **Factitious (self-induced) fever**

IV. **Database**
  A. **Physical examination key points**
     1. **General appearance.** This factor can help determine whether antibiotics should be initiated while awaiting results of diagnostic testing. Should be considered if patient appears toxic.
     2. **Vital signs.** Take both oral and rectal temperatures. (Neutropenia is a contraindication to taking rectal temperature.) A rectal temperature should be taken to make sure the oral temperature is not falsely elevated secondary to recent consumption of a hot liquid or smoking. The rectal temperature is usually 1°F > the oral temperature. Check pulse and blood pressure to make sure the patient is hemodynamically stable. Hypotension suggests sepsis or volume depletion, possibly secondary to the fever. The heart rate should increase 9 bpm for each 1°F increase in temperature. If the heart rate does *not* increase (pulse-temperature dissociation), consider psittacosis (*Chlamydia psittaci*), brucellosis (*Brucella*), typhoid fever (*Salmonella typhi*), atypical pneumonia (*Mycoplasma pneumoniae*) and malaria (*Plasmodium falciparum*).
     3. **Skin.** Check IV sites, if any. Examine skin for rashes; if a rash involves the palms and soles, consider Rocky Mountain spotted fever, secondary syphilis, and Stevens-Johnson syndrome (hypersensitivity drug reaction). Look for splinter hemorrhages under the fingernails, Osler nodes, and Janeway lesions, which suggest endocarditis.
     4. **HEENT.** Look for evidence of sinusitis (can be caused by an indwelling nasogastric tube), otitis, and pharyngitis. Cotton-wool spots and flame hemorrhages on fundoscopic examina-

tion could indicate systemic candidiasis, endocarditis, or cyto-megalovirus. Conjunctival hemorrhages are seen with endocarditis as well as severe thrombocytopenia.

5. **Neck.** Check for meningeal signs, including Kernig's and Brudzinski's signs.

6. **Lymph nodes.** Including cervical, supraclavicular, epitrochlear, axillary, and inguinal nodes. May suggest cause of fever such as lymphoma.

7. **Lungs.** A unilateral increase in tactile fremitus, dullness to percussion, bronchial breath sounds, inspiratory crackles, egophony, and whispered pectoriloquy suggest pneumonia.

8. **Heart.** A murmur, especially a new regurgitant murmur, suggests endocarditis.

9. **Abdomen.** Listen for bowel sounds; palpate and percuss for signs of tenderness. Check for Murphy's sign (while palpating the right upper quadrant, tenderness is elicited and there is inspiratory arrest with deep inspiration), which is seen in cholecystitis. Examine for costovertebral angle tenderness for pyelonephritis.

10. **Genitourinary system.** Exclude pelvic inflammatory disease (PID) or tubo-ovarian abscess in a female and epididymitis or orchitis in a male. Also check prostate for tenderness.

11. **Extremities.** Check intravenous sites for erythema and tenderness. Look for joint effusions or tenderness.

B. **Laboratory data**

1. **Complete blood count with differential.** An elevated WBC count and left shift suggest infectious etiology. Eosinophilia suggests drug reaction or parasitic infection. A low WBC count may suggest overwhelming sepsis, a collagen vascular disease such as SLE, a viral infection, or a process that has replaced the normal bone marrow such as a lymphoma, carcinoma, or a granulomatous disease such as tuberculosis or histoplasmosis.

2. **Blood cultures.** Usually two sets; four sets if endocarditis is suspected.

3. **Culture tips of central lines.** If a patient with a central venous catheter becomes febrile and diagnostic workup fails to reveal a source of infection, the venous catheter must be assumed to be the culprit and must be removed. Be sure to culture the tip of the catheter.

4. **Sputum Gram's stain.** Request a Gram's stain if there is a productive cough.

5. **Urinalysis and culture.** Rule out cystitis, prostatitis, or pyelonephritis. Sterile pyuria suggests tuberculosis or if the white cells are eosinophils possibly a drug reaction.

6. **Miscellaneous tests.** In certain circumstances if clinically indicated: liver function tests, erythrocyte sedimentation rate, hepatitis serologies, PPD and anergy screen, culture for acid-fast

bacillus and fungus, examination of peripheral blood smear, complement fixation, *Legionella* titers, viral titers, fungal serologies, rapid plasma reagin (RPR), antistreptolysin-O (ASO) titer, antinuclear antibody (ANA), lumbar puncture.

C. Radiologic and other studies
1. **Chest x-ray.** CXR should be obtained with a fever of unknown source.
2. **Sinus films.** If sinus tenderness or discharge is present or if a nasogastric tube has been in place.
3. **Acute abdominal series.** Should be considered and obtained if clinically indicated.
4. **Ultrasound.** To assess the gallbladder and biliary tree. Can also be used to detect abdominal, renal, and pelvic masses.
5. **HIDA scan.** If acute cholecystitis is suspected.
6. **Bone scan.** If osteomyelitis is suspected.
7. **CT scans.** To detect subphrenic, abdominal, pelvic, and intracranial lesions.
8. **Echocardiogram.** Especially if blood cultures are positive. Sensitivity is not high enough that a normal transthoracic echocardiogram rules out endocarditis; however, transesophageal echocardiography has a 90% sensitivity.

V. Plan. The plan depends on the clinical setting. Many of the previously mentioned tests should be obtained only in certain circumstances; and only if a previous workup has been unrevealing. The initial workup of a febrile patient late at night will not be as exhaustive as a more leisurely performed FUO evaluation.

A. Initial assessment
1. Rule out hemodynamic instability.
2. Carefully review medications, especially looking for any recent changes.
3. Obtain appropriate cultures.
4. Reduce patient's temperature. Give antipyretics such as acetaminophen 650 mg PO or PR. If the fever is above 40.0°C (104.0°F), consider a cooling blanket. If the patient has underlying cardiac disease, the temperature should be brought down quickly to avoid cardiac decompensation.
5. Maintenance IV fluids need to be increased with a sustained fever because of an increase in insensible fluid losses.
6. Consider antibiotics. If the patient is hemodynamically stable and there is no apparent source of infection, it is often prudent to withhold antibiotics. As noted in the differential, the causes of fever are many and often nonbacterial. Empiric antibiotics will confuse the issue in many cases.

B. Fever with hypotension. *Septic shock is a medical emergency.* Begin fluid resuscitation with normal saline through a large-bore IV, place the patient in Trendelenburg position, begin appropriate antibiotics, and transfer to an ICU. If the patient's blood pressure fails to respond to fluids, begin a dopamine infusion at 2–5 µg/kg/min. The use of IV steroids is not warranted unless you suspect Addisonian crisis.

C. IV catheter infection. Remove the offending IV, apply local heat, use anti-inflammatory agents if it is a peripheral site, and consider antibiotics. If you feel a warm, tender, swollen vein or the patient has a history of IV drug abuse, suspect septic thrombophlebitis. Immediately obtain a surgery consult and begin antibiotics. If a central line is in place, change all line(s) to different site(s), culture the catheter tip(s), and begin antibiotics. Gram-positive organisms are likely causes. Nafcillin or a first-generation cephalosporin are the drugs of choice. If the patient is allergic to these agents, vancomycin is the drug of choice.

D. Pneumonia. Initial treatment of pneumonia should be based on results of Gram's stain and the clinical picture. Community-acquired pneumonia in a normal host requiring hospitalization should be treated with a second- (cefuroxime [Ceftin]) or third- (cefotaxime [Claforan] or ceftazidime [Fortaz]) generation cephalosporin or a beta-lactam/beta-lactamase inhibitor (ampicillin/sulbactam [Unasyn]). A macrolide (erythromycin) can be added to the regimen if *Mycoplasma pneumoniae* or *Legionella pneumophila* is suspected. If Gram's stain reveals gram-positive diplococci, indicating *Streptococcus pneumoniae,* penicillin G 600,000 to 1,000,000 U IV Q 6 hr or penicillin VK 500 mg PO Q 6 hr is preferred unless the patient is intolerant of penicillin. With a severe community-acquired pneumonia (mechanical-ventilation, multi-lobar involvement, shock, vasopressors for > 4 hr, respiratory rate > 30/min at admission, PaO_2/FIO_2 ratio < 250 mm/Hg or urine output < 20 mL/hr), treatment should be a macrolide (erythromycin 1 gm IV Q 6 hr) plus a third-generation cephalosporin with *Pseudomonas* activity, such as ceftazidime (Fortaz) 1–2 gm IV Q 8–12 hr or imipenem/cilastatin (Primaxin) 250–500 mg IV Q 6 hr or ciprofloxacin 400 mg IV Q 12 hr or 500–750 mg PO Q 12 hr. Hospital-acquired pneumonia or pneumonia in an immunocompromised host requires broader coverage. The regimen should include an aminoglycoside such as tobramycin or gentamicin plus an anti-*Pseudomonas* penicillin (ticarcillin, piperacillin, mezlocillin) or ticarcillin/clavulanate (Timentin), or a third-generation cephalosporin such as ceftazidime (Fortaz). Imipenem/cilastatin (Primaxin) or aztreonam (Azactam) may also be used as single agents. Avoid giving aminoglycosides in patients with renal insufficiency. Gram's stain can also be helpful. If there are gram-positive cocci in clusters, the chosen antibiotic regimen should include either nafcillin 1.0–2.0 IV Q 4 hr or vancomycin 1000 mg IV Q 12 hr in a patient with normal renal function. Be sure to adjust the dose of vancomycin with renal insufficiency.

E. **Febrile, neutropenic patient.** Culture completely and empirically begin antibiotics with an anti-*Pseudomonas* penicillin (ticarcillin, piperacillin, mezlocillin) plus a third-generation cephalosporin (ceftazidime [Fortaz]) or an aminoglycoside (tobramycin). If a central line is present, consider adding vancomycin, even if a source of infection is not apparent. Add metronidazole (Flagyl) if anaerobes are suspected, and a first-generation cephalosporin such as cephalothin if a staphylococcal infection is likely.

F. **Meningitis.** *Meningitis is a medical emergency.* A lumbar puncture should be done as quickly as possible, especially if there is no history of a bleeding disorder and no focal neurological deficits or papilledema, and you have no reason to suspect an intracranial abscess. Begin giving antibiotics as you are doing the lumbar puncture. If for any reason there is a delay in performing the lumbar puncture (such as obtaining a CT scan of the head because of papilledema), the antibiotics should be administered immediately and not delayed until after the procedure. A third-generation cephalosporin such as cefotaxime (Claforan) or ceftriaxone (Rocephin) should be given for meningitis of unknown etiology; otherwise, antibiotic therapy should be guided by Gram's stain.

G. **Cholecystitis.** Obtain an ultrasound and/or HIDA scan, begin antibiotics, ticarcillin/clavulanate (Timentin) or gentamicin plus ampicillin plus metronidazole, *or* imipenem/cilastatin, and consult surgery.

H. **Drug-induced fever.** Discontinue all drugs possibly causing a drug fever and substitute appropriate alternatives.

I. **Thyroid storm.** Treat with hydration, apply cooling blanket, and give saturated solution of potassium iodide (SSKI), beta-blockers (specifically propranolol), propylthiouracil, and glucocorticoids.

J. **Addisonian crisis.** Treat immediately with IV steroids (hydrocortisone 100 mg IV push, then 100 mg IV Q 6 hr continuous infusion).

K. **Malignant neuroleptic syndrome.** Treatment consists of discontinuation of the neuroleptics, general supportive measures, and consideration of dantrolene (Dantrium) 50 mg PO Q 12 hr.

L. **Uncertain or unknown diagnosis.** Remember to consider pulmonary infarction and myocardial infarction.

REFERENCES

American Thoracic Society: Guidelines for the initial management of adults with community-acquired pneumonia: Diagnosis, assessment of severity and initial antimicrobial therapy. Am Rev Respir Dis 1993;148:1418.

Gelfand JA, Dinarello CA, Wolff SM: Fever, including fever of unknown origin. In: Isselbacher KJ, Braunwald E, Wilson JD et al, eds.: *Harrison's Principles of Internal Medicine.* 13th ed. McGraw-Hill, Inc;1994:81.

Guze BH, Baxter LR: Neuroleptic malignant syndrome. N Engl J Med 1985;313:163.

Knockaert DC, Vanneste LJ, Vanneste SB et al: Fever of unknown origin in the 1980s—An update of the diagnostic spectrum. Arch Intern Med 1992;152:51.

Littlefield LC: Fever. In: Koda-Kimbal MA, Young LY eds. *Applied Therapeutics: The Clinical Use of Drugs.* 5th ed. Applied Therapeutics, Inc;1992.

Mackowiak PA, LeMaistre CF: Drug fever: A critical appraisal of conventional concepts. Ann Intern Med 1987;106;728.

McGee ZA, Gorby GL: The diagnostic value of fever patterns. Hosp Pract 10/30 1987:103.

McGowan JE, Rose RC, Jacobs NF, et al: Fever in hospitalized patients. Am J Med 1987;82:580.

Petersdorf RG, Root RK: Hypothermia and hyperthermia. In: Isselbacher KJ, Braunwald E, Wilson JD et al, eds.: *Harrison's Principles of Internal Medicine.* 13th ed. McGraw-Hill, Inc;1994:2473.

Pizzo PA: Management of fever in patients with cancer and treatment-induced neutropenia. N Engl J Med 1993;328:1323.

Swartz MN, Simon HB: Pathophysiology of fever and fever of undetermined etiology. In: Dale D, editor-in-chief; Federman DD ed.:*Scientific American.* Sect. 7: Infectious Diseases. vol 2, pt XXIV. Scientific American Inc;1992:1.

22. FEVER IN THE HIV-POSITIVE PATIENT

I. **Problem.** A 35-year-old man presents to the emergency room with a fever to 102.5°F for two days. The patient is known to be HIV-positive but has not yet had an AIDS-defining illness.

II. **Immediate Questions**

A. **Have there been any constitutional symptoms, including headache, anorexia, weight loss, fatigue, or malaise?** Any of these can occur periodically through the course of HIV, and may occur more frequently in the late stages of the disease. Night sweats are sometimes reported but are most often secondary to an infectious process or lymphoma.

B. **What is the fever history? When did it start? How high has the temperature risen?** HIV-related fever is usually no higher than 102.0°F. Symptoms such as chills and rigors are uncommon with HIV-related fever, and are more often associated with bacterial infections. Elevation of temperature above 102°F strongly suggests an opportunistic infection. Remember, however, that nonopportunistic pathogens (eg, *Streptococcus pneumoniae*) are potential causes of pneumonia in an HIV patient, and should be considered as etiologic agents along with opportunistic pathogens.

C. **Are there any specific symptoms?** Your physical examination and further laboratory testing will be directed by specific symptoms, such as a history of visual problems, dysphagia, cough and dyspnea, diarrhea, focal neurologic symptoms, mental status changes, or skin lesions. Headache may be a constitutional symptom or a symptom associated with specific central nervous system (CNS) diseases. About one-half of patients with *Toxoplasma gondii* infections of the CNS complain of headache.

D. Does the patient have AIDS? What was the last CD4 count? If the patient has AIDS, what was the indicator disease? This presentation could be a recurrence since many of the infectious agents associated with AIDS recur, such as *Pneumocystis carinii, Salmonella typhi, Cryptococcus neoformans,* and *Toxoplasma gondii.* Certain infections do not occur until the CD4 count is very low (< 50/mL), such as *Mycobacterium avium-intracellulare.*

III. Differential Diagnosis

There are multiple causes of fever in this setting. The HIV-positive patient is a special problem, in that you must consider not only opportunistic infections seen frequently in this population, but consider also other causes of fever which occur in non-HIV-positive patients. (See Section I, Chapter 21, Fever, p 112). Most opportunistic infections occur when the CD4 count is < 200/mL; and are especially common when the CD4 count is ≤ 50/mL.

A. Drug fever. Anti-retroviral agents rarely cause a fever, but zidovudine (AZT) and zalcitabine (ddC) may cause fever. Antimicrobials, such as sulfonamides, are common causes of fever.

B. Sinusitis. Bacterial sinusitis may occur at any time during the course of HIV infection, but is more severe in the later stages. Presentation may include headache, fever, or congestion. Likely pathogens include: *Streptococcus pneumoniae, Haemophilus influenzae,* and *Staphylococcus aureus.*

C. Eye disease. Retinitis is very common, with the most common pathogen being cytomegalovirus (CMV). This generally occurs in advanced disease, when the CD4 count is < 50/mL. Presentation includes floaters, blurred vision and visual field defects. Pain is not a symptom of CMV retinitis; fever is nonspecific and frequently absent. Patients with the above symptoms should immediately have an ophthalmological exam. CMV retinitis characteristically has a "spaghetti and cheese" appearance (whitish exudate with surrounding edema and hemorrhage). Other organisms that cause retinitis include Varicella-zoster virus, *Toxoplasma,* and *Pneumocystis carinii.* Other eye diseases include optic neuritis, conjunctival Kaposi's sarcoma, and herpetic keratitis.

D. Oral disease. Oral disease rarely causes fever but may signify more widespread disease. For example, darkly pigmented nodular lesions on the hard palate might alert the clinician to widespread Kaposi's sarcoma.

E. Pulmonary disease. Pulmonary disease with fever can be caused by a wide variety of bacteria, fungi, viruses, protozoa, and tumors.

    1. Bacterial pneumonia. Common organisms include *S pneumoniae* and *H influenzae.* In addition to fever, pleuritic chest pain, sputum production, an increased WBC may be present. Focal infiltrates are usually seen on chest x-ray (CXR).

2. **Acid-fast organisms.** Consider *Mycobacterium tuberculosis* (TB) if fever has been present for > 2 weeks. If you suspect TB, but patient has had a negative PPD in the past, place another one with an anergy screen. Keep in mind that TB occurs most frequently at CD4 counts < 500/mL, but can occur at any time during the course of the disease regardless of the CD4 count. CXR findings vary from the classical apical cavitary lesion to hilar adenopathy, nodules or infiltrates in any lung field, or a normal CXR. *Mycobacterium avium-intracellulare* (MAI) may also cause diarrhea as well as fever and pulmonary disease. Often MAI occurs very late in the course of the disease (CD4 counts < 50/mL).

3. **Parasitic infections:** *Pneumocystis carinii* pneumonia (PCP) tends to have a prodromal illness for 1–2 weeks. PCP is the most common indicator disease for AIDS. Progressive dyspnea, nonproductive cough and fever are common symptoms. Diffuse bilateral interstitial pulmonary infiltrates are frequently seen on CXR. An increased LDH may be present.

F. **Cardiac disease.** Consider endocarditis, especially if a new murmur is present on examination.

G. **Gastrointestinal disease**
1. **Esophagitis** generally presents with dysphagia. *Candida* esophagitis may or may not present with fever. Other common causes of esophagitis are CMV and herpes simplex virus (HSV).
2. **Diarrhea.** Often fever and abdominal pain accompany low-volume diarrhea and mucoid stools. Depending on the etiologic agent, blood may be present. *Salmonella typhi* often causes recurrent bacteremia and diarrhea. Other bacterial pathogens may include *Campylobacter jejuni, Shigella flexneri, Clostridium difficile,* and *Mycobacterium avium-intracellulare,* as well as enterotoxigenic *Escherichia coli.* Cytomegalovirus and a variety of parasites including *Cryptosporidium, Isospora belli,* and *Microsporidia* may cause diarrhea and fever. *Histoplasma capsulatum* can also cause diarrhea.

H. **Hepatobiliary/pancreatic disease**
1. **Sclerosing cholangitis-like syndrome**. Fever, RUQ pain, and progressive cholangitis have been described in patients with CMV and *Cryptosporidium* involving the biliary tract.
2. **Hepatitis B or C**.
3. **Cholestatic hepatitis.** Secondary to MAI, TB, *Histoplasma capsulatum, Cryptococcus neoformans.*
4. **Pancreatitis.** May occur as a result of an opportunistic infection, increased triglycerides, or drug toxicity (eg, pentamidine).

I. **Skin.** Bacillary angiomatosis thought secondary to *Bartonella (Rochalimaea) henselae* causes firm purplish-to-reddish papules, subcutaneous nodules or cellulitis-like plaques. Herpes simplex virus type I or II may cause primary or recurrent erythematous/vesicular lesions with ulceration.

    J. Neurologic disease. Many agents can cause a variety of neurologic complications, including meningitis, encephalitis, and mass lesions.

        1. Meningitis. HIV can initially cause an aseptic meningitis. *Cryptococcus neoformans* is a common cause of meningitis; patients present with nonspecific symptoms such as fever, night sweats, and headaches. *M tuberculosis* as well as *S pneumoniae, H influenzae,* and *Neisseria meningitidis* need to be considered as etiologic agents.

        2. Encephalitis. *Toxoplasma gondii* causes altered mental status, headache, fever, and focal neurologic findings.

        3. Mass lesions can be caused by a variety of infectious agents (*Toxoplasma gondii, M tuberculosis, Nocardia asteroides, C neoformans, H capsulatum*) and non-infectious agents (primary CNS lymphoma, metastatic lymphoma, and Kaposi's sarcoma).

    K. Malignant disease. Malignancies, including B-cell non-Hodgkin's lymphoma, Kaposi's sarcoma, and Hodgkin's lymphoma, may have associated fever.

    L. Gynecological complications. Gynecological complications, including sexually transmitted disease (*Neisseria gonorrhoeae, Chlamydia trachomatis*), can cause fever as well as a vaginal discharge and pain.

IV. Database

    A. Physical examination key points

        1. General appearance. The clinician should determine whether the patient appears ill or septic.

        2. Vital signs. Should be evaluated with special attention to hypotension and tachycardia, either of which may be a sign of sepsis.

        3. HEENT. Perform ophthalmologic exam to check for signs of retinitis. Palpate sinuses for tenderness; inspect oral cavity for signs of candidiasis or hairy leukoplakia.

        4. Neck. Check for neck stiffness as a sign of meningitis; however, meningeal signs are often absent in AIDS patients with meningitis. Palpate for lymphadenopathy. Check the jugular veins for distension to help assess fluid status.

        5. Lungs. Percuss the lungs for dullness which may occur with a focal infiltrate. Dullness at one base may indicate a pleural effusion. Auscultate for inspiratory crackles as a sign of consolidation.

        6. Heart. Determine rate and note any murmurs.

        7. Abdominal exam. Note any hepatomegaly or splenomegaly, and look for signs of peritoneal inflammation.

        8. Extremities/skin. Note general appearance of the skin, look for any rashes, papules or nodules.

     9. GU/Rectal. Inspect genitalia, noting presence and characteristic of any discharge. Examine the rectum for perineal abscess.

    10. Neurologic exam. Should be thorough, including mental status examination.

B. Laboratory data. Proceed with your work-up based on findings from the history and physical examination. Many times specific aspects of the patient's history and physical will point you to a specific organ system. When only constitutional symptoms are present, diagnostic testing should include: Complete blood count (CBC) and differential, electrolytes, liver function tests, and blood for bacterial, acid-fast bacteria (AFB) and fungal cultures. A CXR should also be obtained.

    1. CBC with differential. An elevated white blood cell (WBC) count with an increase in banded neutrophils suggests a bacterial infection. The total white count and lymphocyte count will often decrease, especially late in HIV disease. In addition, many medications (eg, AZT) can suppress the white count.

    2. Liver function tests (AST, ALT, bilirubin, GGT, alkaline phosphatase). Look for abnormalities suggesting hepatitis, cholangitis, or liver involvement in a systemic disease.

    3. Arterial blood gases (ABG). Essential in the evaluation of cough and dyspnea. Hypoxemia is almost universally present with *Pneumocystis carinii* pneumonia.

    4. Urinalysis. Pyuria with bacteria suggests a urinary tract infection. Sterile pyuria could result from *M tuberculosis* or fungal involvement of the urinary tract.

    5. Electrolytes, blood urea nitrogen (BUN), and creatinine. To help assess volume status.

C. Other studies

    1. Stool tests. If diarrhea is present, you need to obtain stool for white cells, culture for enteric pathogens, *C difficile* toxin, fungal smear and culture, and AFB stain and culture. In addition, stool will need to be carefully examined for parasites such as *Cryptosporidium*.

    2. Sputum studies. Expectorated sputum should be sent for Gram's stain, culture and sensitivity, AFB stain and culture, and fungal stain and culture. *Pneumocystis carinii* can be diagnosed in about 10% of cases via a silver stain of expectorated sputum. Sputum for AFB smear and culture should be obtained in an HIV patient with a fever and cough even if the CXR is normal.

    3. Blood cultures. Essential in the evaluation of a HIV patient with a fever. Fungi and mycobacteria as well as bacteria are potential isolates.

    4. Serum cryptococcal antigen test. Order this test if meningitis is suspected; 70–90% of patients with cryptococcal meningitis have a positive serum cryptococcal antigen test. May also be helpful in a patient with a fever without neurologic symptoms or signs. Also consider if CD4 count is < 50/mL.

5. **Lumbar puncture.** Should be performed with change in mental status, meningeal signs, or focal neurological findings. An imaging study should be done first to rule out a space-occupying lesion. In addition to the usual studies (See Section III, Chapter 10, Lumbar Puncture, p 364) be sure to obtain CSF for cryptococcal antigen. The sensitivity of AFB smear of CSF for diagnosing *M tuberculosis* will increase with larger amounts of fluid and with repeated lumbar punctures.

6. **CXR.** Essential in the initial evaluation of an HIV patient with a fever or cough and dyspnea. Look for infiltrates, pleural effusions, or cavitary lesions.

7. **CNS imaging.** Necessary with mental status changes and symptoms or signs of CNS disease such as papilledema. Look for a space-occupying lesion which may be secondary to primary lymphoma, metastatic lymphoma or Kaposi's sarcoma, *Toxoplasma gondii,* or *M tuberculosis*. Magnetic resonance imaging (MRI) is more sensitive than computerized tomography (CT) scans and is the preferred modality to image the CNS in this setting.

8. **Bronchoscopy.** With brushings and bronchoalveolar lavage. Essential in the evaluation of an HIV patient with an infiltrate on CXR whose sputum does not reveal the etiology.

V. **Plan.** The treatment of various causes of fever in the HIV patient is beyond the scope of this book. Refer to references specific to this topic. Discussed below are the treatments for the more common causes of fever in the HIV patient and salient points.

A. **General** (See Section I, Chapter 21, Fever, Section V, p 116).

B. **Specific infectious causes**

1. *Pneumocystis carinii* **pneumonia.** First line of treatment is trimethoprim (TMP)-sulfamethoxazole (SMX) PO or IV (15–20 mg/kg/d TMP and 75–100 mg/kg/d SMX in 3–4 divided doses Qd). Pentamidine 4 mg/kg/day as one dose Qd, or dapsone 100 mg/d with trimethoprim can be used. Atovaquone 750 mg TID is reserved for patients who cannot tolerate trimethoprim sulfamethoxazole or pentamidine. Corticosteroids (prednisone 40 mg BID for 5 days followed by a taper) should be given if the initial pO_2 is < 70 mm Hg.

2. *Mycobacterium tuberculosis*. Four first-line drugs should be used initially, including isoniazid (INH) 300 mg once Qd, rifampin 600 mg once Qd, pyrazinamide (PZA) 20–35 mg/kg/d, once Qd, and ethambutol 25 mg/kg or streptomycin 0.5–1 gm Qd to 1 gm twice weekly. There is an increasing incidence of multi-drug-resistant tuberculosis especially in HIV-infected patients. Strict respiratory isolation must be observed. Consider

use of corticosteroids (prednisone 60 mg PO Q d for 1–2 weeks followed by a taper) with tuberculous meningitis.
   3. **Cytomegalovirus retinitis.** Give ganciclovir or foscarnet.
   4. **Cryptococcal meningitis.** Amphotericin B, 0.5–0.7 mg/kg/d with or without flucytosine 150 mg/kg/d initially.
   5. ***Toxoplasma gondii* infection.** Pyrimethamine and sulfadiazine or clindamycin. Will also need folinic acid to prevent myelosuppression from the pyrimethamine.

REFERENCES

Bissuel F, Leport C, Perronne C et al: Fever of unknown origin in HIV-infected patients: A critical analysis of a retrospective series of 57 cases. J Intern Med 1994;236:529.
Sande M, Volberding P: *Medical Management of AIDS*. 4th ed. Saunders;1995.
Sepkowitz K, Talzak E, Carrow M et al: Fever among outpatients with advanced human immunodeficiency virus infection. Arch Intern Med 1993;153:1909.

23. FOLEY CATHETER PROBLEMS

(See also Section III, Chapter 4, Bladder Catheterization, p 347)

I. **Problem.** The Foley catheter is not draining in a patient admitted 2 days previously for congestive heart failure.

II. **Immediate Questions**
   A. **What has the urine output been?** If the urine output has slowly tapered off, then the problem may be oliguria rather than a non-functioning Foley. A catheter that has never drained urine may not be in the bladder.
   B. **Is the urine grossly bloody? Are there any clots in the tubing or collection bag?** Clots or tissue fragments can obstruct the flow of urine in a Foley catheter.
   C. **Is the patient complaining of pain?** Bladder distension often causes severe lower abdominal pain. Bladder spasms are painful and may cause urine to leak out around the catheter rather than run through the catheter.
   D. **Was any difficulty encountered in catheter insertion?** Problematic urethral catheterization should raise the possibility that the catheter is not in the bladder.

III. **Differential Diagnosis**
   A. **Low urine output.** This may be due to volume depletion, hemorrhage, acute renal failure, septic shock, or several other causes. See Section I, Chapter 50, Oliguria/Anuria, p 244.

B. Obstructed Foley catheter
  1. **Kinking of catheter or tubing**
  2. **Clots, tissue fragments.** Most common after transurethral resection of the prostate or bladder. Grossly bloody urine suggests that a clot is obstructing the catheter. "Tea"-colored or "rusty" urine suggests that an organized clot may be present even though the urine is no longer grossly bloody. Bleeding often accompanies "accidental" catheter removal with the balloon still inflated, and in patients with a coagulopathy.
  3. **Sediment/stones.** Chronic indwelling catheters (usually > 1 month) can become encrusted and obstructed. Calculi can lodge in the catheter.
C. Improperly positioned Foley catheter. These problems are much more common in males. In traumatic urethral disruption associated with a pelvic fracture, the catheter can pass into the periurethral tissues. Strictures or prostatic hypertrophy may cause the end of the catheter to be placed in the urethra and not the bladder.
D. Bladder spasms. The patient may complain of severe suprapubic pain, pain radiating to the end of the penis, or urine leaking from around the catheter. Spasms are common after bladder or prostate surgery; they may be the only catheter-related complaint or may be so severe as to obstruct the flow of urine.

IV. Database
  A. Physical examination key points
    1. **Vital signs.** Check for tachycardia or hypotension characteristic of hypovolemia.
    2. **Abdomen.** Determine if the bladder is distended (suprapubic dullness to percussion with or without tenderness). May be indicative of an obstructed Foley catheter.
    3. **Genitalia.** Bleeding at the meatus suggests urethral trauma or partial removal of the catheter with the balloon inflated.
    4. **Rectum.** A "floating prostate" suggests urethral disruption.
  B. Laboratory data. Most problems are usually mechanical in nature so that laboratory data are somewhat limited in this setting.
    1. **Blood urea nitrogen (BUN), serum creatinine.** Elevations may be seen with cases of renal insufficiency.
    2. **Prothrombin time, partial thromboplastin time, platelet count.** Especially if there is severe bleeding present.
  C. Radiologic and other studies. In the acute setting of a Foley catheter problem, radiologic studies are usually not needed. Ultrasound may demonstrate hydronephrosis in cases of obstructive uropathy.

V. Plan
  A. Verify function. A rule of thumb is that a catheter that will not irrigate is in the urethra and not in the bladder. Start by irrigating the

catheter with aseptic technique, using a catheter-tipped 60-mL syringe and sterile normal saline. This may dislodge any clots obstructing the catheter. If sterile saline cannot be satisfactorily instilled and aspirated, the catheter should be replaced.
   B. Oliguria. If the catheter irrigates freely, evaluate the patient for oliguria/anuria. See Section I, Chapter 50, Oliguria/Anuria, p 244.
   C. Spasms. Bladder spasms can be treated with oxybutynin (Ditropan) or propantheline (Pro-Banthine). *Note:* Be sure to discontinue these medications before removing the catheter to allow normal bladder function.

REFERENCE

Andriole UT: Care of the indwelling catheter. In: Kayes D ed. *Urinary Tract Infection and Its Management.* CV Mosby;1973:256.

24. HEADACHE

I. **Problem.** You are called to the emergency room to evaluate a 58-year-old man who complains of a severe headache that has lasted for several hours.

II. **Immediate Questions**
   A. Has the patient experienced similar headaches before? If the headache is similar to previous tension or migraine headaches, then the situation is unlikely to be urgent; however, if the headache is new or deviates from a previous pattern, a number of potentially serious conditions should be considered, including acute glaucoma, sinusitis, subarachnoid hemorrhage, meningitis, neoplasm, and early hypertensive encephalopathy.
   B. What are the patient's vital signs? Although essential hypertension by itself is an infrequent cause of headache, it may exacerbate a preexisting vascular or tension headache. Diastolic blood pressures > 140 can cause severe headache. A fever should alert the clinician to the possibility of subarachnoid hemorrhage, meningitis, temporal arteritis, or acute sinusitis.

III. **Differential Diagnosis.** A detailed, well-focused history is the most important tool for evaluating headache. The great majority of headaches are secondary to either tension-type or migraine headaches. A headache may also be the only symptom of a more serious condition, such as an intracranial mass, temporal arteritis, meningitis, and subarachnoid hemorrhage.

A. Tension-type headache
1. **Episodic tension-type headache.** This is frequently described as a squeezing, "bandlike" tightness that is usually felt bilaterally. It may occur in the occipital, frontal, or bitemporal regions. Occasionally, patients with tension-type headaches may describe a "throbbing" pain. This form of headache may last minutes to days; it is generally described as having a mild to moderate intensity.
2. **Chronic tension-type headache.** This headache is similar to the acute tension-type in quality but its duration may be months or even years. Depression, personality problems, and a history of narcotic abuse are common in these patients.

B. Migraine headache. Although the precise pathophysiology has not been fully ascertained, it is thought to be secondary to cerebral vasoconstriction followed by vasodilation. The initial vasoconstriction may be associated with a variety of neurologic deficits including visual disturbances (scotoma, zig-zag lines, bright lights), dysarthria, hemiparesis, and hemianesthesia. Of these, the visual phenomena are most common. These neurologic features generally last 5–30 minutes and are then followed by headache. The headache is usually pounding or throbbing but may be dull and boring. It is usually unilateral but may also occur bilaterally in any location. Anorexia, nausea, and vomiting are frequently associated. The attack may last several hours to 2–3 days and occasionally longer. Migraines are much more common in women. Three characteristic migraine patterns are recognized:
1. **Migraine without aura.** This vascular headache is not preceded by neurologic deficits or visual disturbances. It is the most frequent type.
2. **Migraine with aura.** The headache is preceded by visual deficits such as scotomata and field deficits.
3. **Complicated migraine.** In this form of migraine, the headache is accompanied by neurologic symptoms including hemiplegia and ophthalmoplegia.

C. Cluster headaches
1. Cluster headaches are excruciating, usually unilateral, and frequently associated with ipsilateral nasal congestion, lacrimation, and conjunctival injection. Nausea and vomiting are unusual. Cluster headaches are not preceded by any neurologic symptoms.
2. Each headache typically lasts < 2 hours; however, multiple attacks can occur within a 24-hour period.
3. Unlike migraine, cluster headaches most often affect men between the ages of 20 and 40. They are not familial.

D. Temporal arteritis
1. Temporal arteritis should be considered in any patient older than 50 years presenting with a recent history of headache.

2. Other symptoms such as malaise, weight loss, fever, and myalgias are frequently present. Jaw claudication may also occur.

3. It is especially important to ask the patient if he or she has experienced any new visual problems such as double or blurred vision. Temporal arteritis can cause sudden blindness as a result of inflammation of the ophthalmic artery. Early diagnosis and treatment with steroids are necessary to prevent this complication.

E. Trigeminal neuralgia. This condition is more common in the elderly. The pain is described as brief, but severe and jabbing. The pain is usually unilateral and localized to one or more divisions of the trigeminal nerve. Precipitants include talking, chewing, or having physical pressure exerted on a specific trigger area. Etiology is unknown.

F. Cerebrovascular disease. Headache can be a presenting complaint in some patients experiencing an acute stroke. When the internal carotid is involved, the headache is usually located in the frontal region; involvement of the vertebrobasilar system generally yields an occipital headache. The headache of a cerebrovascular accident may precede or follow focal neurologic symptoms.

G. Sinusitis

1. Headache is usually dull, aching, and located frontally. Pain is frequently worse in the morning when the patient awakens but improves as the sinuses drain during the day.

2. If the patient displays an altered mental status or complains of a stiff neck, a complicated sinus infection should be suspected (brain abscess, meningitis, septic cavernous sinus thrombosis).

H. Eye disease. Glaucoma, keratitis, and uveitis may all cause headaches. The pain is usually dull and located in the periorbital or retrorbital regions.

I. Dental disease. The teeth are innervated by the second and third divisions of the trigeminal nerve; thus disease involving these structures may cause pain referred to the face or head. Secondary muscle spasm may result.

J. Temporomandibular joint disease. Headache is usually unilateral on side of face and head. It is described as "aching" in quality and is worsened with jaw movement.

K. Mass lesions. Both neoplasm and brain abscess can produce headache as a result of either increased pressure or distension of local structures.

1. Any new neurologic deficit such as visual or motor loss or change in mental status should alert the clinician to the possibility of a mass lesion.

2. Onset of new headache in a patient greater than 50 years old suggests the possibility of a mass lesion.

3. Nonspecific features of headache resulting from a mass lesion include progressive worsening despite administration of anal-

gesics; early-morning headache; headache exacerbated by coughing or sneezing; anorexia; and vomiting without nausea. It is important to note that these features also occur frequently with other types of headache, including chronic tension headache, migraine headache, cluster headache, and sinus headache.

L. Subarachnoid hemorrhage. The rupture of a cerebral aneurysm is associated with acute onset of a violent headache. The patient may also quickly develop neurologic deficits or lose consciousness. Blood in the subarachnoid space may induce fever and nuchal rigidity resembling acute meningitis. Sentinel leaks (warning leaks) from a cerebral aneurysm are more subtle and frequently precede subsequent rupture. These headaches may be difficult to distinguish from tension headaches, and may cause nonspecific symptoms such as myalgias or a stiff neck which may be erroneously attributed to an acute viral illness.

M. Acute febrile illness
1. Fever may cause a vascular-type throbbing headache that remits as the illness resolves.
2. Any febrile patient in whom headache is a major complaint should also be suspected of having meningitis, especially if nuchal rigidity or other signs of meningeal irritation are present.

IV. Database
  A. Physical examination key points
   1. **Vital signs** (See Section II.B.)
   2. **HEENT**
     a. Patients with both migraine and chronic tension headaches frequently complain of scalp tenderness, which may also suggest temporal arteritis.
     b. Palpate the temporal arteries. A diminished pulse or tender temporal arteries suggests arteritis; however, temporal arteries may feel normal to palpation in 30–40% of patients with temporal arteritis.
     c. Examine the eyes for injected conjunctivae and excessive lacrimation, which occur with cluster headaches. Examine the fundi for any signs of papilledema or optic nerve atrophy resulting from an intracerebral mass. Retinal hemorrhage may be observed after subarachnoid hemorrhage. Subhyaloid hemorrhages may be seen trapped behind the vitreous humor at the edge of the optic disc, suggesting a sudden rise in intracranial pressure.
     d. Palpate or percuss the maxillary and frontal sinuses for tenderness.
     e. Examine the ears for any signs of otitis media.
     f. Examine dentition for painful teeth and the temporomandibular joint for any crepitus, pain, or limited jaw opening.

3. **Neck.** Examine for any resistance to passive flexion of the neck, which would suggest meningeal irritation from either subarachnoid hemorrhage or meningitis.
4. **Neurologic exam.** A detailed exam is mandated in any patient with a complaint of headache to identify localizing signs that would suggest a CNS mass lesion, meningitis, or intracerebral hemorrhage.

B. **Laboratory data**
1. **Complete blood count.** An elevated leukocyte count could suggest infection such as sinusitis or meningitis.
2. **Erythrocyte sedimentation rate (ESR).** Almost always greater than 50 mm/h in patients with temporal arteritis; however, on occasion the ESR may be normal. If clinical suspicion is high, a temporal artery biopsy should never be deferred simply because of a normal ESR.

C. **Radiologic and other studies**
1. **Sinus films.** Should be obtained if sinusitis is suspected.
2. **Head CT scan.** Should be obtained in any patient with a chronic headache pattern that has recently changed in frequency or severity; progressive worsening of a headache despite appropriate therapy in any patient greater than 50 years old with a new onset of headache; or if the neurologic exam reveals any focal findings. Additionally, a head CT scan should be obtained in any patient with onset of headache that is exacerbated with exertion, cough, or sexual activity; or in any patient with orbital bruit.
3. **MRI.** Preferable when posterior fossa lesions or craniospinal abnormalities (eg, Arnold-Chiari malformation) are suspected.
4. **Lumbar puncture.** If meningitis is suspected, lumbar puncture should be performed and not delayed for a CT scan when papilledema is absent and the neurologic examination is nonfocal. Lumbar puncture should be performed when subarachnoid hemorrhage is suspected and CT results are negative.

V. **Plan.** The initial goal in the management of headache is to exclude its rare but potentially serious causes, such as brain tumor, subarachnoid hemorrhage, brain abscess,and meningitis. When these conditions have been excluded, treatment can be directed according to the type of headache. Only the management of tension-type headache, migraine headache, and cluster headache is discussed here.

A. **Episodic tension-type headache**
1. Relief of pain can usually be obtained by administration of simple analgesics like aspirin, acetaminophen, or NSAIDs.
2. In general, avoid analgesic combinations containing ergotamines, caffeine, butalbital, and codeine.

B. **Chronic tension-type headache**
1. This condition is notoriously difficult to manage. As with episodic tension-type headache, the physician must attempt to avoid the

chronic use of narcotic analgesics, which frequently results in narcotic dependence.

2. The physician should also inquire about the possibility of overused drugs, as withdrawal of daily analgesics enhances the effect of prophylactic drugs.

3. A tricyclic antidepressant such as amitriptyline (Elavil) 75 mg HS is one of the most useful agents for treating chronic tension headache. This medication should be used regardless of whether depression is overtly present.

4. Nonsteroidal anti-inflammatory drugs (NSAIDs) such as aspirin 325–650 mg PO Q 6 hr, naproxen (Naprosyn) 275–550 mg Q 6 hr, or ibuprofen (Motrin) 400–600 mg PO Q 6 hr may also be beneficial.

5. When suboccipital or cervical muscle spasm is present, massage of the neck and occipital region as well as local application of heat is sometimes useful.

6. Psychotherapy, relaxation therapy, and biofeedback may also be used in those patients who fail to respond to the preceding measures.

C. **Migraine headache.** A number of different medications can now be administered in the management of acute migraine.

1. **NSAIDs.** For an early mild attack, treatment with a NSAID such as ibuprofen 400–600 mg Q 4–6 hr or naproxen (Naprosyn) 500 mg Q 12 hr may be effective. Metaclopramide (Reglan) 10 mg PO can be given at this time to increase drug absorption and reduce nausea and vomiting. In addition, ketorolac, a parenteral NSAID, has been shown to be effective at 60 mg IM.

2. **Ergot alkaloids**
   a. **Ergotamine tartrate** (Cafergot) 1 mg: Two tablets PO at onset of the headache followed by two tablets Q 30 min to a maximum of six tablets in 24 hours. This medication is most effective if taken early in an attack.
   b. **Dihydroergotamine**: 1 mg IV Q 30 min for three doses can also be administered. This regimen is especially useful in patients whose headache has been present for several hours or who cannot tolerate oral drugs because of nausea.
   c. **Caution:** It is important to avoid administration of ergotamines in patients with peripheral vascular disease (PVD), coronary artery disease, hypertension, renal failure, hepatic disease, and hyperthyroidism, and in pregnant patients. Because ergot alkaloids decrease cerebral blood flow, they should be avoided in patients with complicated migraine.

3. **Sumatriptan (Imitrex):** 6 mg SC.
   a. Sumatriptan has been found to be effective in relieving headache symptoms, nausea, vomiting, and photo- and phonophobia. It is effective even when taken late during an attack. A second dose is usually not effective.

    b. Caution: Sumatriptan is contraindicated in patients with a history of angina, ischemic or vasospastic (Prinzmetal's) angina, uncontrolled hypertension, peripheral vascular disease, and hemiplegic or basilar artery migraine.

  4. Isometheptene 65 mg/dichloralphenazone 100 mg/acetaminophen 325 mg (Midrin). Give 2 capsules at onset of headache followed by 1 capsule Q hour to maximum of 5 capsules in 24 hours.

  5. Prochlorperazine (Compazine) 25 mg IV. This medication has been shown in some controlled trials to be superior to dihydroergotamine in migraine relief.

  6. Prophylactic therapy. A number of medications can be used for prophylaxis of migraine, including propranolol (Inderal), amitriptyline (Elavil), and verapamil (Calan). These medications are less useful in the management of an acute attack of migraine and will not receive further discussion here. In addition, naproxen (Naprosyn) has been shown to be effective in migraine prophylaxis.

D. Cluster headaches

  1. Ergotamine is often effective in the treatment of cluster headaches and is administered in the same fashion as described for migraine headache.

  2. Oxygen inhalation by face mask at 7 L/min for 15 minutes has been reported to be successful in aborting a cluster headache. Greatest benefit is obtained in patients younger than 50 years of age with episodic cluster headache.

  3. Sumatriptan has been found to be effective in aborting cluster headache in some patients and is administered as described above for migraine headaches.

  4. Prophylactic therapy is the most effective treatment and involves the use of such medications as verapamil, prednisone with taper, lithium carbonate, and methysergide (Sansert).

REFERENCES

Abramowicz M ed.:*Drugs for Migraine.* Medical Lett Drugs Ther 1995;37:17.
Dalessio DJ: Diagnosing the severe headache. Neurology 1994;44:S6.
Kumar KL, Cooney TG: Headaches. Med Clin North Am 1995;79:261.
Welch KMA: Drug therapy for migraine. N Engl J Med 1993;329:1476.

25. HEART MURMUR

I. Problem. You are asked to see a 50-year-old man complaining of acute shortness of breath. The nursing staff notes a loud murmur.

II. Immediate Questions

A. Is the murmur itself responsible for the problem or is it a sign of some other underlying problem? Acute aortic or mitral regurgitation from endocarditis or acute mitral regurgitation resulting from rupture of a papillary muscle after a myocardial infarction (MI) could explain the patient's condition. Underlying medical conditions such as a severe anemia, hyperthyroidism, and pregnancy can also have associated "innocent" flow murmurs related to increased cardiac output.

B. Does the patient have known valvular disease? Progression of valvular dysfunction may be the cause of deterioration in such a patient.

C. Does the patient have known congenital heart disease? In a patient with a history of a murmur, a bicuspid aortic valve, an atrial septal defect (ASD), a ventricular septal defect (VSD), a patent ductus arteriosus (PDA), and pulmonic stenosis (PS) should always be considered. Often, patients with mild PS or a small ASD will be asymptomatic.

D. Has the deterioration been chronic or acute? Acute decompensation would suggest an acute process such as endocarditis or myocardial ischemia. Chronic deterioration would suggest increasing ventricular dysfunction from preexisting valvular disease.

E. Is there a history of IV drug abuse, recent dental work, invasive procedures such as a sigmoidoscopy or cystoscopy, or a history of fever or chills? These factors would suggest endocarditis.

F. Does the patient have any chest pain? If so, it is important to characterize the chest pain. Chest pain is often seen with angina, aortic dissection, and pericarditis. Ischemic chest pain is a heavy, pressurelike sensation, usually not sharp; radiation to the neck and jaw is very suggestive (radiation to the midscapular area of the back is not uncommon); shortness of breath, nausea, and diaphoresis often accompany the chest discomfort. A sharp, pleuritic, left anterior or substernal pain that improves with sitting up and leaning forward is consistent with pericarditis. A pericardial friction rub may be mistaken as a murmur. Pain associated with dissection usually begins abruptly, reaches maximum intensity quickly, is often continuous, and there is usually a history of hypertension.

G. Does the patient have coronary artery disease, and if so, is this the etiology of the murmur? A recent MI with papillary muscle dysfunction or rupture may result in acute mitral regurgitation. An acute ventricular septal defect or free wall rupture following an MI can cause a new murmur. Previously unrecognized aortic stenosis can also cause classic angina and may result in myocardial ischemia. Hypertrophic obstructive cardiomyopathy (also called idiopathic hypertrophic subaortic stenosis [IHSS]), and aortic dissection can cause angina.

III. Differential Diagnosis
A. Murmur aggravated by an underlying problem
1. **Flow murmur.** A flow murmur may be caused by or aggravated by a significant anemia and resultant high-outflow congestive heart failure (CHF).
2. **Congestive heart failure with "secondary" mitral regurgitation** can result from a variety of etiologies.
3. **Murmur of aortic insufficiency with possible aortic dissection.** In this setting, always consider an underlying connective tissue disorder such as Marfan's syndrome as well as severe hypertension.
4. **Noncardiac murmur.** Thyroid bruits, subclavian artery stenosis, venous hums, and pericardial or pleural friction rubs can all be mistaken for a cardiac murmur.
5. **A new murmur with bacterial endocarditis** is an ominous finding.

B. Coronary artery disease
1. **Acute ischemia/injury with papillary muscle dysfunction.** Can cause reversible mitral regurgitation.
2. **Recent myocardial infarction**
   a. **Acute severe mitral regurgitation secondary to ruptured chordae tendineae or head of a papillary muscle**
   b. **Acute VSD**
   c. **Acute rupture of the ventricular walll**
3. **Acute ischemia.** Leading to immediate, severe left ventricular dysfunction with pulmonary edema and new or worsening mitral regurgitation.

C. Valvular heart disease
1. **Mitral valve prolapse with ruptured chordae/papillary muscle head and CHF.** Arrhythmias (ventricular or atrial) may lead to decompensation.
2. **Mitral stenosis.** New-onset atrial fibrillation can lead to decompensation.
3. **Aortic stenosis.** With progression may result in angina, left ventricular dysfunction, syncope, or arrhythmias (especially ventricular).
4. **Hypertrophic obstructive cardiomyopathy.** Arrhythmias, angina, and dyspnea are common. Sudden death can occur and is often related to exertion.
5. **Prosthetic valve dysfunction**
6. **Severe stenosis or regurgitation of any valve (especially mitral or aortic)** can lead to left ventricular dysfunction and associated symptoms.

D. Congenital heart disease
1. **ASD/VSD with right-to-left shunt, causing systemic hypoxemia.** Occurs with pulmonary hypertension or Eisenmenger's syndrome.

2. **New dysrhythmias in a patient with previously stable congenital defects**. Can cause acute deterioration, especially atrial fibrillation.
   E. **Atrial myxoma.** A rare cause of a murmur; may present with CHF, chest pain, syncope, arrhythmias, or an embolic event.

IV. Database
A. Physical examination key points
1. **General.** Inability to lie flat suggests pulmonary edema or possibly pericarditis.
2. **Vital signs**
   a. **Temperature.** Elevated temperature might indicate infection (endocarditis) although postinfarct patients can have a moderate fever for up to a week. A fever from any etiology can cause or intensify a flow murmur.
   b. **Heart rate and rhythm.** Tachycardia (See Section I, Chapter 58, Tachycardia, p 279) is often associated with CHF, pain, infection, pericarditis, and perhaps arrhythmias. Irregular rhythm may suggest the presence of atrial fibrillation or frequent premature atrial or ventricular beats as well as second-degree atrioventricular block.
   c. **Blood pressure.** Hypertension or hypotension is often associated with angina or MI. Hypotension could reflect sepsis or hemodynamic collapse. Pulsus paradoxus (a difference of 10 mm Hg in systolic blood pressure between tidal inspiration and expiration) suggests pericardial tamponade.
   d. **Tachypnea.** Suggests CHF.
3. **Neck**
   a. Elevated jugular venous distension suggests right-sided ventricular failure or pericardial tamponade.
   b. A decrease in the carotid upstroke suggests significant aortic stenosis. Also, the murmur of aortic stenosis radiates to the carotids bilaterally but should not be confused with bilateral carotid bruits, a venous hum, or a thyroid bruit.
4. **Heart.** Careful cardiac examination is essential. First (S_1) and second (S_2) heart sounds and splitting of S_2 must be characterized. The presence of a fourth heart sound (S_4) may suggest a recent MI, hemodynamically significant aortic stenosis, or long-standing hypertension. A third (S_3) heart sound is consistent with ventricular dysfunction.
   a. **Aortic insufficiency.** A diastolic blowing murmur heard best at the right second intercostal space down to the left lower sternal border with the patient leaning forward in full expiration. This may occur with acute aortic dissection or acute bacterial endocarditis, or may be chronic. The aortic component

of S_2 may be soft or absent. The murmur of acute aortic insufficiency is usually soft in intensity and in duration, is heard best at the left lower sternal border, and can easily be missed.

b. **Aortic stenosis.** The murmur is crescendo-decrescendo and harsh; it is heard best at the right second intercostal space. Critical aortic valve stenosis is characterized by the absence of the aortic component of S_2, a palpable S_4 gallop at the apex, late peaking of the maximal intensity of the murmur, a palpable carotid thrill (usually over the left carotid artery), and a diminished and delayed carotid upstroke.

c. **Mitral regurgitation.** Heard best as a blowing pansystolic murmur at the apex, radiating to the axilla and occasionally into the midback. An intermittent murmur of mitral regurgitation might suggest intermittent papillary muscle dysfunction secondary to ischemia or other causes. The murmur of acute, severe mitral regurgitation may be short in duration and soft in intensity. Other findings associated with severe mitral regurgitation include an S_3 gallop, tachycardia, pulmonary rales, and signs of poor peripheral perfusion.

d. **Mitral valve prolapse.** A mid-systolic click followed by a late systolic murmur suggests mitral valve prolapse. A click or murmur may be present together or singly.

e. **Mitral stenosis.** Heard best with the patient lying in left lateral decubitus position with the bell of the stethoscope positioned over the apical impulse. Mitral stenosis is often missed, particularly in a sick patient. It is *always* an important consideration; a confirmatory echocardiogram is usually indicated. An otherwise stable patient with mitral stenosis will decompensate quickly when atrial fibrillation develops. Control of the heart rate to permit adequate diastolic filling is beneficial.

f. **Hypertrophic cardiomyopathy.** Characteristically causes a systolic murmur that might be confused with aortic stenosis, but actually represents reversible left ventricular outflow tract obstruction secondary to hypertrophy of the interventricular septum. The murmur is a crescendo-decrescendo systolic murmur that increases in intensity with the Valsalva maneuver and standing, and decreases in intensity with squatting. The murmur is best heard at the apex and left lower sternal border. An S_4 gallop is usually present. A bisferiens contour to the carotid pulse is characteristic (double peaking of the pulse). Again, a stable person with this can decompensate rapidly in the face of new atrial fibrillation.

g. **Atrial septal defect/ventricular septal defect.** An ASD murmur may be difficult to hear. Widely fixed splitting of S_2 is a clue to the presence of an ASD. VSDs are usually heard over the entire precordium and the murmur is both systolic and diastolic.

5. **Extremities.** With distal pulses, look for evidence of a pulse deficit that might suggest the presence of dissection or embolic phenomena. **Quincke's sign** (a to-and-fro movement seen in the capillary bed of the fingers when light pressure is applied to the distal finger tip) is seen in chronic severe aortic insufficiency.

6. **Neurologic exam.** Focal neurologic deficits may occur with subacute bacterial endocarditis, myxoma, and thrombus formation with embolus.

7. **Skin.** Look for any evidence of IV drug use that might suggest bacterial endocarditis.

B. **Laboratory data.** Clearly, these depend on the history and exam. The order in which laboratory data are acquired depends on the clinical picture at the bedside.

1. **CBC with differential.** Anemia can be the cause of high-output CHF. A significantly elevated WBC count with an increase in the percentage of banded neutrophils indicates the presence of an infectious process. An elevated WBC count can accompany an acute MI.

2. **Blood culture.** This should be obtained if there is any question of endocarditis. Three sets of two cultures should be obtained over several hours if the patient is stable. If the patient is unstable, at least one set of blood cultures should be obtained before antibiotic therapy is initiated.

3. **Arterial blood gases.** Acidosis (see Section I, Chapter 2, Acidosis, p 9) and hypoxia suggest the presence of significant left ventricular compromise and pulmonary congestion in the sick patient with a new murmur.

4. **Thyroid function tests, electrolytes including magnesium, renal function tests.** May provide clues to reasons for patient's decompensation.

C. **Radiologic and other studies**

1. **Electrocardiogram.** The most useful test to screen for ischemia, MI, or dysrhythmia, particularly atrial fibrillation. Keep in mind that the abrupt onset of atrial fibrillation in a person with compensated CHF, stable hypertrophic cardiomyopathy, or stable valvular disease may cause rapid decompensation.

2. **Chest x-ray.** The cardiac silhouette may give a clue to valvular disease. Increased vascularization, pleural effusion, Kerley A and B lines, and confluent alveolar densities are radiographic evidence of pulmonary edema. Other signs to look for are cardiac chamber enlargement and mediastinal widening.

3. **Echocardiogram.** In evaluating an acutely ill patient with a murmur that is not readily identified, the echocardiogram may be the single best source of information. It can accurately determine

the presence and degree of valvular stenosis or regurgitation. The etiology of the valvular problem can also be suggested. Atrial and ventricular septal defects can be diagnosed.

4. **Swan-Ganz catheterization.** From a diagnostic standpoint, one can obtain right atrial and pulmonary artery blood samples to diagnose a stepup in oxygen saturation, confirming the diagnosis of acute VSD. Acute or severe mitral regurgitation can be suggested by the presence of significant V waves in the pulmonary capillary wedge pressure tracing.

V. Plan. Treatment is generally aimed at the condition that is either causing the murmur (MI, papillary muscle dysfunction, VSD, aortic insufficiency in the face of aortic root dissection) or aggravating the condition for which the murmur is a secondary finding (hyperthyroidism, new-onset atrial fibrillation, endocarditis, thrombus on a mechanical valve or anemia). While initiating therapy, consultation should be considered. When a patient is symptomatic from a cardiac murmur, a cardiology consult is appropriate.

A. **Relieve angina.** This may result in prompt improvement in cases of recurrent pulmonary edema secondary to ischemia. See Section I, Chapter 11, Chest Pain, V, p 62.

B. **Maintain hemodynamic support**
   1. **Dopamine** can be used if an arterial vasoconstricting agent is needed. See Section I, Chapter 41, Hypotension V, p 207.
   2. **Dobutamine** should be used if a positive inotropic drug is required.

C. **ICU monitoring.** Certain pathologic conditions may require arterial pressure monitoring (see Section III, Chapter 1, Arterial Line Placement, p 341) or continuous monitoring of right heart pressures and pulmonary wedge pressure (see Section III, Chapter 12, Pulmonary Artery Catheterization, p 370).

D. **Treatment of acute myocardial infarction**
   1. **Relieve pain with nitroglycerin, IV beta-blockers, and morphine sulfate.** (See Section I, Chapter 11, Chest Pain, Section V, p 62; or Section VII, Commonly Used Medications, p 495, 467, 492 respectively, for doses.)
   2. **Thrombolysis.** If indicated and if the patient is an appropriate candidate.

E. **Treatment of suspected endocarditis.** Initiate antibiotic therapy after obtaining four sets of blood cultures.

F. **Arrange for invasive evaluation if warranted.** The evaluation of an unknown heart murmur in a critically ill patient can be extremely complex. The basic goal is to determine the possible etiologies as quickly as possible. Emergent evaluation with an echocardiogram, aortic root contrast injection, or surgical consultation may be indicated if the patient's condition is unstable.

26. HEMATEMESIS, MELENA

I. **Problem.** A 56-year-old male is admitted to the hospital because of pneumonia; you are called because he "vomited blood."

II. **Immediate Questions**
  A. **What are the patient's vital signs?** Is there supine hypotension (indicates 30% volume loss)? Is there resting tachycardia (indicates 20% volume loss)? Are there orthostatic changes in pulse or blood pressure (indicates 10% volume loss)? If the patient has supine hypotension or resting tachycardia then fluid resuscitation must begin immediately.
  B. **Does the patient have adequate IV access?** With no indication of hemodynamic instability, one 16–18-gauge IV with D5 NS at KVO is adequate. In the presence of hemodynamic compromise, two large-bore (14–16 gauge) IVs should be in place.
  C. **Is there a prior history of gastrointestinal problems? Is there a history of peptic ulcer disease (PUD) or esophageal varices?** A previous history of these disorders may indicate the etiology; however, in only 50% of patients with known esophageal varices can upper GI bleeding be attributed to variceal bleeding.
  D. **Is the patient taking any medications?** Review medications. Note particular use of nonsteroidal anti-inflammatory drugs (NSAIDs), aspirin, steroids, and anticoagulants. Anticoagulants may unmask significant pathology.
  E. **Does the patient smoke, or have a family history of PUD?** Both are risk factors for PUD.
  F. **Does the patient have a history of alcohol abuse?** This suggests gastritis or varices as the source of bleeding. Ethanol alone is not an etiologic factor for peptic ulcer disease, unless there is accompanying cirrhosis. Alcohol use is also a risk factor for a Mallory-Weiss tear.
  G. **Is there a previous hematocrit?** It will be important to establish a baseline with which to monitor the patient.
  H. **Is there a history of abnormal liver function studies?** Suggests occult liver disease.
  I. **What is the volume of hematemesis?** Ask the nurse to save the emesis. This is important to establish the volume of hematemesis as well as to validate the presence of blood. A large amount indicates more urgency.
  J. **Has there been any melena or bright red blood per rectum?** Acute upper GI tract blood loss of about one unit results in melena; two units may cause hematochezia.

III. Differential Diagnosis

A. Peptic ulcer disease. PUD accounts for 50% of upper GI hemorrhages. The use of NSAIDs is the single most important risk factor for PUD and bleeding.

B. Esophageal varices. These account for 10% of upper GI bleeding. Esophageal varices have the highest morbidity and mortality of all causes of upper GI bleeding. (See Section I, Chapter 27, Hematochezia, p 143.)

C. Mallory-Weiss tear. Causes ~5–15% of upper GI bleeding. Associated with recent heavy alcohol intake in 30–60% of cases. A series of vomiting episodes often precedes the hematemesis.

D. Acute hemorrhagic gastritis. Accounts for 15% of community-acquired upper GI hemorrhage. Often associated with alcohol, NSAID use, and stress (severely ill ICU patients).

E. Carcinoma. Very seldom the cause of acute bleeding; almost always found in patients over 50 years old.

F. Arterial enteric fistula. A rare cause of upper GI hemorrhage, but can be quite dramatic. Should be suspected in patients who have had aortic bypass graft surgery. Of these fistulae, 75% communicate with the duodenum (3rd portion). Generally preceded by a self-limited episode of bleeding ("herald bleed").

IV. Database

A. Physical examination key points

1. **Vital signs.** Including orthostatic blood pressure and heart rate. Orthostatic changes are a decrease in systolic blood pressure of 10 mm Hg and/or an increase in heart rate of 20 bpm 1 minute after changing from supine to standing position. Vital signs need to be checked frequently until the patient is stable.

2. **Skin.** Spider telangiectasia, palmar erythema, and jaundice indicate underlying cirrhosis and possible varices. Poor skin turgor and absent axillary sweat may indicate volume depletion. Acanthosis nigricans and Kaposi's sarcoma are associated with GI malignancy.

3. **Eyes.** Scleral icterus suggests chronic liver disease.

4. **Chest.** Gynecomastia suggests cirrhosis.

5. **Abdomen.** An increase in bowel sounds suggests upper GI bleeding. Hepatomegaly or splenomegaly suggests cirrhosis or cancer. An abdominal mass points to cancer. Tenderness in the midepigastric or LUQ suggests PUD. Ascites may be seen with cirrhosis and associated esophageal varices.

6. **Genitourinary system.** Rectal examination to look for melena or bright red blood per rectum. Testicular atrophy may be secondary to cirrhosis/chronic liver disease and may point to varices.

  B. **Laboratory data**
     1. **Stat complete blood count.** This can be done by phlebotomy before your arrival. Differential is not necessary.
     2. **Type and cross-match.** At least four units of packed red blood cells (PRBCs).
     3. **A nasogastric tube for gastric lavage.** This procedure is essential for accurate diagnosis. The possibility of varices is not a contraindication. Lavage until clear or at least pink-tinged.
     4. **Hematocrit.** Serial hematocrits are helpful; however, in acute hemorrhage the hematocrit may not reflect the amount of blood loss. The hematocrit may fall precipitously after aggressive fluid resuscitation.
     5. **BUN and creatinine.** An increased BUN/creatinine ratio is seen in upper GI bleeding and volume depletion.
     6. **PT, PTT, platelet count.** An elevated PT, PTT, or thrombocytopenia can interfere with stabilization of the patient. An elevated PT may be seen in chronic liver disease. Platelets and clotting factors are lost with rapid bleeding.
  C. **Radiologic and other studies.** The source of bleeding must be identified so that specific therapy can be instituted.
     1. **Upper GI endoscopy (EGD).** This is the cornerstone of diagnosis of upper GI tract bleeding; it should be performed as soon as possible after hemodynamic stabilization and adequate lavage.
        a. The optimal timing of EGD is not well established. Most experts believe that EGD should be performed within 24 hours. With the multitude of available therapeutic interventions, however, earlier endoscopy is considered preferable.
        b. The most common situation is a patient with known alcoholic liver disease and upper GI tract bleeding. EGD is necessary to differentiate PUD from varices and to direct therapy.
     2. **Colonoscopy.** Should be performed if EGD is entirely negative and the patient has melena. Necessary to rule out a right-sided colonic lesion.
     3. **Technetium-labeled bleeding scan.** Should be done if the upper GI endoscopy and colonoscopy are negative.

V. **Plan**
   A. **Monitoring.** The first step in management is to determine whether the patient should be monitored in an ICU. The following are guidelines for admission to the ICU.
      1. Clearly documented frank hematemesis.
      2. Coffee-ground emesis *and* either melena or hematochezia.
      3. Hemodynamic instability, either hypotension, tachycardia, or orthostatic hypotension.
      4. A drop in hematocrit of 5 points after fluid resuscitation.

     5. A significant unexplained increase in the BUN when GI bleeding is suspected.

B. Volume resuscitation. If massive bleeding is evident, place two large-bore (14- or 16-gauge) IV lines. Begin IV fluids containing normal saline at a rate to maintain hemodynamic stability. Transfuse packed red cells when available for massive bleeding to keep the hematocrit above 30%. With massive bleeding, consider transfusing typed-uncrossmatched blood.

C. Surgical consult. Essential in the management of upper GI tract hemorrhage; should be obtained within the first few hours of the patient's arrival. If hemodynamic stability cannot be achieved, surgical intervention is necessary.

D. Specific treatment. The management of various sources of upper GI hemorrhage is dependent on the diagnosis.

    1. Peptic ulcer disease. Pharmacologic therapy is ineffective in stopping bleeding or preventing rebleeding. All patients are started, however, on acid reduction therapy, which can include both antacids and H_2-receptor antagonists. Cimetidine (Tagamet) 300 mg IV Q 6 hr, ranitidine (Zantac) 50 mg IV Q 6–8 hr, or famotidine (Pepcid) 20 mg IV Q 12 hr is standard. H_2-receptor antagonists can be given as continuous drips. Omeprazole (Prilosec) 20–40 mg/d is effective in reducing the secretion of acid into the gastric lumen. Endoscopic therapies include thermal probe, electrocoagulation, and laser.

    2. Acute hemorrhagic gastritis or esophagitis. Acid reduction therapy. (See Section V.D.1.)

    3. Mallory-Weiss tear. No specific therapy beyond supportive care. Thermal or electric probes have been used successfully.

    4. Esophageal varices. Give octreotide 25 µg/hr. If octreotide fails, then balloon tamponade should be considered. Endoscopic therapies include injection sclerotherapy and band ligation.

    5. Aortoenteric fistula. Surgical intervention is necessary.

REFERENCES

Besson I, Ingrand P, Person B, et al: Sclerotherapy with and without octreotide for acute variceal bleeding. N Engl J Med;1995:555.

Friedman LS ed: Gastrointestinal Bleeding I. Gastroenterol Clin North Am 1993;717.

Peterson WL, Laine L: Gastrointestinal bleeding. In: Sleisenger MH, Fordtran JS eds.: *Gastrointestinal Disease: Pathophysiology/Diagnosis/Management.* 5th ed. Saunders;1993:162.

27. HEMATOCHEZIA

  I. Problem. A 38-year-old man comes to the emergency room and states "I have just passed a lot of blood from my bowels."

II. Immediate Questions

A. What are the patient's vital signs? Is there supine hypotension (indicates 30% volume loss)? Is there resting tachycardia (indicates 20% volume loss)? Are there orthostatic changes in pulse or blood pressure (indicates 10% volume loss)? If the patient has supine hypotension or resting tachycardia, then resuscitation must begin immediately.

B. Does the patient have IV line access? With no indication of hemodynamic instability, one 16–18-gauge IV with D5 NS at KVO is adequate. In the presence of hemodynamic compromise, two large-bore IVs should be in place.

C. Is there a history of previous gastrointestinal (GI) bleeding? Ask about a history of diseases associated with lower GI bleeding, such as diverticular disease, colon polyps or carcinoma, inflammatory bowel disease, hemorrhoids, and other anal diseases. Inquire about prior upper GI bleeding and also peptic ulcer disease (PUD).

D. What medications is the patient taking? Ask specifically about steroids, nonsteroidal anti-inflammatory drugs (NSAIDs), and anticoagulants.

E. Does the patient have a history of alcohol abuse? This suggests an upper GI source of bleeding such as varices or gastritis.

F. What is the most recent hematocrit? Obtain this information from the chart. This will establish the baseline value with which to compare future hematocrits.

G. What is the volume of bright red blood per rectum? Ask the nurse to save the specimen or specimens for your review. This is important for establishing the presence and volume of blood loss. A large volume of blood suggests need for immediate action.

H. Has there been hematemesis? Acute severe upper GI blood loss may result in hematochezia.

III. Differential Diagnosis

A. Hemorrhoids. These account for 98% of all episodes of hematochezia. Usually not brought to the attention of a physician. Rarely significant but may be of concern in the presence of portal hypertension.

B. Diverticular disease. Most common cause of significant lower GI bleeding. Causes up to 70% of significant lower GI bleeding.

C. Angiodysplasia. This condition is much more common in the elderly, causing approximately 10% of significant lower GI bleeding. Also seen in patients with renal failure.

D. Upper GI bleeding (See Section I, Chapter 26, Hematemesis, Melena, p 140). UGI sources are responsible for 5% of hematochezia. This type represents at least a two-unit bleed and is almost always associated with hemodynamic instability. *Always an indication for ICU monitoring.* Must be ruled out before surgery for hematochezia.

E. **Neoplasia including carcinoma and polyps.** Causes 1–2% of significant lower GI tract bleeding.
F. **Inflammatory bowel disease (IBD).** Infrequent cause of significant lower GI tract bleeding. Bleeding is more likely with ulcerative colitis than with Crohn's disease. Bleeding from IBD is more common in younger patients.
G. **Ischemic colitis.** Seen in elderly patients, often with previous history or signs of vascular disease, such as a history of surgery for peripheral vascular disease or an abdominal bruit or history of atrial fibrillation.

IV. Database

A. Physical examination key points

1. **Vital signs.** Including orthostatic blood pressure and heart rate. A decrease in systolic blood pressure of 10 mm Hg, or an increase in the heart rate by 20 bpm 1 minute after movement from a supine position to standing indicates volume depletion. May need to recheck frequently. An irregularly irregular pulse suggests ischemic colitis caused by emboli secondary to atrial fibrillation.
2. **Skin.** Telangiectasias or melanotic lesions on palms or soles suggest Osler-Weber-Rendu disease and Peutz-Jeghers syndrome, respectively. Look for peripheral stigmata of chronic liver disease and lesions associated with cancer (acanthosis nigricans, Kaposi's sarcoma).
3. **HEENT.** Vascular malformations on lips or buccal mucosa suggest angiodysplasia or Osler-Weber-Rendu disease. Scleral icterus suggests chronic liver disease.
4. **Heart.** Aortic stenosis is associated with angiodysplasia.
5. **Abdomen.** Bruits suggest ischemic colitis. Hyperactive bowel sounds may indicate blood in the upper GI tract. Check for masses (cancer) or tenderness (midepigastric area: PUD). Hepatomegaly and splenomegaly suggest portal hypertension (varices) or cancer.
6. **Rectum.** Check for hemorrhoids and to document blood in the rectal vault (melena, bright red blood, or guaiac-positive stools).

B. Laboratory data

1. **Nasogastric (NG) tube placement.** Obtain a quick aspirate for coffee-ground material (testing for occult blood confirms the presence of bleeding and should *not* be performed if coffee-ground material is not aspirated).
2. **Stat complete blood count; type and cross-match.** These can be done before you arrive if phlebotomy is available. Changes in the indices may also be helpful in differentiating acute from chronic bleeding.
3. **Serial hematocrits.** Can be spun without phlebotomy. Helpful but do not always reflect the amount of blood loss as equilibration with extravascular fluid may take several hours.

   4. **Type and cross-match.** At least four units of packed red blood cells (PRBCs).
   5. **BUN, creatinine.** An increased BUN/creatinine ratio is seen in upper GI bleeding or volume depletion.
   6. **PT, PTT, platelet count.** An elevated PT, PTT, or thrombocytopenia can interfere with stabilization of the patient. An elevated PT may be seen in chronic lever disease. Platelets and clotting factors decrease with brisk bleeding.
C. **Radiologic and other studies**
   1. **Anoscopy and flexible sigmoidoscopy.** Look for bleeding hemorrhoids. Frequently provides the diagnosis.
   2. **Nasogastric tube.** For gastric lavage. Should be done if the NG aspirate is positive for blood.
   3. **Upper GI endoscopy.** An upper GI source must be ruled out prior to surgery. In upper GI bleeds, 10% will have a negative nasogastric aspirate.
   4. **Technetium-labeled bleeding scan.** The next examination to be ordered if upper and lower endoscopy are normal. Can detect very slow bleeding (0.5 mL/min). Localization is only fair and needs to be documented with endoscopy or angiography.
   5. **Angiography.** Localization is very good but patients must be bleeding fairly rapidly (2 mL/min) to detect the source. Can also treat with selective intra-arterial infusion of pitressin.

V. **Plan**
   A. **Monitoring.** The primary question in managing bleeding patients is the necessity of ICU monitoring. The following are guidelines for admission to the ICU:
      1. Clearly documented frank hematochezia (> 100 mL).
      2. Coffee-ground emesis or positive NG aspirate and hematochezia.
      3. Any indication of hemodynamic instability (tachycardia, hypotension or orthostasis).
      4. Drop in hematocrit > five points after fluid resuscitation.
      5. Significant increase in BUN when GI bleeding is suspected.
   B. **Volume resuscitation.** If massive bleeding is evident, place two large-bore (14- or 16-gauge) peripheral or central lines. Begin IV fluids containing NS at a rate to maintain hemodynamic stability. With massive bleeding, transfuse packed red cells when available. Blood should be given to maintain a hematocrit above 30%.
   C. **Surgical consult.** Contact early in the management, especially if brisk bleeding is encountered.
   D. **Establish source of bleeding.** The source of bleeding must be identified in order to institute specific therapy.
      1. If bleeding is brisk: Start with NG aspirate. If positive, evaluate for upper GI source. If negative, proceed with anoscopy and flexible sigmoidoscopy. If sigmoidoscopy is negative and bleed-

ing remains brisk, proceed to bleeding scan and angiography. If all tests fail to reveal the site, and the bleeding remains brisk, then the patient will require laparotomy.
2. If the bleeding has stopped and the nasogastric aspirate is negative, proceed first with colonoscopy after prep. Colonoscopy is rarely helpful during brisk bleeding. If the colonoscopy is negative, do an upper GI endoscopy and then angiography. Remember, if at any point the patient becomes unstable and difficult to stabilize with IV fluids and blood, surgery is indicated.
3. The tempo of the evaluation is dictated by the rate of the patient's bleeding and overall stability.

REFERENCES

Friedman LS ed.: Gastrointestinal Bleeding II. Gastroenterol Clin North Am 1993;1.
Peterson WL, Laine L: Gastrointestinal bleeding. In: Sleisenger MH, Fordtran JS, eds. *Gastrointestinal Disease: Pathophysiology/Diagnosis/Management.* 5th ed. Saunders;1993:162.

28. HEMATURIA

I. **Problem.** A 51-year-old male patient has red blood cells noted on urinalysis 3 days after undergoing a total hip replacement.

II. **Immediate Questions**
A. **Is there a history of gross hematuria?** Microscopic hematuria may have been present for a long time without the patient's being aware of it, suggesting a chronic or acute process. Gross hematuria will not have gone unnoticed by the patient and likely represents an acute process.
B. **Does the patient have a Foley catheter in place?** Irritation of the bladder mucosa by a Foley catheter is a common cause of hematuria, as are trauma during placement and manipulation of the catheter by the patient. Other causes should be investigated if the hematuria does not completely clear after removal of the catheter.
C. **Has the patient had recent abdominal surgery?** This always raises the question of an inadvertently nicked ureter or kidney, and would usually be apparent the night of surgery.
D. **Does the patient have abdominal pain or fever?** Abdominal pain may suggest an inflammatory or infectious cause. Colicky pain radiating from the flank to the groin suggests a renal stone. Infection is often accompanied by fever.
E. **Has there been a significant change in urine output?** A sudden decrease in urine output may indicate acute oliguric renal failure, obstruction, or renal vein thrombosis. See Section I, Chapter 50, Oliguria/Anuria, p 244.

    F. Does the patient have symptoms suggestive of urinary tract infection? Dysuria, frequency, and urgency are common symptoms associated with cystitis.

    G. Is the patient taking anticoagulant medication? Anticoagulation therapy may cause hematuria by unmasking significant urinary tract pathology.

    H. Has the patient been treated with antineoplastic agents such as cyclophosphamide (Cytoxan)? These patients are at risk for developing hemorrhagic cystitis or secondary genitourinary tract tumors.

III. Differential Diagnosis

    A. Blood

        1. Coagulopathy. See Section I, Chapter 12, Coagulopathy, p 64. Inheritable defects such as hemophilia, severe liver dysfunction, and pharmacologic anticoagulation are potential etiologies.

        2. Hemoglobinopathy. Sickle cell disease with crisis is frequently associated with gross hematuria.

    B. Kidneys

        1. Glomerular disease

            a. Primary. Poststreptococcal glomerulonephritis, IgA nephropathy, Goodpasture's syndrome, idiopathic rapidly progressive glomerulonephritis. Characterized by red cell casts.

            b. Secondary. Vasculitis associated with systemic lupus erythematosus (SLE), scleroderma, Wegener's granulomatosis, polyarteritis, hypersensitivity vasculitis, subacute bacterial endocarditis.

            c. Hereditary. Alport's syndrome, associated with sensorineural hearing loss and ocular abnormalities.

        2. Interstitial disease

            a. Consequence of systemic diseases. Diabetic nephrosclerosis, accelerated hypertension, SLE.

            b. Consequence of pharmacologic therapy. Analgesic nephropathy, heavy metals, heroin nephropathy.

        3. Infections

            a. Pyelonephritis

            b. Tuberculosis. Characterized by sterile pyuria.

        4. Malformations

            a. Cystic. Familial polycystic kidney disease, ruptured solitary cysts, medullary sponge kidney.

            b. Vascular. Suggested by findings of hemangiomas or telangiectasias elsewhere.

        5. Neoplasms. Particularly renal cell carcinoma and more rarely transitional cell carcinoma.

        6. Ischemia

            a. Embolism. Aortic atherosclerosis, cardiac arrhythmias, manipulation of the aorta (aortography, coronary angiography).

        b. **Thrombosis.** Nephrotic syndrome, neoplastic disease, co-
agulation disorders (antithrombin III, protein C, or protein S
deficiencies).
   7. **Trauma**
  C. **Postrenal**
    1. **Mechanical**
      a. **Kidney stones.** Nephrolithiasis and urolithiasis.
      b. **Obstruction.** Prostatic hypertrophy, mass effect, posterior
urethral valves, retroperitoneal fibrosis, ureteropelvic junction abnormalities.
    2. **Inflammatory.** Infection or regional inflammation.
      a. **Periureteritis.** Diverticulitis, pelvic inflammatory disease.
      b. **Cystitis.** Infectious or inflammatory, such as cyclophos-
phamide-induced hematuria, which is a medical emergency.
      c. **Prostatitis**
      d. **Urethritis**
    3. **Neoplasm.** Transitional cell carcinoma, adenocarcinoma of the
prostate, squamous cell carcinoma of the penis.
    4. **Exercise.** Especially in marathon runners.
  D. **False hematuria**
    1. **Vaginal/rectal bleeding**
    2. **Factitious.** Most common in patients demonstrating drug-
seeking behavior and requesting narcotics for renal stones.

IV. **Database**
  A. **Physical examination key points**
    1. **Abdomen.** Examine for palpable masses indicative of tumors,
polycystic kidneys, or diverticular abscess. Tenderness will accompany infection, infarction, sickle cell crisis, inflammatory
processes, and obstruction.
    2. **Urethral meatus.** Look for gross blood, especially in trauma
patients, and evidence of recent instrumentation or superficial
lesions.
    3. **Rectum.** Critical in the trauma patient when a "free-floating"
prostate may be found, signifying urethral disruption. More commonly, prostatitis or prostatic carcinoma is uncovered. Attention
should also be given to possible hemorrhoids.
    4. **Pelvis.** Check for another source of bleeding such as vaginitis,
cervicitis, and menorrhagia.
    5. **Skin.** Ecchymoses, petechiae, and rash are suggestive of
vasculitis or a coagulation disorder.
  B. **Laboratory data**
    1. **Urinalysis.** Red cell casts are seen only with glomerulonephri-
tis. White blood cells or bacteria suggest an infectious cause;
WBC casts suggest pyelonephritis. Crystals may be seen in association with stones. Red discoloration without red cells should
suggest myoglobinuria; urine should be checked for myoglobin.

2. **Coagulation studies.** Prothrombin time, partial thromboplastin time, platelets.
3. **Hemogram.** An elevated WBC count will suggest an infectious or inflammatory process. Microcytic anemia may suggest chronic blood loss; however, hematuria is an unusual cause of microcytic anemia.
4. **Urine culture.** Rule out bacterial infection. Cultures for acid-fast bacilli should be done if there is pyuria and bacteria cultures are sterile (assuming the patient is not receiving antibiotics). An acid-fast stain may be helpful; however, some common saprophytes are acid-fast staining.
5. **BUN and creatinine.** To be used for baseline evaluation of renal function or to assess any change in renal function.
6. **Sickle cell screen.** Useful if the patient's status was previously unknown and this is being entertained as a cause of the patient's hematuria.
7. **Urinary cytology.** May diagnose transitional cell carcinoma.

C. **Radiologic and other studies**
   1. **Abdominal plain x-ray (kidney/ureter/bladder [KUB]).** 80% of urinary calculi are radiodense. Also, the KUB may show an inflammatory process (ileus or loss of psoas shadow).
   2. **Excretory urography (IV pyelography).** A part of the evaluation in all patients without an active infection who can receive IV contrast without undue risk.
   3. **Retrograde urethrogram/cystogram.** Second-line study to be used in cases in which tumor, vesicoureteral reflux, posterior urethral valves, or traumatic disruption are suspected.
   4. **Further studies.** Should be directed by clinical suspicion and the results of initial studies. Further studies may include a CT scan of the abdomen, ultrasound, angiography, cystoscopy and renal biopsy. With normal renal imaging, patients with hematuria > 45 years of age should have cystoscopy and if normal a renal biopsy. If < 45 years of age and renal imaging is normal, a renal biopsy should be done without prior cystoscopy.

V. **Plan.** Treatment depends on the etiology. Keep in mind that apart from trauma, severe coagulopathy, and cyclophosphamide-induced hematuria, the causes of hematuria are rarely emergencies; a thoughtful and careful evaluation can therefore be pursued over a period of several days.
   A. **Urinary tract infection.** See Section I, Chapter 19, Dysuria, Section V, p 106. The infection must be eradicated and a repeat urinalysis performed to rule out continued hematuria. If hematuria persists, further evaluation is necessary.
   B. **Urolithiasis.** If the stone is expected to pass spontaneously and there are no complicating factors (infection, obstruction), expectant

therapy with analgesics and hydration is appropriate. The urine should be strained.

C. Neoplasms. Further workup is dictated by the type and location.

D. Tuberculosis. Treat appropriately with antibiotics. Initial therapy is usually with isoniazid (INH) 300 mg PO Q day, rifampin 600 mg PO Q day, and pyrazinamide 15–30 mg/kg with a maximum dose of 2 g Q day and ethambutol 15–25 mg/kg. A four-drug regimen is recommended by the American Thoracic Society and the Centers for Disease Control until the results of drug susceptibility studies are available; or unless there is < 4% primary resistance to INH within the community. If so, an initial three-drug regimen is recommended. Long-term follow-up with IV pyelograms is necessary, as strictures are late sequelae and can lead to obstruction.

E. Collecting system abnormality. Usually requires surgical referral and repair.

F. Coagulopathy. Correct clotting factor deficiencies or adjust anticoagulant dose. Frequently the coagulopathy will induce bleeding from a preexisting abnormality. A thorough evaluation is usually indicated in a patient who has hematuria and a coagulopathy.

G. Glomerulonephritis. Most cases require a biopsy for definitive diagnosis, with therapy as appropriate for the underlying illness.

H. Hemorrhagic cystitis. Treat with continuous saline irrigation and occasionally a 1% alum irrigation.

REFERENCES

Copley JB: Isolated asymptomatic hematuria in the adult. Am J Med Sci 1986;291:101.

Topham PS, Harper SJ, Furness PN et al: Glomerular disease as a cause of isolated microscopic haematuria. Q J Med 1994;87:329.

29. HEMOPTYSIS

I. Problem. A 60-year-old male smoker comes to the emergency room complaining of "spitting up blood" for 1 week.

II. Immediate Questions

A. Is the patient truly experiencing hemoptysis? Blood from a nasal, oral, or gastric source may be aspirated to the larynx and then expectorated.

B. What is the volume of the hemoptysis? Massive hemoptysis (>600 mL/24 h) connotes a life-threatening problem that demands immediate ICU admission as well as a rapid diagnostic evaluation.

C. Has this happened before? If so, how frequently? Patients with recurrent acute bronchitis or with mitral stenosis may have had multiple episodes of minor hemoptysis.

D. **What is the smoking history?** The higher the pack-years, the more likely the patient has chronic bronchitis and/or bronchogenic carcinoma.

E. **Is there a history of productive cough preceding the hemoptysis?** If the answer is yes, then the problem may be an infection such as acute bronchitis.

F. **Has there been any accompanying chest pain?** Pleuritic chest pain may be a symptom of pneumonia or a pulmonary embolism with infarction. Hemoptysis may accompany pulmonary edema from any number of causes.

III. Differential Diagnosis

A. Pulmonary sources

1. **Infection**

    a. **Acute or chronic bronchitis.** Most common cause of hemoptysis.

    b. **Pneumonia.** A necrotizing gram-negative or staphylococcal pneumonia are the usual types of pneumonia to have associated hemoptysis. Symptoms are acute.

    c. **Lung abscess.** Often produces foul-smelling sputum.

    d. **Bronchiectasis.** Think of this in the patient who has had recurrent episodes of respiratory infections, voluminous sputum production, and intermittent hemoptysis.

    e. **Tuberculosis.** Usually apical infiltrates on chest x-ray. Symptoms often chronic or subacute.

    f. **Mycetoma (fungus ball).** A ball of *Aspergillus* fungus may form in a previously formed cavity. Look for the "crescent sign" on the CXR.

2. **Neoplasm**

    a. **Bronchogenic carcinoma.** Usually the CXR is abnormal; but it may be normal in up to 13% of patients with early lung cancer and hemoptysis. You cannot afford to miss it!

    b. **Bronchial adenoma**

    c. **Metastatic disease.** A history of preceding cancers should be uncovered during the history and physical. The CXR will be abnormal.

3. **Vascular**

    a. **Pulmonary embolism (PE) with infarction.** Only 10% of PEs present with hemoptysis; but pulmonary emboli are very common and must not be missed.

    b. **Mitral stenosis.** May arise either from rupture of the pulmonary veins or from frank pulmonary edema.

    c. **Cardiogenic pulmonary edema.** Surprisingly common, especially now that most cardiac patients are on some form of anticoagulation.

    d. **Arteriovenous malformation**

  B. Trauma
  1. **Pulmonary contusion**
  2. **Bronchial or vascular tear**
  3. **Retained foreign body.** Teeth and fillings sometimes find their way down into the bronchi.
  C. Systemic diseases
  1. **Anticoagulation**
     a. **Drugs.** Warfarin (Coumadin), heparin, aspirin, streptokinase (Streptase), urokinase (Abbokinase), tissue plasminogen activator (TPA), and APSAC (anisoylated plasminogen streptokinase activator complex (anistreplase, Eminase).
     b. **Uremia**
     c. **Thrombocytopenia.** Drugs, idiopathic thrombocytopenic purpura, cancer.
     d. **Disseminated intravascular coagulation (DIC)**
     e. **Liver disease.** Severe liver disease can result in thrombocytopenia, and also a decreased production of coagulation factors.
  2. **Autoimmune diseases**
     a. **Wegener's granulomatosis.** Look for renal changes (red cell casts, hematuria, proteinuria) and/or sinus disease. The CXR often is abnormal. Bilateral nodular densities and cavitation are common.
     b. **Goodpasture's syndrome.** This disease also involves the kidney. Proteinuria, hematuria, and red cell casts may be present. Diffuse alveolar infiltrates are often present.
     c. **Systemic lupus erythematosus (SLE).** Lupus more frequently involves the pleura; but patients may develop life-threatening hemoptysis from lupus pneumonitis.

IV. Database
  A. Physical examination key points
  1. **Vital signs.** Imperative! Look particularly for fever and signs of impending respiratory failure: breath rate above 30 per minute, abdominal paradox with inspiration, accessory muscle use.
  2. **HEENT.** Look carefully for a nasal or oropharyngeal source of bleeding.
  3. **Chest.** Inspect and palpate for signs of trauma such as rib or clavicle fractures. Listen carefully for a pleural rub, localized rales, or signs of consolidation.
  4. **Heart.** An irregularly irregular pulse signifies atrial fibrillation and suggests mitral stenosis as a possible source of emboli. An S_3 and jugular venous distension suggest congestive heart failure as a possible etiology. Always listen carefully for the low diastolic rumble of mitral stenosis at the apex with the bell.

    5. **Abdomen.** Palpate the epigastrium, liver, and spleen carefully. Peptic ulcer disease or alcoholic liver disease could certainly cause GI bleeding, which might mimic hemoptysis.

    6. **Extremities.** Examine lower extremities carefully for signs of deep venous thromboses or edema. Look carefully for cyanosis and clubbing. Clubbed fingers associated with hemoptysis would generally implicate either bronchiectasis or a pulmonary neoplasm.

    7. **Skin.** Inspect the skin for petechiae, ecchymoses, angiomata, and rashes.

B. Laboratory data

    1. **Complete blood count.** May reveal an anemia which could be caused by the hemoptysis or, more likely, is related to the hemoptysis. A normocytic anemia with a normal or low reticulocyte count may represent anemia of chronic disease possibly related to cancer. An elevated reticulocyte count indicates a hemolytic anemia possibly secondary to SLE. An iron deficiency may indicate Goodpasture's syndrome.

    2. **Platelet count, prothrombin time, and partial thromboplastin time.** All are indicated to rule out coagulopathy as a cause. See Section I, Chapter 12, Coagulopathy, p 64. If platelet dysfunction is suspected, a bleeding time will be prolonged in the presence of a normal platelet count.

    3. **BUN, creatinine, and urinalysis.** For rapid evaluation of "pulmonary-renal" syndromes (Goodpasture's syndrome, Wegener's granulomatosis, SLE, and vasculitis).

    4. **Arterial blood gases.** Check for adequate ventilation and oxygenation. Most of these patients already have underlying pulmonary disease and may develop respiratory failure at the time of their hemoptysis.

    5. **Sputum examination.** Gram's stain, acid-fast bacillus stain and culture, and cytology are all imperative.

    6. **PPD skin test.** To help rule out tuberculosis and evaluate immune function.

C. Radiologic and other studies

    1. **Chest x-ray.** First and most important test after the history and physical. The pattern and location of any infiltrate, coupled with the history and physical examination, will dictate the remainder of your workup.

    2. **Ventilation/perfusion ($\dot{V}/\dot{Q}$) lung scan.** If pulmonary embolism is highly suspected, a $\dot{V}/\dot{Q}$ scan must be done.

    3. **Angiography.** If pulmonary embolism is suspected and $\dot{V}/\dot{Q}$ scans are not clearly positive or negative, then pulmonary angiography is indicated. Angiography may also be indicated for the diagnosis of pulmonary arteriovenous malformations.

4. **Chest computerized tomography scan.** This will provide a much better anatomic view of pulmonary pathology compared with chest radiographs and will also reveal lesions not seen previously; however, the CT scan is only indicated acutely when looking for an aortic dissection.

5. **Electrocardiogram.** May show atrial fibrillation. An axis change and/or right bundle branch block may suggest a PE. Classically, a PE produces an S wave in lead I, and a Q wave and inverted T wave in lead III ($S_1.Q_3T_3$).

6. **Bronchoscopy.** Patients with unclear sources of hemoptysis, massive hemoptysis, or the suspicion of a neoplasm require fiberoptic bronchoscopy. The earlier it is done, the more likely the source of bleeding will be identified.

V. Plan

A. **Intensive care unit**
   1. **Massive hemoptysis**
   2. **Present or pending hypoxemic or hypercarbic respiratory failure**

B. **Establish IV access.** Death comes from asphyxia rather than hemorrhage, but IV medications will be needed.

C. **Always protect the airway.** This may require early intubation.

D. **Correct any coagulopathy** (See Section I, Chapter 12, Coagulopathy, p 67).

E. **Fiberoptic bronchoscopy.** Arrange for this early if the diagnosis is in doubt or hemoptysis continues.

F. **Consult.** Obtain a thoracic surgery consultation if the patient has massive or continuous hemoptysis. Medical management of massive hemoptysis is associated with a high mortality rate.

G. **Cough suppression.** Retard the cough reflex with codeine-based drugs, and place the patient on quiet bedrest.

H. **Treat the underlying disease state**
   1. Lung cancer can be treated surgically if there are no metastases and the pulmonary reserve is adequate. Otherwise, radiation or laser therapy can rapidly control bleeding.
   2. Treat infections with antibiotics as dictated by Gram's stain and clinical picture.
   3. Treat pulmonary emboli acutely with heparin. See Section I, Chapter 11, Chest Pain, V, p 63.
   4. If diffuse alveolar hemorrhage or a pulmonary-renal syndrome is suspected, 1000 mg methylprednisolone (Solu-Medrol) IV may control bleeding, pending definitive work-up.

REFERENCE

Cahil BC, Ingbar DH: Massive hemoptysis—assessment and management in clinics. Clin Chest Med 1994;15:147.

30. HYPERCALCEMIA

I. **Problem.** A 60-year-old man is admitted for severe back pain and is found to have a calcium of 5.5 mEq/L or 2.75 mmol/L (normal: 4.2–5.1 mEq/L or 2.10–2.55 mmol/L).

II. **Immediate Questions**
   A. **What other symptoms are present?** The classic presentation of primary hyperparathyroidism is "stones, bones, moans, and groans" from renal calculi, osteitis fibrosa, constipation, and neuropsychiatric problems, respectively. Renal calculi and osteitis fibrosa are seldom associated with hypercalcemia of malignancy because both result from long-standing hypercalcemia. Hypercalcemia causes a variety of nonspecific symptoms including polyuria, polydypsia, constipation, nausea, vomiting, anorexia, and mental status changes which can range from confusion to coma. There may also be associated bone pain.
   B. **Does the patient have any condition that could be related to hypercalcemia?** Hypertension, peptic ulcer, and nephrolithiasis are associated with hyperparathyroidism.
   C. **Is the patient on any medications that might cause hypercalcemia?** Thiazide diuretics, vitamin D, and exogenous sources of calcium are possible causes.
   D. **Is there a family history of hypercalcemia?** An unusual cause is familial hypocalciuric hypercalcemia. There are also three syndromes of multiple endocrine neoplasia (MEN) that are inherited in an autosomal dominant pattern. MEN I includes primary hyperparathyroidism and hypersecretion of pancreatic islet hormones and possibly other endocrine tumors. MEN II consists of primary hyperparathyroidism and medullary carcinoma of the thyroid. MEN III includes features of MEN II together with pheochromocytoma.
   E. **Has the patient been noted to have elevated calcium in the past?** Long-standing hypercalcemia suggests primary hyperparathyroidism. Recent-onset hypercalcemia suggests another condition such as malignant disease.

III. **Differential Diagnosis**
   A. **Primary hyperparathyroidism.** About 20% of patients with hypercalcemia suffer from hyperparathyroidism, usually from a single hyperfunctioning adenoma. An elevated calcium, a low phosphate, and elevated or relatively elevated parathyroid hormone are characteristic findings.
   B. **Malignant disease.** From bony metastasis or more often from humoral factors produced by a tumor.

    1. **Metastatic carcinoma to bone.** Breast, lung, and renal cell carcinoma.

    2. **Hematologic malignancies.** Direct bone involvement with multiple myeloma and lymphoma.

    3. **Humoral factors.** Prostaglandins, parathyroid hormone-related protein, and osteoclast-activating factor (OAF). These factors are most commonly seen with squamous cell, renal cell, and transitional cell carcinomas, lymphomas, and multiple myelomas.

C. Medications

    1. **Thiazide diuretics.** These agents increase renal reabsorption of calcium.

    2. **Vitamin D intoxication.** A fat-soluble vitamin that increases intestinal absorption, increases mobilization from bone, and increases renal reabsorption of calcium.

    3. **Vitamin A intoxication.** Another fat-soluble vitamin that is a rare cause of hypercalcemia; causes increased bone reabsorption.

    4. **Exogenous calcium.** Eg, calcium carbonate which is found in certain antacids.

D. Granulomatous diseases—Sarcoidosis. These conditions are marked by increased sensitivity to vitamin D.

E. Milk-alkali syndrome. From increased intake of calcium and alkali. Results in hypercalcemia, hypocalciuria, hyperphosphatemia, renal failure, and metastatic calcifications.

F. Immobilization. Prolonged bed rest increases bone reabsorption resulting in hypercalcemia and osteoporosis.

G. Recovery from acute renal failure. Thought to be from secondary hyperparathyroidism.

H. Endocrinopathies

    1. **Hyperthyroidism.** Bone reabsorption induced by thyroid hormone.

    2. **Acromegaly**

    3. **Adrenal insufficiency**

 I. Paget's disease. Calcium level is usually normal but may increase with immobilization.

IV. Database

A. Physical examination key points

    1. **Vital signs.** There may be associated hypertension.

    2. **Skin.** Excoriations may occur as a result of pruritus from metastatic calcifications in the skin.

    3. **Lymph nodes.** Lymphadenopathy suggests carcinoma, hematologic malignancy, or sarcoidosis.

    4. **HEENT.** An enlarged thyroid gland suggests hyperthyroidism.

    5. **Chest.** Look for evidence of lung carcinoma.

6. **Abdomen.** An enlarged liver or spleen suggests metastatic carcinoma, a hematologic cancer, or sarcoidosis.
7. **Musculoskeletal exam.** Bone pain with palpation or percussion points to carcinoma or Paget's disease. Myopathy from hypercalcemia can cause proximal muscle weakness.
8. **Neurologic exam.** Impaired mentation, weakness, and hyper-reflexia may result from hypercalcemia.

B. **Laboratory data**
1. **Repeat calcium along with a serum albumin or obtain an ionized calcium.** Always confirm an elevated calcium and the severity of the hypercalcemia before initiating therapy. Keep in mind that a high normal total calcium may also signify hypercalcemia in the presence of marked hypoalbuminemia. A calcium value must be corrected in the presence of hypoalbuminemia. Normally, the total calcium decreases by 0.2 mmol/L or 0.4 mEq/L for every 1 g/dL decrease in the serum albumin from normal (4.0 g/deciliter) without changing the ionized calcium level. Symptoms usually develop at 6.5–7.0 mEq/L or 3.25–3.5 mmol/L.
2. **Phosphorus.** The phosphorus level is low in primary hyperparathyroidism; it is elevated in vitamin D intoxication.
3. **Arterial blood gases.** A decrease in the pH will increase the ionized calcium mostly by displacing calcium bound to albumin. A metabolic acidosis may also be seen with adrenal insufficiency, a potential cause of hypercalcemia. An increase in the pH is seen in milk-alkali syndrome and possibly with thiazide diuretics if there is associated volume depletion.
4. **Alkaline phosphatase.** This value is increased in primary hyperparathyroidism with bone disease and in Paget's disease, and may be increased with bony metastases.
5. **BUN and creatinine.** Renal insufficiency will exacerbate hypercalcemia or may be secondary to hypercalcemia.
6. **Total protein and albumin.** An increased total protein-to-albumin ratio suggests multiple myeloma. If there is an elevated total protein-to-albumin ratio, then quantitative immunoglobulins and serum and urine protein electrophoresis should be ordered.
7. **Amylase and lipase.** Hypercalcemia can cause pancreatitis. If abdominal pain is present pancreatitis should be ruled out.
8. **Urinalysis.** Hematuria may arise from renal cell carcinoma or secondary to nephrolithiasis.

C. **Radiologic and other studies**
1. **Chest x-ray.** Bilateral hilar adenopathy implies sarcoidosis. Also, carcinoma or lymphoma may be detected by CXR. Osteopenia of the vertebral column may be evident on the lateral film.
2. **Abdominal x-rays.** May reveal renal calcifications as a result of hypercalcemia; other findings may suggest carcinoma.

3. **Bone films.** These are especially useful if there is localized bone pain; they may reveal osteolytic lesions from carcinoma or multiple myeloma. If present, a bone scan would be helpful to reveal extent of the disease. A bone scan will be negative with multiple myeloma because of the absence of associated osteoblastic activity.

4. **Skull films and skeletal survey.** Obtain if multiple myeloma is suspected. Classically reveals multiple punched-out lesions. May also be helpful in detecting subperiosteal resorption resulting from primary hyperparathyroidism, especially evident on hand films.

5. **Electrocardiogram.** Associated shortening of QT interval and lengthening of PR interval.

V. **Plan.** Lower the calcium level and then treat the underlying disorder. Treat more aggressively with severe hypercalcemia > 7.0 mEq/L or 3.5 mmol/L or when symptomatic. Treatment is directed at decreasing the release of calcium from bone or increasing deposition in bone, decreasing absorption from the gastrointestinal tract, and increasing excretion renally or through chelation.

A. **Restrict calcium intake and encourage mobilization**

B. **Treat underlying causes**

C. **Institute saline diuresis.** Patients with moderate to severe symptomatic hypercalcemia are frequently volume-depleted. It is essential to restore the patient's volume and then to maintain a urine output of at least 2 L/d. Sodium increases calcium excretion by inhibiting proximal tubule reabsorption. Administration of large volumes of normal saline can be hazardous in the elderly or in patients with renal failure or with left ventricular dysfunction.

D. **Administer medications**

1. **Furosemide (Lasix).** Dosage is 20–80 mg IV every 2–4 hours. Furosemide is a calciuric agent; however, calcium excretion is not promoted if volume depletion develops. You must follow urinary output closely as well as monitor the volume of normal saline administered and daily weights. Older patients with tenuous cardiac conditions may need hemodynamic monitoring in an ICU if vigorous saline diuresis is attempted. *Caution:* Thiazide diuretics should *never* be used because they may actually worsen the hypercalcemia through enhanced distal tubular reabsorption of calcium.

2. **Plicamycin (Mithramycin).** Give 25 μg/kg in 1 L of normal saline over 3–6 hours. This agent inhibits bone reabsorption; effect may not manifest for 12–24 hours. The dose can be repeated at 24–48 hours for 3–4 total doses. Nausea and renal, hepatic, and bone marrow toxicity (thrombocytopenia) can occur.

3. **Calcitonin.** This agent is rapid-acting, but weak; it inhibits bone reabsorption and increases urinary excretion of calcium. Usually only a temporary measure as resistance to the calcium-lowering effect often develops. An effective dose is 4–8 units every 6–12 hours, given SC, IM, or IV.

4. **Corticosteroids.** Hydrocortisone 50–75 mg every 6 hours decreases calcium absorption from the GI tract and inhibits bone reabsorption. Also may inhibit growth of lymphoid cancers. Effective for treating hypercalcemia associated with sarcoidosis, vitamin D intoxication, and hematologic cancers (multiple myeloma, lymphoma, leukemia).

5. **Diphosphonates.** These agents inhibit osteoclastic activity. Pamidronate disodium (Aredia) is superior to etidronate (Didronel), the first drug in this class approved to treat hypercalcemia. Pamidronate 15–90 mg is given intravenously over 24 hours, and the lower dosing range (15–45mg/day) can be repeated daily up to 6 days. Hypokalemia, hypomagnesemia, and hypophosphatemia can occur.

6. **Gallium nitrate.** This agent inhibits bone resorption; it can be used to treat hypercalcemia secondary to malignancy. The dose is 200 mg/m^2 continuous infusion via 1 liter of fluid daily for 5 days. Because of its potential nephrotoxicity, gallium nitrate should not be a first-line drug to treat hypercalcemia; it should not be given to patients with renal insufficiency. Concurrent use of other nephrotoxic agents such as aminoglycosides should be avoided; administration in the presence of hypovolemia should also be avoided.

7. **Indomethacin (Indocin).** Dosage is 50 mg PO three times daily. Variable response in treating hypercalcemia of malignancy. Works by inhibiting bone reabsorption caused by prostaglandins.

8. **Intravenous phosphates.** These drugs work by increasing deposition of calcium in bone and soft tissues and decreasing bone reabsorption. Can result in metastatic calcification, renal failure, and death. Their use is contraindicated in patients with renal insufficiency. Should be reserved for life-threatening hypercalcemia resistant to other measures.

E. **Dialysis.** This is a treatment of last resort.

REFERENCES

Bilezikian JP: Management of acute hypercalcemia. N Engl J Med 1992;326:1196.

Edelson GW, Kleerekoper M: Hypercalcemic crisis. In Ober KP, ed. Endocrine Emergencies. WB Saunders Company, Philadelphia; Med Clin North Am 1995;79:79.

Lobaugh B, Drezner MK: Evaluation of hypercalcemia and hypocalcemia. In: Kelly WN, ed-in-chief. *Textbook of Internal Medicine.* 2nd ed. Lippincott; 1992:2115.

Popovtzer MM, Knochel JP, Kumar R: Disorders of calcium, phosphorus, vitamin D and parathyroid hormone activity. In: Schrier RW ed. *Renal and Electrolyte Disorders.* 4th ed. Little, Brown; 1992:287.

31. HYPERGLYCEMIA

I. **Problem.** A 44-year-old man is admitted because of chest pain. His glucose is 428 mg/dL or 23.79 mmol/L.

II. **Immediate Questions**
   A. **What are the patient's vital signs?** Fever may indicate sepsis, which can exacerbate hyperglycemia. Hypotension or tachycardia may indicate volume depletion common in diabetic ketoacidosis (DKA) and hyperosmolar states. Tachypnea may be due to Kussmaul respirations in DKA.
   B. **Is the patient known to be diabetic?** A history of diabetes should make the clinician consider factors such as noncompliance with medication/diet, sepsis, acute stress, glucocorticoid use, and myocardial infarction (MI), which can result in poor control of hyperglycemia. The absence of a prior history of diabetes should make one consider all of the preceding factors as unmasking latent carbohydrate intolerance, as well as the possibility of laboratory error.
   C. **If the patient is diabetic, what medications is s/he taking and when was the last meal in relation to the time of phlebotomy?** Before modifying the regimen it is important to know whether the patient is receiving large or small amounts of insulin, or whether s/he is receiving oral hypoglycemic agents. In addition, it is important to know whether the blood sugar was drawn randomly (and therefore could be postprandial) or whether it represents a fasting level.

III. **Differential Diagnosis**
   A. **Diabetes mellitus**
      1. **Type I (previously called juvenile diabetes or insulin-dependent diabetes).** Type I diabetics require insulin even when not eating (NPO), although in lower doses. They are more likely to be thin or normal in weight, young, and "brittle," and are prone to DKA. Diabetic ketoacidosis may be defined as a blood sugar > 300 mg/dL (16.68 mmol/L), urine ketones that are strongly positive, and a serum bicarbonate < 17 mmol or a pH ≤ 7.30.
      2. **Type II (previously called adult-onset diabetes or non-insulin-dependent diabetes mellitus).** Type II diabetics tend to be obese and older, and are more prone to hyperosmolar states than ketoacidosis. In ideal settings (on a metabolic unit), many of these patients can be managed with diet alone. Weight loss may normalize carbohydrate metabolism; however, in reality a majority of patients require oral hypoglycemic drugs or insulin for adequate control.

    3. **Gestational diabetes.** Glucose intolerance associated with pregnancy. Close monitoring and tight control are important to improve outcome of mother and infant.

B. Acute stress. In patients with mild carbohydrate intolerance, acute events such as sepsis, MI, trauma, and surgery may cause relatively marked hyperglycemia. Some of these patients will not require therapy once the acute event has resolved.

C. Exogenous glucose load. Hyperalimentation and peritoneal dialysis.

D. Glucocorticoids. Either exogenous or endogenous (Cushing's syndrome).

E. Pancreatic disease. Severe acute pancreatitis or long-standing chronic pancreatitis with endocrine pancreatic insufficiency.

F. Spurious hyperglycemia. Drawing blood above an IV line that contains dextrose; mislabeling; or inadvertently switching blood from different patients. When in doubt, immediately repeat the test before treating.

IV. Database

A. Physical examination key points

    1. **Vital signs.** Include orthostatic blood pressure and pulse to evaluate volume status. A decrease in systolic blood pressure of 10 mm Hg and/or an increase in heart rate of 20 bpm indicates volume depletion when going from a supine position to standing after one minute. Fever implies sepsis. Kussmaul respirations (deep, regular respirations whether slow or fast) suggest DKA.

    2. **HEENT.** Fruity odor on breath suggests ketones and DKA. Fundoscopic exam may show diabetic retinopathy, which suggests long-standing disease and increases the likelihood of other diabetic complications such as nephropathy and neuropathy.

    3. **Lungs.** Evaluate for signs of pneumonia.

    4. **Heart.** Listen for associated findings of ischemia/MI such as a third (S_3) or fourth (S_4) heart sound, or murmur of mitral insufficiency.

    5. **Peripheral vascular system.** Listen for bruits.

    6. **Abdomen.** Evaluate for cause of sepsis. Rebound tenderness suggests peritonitis. A positive Murphy's sign (see Section I, Chapter 1, Abdominal Pain, p 1) suggests acute cholecystitis, which is more common in diabetics.

    7. **Extremities.** Check for diabetic foot ulcers and cellulitis.

    8. **Neurologic exam.** A clouded sensorium suggests more severe disease (ketoacidosis or hyperosmolar state).

B. Laboratory data

    1. **Serum glucose.** Significantly elevated fingerstick glucoses should be evaluated with a serum glucose determination.

2. **CBC.** Leukocytosis with a left shift suggests the presence of infection. An elevated WBC count may be seen in DKA without an associated infection or sepsis, but a left shift, toxic granulation, and vacuolization should be absent.

3. **Serum electrolytes, BUN and creatinine, phosphorus, calcium, magnesium, amylase.**

   a. Even though serum potassium may be normal, total body potassium is often depleted and potassium repletion is indicated. An initially normal or elevated potassium will decrease with insulin administration and with correction of acidosis if present.

   b. Serum sodium is spuriously lowered by 1.6 mmol/L for each 100 mg/dL (5.56 mmol/L) rise in glucose concentration.

   c. Serum bicarbonate is low and the anion gap is elevated in DKA.

   d. Creatinine may be falsely elevated in the presence of serum ketones. Both BUN and creatinine may be elevated as a result of profound volume depletion or diabetic nephropathy.

   e. Phosphate may fall with treatment and should be monitored, although routine prophylactic treatment with phosphate is not recommended.

   f. Calcium may be low with acute pancreatitis.

   g. Magnesium may be low, especially in DKA. Magnesium deficiency may contribute to relative insulin resistance.

   h. An elevated amylase may indicate pancreatitis, but ketone bodies may factitiously elevate the serum amylase.

4. **Arterial blood gases.** To evaluate the degree of acidemia. A careful look at the pH, pCO_2, and serum bicarbonate often reveals more than one acid-base disorder. (See Section I, Chapter 2, Acidosis, p 9, and Section I, Chapter 3, Alkalosis, p 17)

5. **Urine or serum for ketones.** This helps to distinguish between DKA and hyperosmolar coma. Acetoacetate is the ketone that is measured on standard tests; however, β-hydroxybutyrate is the predominant ketone in DKA. Initially, the level of ketones may not decrease or may actually increase as β-hydroxybutyrate is metabolized to acetoacetate.

6. **Cultures.** If sepsis is suspected, then appropriate cultures should be ordered.

C. **Radiologic and other studies**

1. **Chest x-ray.** To evaluate for pneumonia and CHF.

2. **Electrocardiogram.** To rule out MI as a cause of recent onset of difficult-to-control diabetes.

3. **Miscellaneous studies.** Depending on clinical suspicion; for example, CT of the abdomen if intra-abdominal abscess is suspected.

V. Plan. Management depends on the clinical setting and severity of hyperglycemia. This section is divided into three parts on the basis of severity.

   A. Type II diabetes with a serum glucose < 450 mg/dL or 25.0 mmol/L (no ketones, no acidosis, and probably asymptomatic)
   1. **Insulin.** May increase usual dose of intermediate-acting insulin plus short-acting insulin Q 6 hr based on results of fingerstick glucoses. For a typical regimen, see Table 1–6.
   2. **Oral hypoglycemic agents.** Some patients with type II diabetes mellitus may be managed with oral hypoglycemic agents, especially those whose glucose is below 300 mg/dL (16.68 mmol/L).
   3. **Diet.** In the short term, an 1800-calorie American Diabetes Association (ADA) diet is useful although other modified diets may be appropriate in certain settings. The importance of diet is controversial. A nutritious diet low in simple sugars and fat will usually suffice. If there is a complicating condition such as a foot ulcer that requires positive nitrogen balance for resolution, be sure the patient receives adequate calories and protein.
   B. Hyperosmolar, hyperglycemic nonketotic coma
   1. **Glucose < 600 mg/dL or 33.35 mmol/L (no ketones, no acidosis).** More aggressive management is indicated, often in the ICU.
   2. **Saline**
      a. Depending on the degree of volume depletion, 500–1000 mL of NS is given in the first hour, after which the rate is decreased to 250–500 mL/h until signs of volume depletion resolve. Obviously, caution is indicated, particularly in smaller or older individuals or those with limited cardiac and renal reserve. These patients need frequent (every 1–2 hours) assessment of volume status with orthostatic blood pressure and pulse, heart exam for S_3, and lung exam for rales. Some patients will need monitoring with a pulmonary artery catheter for optimal fluid management.

TABLE 1–6. SLIDING SCALE OF INSULIN DOSAGE FOR HYPERGLYCEMIA.

Glucose Level	Insulin (Short-Acting/Regular)
<180 mg/dL (10.00 mmol/L)	0 U SC
180–240 mg/dL (10.00–13.34 mmol/L)	3–5 U SC
240–400 mg/dL (13.34–22.23 mmol/L)	8–10 U SC
>400 mg/dL (>22.23 mmol/L)	10–15 U SC[1]

[1] Follow with a stat serum glucose and notify the house officer of result.
SC = subcutaneous.

    b. Some authors prefer switching from NS to half-normal saline after the first liter, or alternating half-normal saline with NS. When the blood sugar reaches 250–300 mg/dL (13.90–16.68 mmol/L), then IV fluids are switched to D5 half-normal saline at a rate based on volume assessment.

  3. Potassium. If serum potassium is < 5.5 mmol/L, add 20–30 mmol/L at a rate not to exceed 10–15 mmol/h. Follow levels Q 4 hr. Keep potassium at 4.0–5.0 mmol/L.

  4. Insulin. There are many ways of giving insulin. Continuous IV infusion drip of short-acting insulin is preferred. An initial dose of 0.15 U/kg of a short-acting insulin is given as a bolus and is followed immediately by a continuous infusion drip at 0.1 U/kg/h. This should be adjusted to ensure that blood glucose is falling at least 10% per hour.

  5. Lab work. Serum glucose measurements are needed Q 1–2 hr. Magnesium should be checked initially and repeated if there are signs of magnesium deficiency. Potassium should be checked Q 4–6 hr, and phosphorus Q 6–12 hr.

  6. When glucose falls to the range 250–300 mg/dL (13.89–16.68 mmol/L), then the insulin drip may need to be decreased and the IV fluids changed to D5 half-normal saline, with the goal of maintaining the glucose at 100–200 mg/dL (5.56–11.12 mmol/L).

C. Diabetic ketoacidosis. This is a medical emergency, often requiring management in the ICU setting. In the setting of profound ketoacidosis, patients are less responsive to insulin and larger doses are required. Volume repletion is essential.

  1. IV fluids. One liter of NS in the first hour followed by 200 mL to 1 L per hour until volume status improves. The same volume assessment parameters should be followed as in hyperosmolar coma described earlier. Some authors prefer switching or alternating half-normal saline with NS. When serum glucose levels reach 250–300 mg/dL (13.89–16.68 mmol/L), change to D5 half-normal saline at a rate based on volume assessment. Some cases may require a pulmonary artery catheter for appropriate fluid management.

  2. Insulin. A continuous infusion drip is initiated by a bolus of 0.2 U/kg of a short-acting insulin initially and is followed by 0.1 U/kg/h as described earlier. If the serum glucose falls by < 10% in the first hour, then the rate is doubled and a repeat bolus of 0.2 U/kg is given. Repeat IV boluses are given Q 1–2 hr if the glucose is not falling by at least 10% per hour, and the rate is doubled Q 2 hr until the serum glucose concentration reaches 250 mg/dL (13.89 mmol/L).

  3. Potassium. If serum potassium is < 5.5 mmol/L, then potassium 20–30 mmol/L is given in IV fluids at a rate not to exceed 15 mmol/h unless the patient's rhythm is being continuously monitored. Potassium 10–15 mmol/h is given to maintain serum potassium at 3.0–5.0 mmol/L. Doses of potassium > 15 mmol/h should not be administered without cardiac monitoring.

4. **Bicarbonate.** Its use is controversial and most authors are more conservative than in the past. One approach is to use bicarbonate to correct the pH to 7.00. For pH 6.90–7.00, give 44 mmol over 1–2 hr; for pH < 6.90, give 88 mmol of sodium bicarbonate over 1–2 hr.

5. **Lab work.** Glucose should be repeated Q 1–2 hr, and electrolytes Q 4–6 hr. Magnesium should be checked initially, and phosphate initially and after 6–12 hr. An ABG should be obtained Q 2–4 hr if acidosis is severe, or if the patient requires sodium bicarbonate. Serum/urine ketones may be of some use, although increasing ketones may be spurious (see IV.B.5, p 163).

6. **Associated conditions.** Treat any associated condition such as sepsis, myocardial infarction, or stress appropriately.

D. **Guidelines for management of hyperglycemia in diabetes.** Accumulating evidence suggests that close management ("tight" control) of diabetes will lower the incidence of complications. Current recommendations for patients with diabetes are to maintain a blood glucose before meals of 80–120 mg/dL and a hemoglobin A_{1c} level < 7%. Such tight control frequently necessitates self-monitoring of finger stick glucoses and multiple insulin injections per day.

REFERENCES

American Diabetes Association: Self-monitoring of blood glucose. Diabetes Care 1995;18:47.
American Diabetes Association: Standards of medical care for patients with diabetes mellitus. Diabetes Care 1995;18:8.
Kitabchi AE, Wall BM: Diabetic ketoacidosis. Med Clin North Am 1995:9.
Lorber D: Nonketotic hypertonicity in diabetes mellitus. Med Clin North Am 1995:39.

32. HYPERKALEMIA

I. **Problem.** A 64-year-old man with diabetes admitted for a myocardial infarction is found to have a potassium of 7.1 mmol/L.

II. **Immediate Questions**
   A. **What are the patient's vital signs?** Hyperkalemia can result in life-threatening ventricular arrhythmias. Obtain an electrocardiogram.
   B. **What is the urine output?** Acute oliguric renal failure is the most common cause of potentially fatal hyperkalemia. Evaluate urine output and renal function tests.

C. **Is the patient receiving potassium in an intravenous solution?** Often a standard IV solution contains 20–40 mEq/L potassium; hyperalimentation solutions may contain more. Stop all exogenous potassium until the problem is resolved.

D. **Is the patient on any medications that could elevate the potassium?** Potential causes include potassium-sparing diuretics such as spironolactone (Aldactone), triamterene (Dyrenium), and amiloride (Midamor); NSAIDs; and angiotensin-converting enzyme (ACE) inhibitors.

E. **Is the lab result correct?** If hyperkalemia is unexpected or inconsistent after the preceding questions are satisfactorily answered, consider pseudohyperkalemia, especially if the ECG shows no changes of hyperkalemia. There are a number of causes of factitious hyperkalemia, the most common being the tourniquet method of drawing blood. A tight tourniquet around an exercising extremity can elevate the potassium as much as 2.0 mmol/L. Hemolysis of a blood sample prior to the chemical determination is another frequent source of error. Extreme leukocytosis ($>70,000$) or thrombocytosis ($>1,000,000$) can also elevate the serum potassium. If there is a question, obtain a plasma potassium.

III. **Differential Diagnosis.** In general, true hyperkalemia results from one of two mechanisms: a shift of potassium from intracellular to extracellular space; or impaired renal excretion of potassium.

A. **Acidosis.** With acidosis, potassium moves out of the cells and hydrogen ions move into the cells. A common example is diabetic ketoacidosis. Although insulin deficiency per se is probably not a cause of hyperkalemia, it may increase the degree of hyperkalemia in response to either an endogenous or an exogenous potassium load.

B. **Tissue breakdown.** Any condition associated with rapid destruction of cells results in the release of potassium into the extracellular fluid. Examples include rhabdomyolysis, burns, massive hemolysis, and tumor lysis.

C. **Digitalis intoxication.** A massive overdose of digitalis is a rare cause of hyperkalemia. This results from inhibition of the sodium/potassium-dependent ATPase pump; intracellular potassium is lost.

D. **Succinylcholine.** Mild increases in serum potassium occur in most patients treated with this commonly used muscle relaxant. In patients with tissue destruction or neuromuscular disease, life-threatening hyperkalemia may occur. Succinylcholine causes cell membrane depolarization, resulting in intracellular-to-extracellular shifts in potassium.

E. **Hyperosmolality.** Administration of hypertonic mannitol or saline results in major increases in serum osmolality, and thus may cause hyperkalemia.

F. Arginine hydrochloride. Intravenous administration of arginine hydrochloride, whether used diagnostically to assess growth hormone reserves, or therapeutically in the treatment of metabolic alkalosis, may lead to hyperkalemia. This is probably due to an arginine-potassium exchange.

G. Hyperkalemic periodic paralysis. This rare, inherited disorder is characterized by spontaneous episodes of hyperkalemia and muscle weakness.

H. Chronic renal failure. Most patients with chronic renal failure maintain normal potassium balance until renal function is severely impaired; however, when these patients are challenged with a potassium load or are treated with potassium-sparing diuretics (spironolactone, triamterene, amiloride), ACE inhibitors (captopril, enalapril), or NSAIDs (indomethacin, ibuprofen), the patient's adaptive mechanisms are inadequate and hyperkalemia may occur.

I. Acute renal failure. Hyperkalemia is most likely to complicate oliguric renal failure because of the flow dependence of distal tubular potassium secretion. Acute renal failure often occurs in the setting of increased potassium load (trauma, blood transfusions, or postoperative hypercatabolic state).

J. Adrenal insufficiency. Adrenal insufficiency, in particular hypoaldosteronism, results in reduced renal ability to excrete potassium.

K. Hyporeninemic hypoaldosteronism. Patients with this condition have hyperkalemia as well as hyperchloremic metabolic acidosis (type IV renal tubular acidosis). They often have mild renal insufficiency secondary to diabetic nephropathy or interstitial nephropathy. This syndrome may be aggravated by administration of NSAIDs or potassium-sparing diuretics.

L. Heparin. Long-term anticoagulation with heparin may lead to hyperkalemia, probably through the inhibition of aldosterone synthesis.

M. Potassium-sparing diuretics. Hyperkalemia secondary to triamterene or spironolactone is usually seen in patients with underlying renal insufficiency. But there have been cases, especially in diabetics, in which patients with normal renal function developed hyperkalemia on these drugs.

N. NSAIDs (See Section III.H).

O. ACE inhibitors (See Section III.H).

P. Systemic lupus erythematosus (SLE), renal transplant, sickle cell disease. Patients with these disorders may demonstrate an isolated defect in renal potassium excretion, thought to result from aldosterone resistance.

Q. Increased exogenous intake. High-potassium foods, potassium salts (salt "substitutes"), or large doses of potassium penicillin are examples of exogenous sources of potassium. Often these patients are also on potassium-sparing diuretics, an ACE inhibitor, or a NSAID.

IV. Database
A. Physical examination key points
1. **Cardiovascular exam.** The conduction system of the heart is most vulnerable to hyperkalemia, which may result in bradycardia, ventricular fibrillation, or asystole.
2. **Neuromuscular exam.** Skeletal muscle paralysis may occasionally dominate. Other findings are weakness, tingling, and hyperactive deep tendon reflexes.

B. Laboratory data
1. **Electrolytes.** A low bicarbonate may indicate a metabolic acidosis. A low sodium may result from aldosterone deficiency.
2. **Plasma potassium.** If the serum level is in doubt.
3. **BUN and creatinine.** Assess renal function.
4. **Arterial blood gases.** Along with a serum bicarbonate, an ABG is essential in establishing the acid-base status.
5. **Platelets and white blood cell count.** Marked elevations may cause factitious hyperkalemia.
6. **Serum creatine phosphokinase (CPK).** To detect rhabdomyolysis.
7. **Digoxin level.** If indicated.
8. **Serum aldosterone level.** Indicated after initial workup. Lack of stimulation with volume depletion is consistent with mineralocorticoid deficiency.

C. Radiologic and other studies.
An electrocardiogram is *a must!* The cardiac abnormalities that occur with hyperkalemia are initially tall, peaked T waves in the precordial leads, followed by decreased amplitude of the R wave, widened QRS complex, prolongation of the PR interval, and then decreased amplitude and disappearance of the P wave. Finally, the QRS blends into the T wave, forming the classic sine wave of hyperkalemia. Ventricular fibrillation and asystole may follow.

V. Plan.
Hyperkalemia should be treated as an emergency if the serum potassium has reached 7 mmol/L, although cardiac or neuromuscular symptoms may mandate urgent treatment at lower potassium levels.
A. Acute hyperkalemia
1. Calcium is initial treatment. Calcium antagonizes the membrane effects of hyperkalemia and restores normal excitability within 1–2 minutes. 10% Calcium chloride 5–10 mL or 10% calcium gluconate 10–20 mL should be given IV over 3–5 minutes.
2. Potassium can be quickly shifted into cells by the administration of alkali or glucose plus insulin.
   a. Sodium bicarbonate (one ampoule [44 mmol] of bicarbonate) may be administered IV over several minutes.
   b. A 50-g ampoule of dextrose and 15 U of IV regular insulin may be given (3 g glucose for every 1 U of regular insulin).

B. Subacute hyperkalemia. It should be noted that calcium, alkali, glucose, and insulin do not lower the total body potassium. Once the patient is stabilized, the total body potassium needs to be reduced.

  1. Potassium-binding resins may be used when the immediate life-threatening cardiac manifestations are under control. Kayexalate may be given orally, 40 g in 25–50 mL of 70% sorbitol every 2–4 hours; or rectally, 50–100 g in 200 mL water as a retention enema for 30 minutes every 2–4 hours.

  2. Hemodialysis and peritoneal dialysis are definitive measures for controlling hyperkalemia in renal failure.

REFERENCES

Black RM: Disorders of acid-base and potassium balance. In: Rubinstein E ed-in-chief; Federman DD ed. *Scientific American*. Vol. 3, Sect 10 *Nephrology*, part 2. Scientific American Inc;1993:10.

Gabow PA, Peterson LN: Disorders of potassium metabolism. In: Schrier RW ed. *Renal and Electrolyte Disorders*. 4th ed. Little, Brown;1992:231.

Tannen RL: Approach to the patient with altered potassium concentration. In: Kelly WN ed-in-chief. *Textbook of Internal Medicine*. 2nd ed. Lippincott 1992;848.

33. HYPERNATREMIA

I. Problem. The clinical chemistry lab calls to tell you that the 65-year-old female patient admitted with pneumonia has a serum sodium of 155 mmol/L (normal 136–145 mmol/L).

II. Immediate Questions

  A. Is the patient awake, alert, and oriented? Or lethargic and confused? The major signs and symptoms of hypernatremia are lethargy, which may lead to coma or convulsions; and neuromuscular irritability, including tremors, rigidity and hyperreflexia. Mortality and symptoms are related to the level and the acuity of the hypernatremia. Mortality in adults is increased with the sodium levels above 160 mmol/L.

  B. What medications is the patient taking? Mannitol can cause an osmotic diuresis, resulting in hypernatremia with low total body sodium. Exogenous steroids and salt tablets can cause an increase in the total body sodium, resulting in hypernatremia.

  C. What are the intake/output values for the past few days? A loss of total body water by fluid deprivation (inadequate thirst mechanism or inadequate administration of fluids) or from sweating can cause hypernatremia.

  D. Are there underlying conditions? Certain diseases, such as central and nephrogenic diabetes insipidus, hyperaldosteronism, and Cushing's syndrome, are associated with hypernatremia.

E. **Does the patient have a condition that prevents access to water?** Dehydration can result from inadequate access to water secondary to being bedridden or inadequate thirst mechanism secondary to CNS dysfunction. These may result in hypernatremia.

F. **Is the lab value accurate?** As with any lab result that is unexpected, the error could be in the lab report itself. It may be of value to repeat the test.

G. **What is the composition of fluids administered?** Check sodium content of fluids; hypertonic solutions (eg, hypertonic dialysate) can cause hypernatremia. If the patient is on tube feedings, be sure there is adequate free water (usually 35 mL/kg/24 h in adults).

H. **Is there a history of polyuria and polydypsia?** Diabetes mellitus and diabetes insipidus can cause hypernatremia.

III. **Differential Diagnosis.** The differential diagnosis is best considered in light of the possible causes of hypernatremia: a loss of water and sodium; a loss of total body water; and rarely, an increase in total body sodium.

A. **Water and sodium loss.** Significant sodium loss with even greater loss of water.

1. **Renal losses** (urine [Na⁺] > 20 mmol/L)

   a. **Osmotic diuresis**

      i. **Mannitol**

      ii. **Hyperglycemia**

      iii. **Urea**

   b. **Diuretics.** Eg, thiazide diuretics and furosemide.

   c. **Post-obstructive diuresis.** Caused by relief of long-standing bilateral renal obstruction and bladder outlet obstruction prostatic hypertrophy).

   d. **Acute tubular necrosis.** Polyuric phase.

2. **Extra-renal losses** (urine [Na⁺] < 20 mmol/L)

   a. **Cutaneous losses**

      i. **Fever.** Losses of 500 mL/24 hr for each degree centigrade increase above 38.3°C (101°F).

      ii. **Burns**

      iii. **Profuse sweating**

   b. **Gastrointestinal losses**

      i. **Vomiting**

      ii. **Nasogastric suction**

      iii. **Diarrhea.** Hypotonic diarrhea in children. Also, with the use of lactulose when the number of stools per day exceeds the recommended 2–3.

      iv. **Fistulae**

B. **Water losses without loss of sodium** (urine [Na⁺] is variable)

1. **Renal losses**

   a. **Central diabetes insipidus.** Results from failure to produce adequate amounts of antidiuretic hormone (ADH). If thirst

mechanism is intact and patient has free access to water, hypernatremia may be minimal. May be idiopathic or caused by CNS surgery, trauma, infection, or tumor (metastatic or primary).
- **b. Nephrogenic.** Antidiuretic hormone is not effective. May be congenital or caused by sickle cell disease, hypokalemia, hypercalcemia, polycystic kidney disease; or by drugs such as lithium, alcohol, phenytoin, and glyburide.
- **2. Extra-renal losses**
  - **a. Pulmonary losses.** Insensible losses, especially in intubated patients who are not receiving adequate humidification or patients with increased respiratory rates.
  - **b. Cutaneous losses.** Fever or sweating.
- **C. Increase in total body sodium without a change in total body water** (urine [Na^+] > 20 mmol/L).
  - **1. Increase in mineralocorticoids or glucocorticoids**
    - **a. Exogenous steroids** (eg, prednisone)
    - **b. Primary aldosteronism**
    - **c. Cushing's syndrome.** Cushing's disease, bilateral adrenal hyperplasia, or ectopic adrenocorticotropin (ACTH) production.
  - **2. Administration of hypertonic sodium**
    - **a. Sodium chloride tablets**
    - **b. Hypertonic dialysate**
    - **c. Hypertonic sodium bicarbonate.** Given during resuscitation after cardiopulmonary arrest.
    - **d. Improper mixed formulas or tube feedings.**

IV. Database
- **A. Physical examination key points**
  - **1. Vital signs.** Check orthostatic changes in blood pressure and heart rate. A decrease in systolic blood pressure of 10 mm Hg and/or an increase in heart rate of 20 bpm 1 minute after moving from a supine to a standing position points to volume depletion. In addition, decreased weight suggests volume depletion.
  - **2. Skin.** Check turgor; poor turgor suggests volume depletion. On the other hand, keep in mind that poor skin turgor can be a normal variant in the elderly.
  - **3. Mouth.** Dry mucous membranes suggest volume depletion.
  - **4. Neurologic exam.** Look for signs of irritability, muscle twitching, hyperreflexia, or seizures; all are signs of hypernatremia. A thorough neurologic examination needs to be done since CNS trauma, infection or tumor can cause diabetes insipidus.
- **B. Laboratory data**
  - **1. Serum sodium.** Normal 136–145 mmol/L. Follow closely, especially if sodium is > 160 mmol/L.

2. **Urine osmolality.** > 700 mosm/L suggests insufficient water intake with or without extra-renal water losses or an osmoreceptor defect. A urine osmolality between 700 mosm/L and the serum osmolality suggests partial central diabetes insipidus, osmotic diuresis, diuretic therapy, acquired (partial) nephrogenic diabetes insipidus, or renal failure. A urine osmolality < serum osmolality suggests complete central diabetes insipidus or nephrogenic diabetes insipidus.
3. **Spot urine sodium.** In hypernatremia with water and sodium loss, a level < 20 mmol/L suggests extra-renal loss. In hypernatremia with water loss without loss of sodium, the spot sodium in extra-renal losses is variable.
4. **Water deprivation/vasopressin.** If you suspect diabetes insipidus (DI). The patient is fluid-deprived until the plasma osmolality is 295 mosm/kg or greater; or on three consecutive hourly urines, the osmolality does not increase; or the patient loses 3% to 5% of his or her body weight. Five units of aqueous vasopressin are then given, either IM or SC.
   a. **Normal subjects.** Urine concentrates with fluid deprivation and no change occurs with vasopressin.
   b. **Complete central DI.** Urine does not concentrate with fluid deprivation. There is a significant increase in urine osmolality after vasopressin.
   c. **Nephrogenic DI.** Urine does not concentrate with deprivation and there is no change in urine osmolality with vasopressin.
C. **Radiologic and other studies.** A CT scan of head may be helpful if central DI is suspected, to rule out a CNS lesion.

V. **Plan.** The overall plan is to slowly decrease the serum sodium toward normal. Only hyperacute hypernatremia (hypernatremia < 12 hr) may be treated rapidly. Too rapid a correction of the sodium in hypernatremia > 12 hr may result in cerebral edema, seizures and herniation leading to death. The rate of correction of the sodium should not exceed 0.7 mmol/L/hr or about 10% of the serum sodium concentration per day. Specific treatment depends on whether there is a loss of sodium and water, a loss of water, or an increase in total body sodium.
A. **Water and sodium loss.** Represents significant volume depletion. If the patient is in shock, replenish volume with normal saline. If patient is hemodynamically stable, replace volume with hypotonic saline (half-normal saline).
B. **Water loss without loss of sodium.** Calculate the free water deficit: weight (kg) $\times$ 0.60 = total body water. Water deficit = total body water $\times$ (1 − [desired [Na^+] / measured [Na^+]]). Give ½ of the calculated free water deficit in the first 12 hours and the remainder in the next 24 hours. Include maintenance fluids.

C. **Increase in total body sodium.** Remove excess sodium, either by giving free water and diuretics, or by dialysis with hypotonic dialysate.
D. **Treatment of underlying cause**
   1. **Central DI.** After correction of free water deficit, begin vasopressin.
   2. **Diabetes mellitus.** Treat with insulin and IV fluids. (See Section I, Chapter 31, Hyperglycemia, p 164)
   3. **Nephrogenic DI.** After correction of free water deficit, begin thiazide diuretic and low salt diet. Remove offending agent if appropriate.

REFERENCES

Avner ED: Clinical disorders of water metabolism: Hyponatremia and hypernatremia. Pediatr Ann 1995;24:23.

Berl T, Schrier RW: Disorders of water metabolism. In: Schrier RW ed. *Renal and Electrolyte Disorders.* 4th ed. Little, Brown;1992:1.

Brown RG: Disorders of water and sodium balance. Postgrad Med 1993;93:227.

Oh MS, Carroll HJ: Disorders of sodium metabolism: Hypernatremia and hyponatremia. Crit Care Med 1992;20:94.

Palvevsky PM, Bhagrath R, Greenberg A. Hypernatremia in hospitalized patients. Ann Intern Med 1996;124:197.

Richardson RMA, Tobe S: Approach to the patient with polyuria or nocturia. In: Kelley WN ed.: *Textbook of Internal Medicine.* 2nd ed. Lippincott;1992:800.

Weisberg LS, Szerlip HM, Cox M: Approach to the patient with altered sodium and water homeostasis. In: Kelley WN, ed-in-chief. *Textbook of Internal Medicine.* 2nd ed. Lippincott;1992:839.

34. HYPERTENSION

I. **Problem.** A 37-year-old patient complains of a severe occipital headache for the past 6 hours. Her blood pressure is 220/140.

II. **Immediate Questions**
   A. **Is there a past history of hypertension?** You want to know if she is being treated for hypertension and regularly sees a physician. Previously, what was the highest blood pressure?
   B. **What is the patient's medical regimen?** You want to know all the medications the patient is taking and whether she is compliant. For example, she may have stopped taking clonidine (Catapres) or a short-acting beta-blocker such as propranolol (Inderal), which can cause severe rebound hypertension. Hypertensive crisis can occur in people taking a monoamine oxidase inhibitor (MAOI), who ingest certain cheeses or wine containing tyramine. Ingestion of street drugs such as cocaine or amphetamines can also cause hypertensive crisis.

C. **Is the patient experiencing any other symptoms besides headache?** A patient with severe hypertension who has a headache with mental status changes may be suffering from hypertensive encephalopathy, which is a medical emergency. Hypertensive encephalopathy is more common in patients whose blood pressure suddenly rises, as with toxemia of pregnancy. Other manifestations of end-organ damage from malignant hypertension include angina, dyspnea (left ventricular dysfunction), visual loss, nausea, vomiting, seizures, focal neurologic deficits, and a decrease in urinary output.

III. **Differential Diagnosis.** Hypertension can be classified as essential or secondary (describes the cause); and as accelerated or malignant (describes urgency). Patients with malignant hypertension often have a secondary cause of hypertension. With malignant hypertension the first concern is to lower the blood pressure.

A. **Essential.** Comprises 90–95% of all hypertension. No underlying cause.

B. **Secondary**

1. **Renovascular.** From fibromuscular dysplasia (usually women 20–30 years old) and atherosclerosis (usually men older than 50).

2. **Primary aldosteronism.** Hypertension with unexplained hypokalemia.

3. **Cushing's disease.** Characteristic findings include moon facies, truncal obesity, purple striae, a buffalo hump, hirsutism, and easy bruising. Hypernatremia and hypokalemic alkalosis are common.

4. **Pheochromocytoma.** Usually episodic hypertension. Often associated diaphoresis, palpitations, and headache.

5. **Coarctation of the aorta.** Should be suspected in anyone young presenting with hypertension. Blood pressures are often higher in the right arm and femoral pulses are often absent.

6. **Primary renal disease.**

7. **Hyperthyroidism.** Systolic hypertension.

8. **Hypothyroidism.** Diastolic hypertension.

9. **Heavy ethanol use or withdrawal.** May cause or aggravate underlying hypertension. Hypertension associated with withdrawal is secondary to hyperadrenergic state.

10. **Drugs**
   a. **Estrogens**
   b. **Other prescription medications.** Cyclosporine, NSAIDs, corticosteroids and erythropoietin can occasionally cause hypertension.
   c. **Over-the-counter medications containing sympatho-mimetics.** For example, phenylpropanolamine or pseu-

doephedrine may or may not elevate the blood pressure when used in excessive amounts.

  d. Illicit drugs. Phencyclidine (PCP), amphetamines, and cocaine.
  11. Postoperative conditions. Multifactorial, including hypoxia, pain, anxiety, volume overload, hypothermia, and medications.
  12. Gestational
  13. Hyperparathyroidism
  C. Miscellaneous diseases. Other diseases can cause a marked elevation in blood pressure; or may be the consequence of long-standing, poorly controlled hypertension.
  1. Cerebrovascular accident. If the patient has suffered a stroke resulting in marked elevation of blood pressure, the physician is not quite as aggressive in lowering the blood pressure. A sudden marked drop in blood pressure can extend a stroke.
  2. Subarachnoid hemorrhage. Patients classically complain of the worst headache of their life.
  3. Aortic dissection. "Tearing" chest pain, often with radiation to the back, and most severe at onset. Usually a previous history of hypertension.
  4. Congestive heart failure/pulmonary edema.
  5. Angina pectoris/myocardial infarction. (See Section I, Chapter 11, Chest Pain, p 55).
  D. Accelerated hypertension. Markedly elevated blood pressure with no current life-threatening problem secondary to the hypertension.
  E. Malignant hypertension. Usually a markedly elevated blood pressure with an associated serious complication, such as hypertensive encephalopathy, angina, myocardial infarction, aortic dissection, or cerebrovascular accident; proteinuria, hematuria, and red blood cell casts may be present.

IV. Database
  A. Physical examination key points
  1. Vital signs. Take blood pressure in both arms; feel both radial pulses and check for a radial-femoral pulse lag. Such maneuvers may point to aortic dissection or coarctation.
  2. Eyes. Look for evidence of papilledema, hemorrhages, exudates, severe arteriolar narrowing, and arteriovenous nicking. Papilledema is usually present with malignant hypertension but can occur in other conditions with increased intracranial pressure.
  3. Lungs. Presence of rales may indicate congestive heart failure.
  4. Heart. Palpate the apical impulse for displacement. Listen for a third heart sound (S_3) indicative of left ventricular dysfunction, and for a murmur of aortic insufficiency, which can occur in aortic dissection.
  5. Neurologic exam. Assess the patient's mental status and look for any focal deficits that may indicate a cerebrovascular acci-

dent. Confusion and somnolence progressing to coma are hallmarks of hypertensive encephalopathy. Be sure to check reflexes; unilateral hyperreflexia may indicate an intracranial event.

B. Laboratory data
   1. **Electrolytes, BUN, glucose, and creatinine.** To rule out evidence of renal insufficiency, hypokalemia, or hyperglycemia. Hypokalemia occurs in Cushing's disease, primary hyperaldosteronism, and renovascular hypertension. Hyperglycemia can be a manifestation of a pheochromocytoma, Cushing's disease, or stress. Mild renal insufficiency points toward hypertensive nephropathy, whereas marked renal insufficiency potentially suggests a secondary cause of hypertension.
   2. **Urinalysis.** To look for proteinuria, hematuria, and red cell casts for evidence of a secondary cause or hypertensive nephropathy.
   3. **Complete blood count (CBC) and examination of peripheral blood smear.** Red blood cell fragments or schistocytes occur in microangiopathic hemolytic anemia resulting from malignant hypertension.

C. Radiologic and other studies
   1. **Chest x-ray.** To look for cardiomegaly, congestive heart failure, and mediastinal widening suggesting proximal aortic dissection. Rib notching and obliteration of the aortic knob suggest coarctation of the aorta.
   2. **Electrocardiogram.** To look for ischemic changes and left ventricular hypertrophy.
   3. **CT scan.** If patient has mental status changes or focal neurologic findings, a CT scan must be performed to exclude a thromboembolic stroke or subarachnoid hemorrhage.

V. Plan
   A. Hypertensive encephalopathy or malignant hypertension. A medical emergency. Treatment must be initiated within minutes if possible.
      1. **Admission to an ICU.** Intravenous and arterial lines should be placed.
      2. **Appropriate therapy.** Initiated once therapeutic goals are established. The goals of immediate therapy should be approximately a systolic pressure of 150–170 and diastolic pressure of 100–120 if the patient is known to have long-standing, severe hypertension. Overly aggressive reduction of blood pressure beyond these levels can lead to cerebral hypoperfusion and worsening neurologic deficits. This is particularly important in patients suffering from a stroke or transient ischemic attack, who are susceptible to abrupt falls in blood pressure.
         a. Nitroprusside is commonly used in hypertensive crises. It reduces preload and afterload when given in a dose of 0.5–10 mg/kg/min as a continuous IV infusion. It has the advantage of immediate onset and is easily titrated. Disadvantages in-

clude the need for constant monitoring; also, prolonged use is associated with thiocyanate toxicity.

b. Intravenous labetalol, an alpha- and beta-blocker, is infused at a rate of 2 mg/min following a 20–80 mg bolus. Potential disadvantages include beta-blocking side effects.

c. For suspected pheochromocytoma, IV labetalol, phentolamine or phenoxybenzamine can be used.

d. Hypertension associated with aortic dissection should be controlled with IV labetalol, esmolol, verapamil, or a combination of nitroprusside and a beta-blocker.

3. Treatment of accelerated hypertension. Can be treated with oral medications. Nifedipine (Procardia) 10 mg orally will decrease blood pressure in 30–60 minutes and seldom causes hypotension. **Caution:** Calcium-channel blocking agents other than sustained-release formulations have fallen into disfavor because of the increased mortality associated with their long-term use. Other oral agents such as beta-blockers and ACE inhibitors can also be used. It is imperative that you closely monitor the blood pressure to be sure that whatever medication is used favorably affects the blood pressure.

4. Treatment of hypertension. A thorough discussion of hypertension is beyond the scope of this book. Please refer to any number of references including those listed here.

REFERENCES

Coates ML, Rembold CM, Farr BM: Does pseudoephedrine increase blood pressure in patients with controlled hypertension? J Fam Pract 1995;40:22.

Joint National Committee on Detection, Evaluation, and Treatment of High Blood Pressure. *The Fifth Report of the Joint National Committee on Detection, Evaluation, and Treatment of High Blood Pressure* Arch Intern Med 1993;153:154.

Kaplan NM: *Clinical Hypertension.* 6th ed. Williams & Wilkins;1994.

35. HYPOCALCEMIA

I. Problem. A 54-year-old man admitted for an acute myocardial infarction (MI) has a calcium of 3.5 mEg/L or 1.75 mmol/L (normal 4.2–5.1 mEg/L or 2.10–2.55 mmol/L).

II. Immediate Questions

A. Are there any symptoms relevant to the low calcium? Asymptomatic hypocalcemia usually does not require emergent treatment. Signs and symptoms of hypocalcemia may include peripheral and perioral paresthesias, Trousseau's sign (carpopedal spasm), Chvostek's sign, confusion, muscle twitching, laryngospasm, tetany, and seizures.

    B. Does the low calcium level represent the true ionized calcium? Most laboratories report the total serum calcium, but it is the ionized calcium level that is important physiologically. The total serum calcium level decreases by 0.2 mmol/L or 0.4 mEq/L for every 1 g/dL decrease in the serum albumin level without changing the ionized calcium level. Calculate the adjusted total calcium level or order an ionized calcium level.

    C. Is there a past history of neck surgery? Surgical removal or infarction of the parathyroid glands is one of the more common causes of hypocalcemia. Look for a scar on the neck.

III. Differential Diagnosis. The causes of low ionized serum calcium can be categorized as parathyroid hormone deficits, vitamin D deficits, and loss or displacement of calcium.

    A. Parathyroid hormone (PTH) deficits
       1. Decreased PTH level
          a. Surgical excision or injury. Including thyroid surgery.
          b. Infiltrative diseases of the parathyroid gland. For example, hemochromatosis, amyloid or metastatic cancer.
          c. Idiopathic
          d. Irradiation. To the neck to treat lymphoma.
       2. Decreased PTH activity
          a. Congenital. Pseudohypoparathyroidism: resistance to PTH at the tissue level.
          b. Acquired. Hypomagnesemia, hypermagnesemia.
    B. Vitamin D deficiency
       1. Malnutrition
       2. Malabsorption
          a. Pancreatitis
          b. Postgastrectomy
          c. Short gut syndrome
          d. Laxative abuse
          e. Sprue
          f. Hepatobiliary disease with bile salt deficiency
       3. Defective metabolism
          a. Liver disease. Failure to synthesize 25-hydroxyvitamin D.
          b. Renal disease. Failure to synthesize 1,25-dihydroxyvitamin D.
          c. Anticonvulsant treatment with phenobarbital or phenytoin (Dilantin). Possibly from an increase in the metabolism of vitamin D in the liver leading to a vitamin D deficiency.
    C. Calcium loss or displacement
       1. Hyperphosphatemia. Increases bone deposition of calcium.
          a. Acute phosphate ingestion
          b. Acute phosphate release by rhabdomyolysis or tumor lysis
          c. Renal failure

2. **Acute pancreatitis**
3. **Osteoblastic metastases.** Especially breast and prostate cancer.
4. **Medullary carcinoma of the thyroid.** Increased calcitonin.
5. **Decreased bone resorption.** Overuse of actinomycin, calcitonin, or mithramycin.
6. **Miscellaneous disorders.** Sepsis, massive transfusion, hungry bone syndrome, toxic shock syndrome, and fat embolism.

IV. Database
A. Physical examination key points
1. **Skin.** Dermatitis with chronic hypocalcemia.
2. **HEENT.** Cataracts with chronic hypocalcemia. Laryngospasm is rare but life-threatening. Look for surgical scars on the neck.
3. **Neuromuscular exam.** Confusion, spasm, twitching, facial grimacing, and hyperactive deep tendon reflexes all indicate symptomatic hypocalcemia.
4. **Specific tests for tetany of hypocalcemia**
   a. **Chvostek's sign.** Present in 5% to 10% of normocalcemic patients. Tapping on the facial nerve near the zygoma will elicit a twitch in hypocalcemic patients.
   b. **Trousseau's sign.** Inflate a blood pressure cuff above the systolic pressure for 3 minutes and watch for carpal spasm.
B. Laboratory data
1. **Serum electrolytes.** Particularly calcium, phosphate, potassium, and magnesium. Calcium must be interpreted in terms of the serum albumin (see II.B., p 179). Hypomagnesemia and hyperkalemia may potentiate the effects of hypocalcemia.
2. **Serum albumin.** As mentioned earlier.
3. **BUN and creatinine.** To rule out renal failure.
4. **Parathyroid hormone level.** A low normal level is inappropriately low in the presence of true hypocalcemia.
5. **Vitamin D levels.** 25-hydroxyvitamin D and 1,25-dihydroxyvitamin D.
6. **Urinary cyclic AMP.** May indicate evidence of PTH resistance.
7. **Fecal fat.** To evaluate for steatorrhea.
C. Radiologic and other tests
1. **ECG.** A prolonged QT interval and T wave inversion can occur with marked hypocalcemia, as can various arrhythmias.
2. **Bone films.** May show bony changes of renal failure or osteoblastic metastases.

V. Plan.
Assess for tetany, which can potentially progress to laryngeal spasm or seizures, and requires immediate treatment. Otherwise, establish the diagnosis by testing blood for calcium, albumin, magnesium, phosphate, and PTH levels, and begin appropriate oral therapy.

    A. Emergency treatment. Emergency treatment is usually needed for a calcium level below 1.5 mmol/L (3 mEq/L) to prevent fatal laryngospasm. Give 100–200 mg of elemental calcium IV over 10 minutes in 50–100 mL of D5W; follow with a 1–2 mg/kg/h infusion for 6–12 hours. Use caution in patients on digitalis as calcium may potentiate its effects (heart block).

      1. 10% calcium gluconate. One 10–mL ampoule contains 23.25 mmol (93 mg) of calcium. Give 10–20 mL initially; follow with the infusion.

      2. 10% calcium chloride. One 10–mL ampoule contains 68 mmol (272 mg) of calcium. Give 5–10 mL IV, being careful to avoid extravasation, which can cause skin to slough; then start an infusion.

    B. Chronic therapy. With primary PTH deficiency the goal is to give 2–4 g of oral calcium daily in four divided doses, adding vitamin D as necessary. With vitamin D disorders, vitamin D must always be supplemented.

      1. Calcium carbonate, 240 mg of calcium per 600-mg tablet.

      2. Calcium lactate tablets and calcium glubionate syrup are also available.

      3. Ergocalciferol (vitamin D_2) 50,000 U/day or dihydrotachysterol (vitamin D_2 analog) 100–400 µg/d or calcitriol (1,25-dihydroxy-vitamin D_3) 0.25–1.0 µg/day.

      4. Patients on parenteral nutrition need at least 4–7 mg/kg/d of magnesium.

    C. Magnesium deficiency (See Section I, Chapter 38, Hypomagnesemia, Section V, p 192).

      1. In an emergency, one can give 10–15 mL of $MgSO_4$ 20% solution IV over 1 minute, followed by 500 mL of $MgSO_4$ 2% solution in D5W over 4–6 hours.

      2. More typically, 6 g (49 mEq or 24.5 mmol) of $MgSO_4$ in 1000 mL of D5W is given IV over 4 hours, followed by 6 g every 8 hours × 2, followed by 6 g every day.

REFERENCES

Reber PM, Heath H: Hypocalcemic emergencies. Med Clin North Am 1995;79:93.
Zaloga GP: Hypocalcemia in critically ill patients. Crit Care Med 1992;20:251.

36. HYPOGLYCEMIA

  I. Problem. A 33-year-old woman was admitted for diabetic ketoacidosis (DKA) 24 hours ago. The patient's fingerstick glucose is now 50 mg/dL or 2.78 mmol/L.

  II. Immediate Questions

    A. What are the patient's vital signs? Is the patient asymptomatic? Assessment of current status and vital signs allows the house officer to evaluate the urgency of the situation; ie, is there time for a repeat fingerstick or blood glucose or should therapy be instituted immediately? Patients with hypoglycemia can have multiple symptoms. Early symptoms include headache, hunger, palpitations, tremor, and diaphoresis. As hypoglycemia progresses, abnormal behavior (such as combativeness) and slurred speech mimicking ethanol intoxication are followed by loss of consciousness, seizures, and even death. Beta-blockers can mask the early adrenergic symptoms of hypoglycemia, except diaphoresis, which is a cholinergic response. Patients with long-standing diabetes mellitus may also lose the ability to perceive hypoglycemia.

B. What medications is the patient taking? Presumably a patient in DKA will be on insulin instead of oral hypoglycemic agents as oral agents are not indicated for the treatment of type I diabetes mellitus.

    1. The dose, route, and type of insulin are important in determining the timing and severity of the hypoglycemia. Patients on intermediate-acting insulin (NPH or Lente) generally have a peak effect between 6 and 16 hours, whereas those on rapid-acting insulin (regular) given subcutaneously peak at 2–6 hours. Only regular insulin is used intravenously. IV bolus insulin produces its maximum effect in 30 minutes. Patients on continuous IV infusion insulin drips and continuous SC insulin (by insulin pump) can show very rapid decreases in their serum glucose although the total dose received may be relatively small.

    2. Some patients have different responses to rapid-acting and intermediate-acting insulin such that the peak effect is extended to 18–24 hours for intermediate-acting insulin and to 6–12 hours or longer for regular insulin.

    3. Knowing the amount, type, and route for administration of insulin will help determine the likelihood of the hypoglycemia's worsening or recurring after treatment, as well as necessary changes in the insulin regimen. If a patient is on an oral hypoglycemic agent, it is important to know which one. Chlorpropamide (Diabinese) has an extremely long half-life (32 hours) and recurrent hypoglycemia may result, especially if the patient is fasting.

C. Is there IV access? It is necessary to determine that IV access is available to administer D50 if needed and to ascertain whether the patient is receiving intravenous fluids containing dextrose.

D. When was the patient's last meal or snack? If the patient has eaten a meal within the hour since the fingerstick was obtained, the situation will be somewhat less urgent since the meal may be treating the hypoglycemia.

III. Differential Diagnosis

  A. Medications

    1. Insulin. Check for accidental overdose, as when insulin is given to the wrong patient; or administration of the wrong type of insulin or by the wrong route; or intentional overdose (eg, Munchausen's syndrome).

2. **Oral hypoglycemic agents.** Especially chlorpropamide (Diabinese) in elderly patients.

3. **Other medications:** Acetaminophen (Tylenol), pentamidine (Pentam), haloperidol (Haldol), para-aminosalicylic acid (PAS), and disopyramide (Norpace) can cause hypoglycemia.

4. **Ethanol.** Ethanol intoxication may cause hypoglycemia; in addition, many alcoholics may be glycogen-depleted prior to alcohol consumption due to inadequate food intake.

5. **Drug interactions.** The activity of oral hypoglycemic agents is increased when taken with NSAIDs, sulfonamides, or MAO inhibitors.

B. **Reactive hypoglycemia.** This is a form of hypoglycemia that occurs after eating. It is found in 5–10% of patients who have undergone partial to complete gastrectomies as well as de novo in the general population.

C. **Severe liver disease.** With massive liver destruction, glycogen stores are easily depleted.

D. **Insulinoma.** Pancreatic islet cell tumor; may be malignant. Serum insulin or C-peptide levels are helpful in establishing the diagnosis.

E. **Endocrinopathies.** These include Addison's disease, pituitary insufficiency, and myxedema.

F. **Renal disease.** This usually occurs in the setting of combined uremia and malnutrition. Insulin clearance decreases in cases of renal failure.

G. **Sepsis.** This is especially likely in the setting of septic shock.

H. **Malnutrition/prolonged fasting.** Hypoglycemia is common in protein calorie malnutrition (kwashiorkor).

I. **Abrupt discontinuation of total parenteral nutrition (TPN).** This diagnosis is more likely if the TPN solution contained insulin.

J. **Factitious hypoglycemia.** This may occur as a result of either a marked elevation in the white blood cell count and metabolism by leukocytes or prolongation of contact of serum with red blood cells. There may be a suspicion of self-induced hypoglycemia if the patient has access to insulin or sulfonylurea drugs.

K. **Neoplasms.** Retroperitoneal sarcoma, hepatocellular carcinoma, and small cell (oat cell) carcinoma can cause hypoglycemia by production of insulin-like hormone, impaired glycogenolysis, or glucose consumption.

IV. Database

A. Physical examination key points

1. **Vital signs.** Hypertension and tachycardia may be caused by increased catecholamines as a response to hypoglycemia. This response may be eliminated in the presence of a beta-blocker.

2. **Skin.** Diaphoresis is a common cholinergic response to hypoglycemia which is not generally eliminated by beta-blockers.

3. **Neurologic exam.** The patient's sensorium and orientation are often altered. (See Section I, Chapter 13, Coma, Acute Mental Status Changes, p 69.) Tremor at rest and with intention may be present. Unconsciousness and seizures indicate need for urgent treatment. Hypoglycemia occasionally presents with focal neurologic findings.

B. **Laboratory data**

1. **Serum glucose.** This is the most critical test; in general, a glucose level below 50 mg/dL *and* the presence of symptoms are diagnostic of hypoglycemia. Fingerstick values should always be confirmed by serum glucose measurements as they are prone to error secondary to strips that have been exposed to air, inappropriate preparation of the finger with betadine, presence of alcohol on the finger, incorrect timing, or an uncalibrated machine. In the presence of symptoms, blood should be obtained immediately but treatment *should not* be withheld pending results or a delay in obtaining blood.

2. **Electrolytes, BUN and creatinine, liver function studies, complete blood count, urinalysis.** In the setting of hypoglycemia with no history available, all are indicated to evaluate for common causes listed in the differential diagnosis.

3. **Drug screens.** Look specifically for oral hypoglycemics as well as for ethanol, acetaminophen, and antipsychotics (eg, haloperidol).

4. **Serum insulin.** Results may indicate either exogenous insulin administration or insulinoma.

5. **C-peptide.** Will help to differentiate between insulinoma and exogenous insulin administration. The C-peptide level will be elevated with an insulinoma and low with the administration of exogenous insulin.

C. **Radiologic and other studies.** These may be indicated in specific circumstances to rule out infection, insulinoma, malignancy, or pituitary lesion.

V. **Plan**

A. **Administer glucose.** Do not wait for the results of the serum glucose if you strongly suspect the diagnosis. It is best to draw blood before administering glucose; however, you should proceed with treatment if there will be a significant delay before blood can be obtained and the patient is markedly symptomatic. If the patient is awake, and able and willing to take fluids, glucose should be given orally. Otherwise, administer IV glucose.

1. Orange juice with added sugar is usually readily available. Specific glucose-containing liquids are being stocked on most hospital floors and may be substituted for orange juice. For mild hypoglycemia, 8 ounces of 2% milk or a package of saltines with juice may be adequate and not result in "overshoot" hyperglycemia.

2. Give one ampoule of 50% dextrose (D50) IV push; repeat in 5 minutes if no response. If there is no response after the second ampoule, the diagnosis should be seriously questioned and other causes for the symptoms should be considered such as hypoxia, transient ischemic attack, and ethanol or drug intoxication or overdose.
3. If the patient is unable to take glucose PO, and IV access is not immediately available, give glucagon 0.5–1 mg IM or SC (may induce vomiting; be prepared to protect the patient's airway) .
4. Start maintenance IV fluids with D5W at 75–100 mL/h, especially if the hypoglycemia may recur, such as that resulting from chlorpropamide or sepsis.
5. Follow serial glucoses frequently. Depending on the severity of the hypoglycemia, repeat glucose after treatment and again in $\frac{1}{2}$–2 hours depending on the results.

B. Adjust medications. Review schedule and dosing of insulin and/or oral hypoglycemics. Consider use of metformin (Glucophage) for Type II diabetics (less likely to cause hypoglycemia). See Section VII, Commonly Used Medications, p 487.

C. Miscellaneous. If the patient is not taking hypoglycemic agents, then consider other causes listed in the differential diagnosis and evaluate accordingly.

REFERENCES

Bailey CJ: Biguanides and NIDDM. Diabetes Care 1992;15:755.
Campbell PJ: Mechanisms for prevention, development and reversal of hypoglycemia. Adv Intern Med 1988;33:205.
Service FJ: Hypoglycemic disorders. N Engl J Med 1995;332:1144.
Service FJ: Hypoglycemia. Med Clin North Am 1995;79:1.

37. HYPOKALEMIA

I. **Problem.** A 72-year-old woman on medication for hypertension develops profound muscle weakness after 3 days of vomiting. Her serum potassium is 2.5 mmol/L (2.5 mEq/L).

II. **Immediate Questions**
   A. What are the patient's vital signs? Premature atrial contractions (PACs), premature ventricular contractions (PVCs), or ventricular arrhythmias may be suggested by examination of the pulse.
   B. What medications is the patient taking? Medications, especially diuretics, can cause renal potassium wasting. Also, digitalis toxicity is potentiated by hypokalemia.

    C. **Has the patient had vomiting, diarrhea, or nasogastric suc-tion?** These are possible sources of potassium loss.

    D. **Is there a history of excessive sweating?** A prolonged, elevated temperature or delirium tremens can result in hypokalemia from sweating.

III. **Differential Diagnosis.** In general, hypokalemia is caused by cellular shifts or by renal and gastrointestinal losses.

  A. **Hypokalemia resulting from cellular shifts**

    1. **Alkalosis.** Both respiratory alkalosis and metabolic alkalosis are associated with hypokalemia. Hyperventilation during surgi-cal anesthesia can cause acute respiratory alkalosis and pro-duce significant hypokalemia.

    2. **Familial periodic paralysis.** This rare, inherited disease is characterized by intermittent attacks of varying severity, rang-ing from muscle weakness to flaccid paralysis.

    3. **Barium poisoning.** Ingestion of soluble barium salts may cause profound hypokalemia, muscle paralysis, and cardiac ar-rhythmias, probably as a result of intracellular shifts, although associated vomiting and diarrhea may also contribute.

    4. **Treatment of megaloblastic anemia.** Hypokalemia may occur within 48 hours of administration of folate or vitamin B_{12}. It results from sequestration of potassium ions by a marked increase in bone marrow activity.

    5. **Leukemia.** Hypokalemia may be produced by sequestration of potassium ions by rapidly proliferating blast cells.

    6. **Insulin.** Intravenous administration of glucose and insulin is an effective treatment of hyperkalemia. The clinical importance of insulin as a cause of hypokalemia is not well established.

    7. **β_2-Adrenergic agents.** Isoproterenol, terbutaline, and other β_2-adrenergic agents can cause potassium ions to shift into cells. This is of uncertain clinical importance and is not sufficient reason to undertreat asthmatics.

  B. **Hypokalemia resulting from normal losses**

    1. **Diarrhea.** Diarrhea from virtually any cause may result in hy-pokalemia. But severe hypokalemia secondary to diarrhea is suggestive of colonic villous adenoma or non-insulin-secreting pancreatic islet cell tumors.

    2. **Excessive sweat.** The sweat glands contain an aldosterone-dependent sodium/potassium exchange mechanism.

    3. **Clay ingestion.** Said to be relatively common in the southeast-ern United States. Clay binds potassium and carries it into the stool.

  C. **Hypokalemia resulting from renal losses**

    1. **Diuretics.** Loop diuretics, thiazides, and acetazolamide (Diamox) may all cause hypokalemia.

2. **Vomiting**

   a. Although gastric contents contain some potassium ions, the major loss through vomiting occurs in the urine. The loss of gastric hydrogen ions generates metabolic alkalosis, which stimulates potassium ion secretion. The sodium and water losses from vomiting cause volume depletion and stimulate aldosterone secretion.

   b. In cases of surreptitious vomiting (bulimia), hypokalemia, metabolic alkalosis, volume depletion, and low urine chloride ion suggest the diagnosis.

3. **Renal losses caused by excess mineralocorticoid**

   a. **Primary aldosteronism.** Should be suspected in hypertensive patients who are hypokalemic prior to institution of diuretic therapy, or in those who become profoundly hypokalemic (< 2.5 mmol/L) with diuretics.

   b. **Cushing's syndrome.** 50% of patients with Cushing's syndrome have hypokalemia. Hypertension and metabolic alkalosis are also common.

   c. **Ectopic ACTH production.** Most commonly seen with small-cell carcinoma of the lung.

   d. **Adrenogenital syndrome.** 11-hydroxylase deficiency is manifested by virilization in the female, precocious puberty in the male, hypokalemia, metabolic alkalosis, and hypertension. 17-hydroxylase deficiency is a rare form of congenital hyperplasia of the adrenal glands associated with hypokalemia and hypertension.

   e. **Licorice ingestion.** Natural licorice contains glycyrrhizic acid, which has potent mineralocorticoid activity. These patients clinically resemble those with primary aldosteronism.

   f. **Hyperreninemic states.** Hypokalemia is accompanied by hypertension and metabolic alkalosis in renal vascular hypertension, malignant hypertension, and renin-producing tumors. It is distinguished from primary aldosteronism by elevated plasma renin.

   g. **Bartter's syndrome.** A rare disorder characterized by hypokalemia, metabolic alkalosis, elevated renin and aldosterone levels, and normal blood pressure.

   h. **Liddle's syndrome.** A rare disorder characterized by hypokalemia, hypertension, metabolic alkalosis, low plasma renin, and low urinary aldosterone.

   i. **Type I (distal) renal tubular acidosis.** Characterized by hyperchloremic metabolic acidosis and hypokalemia. Results from an inability to maintain a hydrogen ion gradient.

   j. **Type II (proximal) renal tubular acidosis.** Impaired proximal bicarbonate reabsorption results in distal delivery of bicarbonate and urinary loss of potassium ions as well as bicarbonate.

   k. **Antibiotics.** Carbenicillin and ticarcillin, administered as sodium salts, enhance potassium ion excretion. Amphotericin B alters distal tubule permeability, resulting in hypokalemia.
   l. **Magnesium depletion.** This may increase mineralocorticoid activity, but the pathophysiology is unknown.
   m. **Ureterosigmoidostomy.** Hypokalemic hyperchloremic metabolic acidosis occurs because of an exchange mechanism in the colon. Ureteral implantation into a loop of ileum is now performed.

IV. **Database**
   A. **Physical examination key points**
      1. **Cardiovascular.** Irregular pulse may represent new arrhythmias (PACs or PVCs), or digitalis toxicity.
      2. **Abdomen.** Look for distension and presence of bowel sounds. Ileus secondary to hypokalemia may be present. Abdominal examination may reveal a cause of vomiting.
      3. **Neurologic exam.** Weakness, blunting of reflexes, paresthesias, and paralysis may be seen.
   B. **Laboratory data**
      1. **Serum electrolytes.** Hypomagnesemia may coexist.
      2. **Arterial blood gases.** Look for alkalosis.
      3. **Urine potassium, chloride, and sodium.** If the patient is not taking diuretics, a low urine sodium or chloride indicates volume depletion. A relatively high urine potassium in the face of hypokalemia indicates renal losses.
      4. **Digoxin level.** A must if the patient is on digoxin. Hypokalemia may potentiate digoxin toxicity.
   C. **Radiologic and other studies.** An electrocardiogram may show digitalis effect or manifestations of hypokalemia ranging from PACs and PVCs to life-threatening ventricular arrhythmias. A U wave is a common finding.

V. **Plan.** The degree of hypokalemia cannot be used as a rigid determinant of the total potassium ion deficit. It has been estimated that in a normal adult, a decrease in serum potassium from 4 to 3 mmol/L corresponds to a 100- to 200-mmol decrement in total body potassium. Each additional fall of 1 mmol/L in serum potassium represents an additional deficit of 200–400 mmol.
   A. **Parenteral replacement**
      1. **Indications.** Should be considered in the following situations: digoxin toxicity or significant arrhythmias, severe hypokalemia (< 3.0 mmol/L), and inability to take oral replacements (NPO,

ileus, nausea and vomiting). Ideally, parenteral solutions should be administered through a central venous catheter. In most other cases, hypokalemia can be safely corrected in a slow, controlled fashion with oral supplementation.

2. **Implementation.** The maximum concentration of potassium chloride used in peripheral veins should generally not exceed 40 mmol/L because of the damaging effects on the veins of high concentrations, although in an emergent situation 60 mmol/L can be attempted. Potassium chloride 20 mmol diluted in 50–100 mL D5W or normal saline can be infused over 1 hour through a central line safely, with doses repeated as needed when severe depletion or life-threatening hypokalemia is present. Special care must be taken to ensure slow infusion of high doses. For lesser degrees of hypokalemia that require parenteral replacement, 10–15 mmol/h can be infused peripherally.

3. **Monitoring.** With large total replacement doses, check serum every 2–4 hours to avoid hyperkalemia. Cardiac monitoring in an ICU is required if arrhythmias are present, or for rapid infusions of potassium chloride. *Caution:* Cardiac monitoring is required for rates that exceed 15 mmol/h.

B. **Oral replacement.** Generally indicated for asymptomatic, mild potassium depletion (potassium usually > 3.0 mmol/L). Oral replacements include liquids and powder. Slow-release pills typically contain 8–10 mmol per tablet and thus are not usually appropriate for repletion therapy. The replacement rate should be 40–120 mmol/d in divided doses, depending on the patient's weight and level of hypokalemia. Maintenance therapy, if needed, should be given in doses of 20–80 mmol daily, using the preparation best tolerated by the patient. In patients with normal renal function, it is difficult to induce hyperkalemia through the oral administration of potassium. An important exception is the use of potassium supplements in patients on potassium-sparing diuretics or angiotensin-converting enzyme (ACE) inhibitors.

C. **Replacement of ongoing losses.** Large amounts of nasogastric aspirate should be replaced milliliter for milliliter, with D5 half-normal saline with 20 mmol/L potassium chloride every 4–6 hours.

D. **Refractory cases.** Rarely, hypokalemia may not be correctable because of concomitant hypomagnesemia.

REFERENCES

Black RM: Disorders of acid-base and potassium balance. In: Rubenstein E ed-in-chief; Federman DD ed. *Scientific American,* Sect 10: *Nephrology,* vol 3, pt II. Scientific American;1993:10.

Gabow PA, Peterson LN: Disorders of potassium metabolism. In: Schrier RW ed. *Renal and Electrolyte Disorders.* 4th ed. Little, Brown;1992:231.

Tannen RL: Approach to the patient with altered potassium concentration. In: Kelly WN ed-in-chief. *Textbook of Internal Medicine.* 2nd ed. Lippincott 1992;848.

38. HYPOMAGNESEMIA

I. **Problem.** A 40-year-old male complaining of chest pain is admitted to rule out myocardial infarction. A magnesium level returns at 0.8 mEq/L (normal 1.5-2.1 mEq/L).

II. **Immediate Questions**
   A. **What are the patient's vital signs?** Magnesium deficiency is associated with cardiac arrhythmias, including atrial fibrillation, supraventricular tachycardia, ventricular tachycardia, and ventricular fibrillation. Determining that the patient is not in any immediate distress and does not have hypotension or a tachyarrhythmia is essential.
   B. **Is the patient tremulous or currently having a seizure?** Tremor, tetany, muscle fasciculations, and seizures are all associated with magnesium deficiency. Determining the presence of these neurologic problems will help guide the urgency of treatment.

III. **Differential Diagnosis.** The diagnosis of magnesium deficiency, in general, rests on a high degree of suspicion, clinical assessment, and measurement of serum magnesium. It is important to recognize that serum magnesium levels do not always correlate well with intracellular magnesium levels. Thus, it is possible to have total body or intracellular magnesium depletion with normal (or even high) serum magnesium levels. For this reason, some experts have suggested that an initial 24-hour urine collection for magnesium, or a 24-hour urine magnesium retention test after parenteral administration of magnesium, be done to determine whether magnesium depletion is really present. Although such tests may be useful in specific settings, an acutely ill patient is generally treated based on the serum level and good clinical judgment.
   A. **Hypocalcemia.** The signs and symptoms of hypocalcemia are similar to those of hypomagnesemia; often both problems are present in a single patient. Hypocalcemia that does not correct with IV supplementation suggests the presence of magnesium deficiency.
   B. **Hypokalemia.** Potassium depletion often coexists with hypomagnesemia and can cause arrhythmias and muscle weakness, similar to hypomagnesemia. Hypokalemia that does not correct appropriately with potassium repletion also suggests magnesium depletion.
   C. **Lab error.** This is more likely if a colorimetric assay has been used. When in doubt, ask the lab to repeat the test and controls.
   D. **Causes of hypomagnesemia**
      1. **Increased excretion**
         a. **Medications.** Especially diuretics, antibiotics (ticarcillin, amphotericin B), aminoglycosides, *cis*-platinum and cyclosporin, may cause hypomagnesemia.

      b. Alcoholism. Very common cause as a result of decreased intake and renal magnesium wasting.

      c. Diabetes mellitus. Commonly seen in patients treated for diabetic ketoacidosis.

      d. Renal tubular disorders. With magnesium wasting.

      e. Hypercalcemia/hypercalciuria

      f. Hyperaldosteronism/Bartter's syndrome

      g. Excessive lactation

      h. Marked diaphoresis

  2. Reduced intake/malabsorption

      a. Starvation. A common cause.

      b. Bowel bypass or resection

      c. Total parenteral nutrition without adequate magnesium supplementation

      d. Chronic malabsorption syndrome. Such as pancreatic insufficiency.

      e. Chronic diarrhea

  3. Miscellaneous

      a. Acute pancreatitis

      b. Hypoalbuminemia

      c. Vitamin D therapy. Resulting in hypercalcuria.

IV. Database

  A. Physical examination key points

    1. Vital signs. Blood pressure and pulse to evaluate for hypotension and tachyarrhythmias. While taking blood pressure, leave cuff inflated above the systolic blood pressure for 3 minutes to check for carpal spasm (Trousseau's sign).

    2. HEENT. Check for Chvostek's sign (tapping over the facial nerve produces twitching of the mouth and eye). Nystagmus may be present.

    3. Heart. Check for regularity of rhythm.

    4. Abdomen. Evaluate for evidence of pancreatitis, such as absent bowel sounds and tenderness. Stigmata of chronic liver disease such as hepatosplenomegaly, caput medusae, ascites, spider angiomas, and palmar erythema suggest chronic alcohol abuse.

    5. Neurologic exam. Hyperactive reflexes, muscle fasciculations, seizures, and tetany can result from hypomagnesemia. Hyperactive reflexes may also be seen with alcohol withdrawal.

    6. Mental status. Psychosis, depression, and agitation may be present.

  B. Laboratory data

    1. Serum electrolytes, glucose, calcium, and phosphorus. Hypomagnesemia frequently accompanies other electrolyte abnormalities, especially hypocalcemia, hypokalemia, and alkalosis. If the patient is an alcoholic, then hypophosphatemia is also likely. Diabetics are prone to develop hypomagnesemia (especially in the setting of diabetic ketoacidosis).

2. **24-hour urine for magnesium.** May be helpful if the diagnosis is in question, or if there is a suspicion of renal magnesium wasting.

3. **Magnesium retention test.** Using either parenteral or oral magnesium. May be helpful in certain subsets of patients in whom either the diagnosis is in question or malabsorption is suspected.

4. **Miscellaneous.** As indicated. Liver function studies in alcoholics and serum amylase if pancreatitis is suspected.

C. **Radiologic and other studies.** Electrocardiographic findings may include prolongation of the PR, QT, and QRS intervals as well as ST depression and T waves. Rhythm disturbances include supraventricular arrhythmias (especially atrial fibrillation) as well as ventricular tachycardia and ventricular fibrillation.

V. **Plan.** The urgency of treatment depends on the clinical setting. The patient who is having neurologic or cardiac manifestations should be treated urgently with parenteral IV therapy. Asymptomatic individuals may be treated with oral magnesium, although many clinicians treat magnesium levels < 1.0 mEq/L with parenteral magnesium even though there is not always a good correlation between serum levels and intracellular levels.

A. **IV magnesium sulfate.** Magnesium sulfate 1 g (2 mL of a 50% solution of $MgSO_4$) equals 98 mg of elemental magnesium, which is equal to 8 mEq $MgSO_4$ or 4 mmol Mg^{2+}. If the patient is in tetany or status epilepticus, or is having significant cardiac arrhythmias, then 2 g of magnesium sulfate can be given IV over 10–20 min. For slightly less urgent situations, 1 g/hr may be given with close monitoring of deep tendon reflexes Q 3–4 hr. Magnesium should be administered only in life-threatening situations in patients with renal insufficiency; monitoring of deep tendon reflexes is required every hour. As long as signs and symptoms of hypomagnesemia are improving, the infusion can be slowed so that the patient receives approximately 10 g of magnesium sulfate in the first 24 hours. Selected patients may require more or less based on clinical findings. Subsequently, 5–6 g of magnesium sulfate may be given over Q 24 hr to replenish body reserves for the next 3–4 days.

In the setting of acute myocardial infarction, some authors feel that therapeutic (rather than replacement) administration of magnesium may prevent arrhythmias, limit damage from reperfusion injury and have a favorable impact on hemodynamics. Other authors dispute these claims. Protocols for administration vary, but one popular regime is to give 2 g magnesium sulfate IV over 5 min followed by 16 g over 24 hr as a constant infusion. Close monitoring of deep tendon reflexes, blood pressure, and respiratory status are essential.

Overdosage of magnesium may occur in the setting of renal failure and also accidentally, since several formulations are available in different concentrations. Treatment of magnesium overdosage complicated by respiratory arrest, shock, or asystole should be initiated with 1–2 g IV calcium gluconate (100–200 mg elemental calcium) over 3 min followed by 15 mg/kg over 4 hr. Physostigmine 1 mg given over 1 min has also been used. Initial treatment can be followed with dialysis, or saline and furosemide diuresis.

B. IM magnesium sulfate. 1–2 g IM Q 4 hr for five doses during the first 24 hours (following the patient's clinical status and serum levels as described earlier). This can then be followed by 1 g IM Q 6 hr for 2–3 days. Many patients complain about pain with the injections.

C. Magnesium oxide PO (20 mEq of magnesium per 400 mg tablet). 1–2 tablets per day for chronic maintenance therapy (may cause diarrhea, especially at higher doses).

D. Miscellaneous. Treat other electrolyte disorders, especially hypocalcemia (see Section I, Chapter 35, Hypocalcemia, V, p 180), hypokalemia (see Section I, Chapter 37, Hypokalemia, V, p 188) and hypophosphatemia (see Section I, Chapter 40, Hypophosphatemia, V, p 202), as well as other underlying illnesses.

REFERENCES

Elin RJ: Magnesium metabolism in health and disease. Dis Mon 1988;34:161.
Flink EB: Magnesium deficiency causes and effects. Hosp Pract 1987; Feb 15:116A.
Heesch CN, Eichorn EJ: Magnesium in acute myocardial infarction. Ann Emerg Med 1994;24:1154.
Reinhart RA: Magnesium metabolism. Arch Intern Med 1988;148:2415.

39. HYPONATREMIA

I. Problem. A 50-year-old man is admitted for evaluation of a right pulmonary hilar mass. Shortly after admission, you are called by the lab with a "panic" lab value. The serum sodium is 118 mmol/L (normal 136–145 mmol/L).

II. Immediate Questions

A. Is the patient symptomatic from the hyponatremia? Patients with hyponatremia may be asymptomatic, or there may be central nervous system (CNS) changes ranging from lethargy, anorexia, nausea, vomiting, agitation, and headache to marked disorientation, seizures, and death. Muscle cramps, weakness, and fatigue are also common symptoms.

B. Are there any recent prior sodium levels to document the chronicity of the hyponatremia? The rate of development and magnitude of hyponatremia correlates directly with the severity of the symptoms. Acute changes in sodium levels are more likely to produce more severe symptoms.

C. **Is there any evidence of volume depletion?** Orthostatic changes in blood pressure and heart rate suggest volume depletion.

D. **Does the patient have a history of vomiting or diarrhea?** Vomiting and diarrhea can cause wasting of sodium and extracellular fluid, resulting in hyponatremia.

E. **Is there any history of renal disease, congestive heart failure (CHF), cirrhosis, or nephrotic syndrome?** Any of these edematous states suggests an excess of sodium accompanied by an even greater excess of total body water.

F. **Is there any history of hypothyroidism or adrenal insufficiency?** Hypothyroidism and hypoadrenalism cause renal wasting of sodium, even in the face of hyponatremia.

G. **Is the patient taking any medications that could cause the hyponatremia?** Diuretics can cause hyponatremia by inducing sodium deficits in excess of water deficits. Chlorpropamide, nicotine, cyclophosphamide, nonsteroidal anti-inflammatory drugs (NSAIDs), antipsychotic medications (eg, haloperidol and thioridazine), and anticonvulsants such as carbamazepine (Tegretol) may cause hyponatremia. Mannitol used to treat elevated intracranial pressure or glaucoma can cause a low serum sodium by shifting water from the intracellular space to the hypertonic extracellular space.

H. **Does the patient suffer from any pulmonary disease?** Pneumonia, tuberculosis, lung carcinoma, and other pulmonary pathology may cause the syndrome of inappropriate antidiuretic hormone secretion (SIADH).

I. **Is there any CNS disease?** Meningitis, encephalitis, brain abscess, tumors, trauma, and a variety of other diseases can cause SIADH.

J. **Is there a history suggesting neoplasm, such as a history of weight loss, cough, and hemoptysis?** SIADH has been associated with bronchogenic carcinoma as well as several other cancers.

K. **Is there any history of hyperlipidemia or hyperproteinemia?** Either can cause a low serum sodium without extracellular fluid hypertonicity. This condition is also called pseudohyponatremia.

L. **Is there a history of diabetes?** A markedly elevated glucose can lower the serum sodium. The serum sodium is diluted by water moving from the intracellular space to the hypertonic extracellular space. Correction of the hyperglycemia will correct the hyponatremia.

M. **Is the lab value correct?** If the sodium level is unexpected, repeat the test.

III. **Differential Diagnosis.** The initial differentiation is between true hyponatremia with hypotonicity and laboratory artifact (pseudohyponatremia), as well as dilutional effects that result in isotonic or hypertonic hyponatremia. True hyponatremia may be classified according to the volume status of the patient: **hypovolemic; euvolemic;** or **hypervolemic** (See IV. A).

- **A. Pseudohyponatremia due to space-occupying compounds.** Lipids are the most common. For every increase in triglycerides of 1 g/dL, sodium will falsely decrease by 1.7 mmol/L. The lab can ultracentrifuge the specimen to find the correct plasma sodium level. Proteins are also a common cause of pseudohyponatremia, such as in Waldenström's macroglobulinemia and multiple myeloma. For accumulation of every 1 g/dL of protein, sodium will be falsely lowered by 1 mmol/L, plus some true reduction that occurs via the accumulation of cationic proteins in multiple myeloma.
- **B. Dilutional.** This is not a true pseudohyponatremia. It is a hypertonic hyponatremia resulting from the intracellular-to-extracellular movement of water. Diabetes mellitus is the most common cause. The expected decrease in serum sodium is 1.6 mmol/L for each 100 mg/dL of glucose > 100 mg/dL. Other non-glucose solutes that can cause the same effects are mannitol or glycerol. If the calculated serum osmolality differs from the measured serum osmolality by > 10 mOsm/kg, then it can be inferred that another solute is present.
- **C. Acute water intoxication.** This is hypotonic hyponatremia, occurring when the patient's water intake exceeds maximal urinary free water excretion. Urine osmolality should be < 120 mOsm/kg (specific gravity < 1.003) if maximal urinary dilution is present. This can occur by inappropriate administration of IV fluids or tube feedings, extensive use of tap water enemas, excessive swallowing of water during swimming or bathing, or abnormal water consumption (eg, in psychiatric patients). Can be treated by restricting patient's water intake.
- **D. Hypovolemic hyponatremia**
    1. **Extra-renal losses** (spot urinary sodium < 10 mmol/L).
        a. **GI fluid losses.** These may occur through vomiting, diarrhea, drainage tubes, fistulae, or gastrocystoplasty. In surreptitious or bulimic vomiting, the urinary chloride is usually < 10 mmol/L.
        b. **Third-space fluid loss.** May occur in pancreatitis, peritonitis, muscle trauma, effusions, or burns.
        c. **Skin.** Fluid may be lost through burns, cystic fibrosis, or heat stroke.
    2. **Renal losses** (spot urinary sodium > 20 mmol/L).
        a. **Diuretic usage.** Caused by thiazides and loop diuretics; often associated with hypokalemia and metabolic alkalosis. With surreptitious diuretic use, urine chloride is > 20 mmol/L.
        b. **Renal disorders.** Renal tubular acidosis, medullary cystic disease, polycystic disease and chronic interstitial nephritis can result in hyponatremia.

      c. Addison's disease. Characterized by mineralocorticoid deficiency. Hyperkalemia, low urinary potassium and metabolic acidosis are also found.

      d. Osmotic diuresis. Most commonly caused by hyperglycemia or mannitol.

E. Euvolemic hyponatremia

  1. SIADH. The diagnosis of SIADH is based on the findings of low serum osmolality, elevated urine sodium (> 20 mmol/L), and concentrated urine (osmolality near normal) after ruling out hypothyroidism and hypoadrenalism in a patient who is euvolemic.

      a. Carcinoma. Small-cell carcinoma of the lung is the most common form, but many others can also cause SIADH.

      b. Pulmonary disease. Pneumonia, tuberculosis, tumor, atelectasis, and pneumothorax.

      c. CNS disorders. These may involve trauma, tumors, cerebrovascular accidents, psychoses, and infections (eg, meningitis and encephalitis).

      d. Stress. Including perioperative stress.

      e. Drugs. Oral hypoglycemics (chlorpropamide), chemotherapeutic agents (cyclophosphamide, vincristine), psychotropic drugs (haloperidol, thioridazine, tricyclic antidepressants), prostaglandin inhibitors (NSAIDs, aspirin), anticonvulsants (carbamazepine), and clofibrate.

      f. Postoperative conditions. Anesthesia and surgical procedures cause an increase in antidiuretic hormone.

  2. Hypothyroidism

  3. Glucocorticoid deficiency

  4. Hypopituitarism

F. Hypervolemic hyponatremia

  1. CHF. Urine sodium is < 10 mmol/L.

  2. Cirrhosis. Urine sodium is < 10 mmol/L.

  3. Renal disease

      a. Chronic renal failure. Urine sodium > 20 mmol/L.

      b. Nephrotic syndrome. Urine sodium < 10 mmol/L.

IV. Database

A. Physical examination key points. The clinician should pay close attention to assessment of volume status.

  1. Vital signs. Evaluate patient for orthostatic blood pressure changes and heart rate changes. A decrease in systolic blood pressure of 10 mm Hg, and/or an increase in heart rate of 20 BPM 1 minute after changing from a supine to a standing position points to volume depletion. Tachypnea may suggest volume overload and pulmonary edema.

  2. Skin. Tissue turgor will be diminished and mucous membranes may appear dry with volume depletion. Poor skin turgor, however, can be a normal variant in the elderly. Edema suggests volume overload. Jaundice, spider angiomas, and caput medusae suggest cirrhosis.

3. **HEENT.** Evaluate the internal jugular veins. Determine the jugular venous pressure. When the patient's bed is elevated at 30 degrees the veins will be flat with volume depletion and markedly engorged with volume overload.

4. **Lungs.** Crackles may be heard with CHF.

5. **Heart.** An S_3 gallop suggests CHF.

6. **Abdomen.** Hepatosplenomegaly and ascites suggest cirrhosis. A hepatojugular reflux may be present in CHF.

7. **Neurologic exam.** Decreased deep tendon reflexes (DTRs), altered mental status, confusion, coma, or seizures may be present after a rapid fall in the serum sodium or from a chronically low serum sodium. If hyponatremia is chronic, the neurologic and mental status exams may be normal, even with levels < 120 mmol/L. Delay in the relaxation phase of DTRs is seen in hypothyroidism.

8. **Extremities.** Clubbing may be present with lung cancer.

B. **Laboratory data**

1. **Electrolytes.** Other abnormalities may coexist. Hypokalemia can potentiate hyponatremia as sodium shifts into cells in exchange for potassium. Hypokalemia and an increase in serum bicarbonate are seen with diuretic use. Hyperkalemia and a decrease in serum bicarbonate are seen in Addison's disease.

2. **Spot urine electrolytes and creatinine.** Obtain prior to any diuretic treatment.

3. **Urine and serum osmolality.** Serum osmolality will be normal in cases of laboratory artifact but decreased in true hyponatremia. Serum osmolality will be increased in hypertonic hyponatremia secondary to mannitol or glucose. Serum osmolality will be low with SIADH.

4. **Liver function test.** To detect liver disease.

5. **Thyroid function.** Hypothyroidism must be ruled out prior to diagnosing SIADH.

6. **Cortisol levels, ACTH stimulation test.** In addition, glucocorticoid deficiency must be ruled out prior to diagnosing SIADH.

7. **Cultures.** Blood and sputum cultures if indicated.

C. **Radiologic and other studies.**

1. **Chest x-ray (CXR).** Look for CHF, lung cancer, pneumonia or tuberculosis.

2. **Head CT scan.** If indicated.

V. Plan. The etiology of the hyponatremia and the presence and severity of symptoms guide therapy. Aggressive treatment of severe symptoms (eg, coma) is discussed below, as are specific therapies for certain diagnoses.

A. **Emergency treatment.** Usually for severe CNS symptoms (eg, seizures or coma).

   1. **Normal saline (NS) or furosemide 1 mg/kg.** Use a combination of NS and diuretics to achieve a net negative free water deficit in hyponatremia associated with euvolemic or hypervolemic conditions. Use NS by itself if the hyponatremia is associated with volume depletion. Carefully document fluid intake and output. Supplement fluids with potassium as needed. Too rapid correction of sodium can be deleterious, resulting in central pontine myelinolysis. Correct sodium level *rapidly* (> 1.0 mmol/L/hr) to 120–125 mmol/L; then *slowly* correct sodium level (< 0.5 mmol/L/hr) over next 24–48 hr to normal. In euvolemic and hypervolemic states, the excess total body water can be calculated from the following formula:

$$\text{weight (kg)} \times 0.60 = \text{total body water (TBW)}$$

$$\text{Water excess} = \text{TBW} \times \left(\frac{\text{desired [Na]}}{\text{measured [Na]}} - 1 \right)$$

     To calculate the total amount of sodium required to increase the sodium to a desired level, use the following formula:

$$\text{sodium required (mmol)} =$$
$$(\text{desired serum [Na]} - \text{actual serum [Na]}) \times \text{TBW}$$

     To estimate the increase in serum sodium concentration for a given amount of saline administered the following equation can be used:

$$\text{Increase in serum [Na]} =$$
$$\frac{(\text{IV fluid [Na]} - \text{serum [Na]}) \times \text{IV fluid volume}}{\text{TBW}}$$

   2. **Hypertonic saline.** (3%: contains 513 mEq of Na per liter). This preparation is rarely needed. Hypertonic saline can replace NS in above treatment regimens. The clinician must be very careful in using hypertonic saline because of the potential for serious complications (eg, pulmonary edema and central pontine myelinolysis) secondary to overly rapid correction of hyponatremia.

B. **Hypovolemic hyponatremia**

   1. For almost all causes, treat by repletion of volume and sodium. Give NS IV.

   2. In cases of diuretic abuse, repletion of lost body potassium is also necessary.

C. **Euvolemic hyponatremia.** (Patient is not edematous.) In cases of SIADH, restrict patient's water intake to 800–1000 mL daily. Give demeclocycline (300–600 mg BID PO) for chronic SIADH, such as that resulting from neoplasms. Onset of medication action may take up to a week.

    D. Hypervolemic hyponatremia. (Patient is edematous). Restrict IV and oral fluids.

        1. CHF. Treat with digoxin, diuretics (eg, furosemide), angiotensin-converting enzyme (ACE) inhibitors, and sodium restriction.

        2. Nephrotic syndrome. Give steroids (if the cause is steroid-responsive); restrict sodium and water intake; increase patient's protein intake. Furosemide is commonly used.

        3. Cirrhosis. Treat with restriction of sodium and water, and diuretics. Initially, give spironolactone 100 mg PO Q day, increasing dose Q 2–3 days up to 400 mg Q day; this regimen is usually effective. A portosystemic shunt is needed in only 5–10% of patients to control ascites.

        4. Renal failure. Treat with sodium and water restriction, loop diuretics, and dialysis if indicated.

REFERENCES

Avner ED: Clinical disorders of water metabolism: Hyponatremia and hypernatremia. Pediatr Ann 1995;24:23.

Bell T, Schrier RW: Disorders of water metabolism. In: Schrier RW, ed. *Renal and Electrolyte Disorders.* 4th ed. Little, Brown;1992:1.

Brown RG: Disorders of water and sodium balance. Postgrad Med 1993;93:227.

Oh MS, Carroll HJ: Disorders of sodium metabolism: Hypernatremia and hyponatremia. Crit Care Med 1992;20:94.

Van Amelsvoort T, Bakshi R, Devaux CV, Schwabe S: Hyponatremia associated with carbamazepine and oxcarbazepine therapy: A review. Epilepsia 1994;35:181.

Weisberg LS: Pseudohyponatremia: A reappraisal. Am J Med 1989;86:315.

40. HYPOPHOSPHATEMIA

I. Problem. A 26-year-old male with type I diabetes was admitted 6 hours ago for treatment of diabetic ketoacidosis and now has a serum phosphate level of 1.0 mg/dL.

II. Immediate Questions

    A. Are there any symptoms related to the low phosphate? Serum phosphate levels below 1.0 mg/dL require prompt treatment regardless of symptoms. Above that level, one should check for symptoms related to low phosphate such as numbness or tingling, muscle weakness, anorexia, confusion, irritability, seizures, and skeletal pain. Muscle weakness, mental status changes, and hematologic abnormalities are the most common findings.

    B. What treatment is the patient receiving? Hypophosphatemia usually results from phosphate shifts within the body. This is most often a consequence of medical treatment, such as hyperalimentation, correction of diabetic ketoacidosis, or refeeding of malnour-

ished or alcoholic patients. Antacids also can cause hypophosphatemia by binding phosphate in the gut.
   C. Does the patient consume alcohol? Chronic alcoholism is a
   common cause of hypophosphatemia secondary to poor intake
   and possible increased renal excretion especially if hypomagnesemia is also present.

III. Differential Diagnosis. A low serum phosphate level usually results
from a combination of increased renal loss, increased intestinal loss,
or intracellular shift of phosphate, the latter being the most common.
   A. Intracellular shift of phosphate. Alkalosis from any etiology. See
   Section I, Chapter 3, Alkalosis, p 17.
   B. Increased intestinal phosphate loss
      1. Phosphate-binding antacids.
      2. Malabsorption, vomiting, diarrhea, malnutrition.
   C. Increased renal phosphate loss.
      1. Acidosis. Including untreated diabetic ketoacidosis (DKA).
      **2. Hyperparathyroidism, renal tubular disease, hypokalemia,
         hypomagnesemia, diuretics.**
   D. Multifactorial.
      1. Alcoholism and liver disease. All three mechanisms.
      2. Vitamin D deficiency or resistance. Renal and intestinal loss.
      3. Treatment of DKA and severe burns. Renal and intracellular
         shift.

IV. Database
   A. Physical examination key points
      1. Vital signs
         a. Temperature. Heat stroke can cause hypophosphatemia
            from intracellular shifts.
         b. Sepsis. Occurs with greater frequency in patients who are
            hypophosphatemic because of leukocyte dysfunction.
         c. Respiratory rate. Hyperventilation with resulting alkalosis is
            a cause of extracellular-to-intracellular shifts of phosphate.
      2. HEENT. Check for thyromegaly. Thyrotoxicosis can also cause
         extracellular-to-intracellular shifts of phosphate.
      3. Heart. A reversible congestive cardiomyopathy may result from
         hypophosphatemia. Look for a laterally displaced apical pulse
         and third heart sound (S_3).
      4. Lungs. Listen for rales as evidence of cardiomyopathy. Acute
         hypophosphatemia can also result in acute respiratory failure
         (ARF).

5. **Neurologic exam.** Confusion and coma may be present. Sensory examination may be abnormal secondary to related paresthesias.
6. **Musculoskeletal exam.** Check for diffuse muscle weakness. Tenderness suggests rhabdomyolysis; however, the phosphate may increase to extremely high levels with rhabdomyolysis.

B. **Laboratory data**
1. **Serum electrolytes.** Especially bicarbonate and potassium. An elevated bicarbonate may suggest a metabolic alkalosis; a low bicarbonate may represent compensation for a chronic respiratory alkalosis. Alkalosis results in extracellular-to-intracellular shifts of phosphate. Hypokalemia can cause hypophosphatemia.
2. **Arterial blood gases and pH.** Alkalosis (either metabolic or respiratory) results in intracellular shifts of phosphate. A metabolic acidosis with an increased anion gap and an elevated glucose suggests diabetic ketoacidosis, which can have associated hypophosphatemia. An elevated pCO_2 also suggests respiratory failure which can occur as a result of hypophosphatemia.
3. **Calcium, magnesium, and glucose levels.** A low calcium may suggest vitamin D deficiency or osteomalacia. A high calcium suggests hyperparathyroidism or thiazide diuretic use, which can cause hypophosphatemia. Hypomagnesemia results in increased phosphate excretion.
4. **Glucose.** There is increased urinary excretion of phosphate in diabetic ketoacidosis.
5. **Uric acid.** Hypophosphatemia can be seen with acute gout; however, the uric acid level may be normal in acute gout.
6. **Liver enzymes, albumin, bilirubin, and creatine phosphokinase (CPK)**. Hypophosphatemia may cause liver dysfunction. A CPK should be checked to rule out rhabdomyolysis from severe hypophosphatemia, especially if muscle tenderness is present or develops.
7. **Complete blood count with differential.** An elevated white blood cell (WBC) count with a left shift suggests a bacterial infection. As a result of white cell dysfunction, patients with hypophosphatemia are susceptible to bacterial infections.
8. **Peripheral smear.** Severe hypophosphatemia can cause hemolysis.
9. **Platelet count.** Thrombocytopenia and platelet dysfunction can result.

C. **Radiologic and other studies**
1. **Bone films.** May show pseudofractures.
2. **Chest x-ray.** Possible complications of hypophosphatemia such as congestive cardiomyopathy and respiratory failure are indications for a CXR.

3. **Electroencephalogram.** An EEG may be needed to evaluate seizures or encephalopathy, which are possible complications of hypophosphatemia.

V. Plan. If the phosphate level is < 1.0 mg/dL, start IV replacement therapy immediately. If the level is 1.0–1.5 mg/dL and the patient is symptomatic, start IV replacement therapy. Otherwise, oral treatment is usually sufficient.

A. **Intravenous treatment**
   1. If the hypophosphatemia is recent and uncomplicated, give 0.08 mmol/kg body weight (2.5 mg/kg) intravenously over 6 hours. Sodium phosphate and potassium phosphate IV solutions both contain 3 mmol of phosphate per milliliter.
   2. If the hypophosphatemia is long-standing or complicated, give 0.16 mmol/kg body weight (5.0 mg/kg) IV over 6 hours.
   3. In either case, consider using 25% to 50% higher doses if the patient is symptomatic, but do not exceed 0.24 mmol/kg (7.5 mg/kg) or 16.9 mmol (525 mg) for a 70-kg patient.
   4. Recheck the phosphate level promptly after the 6-hour infusion, and reassess need for further replacement.

B. **Oral replacement**
   1. Neutra-Phos tablets contain 250 mg phosphorus (8 mmol)/ tablet or Neutra-Phos powder contains 0.1 mmol of phosphate per mL.
   2. Milk contains modest amounts of phosphate. Skim milk has slightly more phosphate and may be better tolerated for those who are lactose-intolerant (Table 1–7).
   3. Fleet enema solution and Fleet Phospho-Soda contain buffered sodium phosphate. Can be administered orally. Fleet enema solution contains 1.4 mmol/mL, administer 15–30 mL, TID–QID (50–150 mmol/24 hr). Fleet Phospho-Soda contains 4.15 mmol/mL of phosphate. It is estimated that 2/3 of orally administered phosphate is absorbed.

C. **Precautions**
   1. It may be necessary to give calcium supplements to hypocalcemic patients who are being given phosphate.

TABLE 1–7. AMOUNT OF PHOSPHATE IN AN 8-OZ SERVING OF MILK.

Milk	Phosphorus[1] (mg/8-oz. serving)
Skim	247
Whole	227

[1] 250 mg of elemental phosphorus = 8 mmol phosphate.

2. Do not give calcium and phosphate through the same IV line.
3. Beware of causing hyperphosphatemia, hypotension, hyperkalemia, osmotic diuresis, and hypernatremia.

REFERENCES

Lentz RD, Brown DM, Kjellstrand CM: Treatment of severe hypophosphatemia. Ann Intern Med 1978;89:941.

Popovtzer MM, Knochel JP: Disorders of calcium, phosphorus, vitamin D and parathyroid hormone activity. In: Schrier RW ed. *Renal and Electrolyte Disorders.* 4th ed. Little, Brown; 1992:287.

41. HYPOTENSION (SHOCK)

I. Problem. A 70-year-old man is admitted for nausea, abdominal pain and weakness. Blood pressure is 70/50.

II. Immediate Questions

A. What are all of the patient's vital signs? Confirm the blood pressure in both arms manually. An arterial line may be useful. A marked bradycardia or tachycardia suggests a cardiac arrhythmia. Tachycardia may accompany hypovolemia, hemorrhage or sepsis. Fever suggests sepsis, but hypothermia can also be seen in sepsis, myxedema, or Addisonian crisis. Tachypnea may be seen in cardiogenic shock, pulmonary embolus (PE), and sepsis.

B. What is the patient's mental status? This is an indicator of adequate perfusion of vital organs.

C. What are the patient's medications and when were they last given? Have any new medications been started? Many medications such as angiotensin-converting enzyme (ACE) inhibitors, direct vasodilators such as minoxidil (Loniten), and central-acting antihypertensive agents such as clonidine (Catapres) lower blood pressure and may do so to an extreme. Other IV medications with similar effects include nitroprusside, nitroglycerin, and phenytoin (Dilantin). Anaphylaxis should be considered, especially if there is respiratory distress. Diuretics can rarely cause sufficiently significant volume depletion to cause hypotension.

D. Does the patient have any other symptoms? The patient's symptoms may indicate where to begin the evaluation, such as a history of bleeding, vomiting, diarrhea, polyuria, or chest pain. Chest discomfort and dyspnea suggest PE or myocardial ischemia/infarction as the cause of the hypotension. Chest discomfort from cardiac ischemia/infarction is not always dull or vise-like; also dyspnea may be the only symptom of cardiac ischemia/infarction.

III. **Differential Diagnosis.** The term **hypotension** is a relative term. For elderly patients with long-standing hypertension, a systolic blood pressure of 100 mm Hg may be inadequate. But in others, a systolic pressure of 90 mm Hg may be normal. Hypotension/shock is defined as a state in which the blood pressure is inadequate to provide adequate tissue perfusion. Subcategories of hypotension/shock include the following:

A. **Hypovolemia**
   1. **Hemorrhagic**
      a. **Traumatic.** Trauma patients may lose a large volume of blood into body cavities such as the chest, abdomen, and pelvis. This loss may not be readily apparent.
      b. **Postoperative or postprocedural.** Blood may be lost following certain procedures such as liver biopsy or central venous line placement.
      c. **Miscellaneous.** Gastrointestinal bleeding, ruptured aneurysm, ruptured ovarian cyst, ectopic pregnancy.
   2. **Fluid losses.** From severe vomiting, diarrhea, perspiration, extensive burns, diuresis, and "third-space losses" (peritonitis or pancreatitis).

B. **Vasogenic.** Inappropriate loss of vascular tone may develop as a result of sepsis, anaphylaxis, adrenal insufficiency, acidosis, central nervous system injury, or from certain medications.

C. **Cardiogenic.** Acute pump failure may develop as a result of myocardial infarction (MI) or decompensated congestive heart failure (CHF). Cardiac arrhythmia (supraventricular, ventricular, or various degrees of heart block), tension pneumothorax, pericardial tamponade, and PE can cause hypotension.

IV. **Database**
A. **Physical examination key points**
   1. **Vital signs.** Temperature, blood pressure, pulse, respiratory rate, including orthostatic blood pressure and heart rate. A decrease in systolic blood pressure of 10 mm Hg and/or an increase in heart rate of 20 bpm on movement from the supine to the standing position after 1 minute is indicative of volume depletion.
   2. **Skin.** Poor skin turgor suggests volume depletion, but may be a normal variant in the elderly. Cool, clammy skin indicates cardiogenic or hypovolemic shock, whereas warm, moist skin signifies vasodilation (sepsis).
   3. **Neck.** Jugular venous distension (JVD) and pulsations may be helpful in determining volume status and cardiac rhythm, as well as in providing clues for the diagnosis of cardiac tamponade or tension pneumothorax. Jugular venous distension with the latter two conditions does not decrease with inspiration.

4. **Chest.** Tracheal deviation suggests tension pneumothorax. Wheezing or stridor may indicate anaphylaxis. (See Section I, Chapter 4, Anaphylactic Reaction, p 23.) Rales and wheezes point to cardiac failure. Abnormalities during chest percussion may indicate pneumothorax, pleural effusion, hemothorax, or pneumonia.

5. **Heart.** Palpate for a thrill or a change in the point of maximal impulse. A new thrill may point to a ventricular septal defect (VSD) or papillary muscle dysfunction complicating an acute MI. Loss of a palpable apical pulse suggests a pericardial effusion. Auscultate for new murmurs suggesting acute mitral regurgitation or a VSD. A third heart sound (S_3) is heard in left ventricular failure; a new fourth heart sound (S_4) suggests an acute MI.

6. **Abdomen.** Rebound tenderness or positive Murphy's sign, and absence of bowel sounds suggest sepsis from an abdominal source. (See Section I, Chapter 1, Abdominal Pain, p 1.) Absent bowel sounds and tenderness may be present with a large GI bleed. A pulsatile mass suggests a leaking aortic aneurysm. Ecchymoses may be seen in retroperitoneal bleeds from a variety of causes such as hemorrhagic pancreatitis.

7. **Rectum.** Presence of hematochezia or occult blood may indicate acute GI blood loss.

8. **Female genitalia.** A gynecologic exam in young females is mandatory to rule out a ruptured ectopic pregnancy.

9. **Extremities.** Instability of pelvis or femurs suggests a fracture, which can result in significant bleeding into either the pelvis or the thigh. Edema may indicate volume overload or venous/lymphatic obstruction. Inspect for inflammation of vascular access sites suggesting iatrogenic infection/sepsis.

10. **Neurologic exam.** Altered mental status may indicate inadequate cerebral hypoperfusion, as well as suggest possible etiologies such as a cerebrovascular accident.

B. **Laboratory data**

1. **Complete blood count.** Serial hematocrits may indicate blood loss. Acute blood loss may not be reflected by an immediate drop in the hematocrit, but will fall as intravascular volume equilibrates. The white blood count and differential may indicate sepsis as the cause. The platelet count will be low in disseminated intravascular coagulation (DIC), suggesting sepsis.

2. **Serum electrolytes.** A low serum bicarbonate could be caused by a lactic acidosis secondary to decreased perfusion. Severe acidosis or hypokalemia may cause an arrhythmia.

3. **Prothrombin time, partial thromboplastin time.** A coagulopathy may indicate DIC, hepatic dysfunction, or excessive anticoagulation.

4. **Arterial blood gases.** Early sepsis may produce a respiratory alkalosis, but usually a metabolic acidosis develops. Metabolic

acidosis also develops in shock as a result of poor perfusion. Severe acidosis (pH < 7.20) may inhibit the effectiveness of vasopressors and cause arrhythmias; it should be corrected. Hypoxemia may also be present and requires ventilatory support.

5. **Lactic dehydrogenase (LDH) and creatine phosphokinase (CPK) with isoenzymes.** Monitor if MI is suspected, as well as to rule out injury secondary to the hypotension.

6. **Type and cross-match.** Blood should be made ready for transfusion for patients in whom hemorrhage is suspected.

7. **Pregnancy test.** To rule out ectopic pregnancy in young females.

8. **Blood, sputum, urine, and wound cultures.** For suspected sepsis.

C. **Radiologic and other studies**

1. **Chest x-ray.** May indicate source of sepsis or congestive heart failure. May be diagnostic for pneumothorax or hemothorax.

2. **Electrocardiogram.** Myocardial infarct or ischemia may be evident and arrhythmias can be evaluated.

3. **Pulmonary artery catheter (Swan-Ganz).** Very helpful in a patient with shock. Hemodynamic measurements may be used to aid the diagnosis and management of the hypotensive patient (see Table 1–8). Also useful when ruling out cardiac tamponade, which results in equalization of pressures. The right atrial pressure equals the elevated right ventricular diastolic pressure in this condition.

4. **Angiography.** Pulmonary angiograms may reveal a PE. Abdominal angiograms are often helpful in detecting the source of GI bleeding, particularly of the lower GI tract.

5. **Nuclear scans.** A ventilation/perfusion ($\dot{V}/\dot{Q}$) lung scan may aid in diagnosing PE. Radiolabeled red blood cell scans may help identify sources of bleeding in the GI tract.

6. **Echocardiogram.** A noninvasive test to evaluate global ventricular function and valvular function, and to rule out mechanical defects such as VSD or ruptured papillary muscle. Pericardial effusion resulting in tamponade can also be excluded.

TABLE 1–8. PARAMETERS USEFUL IN THE EVALUATION OF HYPOTENSION.[1]

Type	CVP	PCWP	CO	HR	SVR
Sepsis	↑ or ↓	↓	↑↑	↑	↓
Hypovolemia	↓	↓	↑ or ↔	↑	↑↑
Cardiogenic	↑	↑	↓	↑ or ↔	↑

[1] CVP (central venous pressure); PCWP (pulmonary capillary wedge pressure); CO (cardiac output); HR (heart rate); SVR (systemic vascular resistance).

    7. Paracentesis, thoracentesis, culdocentesis, pericardiocentesis. As indicated.

V. Plan. Establish adequate tissue perfusion as soon as possible. Generally, a systolic blood pressure > 90 mm Hg is adequate. Signs of adequate perfusion include improved mental status and increased urine output (0.5–1.0 mL/min).

  A. Emergency management

    1. Control external hemorrhage with direct pressure.

    2. Establish venous access, preferably two large-bore (14–16 gauge) peripheral intravenous lines.

    3. Trendelenburg position (supine with feet elevated) or pneumatic antishock garment (PASG or MAST) may be useful in hypovolemic shock.

    4. Insert Foley catheter to monitor urinary output.

    5. Administer supplemental oxygen and ventilatory support as needed.

    6. Severe metabolic acidosis (pH < 7.10) should be corrected with intravenous sodium bicarbonate to a pH > 7.20 or a serum bicarbonate > 12 mmol/L. Remember, an ampoule of sodium bicarbonate is hyperosmolar. After several ampoules, it is prudent to start an isotonic bicarbonate drip for persistent acidosis. A bicarbonate drip is made by adding three ampoules of sodium bicarbonate (50 mmol/50 mL) to one liter of D5W. Respiratory acidosis can be corrected by improving minute ventilation (V_e) to reduce pCO_2.

    7. Central venous pressure (CVP) or Swan-Ganz catheterization will aid in the differential diagnosis of shock as well as with fluid management.

  B. Hypovolemic shock

    1. Administer fluids (intravenous normal saline or lactated Ringer's) and red blood cells if indicated (HCT ≤ 30%), using blood pressure, urine output, and central filling pressures as a guide.

    2. Use vasopressor agents such as norepinephrine and dopamine, if hypotension persists despite a fluid challenge sufficient to achieve adequate filling pressures (PCWP 16–18 mm Hg). Dopamine is started at a dose of 2.5–5.0 mg/kg/min and increased up to 20 mg/kg/min. The dose of norepinephrine is 1–12 µg/min.

  C. Neurogenic shock

    1. Institute moderate IV fluid administration and avoid volume overload.

    2. Low-dose vasopressors may be necessary.

D. Vasogenic shock

   1. Septic shock. Identify and treat the source of the infection.

    a. Administer intravenous fluids and vasopressors as indicated.

    b. Broad-spectrum antibiotics are generally used if a specific source cannot be readily identified. Gram's stain of infected fluid will guide antibiotic choice. An aminoglycoside or a third-generation cephalosporin (ceftazidime or cefopera-zone), and an antipseudomonas penicillin such as pipera-cillin or ticarcillin are good antibiotic combinations to begin with, in the case of sepsis in a neutropenic patient or in a patient with a hospital-acquired infection.

   2. Anaphylactic shock. See Section I, Chapter 4, Anaphylactic Reaction, p 23.

    a. Remove precipitating agent as soon as possible.

    b. Immediately administer epinephrine 0.3 mL of 1:1000 SC.

    c. Maintain an adequate airway.

    d. An antihistamine such as diphenhydramine (Benadryl) 25 mg IM or IV, and corticosteroids such as hydrocortisone 100–250 mg IV, can also be given.

   3. Addisonian crisis. Give hydrocortisone 100 mg IV bolus, then 100 mg IV every 6–8 hours, in any patient in whom this diagnosis is suspected.

E. Cardiogenic shock

   1. This form of shock is usually complicated and more difficult to manage; therefore, hemodynamic monitoring with a Swan-Ganz catheter should always be used to guide therapy.

   2. Initial priority should be given to establishing an adequate perfusion pressure (systolic blood pressure > 90 mm Hg) while hemodynamic monitoring catheters are placed.

   3. Once cardiac hemodynamics have been evaluated, appropriate use of diuretics (IV furosemide), cardiac inotropes (dopamine, dobutamine), vasopressors (dopamine, norepinephrine; see above), antiarrhythmics, and intra-aortic balloon counterpulsation can be instituted.

   4. Pericardiocentesis is indicated if there is hemodynamic compromise secondary to pericardial tamponade.

   5. If a tension pneumothorax is present, a 14- to 16-gauge needle should be placed in the second or third intercostal space just superior to the rib in the midclavicular line until a chest tube can be placed.

42. HYPOTHERMIA

I. Problem. You are called to see a patient in the emergency room with a temperature of 32.0°C (89.6°F).

II. Immediate Questions

A. Does the patient have any possible source of infection? Septic patients may be hypothermic. Look for evidence of pneumonia, urinary tract infection, or any other cause of bacteremia; one study found that 41% of patients admitted for hypothermia had a serious infection.

B. Is there a history of other medical problems? Hypothyroidism, hypoglycemia, hypopituitarism, and hypoadrenalism may all present with hypothermia. Alcohol also predisposes humans to environment-induced hypothermia.

C. What is the clinical setting? Is there a history of exposure to cold weather or inadequate heating or clothing? The very young and very old are susceptible to hypothermia as a result of environmental exposure.

D. Is the patient taking any medications? Barbiturates and phenothiazines impair hypothalamic thermoregulation. Alcohol is a vasodilator and CNS depressant, thus increasing the risk for hypothermia from environmental exposure. The use of insulin, thyroid medication, or steroids may also suggest an etiology.

III. Differential Diagnosis

A. Sepsis. Bacteremia must be ruled out.

B. Environmental exposure. Was the patient found outdoors or in an unheated building?

C. Metabolic abnormalities

   1. **Myxedema.** Thermoderegulation resulting in hypothermia associated with hypothyroidism may have concomitant mental status changes including coma. There is often a precipitating event.

   2. **Hypoglycemia.** This condition has many potential causes (See Section I, Chapter 36, Hypoglycemia, p 181). It may also be associated with overwhelming sepsis or depleted glycogen stores due to chronic alcohol consumption.

   3. **Addison's disease.** May be acute or chronic. Often there is a history of steroid ingestion. May be secondary to metastatic carcinoma or idiopathic.

   4. **Uremia.** Easily ruled out by checking BUN and creatinine.

   5. **Hypopituitarism.** Can result in hypoadrenalism and hypothyroidism. Can also cause hypoglycemia.

D. CNS dysfunction

   1. **Cerebrovascular accident.** Look for focal neurologic findings such as motor weakness or sensory deficit, unilateral hyperreflexia or plantar extension with Babinski reflex.

   2. **Head trauma.** A history and careful examination of head, eyes, ears, nose, and neck should reveal any recent injury.

3. **Spinal cord transection.** Paraplegia or quadriplegia on examination.
4. **Wernicke's encephalopathy.** This condition is characterized by a triad of ophthalmoplegia, mental status changes, and ataxia. It is secondary to thiamine deficiency from decreased intake associated most often in the United States with chronic alcohol ingestion.
5. **Drug ingestion.** (See Section II.D.)
6. **Miscellaneous.** Other diagnoses to consider are generalized erythroderma, protein–calorie malnutrition, and anorexia nervosa.

IV. Database
A. Physical examination key points
1. **Vital signs.** Record the core temperature accurately with a rectal thermometer; make sure that it is a low-recording thermometer. Standard thermometers may not record temperatures lower than 34.4°C (93.8°F). Keep in mind that hypotension and bradycardia frequently occur in hypothermia.
2. **Skin.** Look for evidence of frostbite, diffuse erythroderma, burns, or insulin injection sites. Hyperpigmentation suggests primary adrenal insufficiency.
3. **Heart.** Heart sounds may be distant, slow, or absent.
4. **Lungs.** Respirations may be slow and shallow. Look for signs of pneumonia.
5. **Abdomen.** Ileus may occur with hypothermia.
6. **Neurologic exam.** Look for signs of head trauma. Check pupil reactivity; pupils may be nonreactive but are often sluggish and will react slowly. Mental status may vary from mental slowing to confusion and coma. Check deep tendon reflexes, which may be absent with severe hypothermia. A slow relaxation phase points to hypothyroidism.

B. Laboratory data
1. **Complete blood count.** Hypothermia can cause hemoconcentration and leukocytosis. Leukocytosis or leukopenia with an increase in banded neutrophils suggests sepsis.
2. **Platelet count.** A low platelet count can occur with either secondary sequestration or disseminated intravascular coagulation (DIC) caused by either hypothermia or associated with sepsis. (See Section I, Chapter 58, Thrombocytopenia, p 289)
3. **Prothrombin time, partial thromboplastin time (PT and PTT).** Elevation of the PT and PTT is consistent with DIC, which can be a complication of hypothermia or associated with sepsis. (See Section I, Chapter 12, Coagulopathy, p 64)
4. **Blood urea nitrogen (BUN) and creatinine.** To rule out uremia. The BUN:creatinine ratio may be increased secondary to hemoconcentration.

5. **Glucose.** Hypoglycemia may be the cause of hypothermia or associated with underlying cause.
6. **Thyroxine (T_4) and thyroid-stimulating hormone (TSH).** You will need to rule out hypothyroidism. The T_4 can be low in the euthyroid sick state but the TSH should be normal.
7. **Cortrosyn stimulation test.** (See Section II, ACTH Stimulation Test, p 301) This test is to rule out adrenal insufficiency since a single cortisol level can be misleading. Also, be sure to check adrenal reserve in all patients with severe hypothyroidism.
8. **Arterial blood gases.** Correct pH and pCO_2 findings to allow for changes in body temperature. For each 1°C below 37°C (98.6°F), add 0.015 to the pH. To correct the pCO_2, subtract 4.4% for each 1°C below 37°C (98.6°F). Your clinical lab will make these corrections for you as long as the patient's temperature is known. The pO_2 should also be corrected; however, this function is a nonlinear equation. Refer to the reference listed below for the equation. A metabolic or respiratory acidosis may be present secondary to the hypothermia.
9. **Blood cultures.** Rule out sepsis.
10. **Serum and urine drug screen.** Rule out barbiturates or phenothiazines as possible causes.

C. **Radiologic and other studies**
   1. **Chest x-ray.** Obtain to rule out pneumonia as a source of infection. Pneumonia is also the most common sequela of hypothermia during the recovery period.
   2. **Electrocardiogram.** Hypothermia can promote myocardial irritability and cause conduction abnormalities. The ECG may show T-wave inversion and PR, QRS, and QT prolongation as well as the unique J wave (or Osborn wave), which closely follows the QRS complex. Continuous ECG monitoring is important with a temperature below 32°C (89.6°F) because of the risk of cardiac arrhythmias. Atrial fibrillation is common. Ventricular tachycardia and fibrillation occurs frequently at temperatures below 86.0°F (30°C).

V. **Plan**
   A. **General support**
      1. Make sure the patient is hemodynamically stable. If ventricular fibrillation occurs, cardiopulmonary resuscitation (See Section I, Chapter 9, Cardiopulmonary Arrest, p 42) should be instituted and continued until the core temperature rises. In this clinical setting, the statement "A patient is not dead until they are warm and dead" applies.
      2. If you suspect hypothermia secondary to environmental exposure, place an intravenous line to replace fluids as chronic hypothermia leads to volume depletion. The IV fluids can be warmed to 43°C (109.4°F).
      3. Other therapeutic measures depend on the clinical setting. If sepsis is a possibility, then begin antibiotics immediately.

4. Give IV steroids if you suspect Addison's disease; or IV thyroxine if you suspect possible myxedema coma.

5. Some clinicians advocate administration of 100 mg of thiamine IV, an ampoule (50 mL) of D50, and 2 mg of naloxone (Narcan) to all comatose hypothermic patients.

B. **Rewarming techniques**

1. In cases of environmental exposure, remove the patient from the cold environment and use some insulating material such as blankets.

2. More aggressive rewarming techniques are controversial. Active *external* rewarming with an electric blanket may produce hypovolemic shock through peripheral vasodilation, or cause "afterdrop" in core temperature through movement of the cold blood to the body core. External rewarming may also worsen a metabolic acidosis.

3. Such concerns have led to the use of active *core* rewarming for patients with core temperatures below 32°C (89.6°F), especially in the setting of chronic hypothermia secondary to environmental exposure. Active core rewarming techniques include gastrointestinal rewarming, peritoneal dialysis, inhalation of warmed oxygen, hemodialysis, and use of cardiopulmonary-bypass circuit. Some clinicians favor the latter two techniques in severe accidental hypothermia due to environmental exposure. Gastrointestinal rewarming involves the instillation of warmed normal saline via nasogastric and rectal tubes, removal of the fluid, and repetition of the process.

REFERENCES

Carden DL, Nowak RM: Disseminated intravascular coagulation in hypothermia. JAMA 1982;247:2099.

Danzl DF, Pozos RS: Accidental hypothermia. N Engl J Med 1994;331:1756.

Lewin S, Brettman LR, Holzman RS: Infections in hypothermic patients. Arch Intern Med 1981;141:920.

Reuler JB: Hypothermia: Pathophysiology, clinical settings and management. Ann Intern Med 1978;89:519.

Weinberg AD: Hypothermia. Ann Emerg Med 1993;22:370.

43. INSOMNIA

I. **Problem.** A patient hospitalized for lower-extremity cellulitis complains of lying awake for hours at night.

II. **Immediate Questions**

A. **What is the patient's mental status?** Delirium and dementia can both present with sleep disturbance. Delirium frequently results in a reversal of the normal sleep/wake cycle. It is important to avoid treatment with sedatives/hypnotics as they may actually worsen the symptomatology. Because some causes of delirium are potentially life-threatening, aggressive evaluation of delirious patients is warranted. (See Section I, Chapter 13, Coma, Acute Mental Status Changes, p 69.)

B. **Is the patient kept awake by pain?** Painful stimuli result in a state of increased arousal which interferes with sleep and escalates the cycle of sleep disturbance and pain. Common examples include rheumatoid arthritis, in which a worsening of morning stiffness is associated with sleep disturbance, and fibrositis, in which symptoms can be reproduced by disturbing delta sleep in normal subjects.

C. **What is the patient's daytime sleep pattern?** Certainly, a patient who sleeps for extended periods during the day will not be able to fall asleep readily at night. Sleep hygiene interventions may be of use.

D. **Does the patient take hypnotic medications regularly? What are his or her current medications?** Virtually all hypnotic agents show a tolerance effect with chronic use and a disruption of the sleep patterns that can interfere with normal sleep. Abrupt withdrawal of these agents almost invariably results in sleep disturbance, often termed **rebound insomnia**. It is also important to remember that withdrawal from barbiturates can be associated with convulsions and death. Remember to ask specifically about over-the-counter preparations. In addition to self-administered preparations, many medications prescribed in the hospital can interfere with normal sleep; a thorough review of the patient's medication record is warranted.

E. **What are the patient's food and beverage habits?** Ingestion of stimulant-containing beverages (coffee, tea, some soft drinks) and foods (some cheeses) can interfere with sleep. Cigarette smoking and alcohol consumption both have deleterious effects on normal sleep patterns. Alcohol use and withdrawal are also associated with sleep disturbance and are frequently not reported by patients.

F. **Does the patient have difficulty lying flat?** Most often this is related to a cardiorespiratory condition and is often associated with dyspnea.

G. **What is the patient's customary sleep pattern?** Many clues to the etiology of the patient's sleep disturbance can be derived from a careful history of the sleep/wake cycle, including duration of periods of arousal and associated symptoms. Prolonged sleep latency is frequently associated with chronic or situational anxiety. Early-morning awakening is often seen with major depression, but may also be related to alcohol use. Frequent awakening with urinary urgency may be secondary to prostatic hypertrophy with bladder outlet obstruction, hyperglycemia with polyuria, or mobilization of fluid in a patient with congestive failure or chronic venous stasis and insufficiency. Awakening after a period of sleep with shortness of breath requiring a prolonged upright posture before resumption of sleep would suggest left ventricular failure.

III. Differential Diagnosis
A. Medical causes
1. **Delirium.** Evaluate the patient for systemic illnesses, sepsis, and liver dysfunction; also consider drug toxicities.
2. **Pain.** Control of this symptom frequently relieves the sleep disturbance.
3. **Cardiac disorders.** Ventricular dysfunction with congestive heart failure symptoms, arrhythmias, and ischemia can all result in sleep disturbances. Frequent symptoms include orthopnea, paroxysmal nocturnal dyspnea, palpitations, and angina.
4. **Respiratory disorders.** Asthma, chronic obstructive airway disease, cystic fibrosis, sarcoidosis, pneumonia, and sleep apnea are among the many respiratory disorders that can result in sleep disturbance. Sleep apnea is most frequently seen in patients who are morbidly obese. Central apnea syndrome is not necessarily related to body habitus. These patients are frequently unaware of their frequent arousals and instead complain of excessive daytime drowsiness.
5. **Hyperthyroidism.** Associated symptoms and signs include weight loss, hyperdefecation, heat intolerance, anxiety, tachycardia and tremor.

B. Drugs/toxins
1. **Tolerance to sleep medications from chronic usage**
2. **Abrupt withdrawal of sedative/hypnotics or antidepressant medications**
3. **Alcohol abuse.** There may be secondary disruption of appropriate sleep patterns as a result of chronic consumption. Sudden withdrawal also causes sleep disturbance.
4. **Tobacco use**
5. **Caffeine ingestion.** When inquiring about the patient's beverage consumption, keep in mind that many soft drinks also contain caffeine.
6. **Stimulant use or abuse**

C. Psychiatric causes
1. **Depressive illness.** Either bipolar or unipolar. Hallmarks are decreased sleep with no perception of sleep deficiency and early-morning awakening, respectively.
2. **Anxiety disorders.** Generally manifested by a prolonged sleep latency.

D. Situational causes. Frequently related to hospitalization.
1. **Noise.** The ICU environment and talkative or emotionally distressed roommates are cited as common offenders.
2. **Frequent disruptions.** Nursing duties such as administration of medications, recording of vital signs, and hygienic activities often interrupt patients' sleep.

3. **Anger.** The patient may be troubled by unexpressed anger over illness or toward staff or family.
4. **Anxiety.** This is a short-term response, usually related to the patient's medical condition or disorienting environment.

IV. Database. The most important components of the database in evaluating insomnia are the patient's history and an evaluation of his or her mental status.

A. **Physical examination key points**
   1. **Cardiopulmonary exam.** Rales, elevated jugular venous pressure, displaced point of maximal impulse, S_3 gallop, and peripheral edema all suggest congestive heart failure.
   2. **Respiratory exam.** Wheezing suggests obstructive airway disease but can be seen with pulmonary edema.
   3. **Neurologic exam.** Conduct a mental status examination for evidence of anxiety, depression, delirium, and dementia.

B. **Laboratory data.** The cause of insomnia is very often determined without the use of laboratory tests.
   1. **Screening chemistries.** Include hepatic and renal function tests, which are most useful as part of the evaluation of possible delirium.
   2. **Thyroid hormone levels.** If indicated by clinical presentation. (See Section III.A.5.)
   3. **Urine drug screen.** To be obtained in cases where drug use is strongly suspected but denied.

C. **Radiologic and other studies.** CXR is indicated if congestive heart failure or pneumonia is suspected.

V. Plan. It is most important to determine the medical, psychologic, or situational causes of the patient's sleeplessness. Most cases are secondary to a situational cause and do not represent a pathologic situation. In cases where there is no contraindication to their use, it is reasonable to include a sleeping medication to be taken as needed with admission orders. When a specific cause is determined, it should be remedied if possible rather than treating the sleeplessness symptomatically.

A. **Nonmedical treatments.** These measures are often as effective as medical treatment and lack side effects. They include minimizing disturbances, trying to maintain the patient's normal waking and sleeping times, eliminating roommate problems when possible, eliminating caffeine and tobacco from the diet, and minimizing noise from monitors or other hospital equipment.

B. **Symptomatic treatment**
   1. **Oral sleeping medication.** Choices include the benzodiazepines, chloral hydrate, and antihistamines. Barbiturates are not recommended.

a. **Benzodiazepines.** These are most frequently used for short-term treatment of insomnia. Newer hypnotics such as estazolam (ProSom) 0.5–2.0 mg or zolpidem (Ambien) 5–10 mg PO nightly are effective; reports suggest less disturbance of rapid eye movement (REM) sleep and lower abuse potential than with older benzodiazepines. Other older, rapidly absorbed, short half-life agents such as triazolam (Halcion) 0.125–0.25 mg PO every night; or temazepam (Restoril) 15–30 mg PO and flurazepam (Dalmane) 15–30 mg PO every night can be used.

b. **Chloral hydrate.** Available in both oral and rectal forms; the dose is 500–1000 mg by either route. Do not use in patients with hepatic or renal failure.

c. **Antihistamines.** Be conscious of anticholinergic side effects, particularly in the elderly.

    i. **Diphenhydramine (Benadryl)** 25–50 mg PO or IM.

    ii. **Hydroxyzine (Vistaril)** 25–50 mg PO or IM.

d. **Antidepressants.** Many have significant anticholinergic side effects and should be used with caution in the elderly. Also be aware of cardiac side effects.

    i. **Amitriptyline (Elavil)** 25–50 mg PO every night. Has significant anticholinergic side effects; most useful when chronic pain syndromes accompany sleep disturbance.

    ii. **Imipramine (Tofranil)** 75 mg PO every night. Requires the same precautions as with amitriptyline but is less useful in chronic pain.

    iii. **Desipramine (Norpramin)** 50 mg PO every night. May have fewer anticholinergic side effects.

REFERENCES

Erman MK: Insomnia. Psychiatr Clin North Am 1987;10:525.

Gillin JC, Byerley WF: The diagnosis and management of insomnia. N Engl J Med 1990;322:239.

Schmidt PJ: Evaluation and treatment of sleep disorders in the medical setting. Gen Hosp Psychiatry 1988;10:10.

44. IRREGULAR PULSE

(See also Section I, Chapter 58, Tachycardia, p 279, and Section I, Chapter 8, Bradycardia, p 37.)

I. Problem. A 77-year-old man being transferred to the hospital with mental status changes is reported to have an irregular pulse.

II. Immediate Questions

    A. What is the patient's heart rate? The heart rate, as well as the frequency of irregularity, can assist the physician in developing a differential diagnosis of the irregular heart rhythm. For example, an irregularly irregular rhythm with an apical pulse of 130 beats per minute (bpm) suggests atrial fibrillation.

B. What are the patient's other vital signs? Low systolic blood pressure would signify an urgent situation. (See Section I, Chapter 41, Hypotension, p 203.)

C. Has the patient been noted to have an irregular pulse before? A previous history of "skipped heart beats" suggests a chronic problem. The occurrence of isolated premature atrial contractions (PACs) or premature ventricular contractions (PVCs) may be chronic. It is a common benign condition associated with a number of medical problems or the use of a variety of medications, and can be seen occasionally in otherwise healthy individuals.

D. Is there any history of previous cardiac disease? A history of mitral stenosis points to atrial fibrillation related to left atrial enlargement; whereas a history of previous myocardial infarction or long-standing hypertension with left ventricular hypertrophy or dilated cardiomyopathy might suggest PVCs.

E. What medications is the patient taking? Ask specifically about cardiac medications (eg, digitalis, antiarrhythmic agents, diuretics) and other medications such as bronchodilators (especially theophylline) and tricyclic antidepressants. Digitalis can cause atrioventricular heart block with variable conduction. Diuretic-induced hypokalemia and hypomagnesemia as well as the use of antiarrhythmic drugs can cause both PACs and PVCs, which, if frequent, may be responsible for an irregular rhythm. Many asthma drugs and other stimulants can cause an irregular heart beat.

III. Differential Diagnosis
A. Premature contractions
1. **Premature atrial contractions (PACs).** PACs can be seen in almost any patient with illness-related stress, severe infection, inflammation, or myocardial ischemia; or in patients with a significant history of tobacco, alcohol or caffeine use. PACs may occasionally lead to sustained supraventricular tachycardia (SVT), but usually PACs do not require acute therapy in the absence of a sustained supraventricular tachyarrhythmia.

2. **Premature ventricular contractions (PVCs).** The prevalence of benign, asymptomatic, isolated PVCs increases with age. PVCs are also seen, however, with serious infections or illnesses; during acute myocardial ischemia; with stress; with use of many types of anesthetic drugs; with excessive use of tobacco, alcohol, caffeine, or other cardiac stimulants. PVCs may also be seen in patients with hypoxemia, metabolic or respiratory acidosis or alkalosis, hypokalemia, and hypomagnesemia. Patients with hypertrophic cardiomyopathy and mitral valve prolapse may have frequent multifocal nonsustained runs of ven-

tricular ectopy that are considered risk factors for sudden cardiac death. In the absence of underlying organic heart disease, the presence of isolated PVCs does not affect the patient's life span and therefore does not require any specific therapy.

B. Sinus arrhythmia. Occurs in almost every age group and is usually a normal variant. Treatment is rarely indicated or required. Sustained tachyarrythmias rarely occur in otherwise healthy patients with sinus arrhythmia. The P wave and QRS morphologies will appear normal.

C. Sinoatrial exit block. This is defined by the absence of a normally timed P wave, resulting in a pause that is a multiple of the P-to-P interval. This rhythm can be seen with vagal nerve stimulation; during acute myocarditis or acute myocardial infarction (MI); or with fibrosis of the conduction system. It can be related to the use of several cardiac drugs such as quinidine, procainamide, and digitalis. Syncope is a rare result.

D. Atrial fibrillation. Defined as chaotic atrial depolarizations and a grossly irregular ventricular response. Atrial fibrillation can be seen in patients with apparently normal hearts; or in patients with rheumatic heart disease, acute myocardial ischemia/infarction, myocarditis, pericarditis, hypertrophic and dilated cardiomyopathies, hypertensive heart disease, pulmonary embolism (PE), and thyrotoxicosis. The ventricular response is usually between 100–160 bpm. It may, however, be < 100 bpm in the presence of AV node disease or certain medications.

E. Atrial flutter. The pulse may be irregular if the atrioventricular node conduction varies; however, the pulse during atrial flutter is frequently rapid and usually regular. Atrial flutter is associated with the same diseases as atrial fibrillation.

F. Second-degree atrioventricular block. With variable block, both Mobitz type I (Wenckebach) and Mobitz type II second-degree heart block can cause an irregular pulse, and can be seen in patients with acute MI, degenerative disease of the cardiac conduction system, viral myocarditis, acute rheumatic fever, and Lyme disease. Mobitz type I can also be seen during times of increased parasympathetic tone; it does not necessarily indicate disease of the intracardiac conduction system.

IV. Database
A. Physical examination key points
1. **Vital signs.** Palpate the brachial or carotid pulses to determine the heart rate and assess the degree of cardiac irregularity. The brachial and carotid pulses are better for palpation than more peripheral pulses. Be careful to avoid mistaking a heart beat with a variable pulse amplitude from an irregular cardiac rhythm. Variations in pulse amplitude can be seen during severe pul-

monary bronchospasm, during a large MI, with decompensated congestive heart failure, with acute aortic insufficiency, or with pericardial tamponade. Quick action must be taken if hypotension is present. A fever may suggest an infection, which can have associated PVCs or PACs. Several specific infections (eg, acute rheumatic fever and acute Lyme disease) can cause atrioventricular node block.

    2. Heart. A complete cardiac examination is indicated. Atrioventricular node block with an associated murmur might suggest acute rheumatic fever. A fourth heart sound (S_4) might suggest acute MI. A number of cardiac arrhythmias may be present with an acute MI, including PVCs and PACs, variable degrees of atrioventricular block, atrial fibrillation, and atrial flutter. If atrial fibrillation is present, listen for the diastolic murmur of mitral stenosis, characteristically a diastolic rumble at the cardiac apex. It is best heard with the bell of the stethoscope, with the patient in the left lateral decubitus position.

B. Laboratory data

    1. Electrolytes. Rule out hypokalemia. In addition, a low serum bicarbonate suggests metabolic acidosis.

    2. Arterial blood gases. If PVCs are present, exclude hypoxemia and severe acidosis or alkalosis as the cause.

    3. Medications. A recent serum digoxin level is imperative if the patient is taking this medication. Digitalis intoxication can cause PVCs, sinoatrial exit block, or second-degree heart block. Consider measuring serum levels of other medications, such as quinidine, procainamide and theophylline.

C. Electrocardiogram and rhythm strip

    1. Be sure to include a long rhythm strip in order to catch the responsible arrhythmia.

    2. Identify all of the P waves that are present and note their timing and relationship to the QRS complexes. P waves are best seen in leads I, II, aVR, aVF and V1. You may need to examine several rhythm strips from different leads in order to correctly identify the cardiac rhythm.

    3. Be certain to examine the ECG for evidence of myocardial ischemia; drug effects such as prolongation of the QT interval; and for the electrocardiographic changes of pulmonary embolism (S_1, Q_3, T_3, acute right bundle branch block, acute right-axis deviation), and for pericarditis (diffuse ST elevation with upward concavity, T wave inversion, and PR segment depression).

V. Plan. Most of the cardiac arrhythmias that result in a detectable irregular pulse do not need emergent therapy; however, they should be identified and the predisposing condition treated appropriately. Possible exceptions to this statement include the following:

A. **Frequent or multifocal PVCs following a myocardial infarction or with impaired left ventricular function.** Be sure to exclude predisposing conditions, such as hypokalemia, hypoxemia, hypomagnesemia, acidosis, alkalosis, and myocardial ischemia. Beta-blockers are the agents of choice because they are the only class of drugs proven to decrease the incidence of sudden cardiac death in post-infarction patients. Beta-blockers may cause or worsen congestive heart failure (CHF) in patients with impaired left ventricular function; therefore, proceed cautiously when starting patients with CHF on beta-blockers. If treatment with an antiarrhythmic drug is considered, it is recommended that consultation with a cardiac electrophysiologist be obtained prior to starting the patient on any long-term antiarrhythmic drug. This recommendation is based on the results of the Cardiac Arrhythmia Suppression Trial (CAST) study, which showed that the pro-arrhythmic side effects of some of these medications (eg, encainide, flecainide, moricizine) may raise the risk of sudden cardiac death rather than decrease it.

B. **Mobitz type II second-degree atrioventricular block.** This condition frequently progresses to third-degree heart block; therefore, exclusion of reversible causes and placement of a temporary transvenous pacemaker should be considered.

C. **Atrial fibrillation and flutter.** (See Section I, Chapter 58, Tachycardia, p 286.)

REFERENCES

Cardiac Arrhythmia Suppression Trial (CAST) Investigators: Preliminary report: Effect of encainide and flecainide on mortality in a randomized trial of arrhythmia suppression after myocardial infarction. N Engl J Med 1989;321:406.

Wagner GS ed: *Marriott's Practical Electrocardiography.* 9th ed. Williams and Wilkens;1994.

Zipes DP: Specific arrhythmias: diagnosis and treatment. In: Braunwald E ed. *Heart Disease: A Text Book of Cardiovascular Medicine.* 4th ed. Saunders;1992:667.

45. JAUNDICE

I. **Problem.** A 66-year-old woman is admitted because of icteric sclerae and abdominal pain.

II. **Immediate Questions**
   A. **What are the patient's vital signs?** Fever and tachycardia with or without hypotension could indicate sepsis associated with ascending cholangitis. This is a medical emergency and requires immediate aggressive attention.
   B. **Does the patient have diabetes?** Diabetes is a significant risk factor for ascending cholangitis.

C. **Is there a history of alcoholism or chronic alcohol use?** Cirrhosis may be a source of jaundice.

D. **Is there a history of intravenous drug abuse, homosexual activity, or exposure to hepatitis?** Viral hepatitis could be the source of the jaundice. A viral prodrome is often elicited.

E. **Is there associated abdominal pain?** A history of postprandial right upper quadrant or epigastric pain, especially with radiation to the back, may represent biliary colic. Abdominal pain can be also associated with cancer.

F. **Is there a history of previous biliary surgery?** Jaundice may occur as a result of a retained common duct stone or biliary stricture.

III. **Differential Diagnosis.** The differential diagnosis of jaundice is based on metabolism and excretion of bilirubin. Knowledge of that process leads to three major subcategories of problems leading to jaundice: prehepatic; hepatic; and posthepatic.

A. **Acute biliary obstruction.** This category includes carcinoma and common bile duct stones. Biliary obstruction may lead to cholangitis and potentially life-threatening sepsis.

B. **Alcoholic liver disease (alcoholic hepatitis or cirrhosis).** Alcoholic cirrhosis is usually seen after at least 10 years of heavy ethanol ingestion. Check for stigmata of chronic liver disease (palmar erythema, spider telangiectasias, and gynecomastia).

C. **Viral hepatitis.** Consider with a history of IV drug abuse, exposure to persons with jaundice, male homosexual activity, travel to endemic areas, or recent history of transfusion.

D. **Other causes of hepatitis.** Autoimmune disorders or drugs such as isoniazid and halothane.

E. **Hemolysis.** This rarely raises the bilirubin over 5 mg/dL. Look for an increased indirect bilirubin.

F. **Primary biliary cirrhosis.** Usually found in middle-aged women who present with jaundice, fatigue, and pruritus.

G. **Drugs.** May cause hepatitis, cholestasis, or hemolysis. Phenothiazines and estrogens are common causes of cholestasis.

H. **Total parenteral nutrition (TPN).** Associated with high carbohydrate loads. Usually from long-term TPN.

I. **Pregnancy.** An unusual cause of jaundice, but can be life-threatening.

J. **Postoperative cholestasis.** Diagnosis of exclusion.

K. **Sepsis.** Diagnosis of exclusion.

IV. **Database.** An experienced clinician can make an accurate diagnosis with history, physical examination, and simple laboratory tests 85% of the time.

A. Physical examination key points

1. **Vital signs.** A fever with rigors may suggest ascending cholangitis.

2. **Skin.** Palmar erythema and telangiectasia points toward chronic liver disease. Look for needle marks or "tracks" suggestive of IV drug abuse.

3. **Breasts (in males).** Gynecomastia is consistent with chronic liver disease.

4. **Abdomen.** The physical exam should be centered on the abdomen. Look for hepatomegaly or palpable gallbladder (Courvoisier's sign), which may indicate malignant obstruction. The presence or absence of abdominal tenderness, particularly right upper quadrant tenderness and Murphy's sign (tenderness in the right upper quadrant with palpation during inspiration), should be documented. Ascites may be present in patients with cirrhosis.

5. **Rectum/genitourinary system.** A rectal exam should be done looking for occult blood. Testicular atrophy may be present in patients with chronic liver disease.

B. Laboratory data

1. **Liver function studies.** Including transaminases (AST [SGOT] and ALT [SGPT]), bilirubin total and fractionated, alkaline phosphatase, and γ-glutamyl transpeptidase (GGT). There are two basic patterns in liver function tests, hepatocellular and hepatocanalicular. The hepatocellular pattern is characterized by AST and ALT 10 $\times$ the upper limits of normal with much smaller increases in alkaline phosphatase or GGT and bilirubin. Conversely, the hepatocanalicular pattern is suggested when the alkaline phosphatase or GGT is 5–10 $\times$ > normal with relatively normal transaminases. Bilirubin is also more commonly elevated. Transaminases > 300 virtually never occur in alcoholic liver disease without the combined effect of some other toxin such as acetaminophen (Tylenol). Bilirubins > 20 are very suggestive of extrahepatic cholestasis. An elevated indirect bilirubin suggests hemolysis; a total bilirubin secondary to hemolysis seldom exceeds 5 mg/dL.

2. **Amylase.** Significant elevations in amylase (> 10 $\times$ the upper limits of normal) are suggestive of biliary disease.

3. **Prothrombin time.** Elevation which corrects with vitamin K is caused by extrahepatic obstruction, while failure to correct is seen in fulminant hepatitis or cirrhosis.

4. **Hepatitis serology.** Hepatitis B surface antigen, hepatitis B IgM core antibody, hepatitis A IgM antibody and hepatitis C antibody. (See Section II, Laboratory Tests: Hepatitis, pp 318–319.)

5. **Other serology.** Antinuclear (ANA), antimitochondrial, and antismooth muscle antibodies may be helpful. The triad of antimitochondrial antibody, elevated alkaline phosphatase, and an elevated Class M immunoglobulin is consistent with primary bil-

iary cirrhosis. A high ANA titer suggests autoimmune hepatitis. High titers of anti-smooth muscle antibodies are seen in chronic active hepatitis.

C. **Radiologic and other studies**
1. **Ultrasound and computerized tomography.** First examination in patients with intermediate or low risk for extrahepatic biliary obstruction. Ultrasound and CT are good primarily for detecting dilated ducts, pancreatic masses, and stones in the gallbladder. Detection of stones in the common bile duct is uniformly poor with both of these tests.
2. **Endoscopic retrograde cholangiopancreatography (ERCP) and percutaneous transhepatic cholangiogram (PTC).** Tests of first choice for extrahepatic obstruction. Selection of ERCP or PTC is based on local expertise and the clinical situation. ERCP is recommended in patients with ascites; coagulation abnormalities; a previous history of failed percutaneous transhepatic cholangiography; a suspicion of sclerosing cholangitis; and a planned sphincterotomy. It is also the test of choice when carcinoma of the pancreas is suspected, as a biopsy can be done. Indications for PTC are given in the following section.
3. **Percutaneous transhepatic cholangiogram (PTC).** Test of choice when the patient has dilated ducts, previous gastric surgery with Bilroth II anastomosis, a previous failed ERCP, or a mass involving the proximal bile duct.
4. **Liver biopsy.** Generally not useful in the diagnosis of jaundice. Occasionally reveals an unsuspected medical cause such as metastatic tumor. Liver biopsy is sometimes performed in the evaluation of alcoholic liver disease or viral hepatitis.
5. **Nuclear scan (HIDA).** This scan is generally of low utility in the diagnosis of jaundice. It is very helpful when the diagnosis of acute cholecystitis is suspected.

V. **Plan.** The tempo of diagnostic evaluation is dictated by the severity of the patient's illness. If acute cholangitis is suspected, then the evaluation must proceed emergently. Patients with signs of liver failure, specifically significant coagulopathy and hepatic encephalopathy, need ICU monitoring and aggressive supportive care.

A. **Hepatocellular cholestasis**
1. **Viral hepatitis.** Patients who are dehydrated, vomiting, or have significant coagulopathy will need admission for treatment with IV fluids and fresh-frozen plasma.
2. **Alcoholic liver disease.** Requires aggressive supportive care, entailing dietary restriction of protein, full evaluation of any coagulopathy (see Section I, Chapter 12, Coagulopathy, p 64), and treatment of associated electrolyte deficiencies that are

often encountered in alcoholics (eg, hypokalemia, hypomagnesemia, and hypophosphatemia). Thiamine, folate, and multivitamins may be needed. Prophylactic antibiotics are recommended to prevent peritonitis (norfloxacin 400 mg Q day).
   B. Extrahepatic cholestasis
      1. If there is a strong clinical suspicion of extrahepatic obstruction, proceed at once with ERCP or PTC.
      2. If extrahepatic obstruction is possible but not definite, obtain a biliary ultrasound or CT scan first. If obstruction is confirmed, then proceed with ERCP or surgery. If ascending cholangitis is suspected and confirmed by ultrasound or CT scan, begin antibiotics (ampicillin and gentamicin) and request immediate surgical consultation.
   C. Hemolysis. Treat underlying cause.

REFERENCES

Frank BB: Clinical evaluation of jaundice. JAMA 1989;262:3031.
Lidofsky SD, Scharschmidt BF: Jaundice. In: *Gastrointestinal Disease: Pathophysiology/ Diagnosis/Management.* Sleisenger MH, Fordtran JS, eds. Saunders;1993:1765.

46. JOINT SWELLING

   I. Problem. A 35-year-old woman is admitted with right knee swelling and pain.

   II. Immediate Questions
      A. Is there a previous history of joint swelling? A history of multiple joint involvement suggests an etiology resulting in polyarthritis rather than monarthritis. Remember, many diseases causing a polyarthritis can present initially as a monarthritis. The pattern of joint involvement may suggest the cause; for example, the first metatarsophalangeal (MTP) joint in gout, or metacarpophalangeal (MCP) and proximal interphalangeal (PIP) joints in rheumatoid arthritis. The history of onset, such as acute, chronic, or migratory, may be helpful in diagnosis.
      B. Is there a history of trauma? Trauma to the joint would lead the clinician to consider fracture, ligamentous tear, loose body, or dislocation. A sport and occupational history is essential.
      C. Does the patient have any constitutional symptoms? The presence of fever suggests septic arthritis, although infection must be considered in any case of monarticular arthritis even in the absence of fever. Malaise, fatigue, and weight loss suggest a systemic arthritis. Morning stiffness of significant duration (> 1 hour) suggests inflammatory arthritis.

D. Are there any other systemic symptoms? It is important to obtain a full rheumatic disease systems review. A photosensitive rash suggests systemic lupus erythematosus (SLE), whereas diarrhea may occur with inflammatory bowel disease (IBD) or reactive arthritis. A partial list of systemic symptoms would include rash, alopecia, Raynaud's phenomenon, oral or genital ulcers, urethritis or cervicitis, diarrhea, eye inflammation, sicca symptoms, weakness, and CNS disturbances.

E. What is the patient's past medical and family history? Inquire about recent febrile illnesses, tick bites, and other events, as the patient may not associate these symptoms with the onset of arthritis. A medication history may provide a clue to diagnosis (eg, hemarthrosis associated with warfarin therapy); or a positive family history may suggest arthritis associated with psoriasis, hemoglobinopathies, or coagulopathies.

III. Differential Diagnosis. Arthritis is classified as being either monarticular or polyarticular. Subclassification is often based on the joint fluid analysis (see Section IV). Remember that an arthritis that is generally polyarticular can present as a monarticular arthritis.

A. Monarticular arthritis

1. **Infection.** May be bacterial, viral, fungal, or tuberculous.
2. **Trauma.** Etiologies include loose foreign bodies, fracture, plant thorn synovitis, and internal derangement.
3. **Hemarthrosis.** Causes include hemoglobinopathy, coagulopathy, warfarin therapy, and pigmented villonodular synovitis.
4. **Tumors.** Consider osteogenic sarcoma, metastatic tumor, synovial osteochondromatosis, and paraneoplastic syndromes.
5. **Crystals.** Types of crystal associated with arthritis include gout (first MTP involvement characteristic), pseudogout (may be secondary to hyperparathyroidism and hemochromatosis), and hydroxyapatite.
6. **Noninflammatory diseases.** These include avascular necrosis, which is often associated with a history of trauma, steroid use, alcohol use, or sickle cell anemia; osteoarthritis; endocrine disorders; amyloid; osteochondritis dissecans; and neuropathy.
7. **Inflammatory-connective tissue diseases.** Rheumatoid arthritis or Reiter's syndrome.

B. Polyarticular arthritis

1. **Infection or associated with infection**
   a. **Gonococcal infection.** Frequently associated with a migratory arthritis, tenosynovitis, and a pustular rash.
   b. **Lyme disease.** Associated with both an acute arthritis and a late chronic destructive arthritis.
   c. **Rheumatic fever.** Primarily lower-extremity large joints. In the adult, arthritis is rarely migratory.

   d. AIDS. Septic arthritis, Reiter's syndrome, and a lupus-like presentation with nondestructive polyarthritis, rash, pleuritis, and CNS symptoms have all been described.
   e. Subacute bacterial endocarditis
   f. Chronic active hepatitis. Chronic hepatitis B and C infections are associated with arthritis alone, or with polyarteritis nodosa or mixed essential cryoglobulinemia.
2. **Crystals.** Eg, gout, pseudogout, and hydroxyapatite.
3. **Metabolic disorders.** Etiologies include hypothyroidism, acromegaly, hemochromatosis, ochronosis, (alkaptonuria—associated with osteoarthritis primarily of the spine and hips), hemophilia, and hyperparathyroidism. Hyperparathyroidism and hemochromatosis are associated with pseudogout.
4. **Noninflammatory diseases**
   a. Osteoarthritis. Consider when distal interphalangeal (DIP) and carpal-metacarpal joints of hands are involved.
   b. Intestinal bypass surgery
5. **Spondyloarthropathies.**
   a. Associated with involvement of spine and/or sacroiliac joints. Peripheral arthritis is often asymmetric, involving joints in only one of the arms and/or one of the legs.
   b. Psoriatic arthritis can involve joints in both arms or legs but the joints tend to be different, unlike rheumatoid arthritis which involves the same joints on both sides of the body. Psoriatic arthritis, unlike rheumatoid arthritis, can affect the DIP joints.
6. **Inflammatory disease**
   a. Juvenile rheumatoid arthritis (JRA). Also called adult Still's disease. Fever, sore throat, and often systemic complaints (myalgias) are present. Rheumatoid factor (RF) is negative.
   b. Rheumatoid arthritis. A symmetric arthritis characteristically involves the MCP and PIP joints of the hands.
   c. Systemic lupus erythematosus (SLE). Resembles rheumatoid arthritis but is rarely an erosive arthritis.
   d. Scleroderma. Significant joint swelling is uncommon.
   e. Polychondritis
   f. Mixed connective tissue disease. Defined by a positive anti-ribonuclear protein (anti-RNP) antibody. Includes features of rheumatoid arthritis, scleroderma, polymyositis, and SLE.
   g. Sarcoidosis. An acute migratory arthritis frequently associated with tenosynovitis and erythema nodosum, and a chronic pauciarticular form involving the knees and ankles.
   h. Vasculitis. Leukocytoclastic vasculitis and larger vessel vasculitides such as Churg-Strauss syndrome, Wegener's granulomatosis, polyarteritis nodosa, and Behçet's syndrome can rarely present with arthritis.

IV. Database

A. Physical examination key points.
Physical exam must be complete. Systemic disease must be ruled out as the cause of the arthritis; there can be no shortcuts.

1. **Skin.** A rash may indicate the etiology. For evidence of psoriasis, frequently overlooked areas include under the hairline or rectum. Telangiectasia, nailfold infarcts, palmar erythema, and livedo reticularis suggest connective tissue disease or vasculitis. Nodules are seen in rheumatoid arthritis and gout.
2. **Eyes.** Retinal abnormalities (hemorrhages) may suggest an infectious etiology such as subacute bacterial endocarditis.
3. **Mouth.** Oral and nasal ulcers point to SLE or Behçet's syndrome.
4. **Musculoskeletal system.** All major joints should be examined for range of motion, tenderness, deformity, and swelling. The clinician must ensure that there is true swelling (arthritis) rather than bone pain, muscle pain, or pain from bursitis, tendinitis, or torn ligaments or menisci.

B. Laboratory data

1. **CBC with differential.** To rule out infection and to identify anemia or thrombocytopenia if a systemic arthritis is considered.
2. **Joint fluid analysis**
   a. Any initial presentation of arthritis should be worked up with a joint aspiration if possible. (See Section III, Chapter 3, Arthrocentesis, p 343.) Fluid should be sent for Gram's stain, as well as bacterial, acid-fast bacillus, and fungal cultures if indicated. You should also obtain a crystal exam, and cell count with differential. A WBC count of 0–300 is normal, 300–2000 is noninflammatory, 2000–75,000 indicates an inflammatory process, and > 100,000 indicates septic arthritis; however, cell counts from a bacterial source may be as low as 5000 WBC/mL. A differential count with a predominance of neutrophils suggests septic arthritis, whereas lymphocytosis suggests leukemia or tuberculosis. These values are only guidelines as there is considerable overlap in all of these diseases.
   b. **Gram's stain smears** are positive in only 66% of subsequent culture-proven cases of septic arthritis. A negative result does not therefore exclude the possibility of infection. The monosodium urate crystals of gout are rod-shaped, negatively birefringent crystals (3–10 μm) seen within white cells during active disease and often extend beyond the cell wall. The crystal is yellow when parallel to the slow ray of the compensator. Calcium pyrophosphate dihydrate (CPPD) crystals are rhomboid-shaped, positively birefringent crystals that are blue when parallel to the slow ray of the compensator. The crystal is usually contained within the white cell. Calcium hydroxyapatite crystals are small (< 1 μm), minimally birefrin-

gent, irregularly shaped cytoplasmic inclusions that appear under light microscopy as "shiny coins" when extracellular. Calcium hydroxyapatite crystals are more commonly associated with acute episodes of bursitis, tendinitis, or periarthritis seen in chronic renal failure patients or in older women with the progressive destructive arthritis of Milwaukee shoulder syndrome.

3. **Other cultures.** Cultures of urine and blood should be obtained if septic arthritis is considered. If gonorrhea is considered, obtain cervical/urethral, rectal, and pharyngeal specimens.

4. **Creatinine.** Often obtained because many drugs, especially nonsteroidal anti-inflammatory drugs (NSAIDs), used in treatment are contraindicated if creatinine is elevated.

5. **Urinalysis.** Proteinuria, red cells, and casts may indicate a systemic cause such as SLE.

6. **Rheumatic disease workup.** If a collagen vascular disease is suspected, obtain a Westergren erythrocyte sedimentation rate (ESR), C-reactive protein (CRP), antinuclear antibodies (ANA), and RF. Tests for anti-double-stranded DNA (anti-DSDNA), extractable nuclear antigens (anti-RNP, anti-Smith, anti-SSA(Ro), anti-SSB(la), complement (CH50, C3, C4), and cryoglobulin are usually not obtained initially. Measurement of Hepatitis B and C serologies or anti-neutrophil cytoplasmic antibody (ANCA) may be considered if the history is suggestive. A positive C-ANCA is highly suggestive of Wegener's granulomatosis. HLA-B27 is rarely helpful.

C. **Radiologic and other studies.** Plain films of the involved joints are often helpful, especially if the arthritis is chronic. If normal, they can serve as a baseline as the arthritis progresses. Films of the hands and feet are particularly helpful when RA is considered.

V. **Plan.** Treatment is dependent on the type of arthritis diagnosed. An individual discussion of each type is beyond the scope of this book.

A. **Drug therapy.** Ensure from the patient's history and laboratory tests that there are no contraindications to the medication chosen. The patient must be informed of side effects. The most commonly prescribed medications (NSAIDs) are contraindicated in patients with elevated creatinine, a history of hypersensitivity reaction to aspirin or NSAIDs, platelet abnormalities, and possibly peptic ulcer disease. In the elderly, one must be aware of the CNS side effects.

B. **Supportive measures.** Dependent on the diagnosis, heat or ice therapy, specific exercises, splinting, and physical therapy may be indicated.

C. **Septic arthritis**

1. Daily drainage of joint fluid is absolutely necessary. If the joint is not easily drained, open drainage may be necessary. Gram's

stain will help direct the initial choice of antibiotic pending cultures.

2. If gonococcal arthritis is suspected, penicillin is effective unless the patient is at risk of having a penicillinase-producing strain, as may be seen in IV drug abusers. A third-generation cephalosporin is then indicated. (See Section VII, p 405.)

3. In nongonococcal bacterial arthritis, gram-positive cocci on gram stain should be treated with a penicillinase-resistant penicillin or vancomycin if methicillin-resistant *Staphylococcus aureus* is prevalent or if *S epidermidis* is suspected. An aminoglycoside and an antipseudomonal penicillin or third-generation cephalosporin would be used for gram-negative bacilli. If the gram strain is negative in a compromised host, use broad-spectrum coverage for both gram-positive and gram-negative organisms.

REFERENCES

Baker DG, Schumacher HR: Acute monarthritis. N Engl J Med 1993;329:1013.
Kelly WN, Harris ED, Ruddy S et al, eds. *Textbook of Rheumatology.* 4th ed. WB Saunders;1993.
Klippel JH, Dieppe PA eds. *Rheumatology.* Mosby;1994.
McCarty DJ, Koopman WJ. *Arthritis and Allied Conditions: A Textbook of Rheumatology.* 12th ed. Lea and Febiger;1993.

47. LEUKOCYTOSIS

I. **Problem.** A 63-year-old woman is admitted for hypoxemia, diffuse bilateral pulmonary infiltrates and fever. She is placed on broad-spectrum IV antibiotics after appropriate cultures are obtained. Her white blood cell count (WBC) remains about 25,000–30,000/µL.

II. **Immediate Questions**
   A. **What is the patient's current clinical status?** Elevated WBC counts may be associated with other evidence of infection including fever, rigors, hypotension, or tachycardia.
   B. **Have any intervening clinically relevant episodes of physical stress occurred since admission?** Hypotension and other signs of shock can certainly be associated with a leukocytosis. The use of mechanical ventilation or resuscitative measures can stimulate a leukocytosis.
   C. **Is there a history suggestive of prior underlying systemic illness?** Symptoms such as weight loss, prior sustained fevers, night sweats, chronic cough or dyspnea, hemoptysis, myalgias, and bone pain are all suggestive of chronic illnesses such as my-

cobacterial or fungal infections, connective tissue diseases, or possibly a neoplastic disorder. A history of new symptoms argues against a chronic or subacute illness.

D. Are there any prior complete blood counts with which to compare to this leukocyte count? Again, the presence or absence of prior leukocytosis critically aids the evaluation. Sustained leukocytosis over weeks or months strongly implies a chronic or subacute process, whether it be an infection such as an abscess or tuberculosis (TB), or a neoplasm or some other process.

E. Is there evidence of infection that has not been addressed, such as intra-abdominal infection (abscess), genitourinary infection, or CNS infection? Pulmonary infiltrates may represent adult respiratory distress syndrome (ARDS) occurring as a reaction to underlying sepsis, especially from an abdominal infection. Acute infectious causes of leukocytosis must be excluded since they are so readily treatable.

F. Is the patient currently on any medication such as granulocyte colony-stimulating factor (G-CSF), granulocyte-macrophage colony-stimulating factor (G-M-CSF), or any other growth factors used to stimulate white cell production that are now commonly used in a variety of oncologic or hematologic conditions? Has the patient received one of these growth factors recently? In addition, other medications such as vasopressors and glucocorticoids can cause demargination and subsequent leukocytosis. Lithium also causes a benign reversible leukocytosis.

G. Does the patient have a history of an underlying hematologic disorder? Symptoms such as paresthesias, cyanosis in response to changes in ambient temperature, and easy bruising or bleeding are all suggestive of a primary bone marrow pathology.

H. Does the patient have a history of prior abdominal trauma or surgery or, specifically, splenectomy? The postsplenectomy state is often associated with a baseline WBC count that is above normal. In addition, the splenectomized patient is at greater risk of developing sepsis, especially from encapsulated organisms.

III. Differential Diagnosis. There are numerous causes of leukocytosis. It is a normal response to many noxious emotional and physical stimuli. Leukocytosis is defined as a WBC count greater than 10,000/μL. A broad division of causes separates leukocytosis into acute and chronic.

A. Acute
   1. **Acute bacterial infection.** Either localized or generalized (sepsis).
   2. **Other infections.** Mycobacteria, fungi, certain viruses, rickettsiae, or even spirochetes.
   3. **Trauma**

  4. **Myocardial infarction (MI), pulmonary embolism/infarction, mesenteric ischemia/infarction, or peripheral vascular disease with ischemia.**
  5. **Vasculitis, antigen-antibody complexes, and complement activation.**
  6. **Physical stimuli.** Extremes of temperature, seizure activity, and intense pain are associated with increased WBC counts.
  7. **Emotional stimuli.** Occasionally can trigger acute leukocytosis.
  8. **Drugs.** Can often cause or contribute to leukocytosis, especially vasopressor agents, corticosteroids, lithium, G-CSF, and GM-CSF.
B. **Chronic**
  1. **Persistent infections.** Often the same infection that caused the acute leukocytosis.
  2. **Partially treated or occult infections.** Osteomyelitis, subacute bacterial endocarditis (SBE), and intra-abdominal abscess can often present as chronic leukocytosis.
  3. **Mycobacterial or fungal infections.** These are notorious for promoting a sustained leukocytosis, often with little other clinical pathology at initial evaluation.
  4. **Chronic inflammatory states.** Rheumatic fever, connective tissue disease such as systemic lupus erythematosus (SLE), thyroiditis, myositis, drug reactions, and pancreatitis can all chronically elevate the WBC count.
  5. **Neoplastic processes.** Solid tumors and lymphoproliferative disorders can have an associated chronic leukocytosis.
  6. **Primary hematologic disorders.** These include myeloproliferative disorders, myelodysplasia, leukemias, chronic hemolysis, and asplenic states.
  7. **Congenital disorders (including Down's syndrome).** May be associated in rare cases with chronic leukocytosis.
  8. **Drugs.** These are less common causes. Potential offending agents include vasopressor agents, glucocorticoids, and lithium.
  9. **Overproduction of ACTH or thyroxine.** May cause chronic elevation of the baseline WBC count.

IV. **Database**
  A. **Physical examination key points**
    1. **Vital signs.** Be especially careful to check for the presence of fever or hypothermia, which suggests infection or sepsis. Fever can also indicate a neoplastic process, infarction of various tissues, or a connective tissue disorder. (See Section I, Chapter 21, Fever, p 112.) Hypotension may occur in patients who are septic.

2. **General.** Look for evidence of acute distress or a chronic disease state (cachexia, digital clubbing, bitemporal wasting).
3. **Lymph nodes.** Check for palpable lymph nodes and note their character. Soft and tender nodes are most consistent with an infectious etiology. Rubbery and generalized nodes are most often seen with lymphoreticular disorders such as lymphoma. Hard, fixed, and localized nodes suggest carcinoma.
4. **Skin/mucosa.** Petechiae or ecchymoses suggest sepsis with disseminated intravascular coagulation (DIC), primary bone marrow pathology with altered platelet number or function and/or clotting dysfunction, or vasculitis.
5. **Lungs.** Inspiratory rales imply pneumonitis or pneumonia. Diminished breath sounds and dullness to percussion suggest a pleural effusion or abscess. A pleural rub may accompany infectious processes, malignant pathology, or other processes such as thromboembolism and SLE, all of which are commonly associated with leukocytosis.
6. **Heart.** Tachycardia is consistent with acute stress. The presence of a new murmur, particularly with fever, is suggestive of bacterial endocarditis. Look for evidence of volume overload, sometimes triggered by infection or occasionally associated with leukemias or myeloproliferative disorders.
7. **Abdomen.** Tenderness on rebound suggests an acute abdominal process such as perforation or infarction of a viscus.
8. **Genitourinary/gynecologic exam.** Flank, pelvic, or prostate tenderness is suggestive of acute infection.
9. **Neurologic exam.** Altered mental status, confusion, seizures, and focally abnormal deep tendon reflexes can all be seen in a variety of situations associated with leukocytosis, including meningitis (infectious or neoplastic), sepsis, leukemias, lymphomas, and solid malignancies.

B. **Laboratory data**
1. **Blood.** *Personal evaluation of the peripheral blood smear is absolutely critical.* Look for a coexisting anemia, polycythemia, or abnormal platelet count. Leukocytosis with a "left shift," Döhle bodies, and toxic granulation suggest an acute infection, whereas a normal differential pattern implies a nonbacterial cause. A lymphocytosis points to a viral illness, lymphoma, or leukemia. An increase in monocytes is often seen with carcinoma or TB. Eosinophilia suggests connective tissue disease, possible drug reaction, or possible parasitic infection. Promyelocytes, myelocytes, or an increase in basophils are consistent with myeloproliferative disorders (leukemias most commonly), although severe infections, toxic insults, and inflammation can result in the release of early myeloid forms.

2. **Liver function tests.** Can be elevated in acute hepatitis, sepsis, leukemia, lymphoma, or metastatic carcinoma.
3. **Electrolytes.** Acute infection (especially pneumonia) and chronic infection involving the lung (tuberculosis) or central nervous system (tuberculous or fungal meningitis) can cause the syndrome of inappropriate antidiuretic hormone (SIADH) release, as well as hyponatremia.
4. **Arterial blood gases.** A metabolic gap-acidosis can accompany sepsis, leukemia, or solid tumors.
5. **Cultures.** Blood, urine, cerebrospinal fluid, sputum, and other cultures and skin tests are vital to rule in or exclude an infectious etiology.

C. **Radiologic and other studies**
   1. **Chest x-ray.** Check CXR for evidence of acute pneumonic process as well as a mass lesion or a mediastinal abnormality.
   2. **CT scan.** Can be used to localize an abscess, define the extent of any suspicious masses or adenopathy, and determine the presence or extent of organomegaly.
   3. **Tumor markers.** Tests like terminal deoxynucleotidal transferase (TdT), leukocyte alkaline phosphatase (LAP), and vitamin B_{12} level, as well as tests for monoclonal antibodies to carcinomas, can be quite useful. Frequently in a patient with a sustained leukocytosis, the LAP score can be one of the most useful initial lab tests to distinguish between an infectious/inflammatory etiology and a myeloproliferative disorder. The LAP score is usually elevated in infectious processes, whereas it is classically low in chronic granulocytic myelogenous leukemia (CML) and variable in the other myeloproliferative disorders. The LAP score is also elevated in polycythemia vera.
   4. **Bone marrow aspiration and biopsy.** May be required to rule in or exclude primary marrow pathology, metastatic tumor, or chronic infections. Cytogenic studies can be performed to look specifically for myelodysplasia, and myeloproliferative disorders such as leukemias or lymphomas. At times, this is the only way to differentiate between a reactive bone marrow and chronic myelogenous leukemia.

V. **Plan.** The etiology of the increased WBC count, of course, guides therapy. When obvious acute stress (infection, trauma, inflammation) is not present, chronic infections, inflammation, carcinoma, or primary marrow pathology must be considered. As mentioned, strict attention to history, clinical presentation, and physical examination together with personal review of the peripheral blood smear are absolutely vital for the initial evaluation of leukocytosis. The overlooked or inappropriately treated infection can be catastrophic. For specific treatment of the various etiologies of leukocytosis, please refer to any general reference.

REFERENCES

Bunn PA, Ridgeway EC: Paraneoplastic syndrome. In: Devita VT, Hellman S, Rosenberg SA, et al eds. *Cancer: Principles and Practice of Oncology.* 4th ed. Lippincott; 1993:2046.

Coates TD, Baehner R: Leukocytosis and leukopenia. In: Hoffman R, Benz EJ, Shattil SJ et al eds. *Hematology: Basic Principles and Practice.* 2nd ed. Churchill Livingstone;1995:769.

Dale DC: Neutrophilia. In: Beutler E, Lichtman MA, Coller BS et al eds. *William's Hematology.* 5th ed. McGraw-Hill;1995:824.

48. LEUKOPENIA

I. **Problem.** An 18-year-old woman is placed on phenytoin (Dilantin) for seizure control. Two weeks later, she returns with complaints of fever, chills, and productive cough. She is admitted with a temperature of 102°F; the white count is 2000/μL.

II. Immediate Questions

A. **What is the absolute neutrophil count (ANC)? Neutropenia** is defined as an absolute neutrophil count (% of segmented and banded neutrophils × total white count = ANC) < 1800/μL. At ANCs < 1000/μL, the risk of infection begins to increase. At values of 500/μL or less, there is a further dramatic increase in the likelihood of a serious infection.

B. **What is the patient's occupation? Has she been exposed to any chemicals?** Farmers and gardeners may be exposed to insecticides (DDT, lindane, chlordane) that can cause leukopenia. A painter, dry cleaner, or chemist may be exposed to benzene (another myelosuppressive chemical).

C. **Has the patient received any antineoplastic drugs or radiation therapy?** Myelosuppression is often an expected result of chemotherapy. Radiation is a direct myelosuppressant.

D. **What are the patient's medications?** Several commonly used drugs have been documented to cause neutropenia, including β-lactams, phenothiazines, sulfonamides, phenytoin, cimetidine (Tagamet), and ranitidine (Zantac).

E. **Has the patient noted any tea-colored urine?** Paroxysmal nocturnal hemoglobinuria (PNH) and hepatitis may be associated with aplastic anemia.

F. **Has the patient reported any fever, gastrointestinal complaints, or viral symptoms?** Several viral (infectious hepatitis, mononucleosis) and bacterial (salmonellosis, bacillary dysentery) illnesses and rickettsialpox have been associated with neutropenia.

G. **Does the patient have a history of alcohol abuse or any history of cirrhosis?** Ethanol is a direct myelosuppressant and can cause leukopenia. Folate deficiency, which can occur in alcoholics, may also cause leukopenia. Cirrhotics can develop hypersplenism and sequestration of white cells as well as platelets can occur.

H. **Is there any psychiatric history or history of anorexia nervosa?** Several medications (eg, phenothiazines) used in the treatment of psychiatric disorders can cause leukopenia. Anorexia nervosa and starvation can cause leukopenia; however, the mechanism is unknown.

I. **Does the patient have rheumatoid arthritis?** Felty's syndrome is a constellation of splenomegaly, neutropenia, and rheumatoid arthritis.

J. **What is the patient's ethnic background?** African Americans and Yemenite Jews may have a normal racial variant of leukopenia; their neutrophil count may be as low as 1500 cells/μL.

K. **What is the patient's sexual and drug history?** Homosexuals, bisexuals, and IV drug users are at increased risk for human immunodeficiency virus infection, which can cause leukopenia; the exact mechanism is unknown.

L. **Has the patient experienced recurrent, cyclic fevers?** Cyclic neutropenia is a rare form of neutropenia that has fluctuations of the neutrophil count at fairly regular 3-week intervals. The only clue may be unexplained recurrent fevers every 3 weeks.

III. **Differential Diagnosis.** The causes of neutropenia can be grouped in three broad categories: (1) bone marrow failure (defective neutrophil production or maturation); (2) accelerated neutrophil removal; and (3) neutrophil redistribution. This classification is useful because it helps direct the choice of laboratory studies.

A. **Inadequate bone marrow production**

1. **Leukemia (acute).** About 25% of acute cases of leukemia present with pancytopenia.

2. **Myelodysplastic syndromes.** Eg, refractory anemia. The bone marrow is normally hypercellular or normocellular but the white cells fail to reach the circulation.

3. **Megaloblastic syndromes.** Both vitamin B_{12} and folate deficiencies can result in neutropenia and increased intramedullary hemolysis.

4. **Marrow infiltration**
   a. **Metastatic cancer**
   b. **Granulomatous diseases**

5. **Drugs.** Benzene, alkylating agents (melphalan), vinca alkaloids (vincristine or vinblastine), doxorubicin (Adriamycin), and antimetabolites (methotrexate).

6. **Radiation.** A direct marrow toxin.

7. **Aplastic anemia**

   8. **Cyclic neutropenia**
   9. **Racial or familial neutropenia**
  10. **Infections.** In cases of infectious mononucleosis, 20–30% have moderate neutropenia. Other viral infections (HIV, hepatitis A or B) and bacterial illnesses may have a direct myelosuppressive effect.
  11. **Starvation/anorexia nervosa**
  12. **Paroxysmal nocturnal hemoglobinuria (PNH)**
  B. **Accelerated removal/consumption**
   1. **Drug induction**
      a. **Immune.** Such as hydralazine (Apresoline), quinidine, quinine, cefoxitin (Mefoxin), and nafcillin.
      b. **Nonimmune.** Such as phenacetin, indomethacin (Indocin), phenytoin, chloramphenicol, cimetidine, ranitidine, and phenothiazines.
   2. **Hemodialysis and cardiovascular bypass.** Exposure of blood to a dialysis coil of cellophane or nylon fiber appears to activate the complement pathway. This increases neutrophil adhesion, causing them to sequester in pulmonary capillaries.
   3. **Felty's syndrome.** Neutropenia associated with seropositive rheumatoid arthritis and splenomegaly suggests this diagnosis.
   4. **Infection**
      a. **Nonimmune.** At times, the peripheral requirements for neutrophils during overwhelming sepsis can exhaust the marrow reserves. This is particularly true in the debilitated patient, such as a patient with chronic alcohol abuse.
      b. **Immune.** Tests for antineutrophil antibodies are not routinely available. Consequently, this is a diagnosis of exclusion.
  C. **Redistribution of neutrophils**
   1. **Enhanced neutrophil margination.** Endotoxemia in gram-negative sepsis can give rise to rapid margination of neutrophils to the tissue.
   2. **Hypersplenism.** Refers to the clinical situation in which, in the presence of splenomegaly and a relatively normal bone marrow, there is a decrease of one or more cell lines in the peripheral blood because of sequestration in the spleen.

IV. **Database**
   A. **Physical examination key points**
      1. **Vital signs.** Fever suggests infection. Hypotension may be a sign of sepsis.
      2. **Skin.** Petechiae are consistent with Rocky Mountain spotted fever or disseminated intravascular coagulation (DIC). Rash may be seen in connective tissue diseases, or with certain bacterial infections such as *Neisseria gonorrhoeae* or *N meningitidis*.

3. **HEENT.** Temporal wasting and oral thrush may occur in acquired immunodeficiency syndrome (AIDS). Nuchal rigidity suggests meningitis.
4. **Lymph nodes.** Lymphadenopathy can be seen in both malignant and infectious processes, including HIV infection.
5. **Lungs.** Pneumonia with overwhelming sepsis may cause or be secondary to neutropenia. Inspiratory crackles, increased tactile and vocal fremitus, and egophony may be present.
6. **Abdomen.** Hepatosplenomegaly can be a sign of malignancy (leukemia or lymphoma), infection, or hypersplenism.
7. **Joints.** Look for classic findings of rheumatoid arthritis, such as symmetric swelling of the proximal interphalangeal (PIP) and metacarpophalangeal (MCP) joints. Rheumatoid nodules on the extensor surface of the arms near the elbows are also a classic sign of rheumatoid arthritis.

B. **Laboratory data**
1. **CBC with differential.** Presence of anemia and thrombocytopenia along with leukopenia may suggest B_{12} or folate deficiency, aplastic anemia, PNH, ethanol abuse, or leukemia. The mean corpuscular volume (MCV) will be increased with B_{12} or folate deficiency.
2. **Blood and urine cultures.** If an infectious process is suspected.
3. **Liver function test and hepatitis serologies.** If hepatitis is suspected. Elevated LDH may suggest B_{12} deficiency or lymphoma.
4. **Peripheral blood smear.** Dysplastic, degranulated neutrophils with pseudo-Pelger-Huet anomaly (a bilobed neutrophil) may suggest a myelodysplastic syndrome. Toxic granulation and Döhle bodies suggest infection. Neutrophils with five and six lobes point toward B_{12} deficiency. Blasts are consistent with leukemia.
5. **Leukocyte alkaline phosphatase (LAP) score.** Is increased in certain infectious and inflammatory diseases and polycythemia vera. In contrast, it is decreased in chronic myelogenous leukemia.
6. **Rheumatoid factor and antinuclear antibodies (ANA).** Obtain these values if collagen vascular disease is suspected.
7. **Carotene (serum).** Elevated in anorexia nervosa and decreased in starvation.
8. **Vitamin B_{12} and folate levels.** To rule out megaloblastic anemia.
9. **Sucrose water test/Ham test.** Useful in making the diagnosis of PNH. The sucrose water test involves mixing the patient's red blood cells in an isotonic solution of sucrose dissolved in water. The Ham test is performed by mixing the patient's red blood cells with acidified serum. Both tests promote the binding of a

small amount of complement to the surface. This results in hemolysis in patients with PNH.
- **C. Radiologic and other studies**
  1. **Chest x-ray.** To rule out pneumonia if suspected.
  2. **Sinus films, dental Panorex.** As indicated when looking for source of fever in a neutropenic patient.
  3. **Lumbar puncture.** Indicated when meningitis (acute or chronic) is suspected.
  4. **Bone marrow biopsy and aspiration.** (See Section III, Chapter 5, Bone Marrow Aspiration and Biopsy, p 348.) These procedures can provide critical information about granulocyte aplasia, hypoplasia or dysplasia, infiltration, cellularity, and cellular maturation. A bone marrow is essential in all patients with neutropenia except when it is mild, stable, or clinically associated with a drug known to cause neutropenia. Even in the setting of a drug-induced process, it is good management to document suspected marrow findings.

V. Plan. The major consequence of neutropenia is vulnerability to infection. The usual clinical manifestations of infection are often absent because of the lack of granulocytes (neutrophils). Thus, pneumonia may be present without significant infiltrate on CXR; meningitis may occur without pleocytosis or meningeal signs; and pyelonephritis may be present without pyuria. A heightened awareness for infection is extremely important in the neutropenic patient, as an untreated infection can be fatal.
- **A. Emergent management**
  1. If there is evidence of infection or fever (higher than 100.5°F) with an ANC below 500/μL, the patient should be immediately pancultured (cerebrospinal and other body fluid cultures as indicated) and broad-spectrum antibiotics initiated (third-generation cephalosporin (ie, ceftazidime) + an aminoglycoside, depending on how toxic the patient appears) and/or vancomycin if the patient has a central line, prosthesis in place, or a gram-positive organism is highly suspected). Neutropenia with infection is a medical emergency requiring immediate investigation and treatment.
  2. Identify any potential drugs or chemicals that may have induced the neutropenia; stop or remove them.
  3. Always wash your hands prior to touching the patient. Keep the patient away from visitors with active infections, fresh fruits or vegetables, flowers, and live plants. Avoid rectal manipulation such as with digital examination or rectal temperature.
- **B. Definitive care.** After a complete history and physical exam, the etiology of the neutropenia can usually be placed in one of the three broad categories discussed earlier. Subsequent tests can be ob-

tained to confirm a specific diagnosis. In general, regardless of the etiology, supportive care is indicated for most of these patients. This includes antibiotics for infections and blood products for associated severe anemia or thrombocytopenia.

1. **Bone marrow failure.** For drug-induced neutropenia, remove the offending agent and give supportive care until the counts return (generally within 1–2 weeks). Now available colony-stimulating factors (CSFs) *can be* used for drug-induced (ie by chemotherapy) neutropenia to speed recovery. Data thus far does not support the routine use of CSFs to treat non-febrile neutropenia or febrile neutropenia, although their use in "high-risk" patients (eg, those with pneumonia or sepsis) may be reasonable. Treatment for viral etiology or myelodysplastic syndromes is generally supportive care. The use of CSFs can be considered in myelodysplastic patients if they are experiencing neutropenic infections.

2. **Consumption.** Treat bacterial infections as indicated. Immune consumption may require steroids. Felty's syndrome generally requires no treatment unless the patient suffers recurrent infections. Then, splenectomy may be required.

3. **Redistribution.** Patients with hypersplenism are generally able to immobilize the sequestered neutrophils and thus fight off infection; subsequently, they do not require any specific therapy.

REFERENCES

American Society of Clinical Oncology. Recommendations for the use of hematopoietic colony-stimulating factors: Evidence-based, clinical practice guidelines. J Clin Oncol 1994;11:2471.

Schrier SL: Leukocyte function and nonmalignant disorders. In: Dale DC, ed-in-chief; Federman DD, ed. *Scientific American*, vol. 1, sect 5: Hematology. pt VII: Leukocyte Function. Scientific American Inc;1989:5.

49. NAUSEA AND VOMITING

I. **Problem.** A 39-year-old man is admitted with diffuse abdominal pain and fever. Later that evening, you are called because the patient has severe nausea and vomiting.

II. **Immediate Questions.** When evaluating a patient with nausea and vomiting, a careful history and a complete physical exam are important to rule out serious causes that require prompt intervention such as peritonitis or intracranial lesions.

  A. **What are the patient's vital signs?** Fever suggests an inflammatory process such as gastroenteritis, peritonitis, or cholecystitis.

Hypotension may be secondary to volume depletion or associated sepsis. Hypertension and bradycardia may reflect increased intracranial pressure.

B. When do the nausea and vomiting occur? Are they related to meals? Vomiting during or soon after a meal suggests psychogenic causes or may be seen with pyloric channel ulcer, pancreatitis, or biliary tract disease. If abdominal pain is relieved with vomiting, an ulcer becomes more likely. Vomiting an hour or more after a meal is more characteristic of gastric outlet obstruction, pancreatitis, or motility disorders, such as diabetic gastroparesis and postvagotomy. Nausea and vomiting early in the morning on arising are often associated with alcoholism, pregnancy, uremia, and increased intracranial pressure.

C. What are the appearance and volume of the vomitus? Large amounts of vomitus or secretions usually indicate partial or complete bowel obstruction, gastric atony, or, in rare cases, Zollinger-Ellison syndrome. Vomiting of undigested food suggests the presence of esophageal disorders, such as achalasia or a diverticulum, as well as gastric outlet obstruction. The presence of bile indicates a patent pyloric channel. A fecal smell suggests lower abdominal obstruction. Occasionally, this can be seen with bacterial overgrowth in the proximal small intestine. Blood or coffee-ground-appearing material points to an upper GI bleed. Vomiting can also induce hematemesis secondary to a Mallory-Weiss tear. (See Section I, Chapter 26, Hematemesis, Melena, p 140.)

D. Does the patient consume alcohol? Are they taking any non-steroidal anti-inflammatory drugs (NSAIDs)? Pancreatitis or acute gastritis can be caused by ethanol and result in nausea and vomiting. A NSAID such as ibuprofen (Motrin) may induce gastritis.

E. Is there associated abdominal pain? This can be seen with most abdominal causes of nausea and vomiting. The location of the abdominal pain will help in deciding the etiology of the nausea and vomiting. (See Section I, Chapter 1, Abdominal Pain, p 1.)

III. Differential Diagnosis. Those disorders that are associated with nausea and vomiting, and require immediate attention can be grouped as follows:

A. Intra-abdominal or thoracic etiology

    1. Gastric outlet obstruction. Occurs in patients with a history of peptic ulcer disease (PUD), prior abdominal surgery, or neoplasms.

    2. Small or large bowel obstruction. May be caused by fibrous bands and adhesions (usually after surgery), primary or secondary metastatic neoplasms, impacted feces, strictures from active inflammatory bowel disease (IBD), intestinal parasites, gallstones, incarcerated hernia, or a volvulus.

3. **Pseudo-obstruction or functional (paralytic) ileus.** Results from failure of normal intestinal peristalsis. Causes include abdominal surgery; retroperitoneal or intra-abdominal hematomas; severe infections; renal disease; metabolic disturbances such as hypokalemia; or drugs, particularly anticholinergics.

4. **PUD.** Results from local irritation or edema surrounding a pyloric channel ulcer, causing a mechanical obstruction.

5. **Pancreatitis.** Usually associated with abdominal pain that frequently (in > 50% of cases) radiates to the back. A CT scan is helpful in demonstrating inflammation and pseudocyst formation. Retroperitoneal abscess formation can complicate pancreatitis.

6. **Biliary colic.** From distension of smooth muscle in bile ducts secondary to stones, inflammation, or neoplasms.

7. **Intestinal ischemia.** From local vascular compromise or from reduced cardiac output. Guaiac-positive stools are common findings.

8. **Pyelonephritis or nephrolithiasis.**

9. **Hepatitis.** May be either viral or drug-induced.

10. **Appendicitis.** Often associated with right lower quadrant pain, fever, and leukocytosis with a left shift.

11. **Diverticulitis.** Lower abdominal pain and fever are common.

12. **Perforated viscus.** Usually presents as an acute abdomen.

13. **Pelvic inflammatory disease (PID).**

14. **Acute myocardial infarction (MI).** MI, especially involving the inferior wall, can present with nausea and vomiting; chest pain may be absent.

B. **Intracranial etiology**

1. **Tumor or mass lesions leading to increased intracranial pressure.** Consider an acute cerebral vascular accident, neoplasm, or subdural hematoma.

2. **Bacterial and viral meningitis**

3. **Migraine headache.** Usually unilateral headache, with photophobia and previous history of headache. May have prodrome (eg, aura).

4. **Labyrinthitis**

C. **Metabolic etiology**

1. **Uremia.** Often associated with weight loss, lethargy, and intense pruritus. The BUN is usually > 100.

2. **Hepatic failure.** From a variety of causes including cirrhosis, hypoxic injury, and drug-induced states such as acetaminophen overdose.

3. **Adrenal insufficiency.** Can occur in patients on chronic corticosteroid therapy which is suddenly discontinued. Adrenal insufficiency may also occur if the patient is stressed (surgery, serious infection) and the steroid dose is not increased. Associated symptoms include weakness, fatigue, hypotension, and abdominal pain.

   4. **Metabolic acidosis** (See Section I, Chapter 2, Acidosis, p 9.)
   5. **Electrolyte abnormalities.** Hypercalcemia and hyperkalemia as well as hypokalemia can cause nausea.
   6. **Hypothyroidism secondary to decreased intestinal motility or thyroid storm.** Weight gain, constipation, mental status changes, and dry skin suggest hypothyroidism. Weight loss, hyperdefecation, moist skin, hyperthermia, and mental status changes as well as a precipitating event are consistent with thyroid storm.
 D. **Miscellaneous etiology**
   1. **Drug-induced.** Major offenders are dopamine agonists such as l-dopa and bromocriptine (Parlodel), opiate analgesics such as morphine, digoxin (Lanoxin), and certain chemotherapy agents such as cisplatin (Platinol). Also consider alcohol, NSAIDs, and aspirin.
   2. **Acute gastroenteritis.** Common in the outpatient setting with "food poisoning" from bacterial endotoxins. Diarrhea is often present. (See Section I, Chapter 17, Diarrhea, p 17.)

IV. **Database**
 A. **Physical examination key points**
   1. **Vital signs.** Hypotension may result from volume depletion or sepsis. Orthostatic blood pressure changes suggest volume depletion. An orthostatic decrease in blood pressure without an increase in heart rate suggests autonomic neuropathy, which may accompany diabetes with gastroparesis. Fever points to an inflammatory component, possibly infection. Tachycardia can result from associated pain.
   2. **HEENT.** Look for signs of head trauma which would point to an intracranial process. Scleral icterus suggests hepatic failure/hepatitis. Papilledema is consistent with an intracranial process or a hypertensive emergency. An enlarged thyroid gland points toward hypothyroidism or hyperthyroidism.
   3. **Skin.** Check the patient's skin turgor and mucous membranes to estimate volume status. Yellowing of the skin may signify jaundice. Hyperpigmentation may be caused by adrenal insufficiency (Addison's disease).
   4. **Chest.** Inspiratory crackles secondary to atelectasis can be associated with any intra-abdominal process limiting deep inspiration because of pain. They may also suggest left ventricular dysfunction associated with MI.
   5. **Abdomen.** (See Section I, Chapter 1, Abdominal Pain, p 1.)
   6. **Rectum.** Check for fecal impaction, rectal masses, and occult blood. Tenderness on the right side is consistent with appendicitis. Blood can be secondary to diverticulitis, IBD, PUD, and gastritis; or may result from vomiting (Mallory-Weiss tear).

7. **Female genitalia.** Helpful in diagnosing PID. A discharge is often present.
8. **Neurologic exam**
   a. **Mental status changes** may signify central nervous system (CNS) lesions, encephalopathy, or severe electrolyte disturbances.
   b. **Focal neurologic findings** such as weakness, unilateral hyperreflexia, or a positive Babinski on one side suggest an intracranial process.
   c. **Pain with flexion of the neck** is consistent with meningeal inflammation secondary to either a subarachnoid bleed or meningitis. A positive Kernig's sign also indicates meningeal irritation; it is obtained by flexing the patient's hip and knee to a 90-degree angle. Attempts to extend the leg at the knee will result in hamstring pain and resistance to movement.

B. **Laboratory data**
1. **Electrolytes.** Severe vomiting may lead to various electrolyte disturbances, such as hypokalemia, hypochloremia, and metabolic alkalosis.
2. **CBC with differential.** A leukocytosis with an increase in banded neutrophils suggests an infection. An elevated hematocrit can be associated with volume depletion. Anemia suggests chronic GI blood loss or massive acute bleeding.
3. **BUN and creatinine.** To rule out renal failure.
4. **Urinalysis.** Look for white blood cells and casts suggesting pyelonephritis. Red blood cells, especially with flank pain, point to nephrolithiasis.
5. **Liver function tests, transaminases (AST and ALT), total bilirubin, and alkaline phosphatase.** To rule out hepatic failure and hepatitis.
6. **Amylase and lipase.** If pancreatitis is suspected.
7. **Arterial blood gases.** Needed to evaluate the presence of an acid-base disturbance as a cause or consequence of vomiting.
8. **Serum intact human chorionic gonadotropin (HCG) serum.** If pregnancy is suspected.

C. **Radiologic and other studies**
1. **Acute abdominal series (KUB).** Air-fluid levels are seen in obstruction; free air under the diaphragm indicates perforation. If the patient may be pregnant, defer KUB until the result of HCG is known.
2. **Electrocardiogram.** Helpful in evaluating for acute myocardial infarction. ST segment depression or elevation, T wave inversion, or Q waves suggest myocardial ischemia or infarction.
3. **Abdominal ultrasound or HIDA scan.** These may aid in the diagnosis of cholecystitis, biliary duct obstruction, or abscesses. Biliary colic cannot be ruled out with a normal ultrasound. A HIDA scan is important as a means of assessing cystic duct function.

4. **Endoscopy.** Important in the diagnosis of PUD or esophageal diverticula.
5. **Gastric emptying scan.** Useful in suspected gastroparesis, especially in patients with long-standing diabetes who have nausea and vomiting.

V. **Plan.** Treatment of the underlying etiology is essential in the management. A nasogastric tube should be used for decompression if obstruction is present. Separate treatment of each cause is beyond the scope of this section. Commonly used medications are listed here.
   A. **Phenothiazines.** Most commonly used antiemetics. Principal mode of action is via depression of CNS dopamine receptors. Prochlorperazine (Compazine) 10 mg PO Q 4–6 hr or 25 mg PR; chlorpromazine (Thorazine) 25 mg PO Q 8 hr, and promethazine (Phenergan) 12.5–25 mg PO, PR, or IM Q 6–12 hr PRN are effective agents. Extrapyramidal side effects can be treated with diphenhydramine (Benadryl) 25 mg IV or IM Q 4–6 hr.
   B. **Butyrophenones.** These agents also block CNS dopamine receptors. Give haloperidol (Haldol) 2 mg PO or IM Q 4–6 hr; or droperidol (Inapsine) 2–5 mg IV or IM Q 4–6 hr.
   C. **Miscellaneous drugs.** High doses of metoclopramide (Reglan), 1–2 mg/kg Q 4–6 hr, constitute a useful and very effective adjunct with cancer chemotherapy to prevent nausea and vomiting. Benztropine (Cogentin) 2 mg PO or IV or diphenhydramine 25–50 mg PO or IM should be given prophylactically to prevent extrapyramidal reactions with high doses of metoclopramide.

REFERENCES

Lee M, Feldman M: Nausea and vomiting. In: Sleisenger MH, Fordtran JS, eds. *Gastrointestinal Disease: Pathophysiology/Diagnosis/Management.* 5th ed. WB Saunders;1993:510.
Malagelada JR, Camilleri M: Unexplained vomiting: A diagnostic challenge. Ann Intern Med 1984;101:211.

50. OLIGURIA/ANURIA

I. **Problem.** A 72-year-old man admitted for pneumonia and altered mental status has had steadily declining urinary output. On morning rounds, his nurse reports that he did not void during the previous shift.

II. **Immediate Questions**
   A. **Does the patient have any symptoms or predisposing conditions that suggest hypovolemia?** Hypovolemia is a common

cause of oliguria. Diarrhea, vomiting, gastrointestinal (GI) bleeding, high fever, and low oral intake are possible causes. Positional dizziness suggests hypovolemia.

B. Is there any previous history of symptoms to suggest bladder outlet obstruction from prostatic hypertrophy? A history of hesitancy, difficulty initiating voiding, and dribbling suggests prostatic hypertrophy, which can result in postrenal obstruction.

C. Is there a history of hematuria? Bilateral nephrolithiasis or carcinoma can cause obstruction resulting in anuria or oliguria.

D. Is the patient likely to be suffering from acute renal insufficiency? Acute renal insufficiency can cause oliguria, although it is an uncommon etiology of complete anuria. Clues to the presence of acute renal insufficiency include baseline renal insufficiency (which amplifies the effects of ischemic or toxic insult); documented episodes of hypotension; medications known to adversely affect renal function (eg, aminoglycoside antibiotics and nonsteroidal anti-inflammatory agents [NSAIDs]); and exposure to nephrotoxic agents, especially contrast dye and some chemotherapeutic agents such as cisplatin.

E. Are there any underlying diseases that could result in oliguria/anuria? Congestive heart failure (CHF) and cirrhosis can cause oliguria/anuria by reducing effective arterial blood volume.

F. Does the patient have any symptoms suggestive of uremia? Nausea, vomiting, anorexia, insomnia, and mental status changes are seen with increasing renal insufficiency. Uremic symptoms are an indication for immediate dialysis.

III. **Differential Diagnosis.** Oliguria is defined as a urine output < 500 mL/d and anuria as an output < 100 mL/d. The differential diagnosis for acute oliguria is identical to that for acute renal failure, and may be divided into prerenal, renal, and postrenal causes.

A. **Prerenal causes.** Relating to renal hypoperfusion.
   1. **Shock/hypovolemia**
      a. **Hemorrhage.** From GI bleeding or trauma, or as a postoperative complication.
      b. **Inadequate fluid administration.** Fever, diarrhea, vomiting, poor oral intake without adequate fluid administration.
      c. **Sepsis.** Causing decreased renal perfusion as a result of decreased systemic vascular resistance.
   2. **Apparent intravascular hypovolemia.** A relative decrease in the effective circulating volume.
      a. **"Third-space" losses.** Very common in pancreatitis, major burns and after major operations.
      b. **CHF**
      c. **Cirrhosis.** May have associated hepatorenal syndrome.
      d. **Nephrotic syndrome**

3. **Vascular**
   a. **Renal artery occlusion (acute or chronic)**
   b. **Aortic dissection**
   c. **Emboli (such as cholesterol)**
B. **Renal causes**
   1. **Acute tubular necrosis**
      a. **Ischemia.** Secondary to shock from any cause, including sepsis.
      b. **Toxins.** These may include medications (aminoglycosides, amphotericin B), contrast media, and heavy metals.
      c. **Transfusion reaction**
      d. **Myoglobinuria.** Secondary to rhabdomyolysis; often seen in alcoholics. Muscle tenderness, elevated creatine phosphokinase, and pigmented casts point to myoglobinuria.
   2. **Acute interstitial nephritis**
      a. **Drugs.** β-lactamase-resistant penicillins (eg, methicillin); also sulfonamides, fluoroquinolones, and NSAIDs.
      b. **Hypercalcemia.** Can cause nephrocalcinosis.
      c. **Uric acid.** Gouty nephropathy or tumor lysis (chemotherapy for leukemia or lymphoma).
   3. **Acute glomerular disease**
      a. **Malignant hypertension**
      b. **Emboli, thrombosis, disseminated intravascular coagulation (DIC)**
      c. **Rapidly progressive glomerulonephritis**
      d. **Systemic diseases.** Wegener's granulomatosis, Goodpasture's syndrome, thrombotic thrombocytopenic purpura, systemic lupus erythematosus (SLE), scleroderma.
C. **Postrenal causes**
   1. **Urethral obstruction.** Prostatic hypertrophy, catheter obstruction. Prostatic carcinoma is an unusual cause of postrenal obstruction.
   2. **Bilateral ureteral obstruction.** Most often as a result of carcinoma or retroperitoneal fibrosis. Common cause of death in women with cervical carcinoma.

IV. **Database**
A. **Physical examination key points**
   1. **Vital signs**
      a. A decrease in weight suggests volume depletion.
      b. Hypertension can result from volume overload associated with anuria. Also long-standing hypertension can be a cause of renal insufficiency.
      c. Fever points to an infection (possibly sepsis) or acute interstitial nephritis.

    d. Most importantly, assess the patient for orthostatic blood pressure and pulse changes (a decrease in systolic blood pressure of 10 mm Hg or an increase in heart rate by 20 BPM 1 minute after movement from supine to standing position). Orthostatic hypotension without a change in heart rate can be found in elderly patients secondary to autonomic insufficiency. An imbalance in intake and output (I&O) or weight loss can cause volume depletion resulting in orthostatic changes in heart rate and blood pressure.

    e. An irregularly irregular pulse is consistent with atrial fibrillation, a common cause of emboli.

  2. Skin. Decreased tissue turgor and dry mucous membranes occur with volume depletion.

  3. HEENT. Flat neck veins with the patient supine suggest volume depletion. There may be an increase in jugular venous pressure secondary to volume overload from oliguria/anuria.

  4. Chest. Rales suggest CHF, possibly from volume overload.

  5. Abdomen. Determine if there is ascites or a distended bladder. An enlarged bladder suggests bladder outlet obstruction such as from prostatic hypertrophy.

  6. Genitourinary system. Examine males for an enlarged prostate. Keep in mind, however, that bladder outlet obstruction can occur even when the gland feels normal in size. In females, rule out a pelvic mass.

  7. Extremities. Assess perfusion by color and temperature of skin.

B. Laboratory data (See Section II, Table 2–6, p 328, for urinary indices useful in the evaluation of renal failure.)

  1. Urinalysis. This is useful because it can be performed immediately in a housestaff laboratory.

    a. Look specifically for high specific gravity suggesting volume depletion or recent dye administration.

    b. Large amounts of protein or red blood cell casts suggest glomerular disease.

    c. Significant hematuria points toward renal embolization or ureteral calculi and white blood cell casts suggest infection or severe inflammation. Eosinophils are seen with allergic interstitial nephritis; frequent granular casts are consistent with acute tubular necrosis.

  2. Serum chemistries. Compare the blood urea nitrogen (BUN) and creatinine. If their ratio is > 20:1, a prerenal cause is likely, although obstruction may also cause a high ratio, as can GI bleeding and severe catabolic states. If the ratio is < 15:1 and the BUN and creatinine are elevated, a renal cause is likely. Note the presence of hyponatremia or hypernatremia and hyperkalemia, any of which may complicate acute renal insufficiency.

  3. Urine electrolytes and creatinine. A urinary sodium < 15 mmol/L suggests a prerenal cause; a urinary sodium > 20 mmol/L suggests renal causes. The fractional excretion of sodium (FE_{Na}) is calculated as [urinary sodium $\times$ serum creatinine/urine creatinine $\times$ serum sodium] $\times$ 100. A $FE_{Na} < 1$ suggests volume depletion; a $FE_{Na} > 1$ suggests renal causes. Acute urinary tract obstruction and dye nephrotoxicity may also reduce the FE_{Na} to < 1.

C. **Radiologic and other studies**

1. **Ultrasound.** An accurate means of examining the collecting system for signs of obstruction, particularly ureteral obstruction that cannot be relieved by simple insertion of a urinary catheter.

2. **Central venous pressure line or pulmonary artery catheter.** Will give a more accurate assessment of volume status.

3. **IV pyelogram.** For practical purposes, ultrasound is as accurate for detecting obstruction and avoids the nephrotoxicity and volume-expanding properties of radiographic dye. Avoid IV pyelograms if creatinine > 2 mg/dL.

4. **Retrograde pyelogram (RPG).** If obstruction is suspected, an RPG can reveal the cause and specific location of the obstruction. In addition, the urologist can place ureteral stents at the time of the procedure to bypass the obstruction.

5. **Renal scan.** Technetium-labeled diethylenetriaminepentacetate (DTPA) nuclear medicine study can assess blood flow to the kidneys if renal artery embolization or thrombosis is suspected.

6. **Angiogram.** Provides better detail of renal anatomy but is rarely acutely needed.

7. **Renal biopsy.** Useful in determining specific causes of renal insufficiency, particularly allergic interstitial nephritis, although not needed acutely.

V. **Plan.** As a general rule, the minimal acceptable urine output is 0.5–1.0 mL/kg/h. Accurate records of fluid intake and output are essential. Review the patient's medications and stop all nephrotoxic drugs. Doses of renally excreted drugs should be adjusted and potassium removed from all IV fluids.

A. **Post-renal causes.** Place a Foley catheter. If immediate flow of urine is obtained, the diagnosis of urethral obstruction is very likely and a catheter can be placed at least temporarily. If no urine is obtained, there may still be bilateral ureteral obstruction (or obstruction of a congenital or surgical single ureter). If the patient is already catheterized, assess the patency of the current catheter, and, if in doubt, replace it. See Section I, Chapter 23, Foley Catheter Problems, p 125. Make sure the Foley catheter is working by irrigating with 50 mL normal saline (NS), using a catheter tip syringe. The fluid should pass easily and the entire amount should be aspirated. If a catheter problem is noted, correct it or consult a urologist.

B. Management of prerenal causes

1. **Volume challenge.** In almost every case, it is appropriate to give a potassium-free volume challenge such as with 500 mL of NS for 30 minutes. In patients with fragile cardiorespiratory status, smaller boluses should be given and central venous catheters used to monitor volume status. Then adjust the IV rate accordingly.

2. **Monitor volume replacement.** Give crystalloid to increase central venous pressure above 10 mm Hg or pulmonary capillary wedge pressure above 12–14 mm Hg. A hematocrit > 25–30% is adequate.

3. **Follow hourly urine output.** Give specific criteria so as to keep apprised of the patient's condition. For example, have the house officer called if urine output is < 25 mL/h. A typical limit is 0.5 mL/kg/h.

4. **Remove potassium and magnesium from IV solutions** unless abnormally low.

5. **Consider additional measures** to increase urine output once volume status is corrected, although this is rarely useful unless the renal insult has been recent (within several hours). These additional methods of increasing urine output carry with them the risk of hypovolemia and ototoxicity, as in the case of high doses of furosemide (Lasix).

   a. **Furosemide.** Use escalating doses in an attempt to obtain increased urine output. One method is to start with 80 mg IV, then increase to 160 mg IV and then 320 mg IV. Check urine output over 1–2 hours before proceeding to the higher dose.

   b. **Mannitol.** A dose of 12.5–25 g (50–100 mL of a 25% solution) IV may induce an osmotic diuresis.

6. **Review medications.** Adjust doses or stop nephrotoxic drugs.

C. Management of renal causes

1. **Consider increasing the urine output** as in V.B.5. It is easier to manage a patient with nonoliguric renal insufficiency than one with oliguric or anuric renal failure.

2. **Emergent dialysis** should be considered in the following circumstances: severe hypervolemia unresponsive to diuretics, intractable acidosis, severe hyperkalemia, pericarditis thought secondary to uremia, and severe uremic symptoms or encephalopathy.

D. Postrenal management. Usually requires urologic consultation. Most causes can be acutely managed with a Foley catheter, ureteral catheters, or percutaneous nephrostomy tubes.

REFERENCE

Conger JD, Briner VA, Schrier RW: Acute renal failure: Pathogenesis, diagnosis, and management. In: Schrier RW ed. *Renal and Electrolyte Disorders*. 4th ed.; Little, Brown 1992;495.

51. PACEMAKER TROUBLESHOOTING

I. **Problem.** A 44-year-old man was admitted earlier today to the CCU for an acute myocardial infarction (MI) complicated by third-degree heart block, and a pacemaker was inserted. The CCU nurse calls to report seeing pacemaker spikes but no capture.

II. **Immediate Questions**
  A. **What is the patient's condition and what are his or her vital signs?** Bradycardia with hypotension warrants immediate attention, as does the development of symptoms of hypoperfusion (confusion, pre-syncope or syncope, chest pain, and dyspnea).
  B. **What were the circumstances surrounding pacemaker insertion?** Prophylactic insertion of a temporary pacemaker wire in the setting of an acute MI and Mobitz type II second-degree heart block carries a different set of implications than the development of third-degree heart block and hypotension. The latter situation may rapidly deteriorate to cardiac arrest; whereas the former may require no intervention other than close observation.

III. **Differential Diagnosis.** Most problems encountered with pacemakers are generally classified into one of two categories: failure to capture a pacing impulse, or failure to sense a cardiac depolarization. Temporary pacemaker output is programmed to be inhibited by cardiac depolarization.
  A. **Failure to capture.** Failure to capture occurs when the temporary intravenous (or transcutaneous) pacemaker generates an impulse (as evidenced by a narrow, vertical pacemaker "spike"), but there is no evidence of ventricular depolarization. Keep in mind that a transvenous pacing wire placed appropriately in the apex of the right ventricle should produce a wide complex depolarization immediately after the pacemaker spike. A 12-lead ECG will reveal a superior axis (~ −90) with a left bundle branch block morphology. See Figure 1–4 for an example of failure to capture. Fail to capture represents one of the most common problems encountered in temporary transvenous pacing.
    1. **Problems intrinsic to the pacemaker**
      a. **Malposition of the catheter** resulting in loss of contact between the catheter tip and the endocardium. This can occur when the patient is repositioned in bed. Malposition will result in raising the pacing threshold, and thus will fail to capture.
      b. **Inappropriate lead placement**
      c. **Inappropriate generator settings.** Be sure that the heart rate and output settings have not been changed.

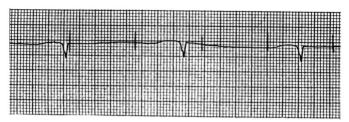

Figure 1–4. Failure to capture. The rhythm is a nodal rhythm at 40 beats per minute. The pacemaker spikes occur at 72 per minute. The pacemaker spikes are not associated with the ventricular depolarizations.

        d. Malfunction of the generator. This is an uncommon reason; however, generators run on alkaline batteries which sometimes fail. Be sure to check the generator battery regularly.
        e. Fractured pacing electrode
        f. Poor connection between the electrodes and the generator
    2. Local factors
        a. Profound hypoxemia
        b. Severe acidemia
        c. Marked hyperkalemia
        d. Fibrosis at the electrode
        e. Myocardial infarction that includes the right ventricular apex.
        f. Myocardial edema at the catheter tip
        g. Drugs. Type IIC antiarrhythmic agents (eg, flecainide, encainide) can raise the myocardial threshold for depolarization.
  B. Failure to sense. Failure to sense occurs when the pacemaker fails to recognize a native depolarization and subsequently generates a pacemaker spike shortly after the native depolarization. See Figure 1–5 for an example of failure to sense. Often, this inappropriate pacemaker spike will fall somewhere between the QRS complex and the T wave of the native depolarization, and a ventricular depolarization will *not* follow this pacemaker spike. This is because the pacemaker spike is occurring during the refractory period of the ventricle (the native depolarization was not sensed by the pacemaker). Failure to sense should not be interpreted as failure to capture; even though failure to capture often accompanies failure to sense, especially when the problem results from pacing electrode displacement and poor endocardial contact. In essence, the same

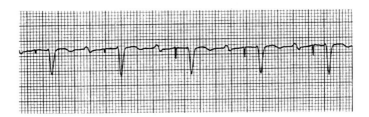

Figure 1–5. Failure to sense. A pacemaker spike is seen immediately after the 3rd, 4th, 5th and 6th QRS complexes. The pacemaker should have been inhibited by the QRS complexes. (Photograph courtesy of Alberto Mazzoleni, MD.)

circumstances that cause failure to capture can also cause failure to sense. If the timing of the pacemaker spike is right (on the T wave), sustained ventricular tachycardia can occur.

  C. Other complications of transvenous pacemakers
    1. Oversensing of P waves and T waves
    2. Myocardial perforation with pericardial effusion and tamponade (rare).
    3. Ventricular ectopy
    4. Tricuspid valve dysfunction
    5. Line sepsis
    6. Venous thrombosis

IV. Database
  A. Physical examination key points
    1. Vital signs. Heart rate and blood pressure are essential to determine the need for immediate intervention.
    2. Cardiopulmonary examination. An elevated jugular venous pressure, inspiratory rales at the bases, and an S_3 indicate congestive heart failure (CHF), possibly secondary to hypoperfusion. An elevated jugular venous pressure, new pericardial friction rub, and loss of a palpable apical impulse could indicate a pericardial effusion from myocardial perforation by the pacemaker wire.
    3. Neurologic examination. A change in mental status or confusion may indicate hypoperfusion.
  B. Laboratory data
    1. Portable chest x-ray. To check placement of the catheter tip. This will help if catheter displacement or myocardial perforation is the problem. In addition, comparison to post-insertion chest x-rays can be helpful. Unfortunately, the most relevant information is obtained from the lateral projection, which often is not obtained after insertion and is often not feasible to obtain at the time of malfunction.

2. **Electrocardiogram and rhythm strip.** To rule out myocardial infarction as a cause of the problem and to rule out myocardial ischemia as another possible indicator of hypoperfusion. Clues as to the current location of the catheter can be obtained from the surface ECG. For instance, a pacemaker in the right ventricular apex will result in a QRS configuration with a left bundle branch morphology. If a right bundle branch morphology is present, the clinician should suspect interventricular septum rupture and subsequent pacing from the left ventricle.

3. **Arterial blood gases.** To rule out acidemia or hypoxemia as a cause.

4. **Electrolytes..** To rule out hyperkalemia as a cause of the pacemaker's failure to sense or capture.

V. Plan

A. **Electrode placement.** If there has been any decline in the patient's condition or significant change in vital signs, ask the nurse to place anterior and posterior transcutaneous pacing electrodes on the patient in preparation for possible use until the problem with the transvenous pacing wire can be resolved. In addition, have the "crash cart" readily available in case of cardiopulmonary arrest.

B. **Obtain back-up.** There are few problems in internal medicine more anxiety-provoking than a dysfunctional pacemaker in a pacemaker-dependent patient. If a senior resident or cardiology fellow supervises you in the CCU, give him/her a call.

C. **Inspect the generator and connections to the pacing wire.** Care must be taken to avoid "short-circuiting" the system. Be sure you are wearing rubber gloves. Empiric replacement of a new generator "box" is generally preferred over attempts to replace batteries. In addition, replace the generator if something appears to be wrong with it.

The pacing wire can be tested for electrode fracture by connecting the distal cathode to the V lead on the ECG machine, and then connecting the proximal anode to the V lead. If an ECG can be recorded from each electrode, the pacing wire has not fractured. When you cannot see a pacemaker spike, the problem usually lies with either the generator or the pacing wire. Pacemaker spikes are more easily seen with unipolar pacing (eg, the proximal anode is usually a subcutaneous wire). Also, a unipolar pacing configuration is more sensitive than a bipolar pacing configuration. Thus, changing from a bipolar to a unipolar configuration may help to restore both capture and sensing.

D. **Adjust the pacemaker settings.** Check the settings to be certain that the output, heart rate, and sensitivity settings are appropriate.

1. **Check the pacing threshold of the electrode**. First raise the pacing rate on the generator to a level at which the patient's rhythm is completely paced. Second, turn down the pacing out-

put until pace beats no longer appear. This is the pacemaker's pacing threshold. Acceptable threshold values are usually < 2 mAmps. *Caution:* Raise the pacing output back to its original setting before leaving the patient's bedside.

2. **For failure to capture:** Increase the output until capture reappears. A high pacing threshold may be related to electrode displacement or other problems as listed above.

3. **For failure to sense:** Increase the sensitivity until it reliably detects and is inhibited by cardiac depolarization.

E. **Consider repositioning the catheter** if adjusting the pacemaker settings does not solve the problem. Pacemaker wires can be advanced and repositioned blindly by following the configuration of the ECG tracing recorded from the endocardium. *This should be done only by someone experienced in this technique.* It is much safer to use fluoroscopy, if available, or to rely temporarily on transcutaneous pacing until someone skilled in pacemaker insertion arrives. Many hospitals have fluoroscopy either available in a CCU procedure room or have portable fluoroscopy on a "C-arm." If either is available, repositioning of transvenous pacing electrodes under fluoroscopic visualization is advised.

REFERENCES

Emergency cardiac pacing. In: Cummins RO ed. *Textbook of Advanced Cardiac Life Support.* American Heart Association;1994:5.

Narula OS: Clinical concepts of spontaneous and induced atrioventricular block. In: Mandel WJ ed.: *Cardiac Arrhythmias: Their Mechanisms, Diagnosis and Management.* Lippincott;1995:441.

Watanabe Y, Dreifus LS, Mazyalev T: Atrioventricular block: Basic concepts. In: Mandel WJ ed.: *Cardiac Arrhythmias: Their Mechanisms, Diagnosis and Management.* Lippincott;1995:417.

Wood M, Ellenbogen KA, Haines D: Temporary cardiac pacing. In: Ellenbogen KA ed. *Practical Cardiac Diagnosis and Cardiac Pacing.* Blackwell;1992:162.

52. PAIN MANAGEMENT

I. **Problem.** A 72-year-old man admitted to the oncology service for metastatic prostate cancer cannot sleep because of persistent back pain.

II. **Immediate Questions**

A. **Has the patient experienced this pain before?** The initial temptation is to assume that his pain results from metastatic disease; however, if the pain is of recent onset, the patient will require a full evaluation to ensure that a cause other than cancer is not responsible. For example, the pain may be from herpes zoster, pyelonephritis, renal colic, or an epidural abscess. Clearly, these

causes of low back pain require different management than
metastatic disease.

B. Is the patient currently receiving pain medication, and if so, what is the drug, dosage, and dosing interval? If the patient has previously received narcotics, the pain may represent development of tolerance and therefore an inadequate dose of medication. Similarly, physicians frequently prescribe an inappropriately long interval between doses of narcotics. Determine the interval since the last administration of medication.

III. Differential Diagnosis. Clearly, it is not within the scope of this chapter to provide a comprehensive differential diagnosis for all causes of pain. The following discussion pertains chiefly to the management of pain in terminally ill cancer patients. The management of chronic pain (pain that has lasted longer than three months) is not discussed here. Pain in a patient with cancer may be caused by the malignancy itself, may occur as a complication of treatment, or may result from a psychologic disorder.

A. Pain caused directly by tumors
1. **Tumor invasion of bone and pathologic fracture**
2. **Infiltration/compression of nerves**
3. **Obstruction of a hollow viscus**
4. **Expansion of a viscus or its capsule.** Eg, liver metastases.
5. **Tissue ischemia after tumor invasion of lymphatics and blood vessels**
6. **Paraneoplastic syndromes.** Eg, arthritis and neuropathy.

B. Iatrogenic causes of cancer pain
1. **Surgery.** Incisions; phantom limb pain.
2. **Chemotherapy.** May cause a variety of infectious, gastrointestinal and neurologic causes of pain.
3. **Radiation.** In the short term, radiation may cause inflammation (colitis, esophagitis). Over the long term, radiation can result in fibrosis.

C. Psychological pain. Anxiety and depression are frequently associated with malignancy and may intensify the patient's perception of pain.

IV. Database
A. Physical examination key points
1. **Vital signs.** Tachycardia occurs with a variety of causes of acute pain and therefore is too nonspecific to suggest a specific etiology. Fever, however, points in the direction of an infectious etiology.
2. **Skin.** Chemotherapy and hematologic malignancies can predispose to herpes zoster infections; therefore, ascertain if the

pain is in the distribution of a specific dermatome. Look for vesicular lesions that would also suggest shingles. Pain may precede the development of the typical vesicular rash by 2 days.

3. **HEENT.** In a cancer patient complaining of a headache, be sure to examine for papilledema, which would suggest increased intracranial pressure from cerebral metastases.

4. **Neck.** A stiff neck could indicate bacterial or carcinomatous meningitis causing back or neck pain.

5. **Chest.** In addition to auscultating the lungs for evidence of pneumonia, palpate the ribs and sternum for evidence of bone pain suggesting metastases.

6. **Abdomen.** In a patient with abdominal pain, examine for hepatomegaly, which could indicate liver metastases. Bowel obstruction could result from the underlying malignant process itself, or could occur as a result of decreased bowel motility from the administration of narcotics.

7. **Extremities.** Examine for evidence of bone pain or arthropathy, which may occur with underlying malignancy.

8. **Neurologic exam.** In a patient complaining of headaches, perform a careful neurologic exam looking for localizing findings that could indicate the presence of cerebral metastases. Stocking-glove distribution of pain may result from a peripheral neuropathy caused by underlying cancer or chemotherapeutic agents such as vincristine.

B. **Laboratory data**

1. **Complete blood count (CBC).** Obtain if infection is suspected.

2. **Alkaline phosphatase and serum calcium.** Order if bone metastases are suspected. Remember to correct the total calcium in the face of hypoalbuminemia or check an ionized calcium. See Section I, Chapter 35, Hypocalcemia, p 178.

3. **Alkaline phosphatase, γ-glutamyl transpeptidase (GGT), and transaminases (AST and ALT).** Obtain liver function tests on patients with suspected hepatic metastases.

C. **Radiologic and other studies.** Specific radiographs should be directed by findings from history and physical examination. Keep in mind that bone scintigraphy is more sensitive for bony metastases than plain films. Bone scintigraphy may be falsely negative if there is bone destruction without accompanying osteoblastic response, such as in multiple myeloma.

V. **Plan.** Fear of uncontrolled pain is one of the greatest concerns of a patient with malignancy. Attempts by the physician to allay the patient's anxiety regarding pain, and assurance that everything will be done to alleviate that pain may help significantly in achieving pain control. A frequent mistake made by physicians is reluctance to administer narcotics sufficient to control pain for fear of subsequent addiction. This is an unfounded fear in patients with acute pain, especially those patients with pain related to malignancy, as the great majority will *not* develop addiction or psychologic dependence. Physical dependence and tolerance may occur in patients who receive narcotics for long periods. After the initial history and physical examination, and exclusion of potentially reversible causes of pain, the management of presumed cancer pain can proceed.

A. **Mild pain.** Non-narcotic analgesics may be tried initially.
   1. **Aspirin** 650 mg by mouth (PO) Q 4 hr
   2. **Acetaminophen (Tylenol)** 650–1000 mg PO Q 4 hr (up to a maximum of 4 gm/day).
   3. **NSAIDs** such as ibuprofen (Motrin) 600 mg PO Q 6 hr or 800 mg PO Q 8 hr. Use cautiously in patients with underlying renal insufficiency.

B. **Moderate pain.** For patients whose pain persists despite the preceding measures, a weak narcotic-analgesic may be administered. Usually, these are administered in combination with either acetaminophen or aspirin, as the analgesic effect is greatly heightened by adding these agents.
   1. **Tylenol #3** (acetaminophen 300 mg with codeine phosphate 30 mg) PO Q 3 hr.
   2. **Percodan** (aspirin 325 mg with oxycodone 5 mg) PO Q 3 hr.
   3. **Percocet** (acetaminophen 325 mg with oxycodone 5 mg) PO Q 3 hr.

C. **Severe pain.** Although a variety of drugs may be used for more severe pain, morphine sulfate still remains the gold standard for management. It is important to emphasize that narcotics should be administered on a round-the-clock basis rather than on an as-needed basis. This provides a more sustained effect, reduces the overall narcotic requirement, and lessens overall patient suffering, as the goal is to circumvent the development of pain rather than to allow the patient to feel pain first and then request narcotics.
   1. **Morphine sulfate** initially 20 mg PO Q 4 hr. After initial titration with the immediate-release form of morphine, one of the newer longer-acting preparations such as MS Contin may be administered on an every-8-hour schedule. This preparation comes in 30- and 60-mg tablets. For patients unable to take morphine PO, consider use of transdermal fentanyl (Duragesic transdermal patch).
   2. **Demerol.** The use of this agent is discouraged in the management of acute pain because of its short half-life, requiring every-3-hour dosing. Use of Demerol may also result in accumulation of toxic metabolites that can cause CNS agitation and confusion, especially in patients with renal insufficiency. Also, avoid use of this agent in patients taking monoamine oxidase inhibitors (can cause encephalopathy and death).

D. Adjunctive measures. The majority of cancer patients (85–90%) obtain relief with one of the preceding regimens. For those with persistent pain, a variety of measures can be used.
1. **Intraspinal opioids**
2. **Patient-controlled IV analgesia (PCA)**
3. **Corticosteroids.** Effective for neurologic compression syndromes due to tumor infiltration.
4. **Antidepressants.** Amitriptyline (Elavil) has some analgesic effect, especially for neuropathic pain.
5. **Hydroxyzine (Vistaril)** 50–100 mg IM. Adds to analgesic effect of opioids and reduces nausea.

REFERENCES

Driscoll CE: Pain management. Prim Care 1987;14:337.
Drugs for pain. In: Abramowicz M ed. Med Lett Drugs Ther 1993;35;1.
Mather LE, Cousins MJ: The pharmacological relief of pain: Contemporary issues. Med J Aust 1992;156:796.

53. PHLEBITIS

I. **Problem.** A 60-year-old man is being treated for pneumonia. An intravenous catheter in the arm has not been changed for 5 days, and the site is now red and painful.

II. **Immediate Questions**
A. **What are the vital signs?** Fever can develop from both superficial thrombophlebitis and deep venous thrombosis. Hypotension as well as fever can occur with bacteremia (sepsis) from an infected vein.
B. **Can pus be expressed from the site?** Pus indicates a local infection, but is present in only 50% of cases of suppurative thrombophlebitis. Pus and hypotension strongly suggest suppurative thrombophlebitis.
C. **What medications are being administered into the intravenous line?** Many antibiotics, chemotherapeutic agents, potassium, and calcium can cause irritation, especially with extravasation into the surrounding tissue.

III. **Differential Diagnosis.** Acute venous inflammation or occlusion can occur in superficial or deep veins, and may or may not involve infection. The presence of an indwelling catheter or history of intravenous drug use, or an immunocompromised state (burns, cancer, steroid treatment) will increase the likelihood of infection. Both inflammation and infection of superficial veins are discussed under the heading of this problem.

A. **Superficial thrombophlebitis.** Acute inflammation without infection is the most common presentation.
   1. Especially in an upper extremity, the site of an intravenous catheter is the cause.
   2. Extravasation of irritant medications, such as hemotherapeutic agents, may cause superficial thrombophlebitis.
   3. The etiology may be unknown, especially in the lower extremities.
B. **Superficial suppurative thrombophlebitis.** Persistent fever, hypotension, expressible pus, and positive blood cultures indicate significant infection of the affected vein. Septic pulmonary embolization with pneumonia and abscess formation are rare complications.
C. **Other causes**
   1. **Deep venous thrombosis**
   2. **Septic thrombophlebitis of subclavian vein**
   3. **Migratory thrombophlebitis.** May be the first sign of an occult malignancy.

IV. Database
A. **Physical examination key points**
   1. **Vital signs.** Fever may indicate sepsis or thrombosis.
   2. **Lungs.** Examine for crackles or consolidation of pneumonia resulting from septic embolization.
   3. **Heart.** Listen for regurgitant murmurs that might suggest acute bacterial endocarditis in patients with bacteremia.
   4. **Extremities.** Examine intravenous sites for erythema, warmth, or tenderness in all febrile patients. Attempt to express pus if the site is erythematous. Palpate the calves for tenderness. Examine for edema, which could indicate deep vein thrombosis.
B. **Laboratory data**
   1. Leukocytosis is present in suppurative superficial thrombophlebitis.
   2. Order culture, sensitivity, and gram stain of purulence to identify specific bacterial agent.
   3. Remove catheter and culture the tip.
C. **Radiologic and other studies**
   1. **Chest x-ray.** To exclude septic pulmonary embolization, or empyema.
   2. **Venography, or venous Doppler studies.** Indicated only if central vein infection or deep vein thrombosis is suspected. May be necessary in a septic patient.
   3. **Echocardiogram.** To exclude presence of valvular vegetations if blood cultures are positive.

V. Plan. Thrombophlebitis can be prevented by periodic rotation of intravenous sites every 48 hours. Any intravenous site that appears infected must be changed.
  A. Superficial thrombophlebitis
    1. Dry or moist local heat
    2. Limb elevation
    3. Nonsteroidal anti-inflammatory agents (NSAIDs). For example, ibuprofen (Motrin) may be given, 600 mg PO Q 6 hr or 800 mg PO Q 8 hr.
  B. Suppurative thrombophlebitis
    1. Intravenous antibiotics. Must have good antistaphylococcal coverage as well as for gram-negative bacteria, including *Pseudomonas*. Nafcillin and gentamicin provide adequate initial coverage pending cultures.
    2. Local wound care. Such as wet-to-dry dressings.
    3. Analgesics or NSAIDs
    4. Exploratory venotomy or venectomy of involved vein
  C. Other measures. Suppurative thrombophlebitis of the subclavian vein requires resection and intravenous antibiotics as above.

REFERENCES

Arnow PM, Quimosing EM, Beach M: Consequences of intravascular catheter sepsis. Clin Infect Dis 1993;16:778.
Scheld WM, Sande MA: Endocarditis and intravascular infections. In: Mandell GL, Bennett JE, Dolin R, eds. *Principles and Practices of Infectious Diseases.* 4th ed. Churchill Livingstone;1995:740.

54. POLYCYTHEMIA

I. Problem. A 65-year-old male is admitted to your service with a hematocrit of 62%.

II. Immediate Question. Are there any medical conditions that require the prompt institution of therapy directed at the elevated hematocrit? Usually the finding of an elevated hematocrit is incidental, or it is discovered during the evaluation of a nonacute problem. You should determine that there is no evidence of decompensated congestive heart failure (CHF) and cardiac or cerebral ischemia that might benefit acutely from phlebotomy. Evidence of profound intravascular volume depletion requiring fluid replacement should be noted.

III. Differential Diagnosis. When you are confronted with an elevated hematocrit (> 50% for men, > 45% for women), you can simplify the differential diagnosis by separating polycythemia into three broad diagnostic categories.

A. **Relative polycythemia.** This condition is generally asymptomatic. Patients can, however, present with venous thrombosis, which can occur in any individual who becomes severely volume-depleted for any reason (eg, profuse diarrhea or vomiting).

B. **Polycythemia vera.** Onset is usually insidious, often found on routine blood counts for other reasons. Polycythemia vera may present with major venous thrombosis or hemorrhage. Symptoms may include headache, dizziness, vertigo, tinnitus, diplopia, blurred vision, claudication, angina, symptoms of peptic ulcer disease (PUD), pruritus, mucosal bleeding, epistaxis, ecchymoses, symptoms of deep venous thrombosis, pulmonary embolism, or symptoms of cerebral vascular thrombosis. It is usually a disease of middle and later years of life with a peak incidence in the sixth and seventh decades. There is a slight male predominance.
   1. **The diagnosis is made by meeting three major criteria; or the first two major criteria and two minor criteria.**
      a. **Major criteria**
         - **Elevated red blood cell mass** ($\geq$ 36 mL/kg in a male; $\geq$ 32 mL/kg in a female)
         - **Arterial oxygen saturation > than 92%**
         - **Splenomegaly**
      b. **Minor criteria**
         - **Platelet count > 400,000/mL**
         - **Elevated leukocyte alkaline phosphatase (LAP) score**
         - **Elevated vitamin B$_{12}$**
         - **Leukocytosis > 12,000/mL**

C. **Secondary polycythemia.** This condition has numerous causes. May be classified from the standpoint of whether the polycythemia is physiologically appropriate (response to tissue hypoxia) or physiologically inappropriate (inappropriate stimulation or secretion of erythropoietin).
   1. **Physiologically appropriate polycythemia**
      a. **High-altitude acclimatization**
      b. **Chronic obstructive pulmonary disease (COPD).** Caused by a pO$_2$ below 90% saturation. May occur as a result of desaturation at night or with exercise.
      c. **Cardiovascular disease (right-to-left shunts).** Most commonly as a result of congenital heart disease.
      d. **Alveolar hypoventilation.** Sleep apnea.
      e. **High-oxygen-affinity hemoglobins.** The patient may have a positive family history for this condition.
      f. **Congenital deficiency of 2,3-diphosphoglyceric acid**
      g. **Carboxyhemoglobinemia**
   2. **Physiologically inappropriate polycythemia**
      a. **Renal vascular disease**

   b. **Hepatic tumors**
   c. **Uterine leiomyomas**
   d. **Cerebellar hemangioblastomas**
   e. **Renal transplantation**
   f. **Renal cell carcinoma**
   g. **Ovarian carcinoma**
   h. **Renal cysts.** Flank pain or hematuria may be present.
   i. **Pheochromocytoma**

IV. **Database**
   A. **Physical examination key points**
      1. **Vital signs.** Hypertension is indicative of possible renal vascular disease or pheochromocytoma. Respiratory rate helps to assess presence of cardiac or pulmonary disease. Fever may indicate underlying systemic illness that may have caused volume depletion or be a sign of underlying malignancy.
      2. **General appearance.** Plethora is not helpful in the distinction of polycythemia vera from secondary polycythemia. Clubbing should be noted as a sign of underlying pulmonary or cardiac disease. Cyanosis is usually an indicator of hypoxemia and might be more suggestive of a secondary polycythemia.
      3. **HEENT.** Look for conjunctival injection and, on fundoscopic exam, hemorrhages and engorged vessels. Congested mucous membranes are often present and are nonspecific. All these symptoms would be more in favor of a true polycythemia.
      4. **Heart.** The presence of any murmurs or an S_3 might either suggest a cardiac etiology or be a sign of cardiac dysfunction caused by polycythemia.
      5. **Lungs.** Rales, barrel chest, or diminished breath sounds suggest COPD.
      6. **Abdomen.** Hepatomegaly and abdominal masses suggest a secondary cause, whereas splenomegaly is expected with polycythemia vera.
      7. **Extremities.** Clubbing, cyanosis, and edema point to secondary physiologically appropriate causes. Evidence of deep vein thrombosis may be a complication of polycythemia.
      8. **Neurologic exam.** Look for evidence of focal findings consistent with cerebrovascular accident or tumor. Global findings consistent with hypoxic encephalopathy suggest a secondary cause of polycythemia.
   B. **Laboratory data.** If there are obvious clues from the history and/or physical exam, an extensive lab evaluation may not be indicated. For example, a patient with a history of vomiting and diarrhea, poor oral intake, and marked orthostasis and tachycardia with a hematocrit of 55% would be appropriately treated with fluid resuscitation and evaluation of the etiology of the volume loss. Unfortu-

nately, the diagnosis is not obvious in most cases and further evaluation is indicated.

1. **Hematocrit.** Generally, a hematocrit $> 60\%$ predicts a true increase in the red cell mass; hematocrits $< 60\%$ may result from either true or relative increases in the red cell mass.

2. **Platelet count.** A count $> 400,000/\mu L$ suggests polycythemia vera.

3. **White count.** Leukocytosis $> 12,000/\mu L$ suggests polycythemia vera.

4. **Arterial blood gases.** Oxygen saturation $< 90\%$ points to a physiologically appropriate secondary cause.

5. **LAP score.** An elevated LAP score is consistent with polycythemia vera.

6. **Vitamin B_{12}.** Elevated B_{12} or unbound B_{12} binding capacity is seen with polycythemia vera.

7. **p50 (Oxygen affinity of hemoglobin).** This test evaluates the presence of abnormal hemoglobins with high oxygen affinity.

8. **Carboxyhemoglobin level.** The presence of an elevated carboxyhemoglobin level points to a physiologically appropriate secondary cause.

9. **Erythropoietin level.** This value will be elevated with physiologically inappropriate causes (eg, hepatoma) as well as with physiologically appropriate causes.

C. **Radiologic and other studies**

1. **Red cell mass.** A nuclear medicine study to distinguish between relative and true polycythemia. A normal red cell mass with a diminished or low normal plasma volume is characteristic of relative polycythemia. If this is found, no further evaluation of the elevated hematocrit is needed. An elevated red cell mass with a normal or increased plasma volume is found in true polycythemia. If this is the case, then further evaluation is indicated to determine if this represents a primary (polycythemia vera) or secondary polycythemia.

2. **Abdominal and pelvic CT scan.** To look for evidence of benign or malignant neoplasms of the liver, kidney, adrenals, and endometrium.

3. **CT scan or MRI scan of the brain.** To rule out cerebellar tumor.

4. **Echocardiogram.** Look for right-to-left shunts. May also show left ventricular dysfunction, a possible complication of polycythemia.

5. **Pulmonary function studies.** These may reveal severe obstructive lung disease.

V. **Plan.** Treatment depends on the type of polycythemia.

A. **Relative polycythemia.** This condition requires no therapeutic intervention directed specifically at reduction of the hematocrit, although the underlying disorder needs to be addressed (eg, volume depletion; or the impact of stress-related disorders such as obesity, hypertension, and nicotine addiction). Isovolemic phlebotomy can be used but has not been shown to affect morbidity or mortality.

B. True polycythemia of secondary cause

    1. In physiologically appropriate secondary polycythemia, it may be difficult to determine if symptoms are due to the underlying disease or the elevated hematocrit. Remember that the elevated hematocrit is a physiologically important compensatory mechanism; you must prove that the erythrocytosis is detrimental prior to phlebotomy. In physiologically inappropriate polycythemia, therapy should be directed at the underlying cause.

    2. Therapeutic phlebotomy is performed in physiologically appropriate polycythemia if the patient is clearly symptomatic from the elevated hematocrit. If phlebotomy is indicated, the goal should be to maintain the hematocrit between 50–60%. In patients with physiologically inappropriate polycythemia, phlebotomy is reasonable and can be done safely. The goal should be to maintain a hematocrit of 45%, especially if surgery is contemplated.

    3. Cytotoxic therapy is contraindicated in any type of secondary polycythemia.

C. Polycythemia vera. Therapy is directed at overproduction of red cells and frequently accompanying platelet disorders.

    1. Phlebotomy. This procedure is quite effective in lowering the hematocrit. It is essentially free of complications as long as the patient is monitored for signs of hypovolemia during the phlebotomy and treated appropriately with crystalloid infusion should hypotension occur; or be replaced prophylactically if there is risk that a brief period of hypotension would be dangerous in a given patient. An expected long-term complication with frequent phlebotomy is iron deficiency. It has been debated whether or not iron repletion should be undertaken in this setting as this will increase the phlebotomy requirements. At least two reasons are commonly cited for iron replacement therapy.

        a. As red cells become progressively more microcytic, there is an actual increase in the whole blood viscosity, which is the reason for doing therapeutic phlebotomy in the first place.

        b. There is a need for iron as a cofactor in many enzyme systems, the effects of iron depletion at this level are uncertain.

    2. Cytotoxic therapy. In patients with a history of thrombotic or bleeding problems, phlebotomy may be inadequate therapy. These patients benefit from therapy with chemotherapeutic agents or radioactive phosphorus injections.

        a. Hydroxyurea has been shown to be effective, appearing to have minimal, if any, risk of induction of leukemia.

   b. Alkylating agents have been associated with an increased risk of secondary leukemias, especially in younger patients.
   c. ^{32}**P** is also associated with an increased risk of secondary leukemias.
3. **Antiplatelet agents.** These cannot be recommended as they were not found to be effective in prevention of thrombosis by the Polycythemia Vera Study Group. These agents *have* been found to be associated with a significant risk of GI bleeding, especially with platelet counts above 1,000,000/μL.
4. The most recent recommendations for therapy in polycythemia by the Polycythemia Vera Study Group are as follows:
   a. Patients older than 70 years are most effectively treated with radioactive phosphorus and phlebotomy because of the increased risk of thrombosis associated with increasing age.
   b. Patients younger than 50 years should be treated with phlebotomy alone unless there are risk factors for thrombosis or a history of prior thrombotic event. In these cases, hydroxyurea would appear to be a safe alternative to radioactive phosphorus and alkylating agents.
   c. In patients between 50 and 70 years of age, the role of myelosuppressive agents is unclear. But management similar to that in the younger-than-50 age group seems appropriate.
   d. Patients with other symptoms such as pruritus, bone pain, and troublesome splenomegaly are best managed by a myelosuppressive agent.

REFERENCES

Berk PD et al: Therapeutic recommendations in polycythemia vera based on Polycythemia Vera Study Group Protocol. Semin Hematol 1986;23:132.

Beutler E. Polycythemia vera. In: Beutler E, Lichtman MA, Coller BS et al eds. *William's Hematology* 5th ed. McGraw-Hill, Inc;1995:324.

Erslev AJ: Clinical manifestations and classification of erythrocyte disorders. In: Beutler E, Lichtman MA, Coller BS et al eds. *William's Hematology.* 5th ed. McGraw-Hill, Inc;1995:441.

Erslev AJ: Secondary polycythemia (erythrocytosis). In: Beutler E, Lichtman MA, Coller BS et al eds. *William's Hematology* 5th ed. McGraw-Hill, Inc;1995:714.

Gruppo Italiano Studio Policitemia. Polycythemia Vera: The natural history of 1213 patients followed for 20 years. Ann Intern Med 1995;123:656.

55. PULMONARY ARTERY CATHETER PROBLEMS

(See also Section I, Chapter 10, Central Venous Line Problems, p 51.)

  I. **Problem.** A 50-year-old man is admitted to the coronary care unit (CCU) with an anterior myocardial infarction (MI). A pulmonary artery catheter is placed. You are notified 24 hours later by the CCU nurse that he is having trouble interpreting the pressure tracings.

II. Immediate Questions

A. What does the waveform look like? The pulmonary artery waveform varies with inspiration and expiration and has a characteristic systolic/diastolic waveform. (See Figure 3–10, p 374; and Section III, Chapter 12, Pulmonary Artery Catheterization, p 374.)

B. Is there a waveform when the catheter is tapped? The absence of a waveform or a "dampened" tracing suggests that the catheter is not patent; or that there are technical difficulties including transducer malfunction, cracked hub, loose connections, incorrect stopcock positions, too-tight skin sutures, and too-tight plastic sleeve diaphragms.

C. Can the catheter be flushed? Can blood be withdrawn? If the catheter cannot be flushed or blood withdrawn, the catheter may not be patent. The catheter may be kinked, or there may be a venous thrombus obstructing the catheter. (See Section I, Chapter 10, Central Venous Line Problems, p 51.)

D. Is the catheter in permanent wedge? After a period of time within the patient's circulation, pulmonary artery catheters tend to become softer and more pliable, and may migrate distally. With a decreasing pulmonary pressure, the same effect may occur as the pulmonary vascular bed shrinks relative to the catheter position. The catheter may end up wedged with its balloon deflated, a situation analogous to a pulmonary embolus. The catheter position must be corrected as soon as possible. Careful evaluation is needed to ensure that the problem is really a case of permanent wedge and not a kink or system malfunction. If all else fails to help distinguish the various causes of a flat tracing, wedge position can be confirmed with blood gas sampling, showing saturation in the arterial range, as opposed to the mixed venous range usually found when blood gases are sampled from the pulmonary artery position.

E. Can a wedge tracing be obtained with the balloon inflated? If not, the balloon may have ruptured or the catheter may have been partially removed. *Do not continue to inject air if the balloon has ruptured*, because the air is injected directly into the pulmonary artery.

F. Are there any associated symptoms? Chest pain may result from a pulmonary artery catheter in permanent wedge, resulting in a pulmonary infarction. Hemoptysis can result from pulmonary infarction or from pulmonary artery rupture or erosion. This is usually associated with inflation of the balloon in a vessel smaller than the balloon, rupturing the pulmonary artery with entry of blood into the airways. Hemoptysis usually results and can sometimes be severe, but is rarely life-threatening. A fever may be secondary to catheter infection, catheter sepsis, or pulmonary infarction.

G. What is the relative necessity of the pulmonary artery catheter? If critical measurements are being made, such as hourly pulmonary artery wedge pressure readings, the situation is more serious than if the line has outlived its usefulness and can be removed.

III. Differential Diagnosis. Problems with pulmonary artery catheters (Swan-Ganz) can be conveniently divided into problems occurring inside the patient and outside the patient.

  A. Outside the patient

    1. Transducer error. This type of error often results in a "dampened" or flattened tracing. It is probably the most common source of problems, particularly with aging, nondisposable transducers. Bubbles within the transducer and any improper mounting will result in a low-quality pressure tracing.

    2. Cables. As with most electrical systems, particularly nondisposable systems, cables are a common source of problems.

    3. Monitor-related problems. Perhaps the most common monitor-related problems arise when the monitor is set on an improper scale or is not properly balanced.

  B. Inside the patient

    1. Catheter migration. The catheter may have moved from its original insertion position, migrating either distally or proximally. Distal migration may result in a permanent wedge.

    2. Thrombosis. A blood clot in the pressure-monitoring lumen may preclude good-quality pressure recordings.

    3. Kinks. The most common sites for kinking are at the skin surface, under the clavicle, and at the proximal and distal ends of the sheath. Kinks are another cause of poor-quality tracings.

    4. Malfunctioning balloon. If the catheter will not wedge, the balloon may have ruptured or the catheter may have migrated proximally. *Do not continue to inject air into the catheter system if a wedge tracing does not appear,* as a ruptured balloon may be the cause.

IV. Database

  A. Physical examination key points

    1. General exam. As in most technical areas of medicine, be sure that the information provided by your technology correlates with your clinical assessment.

    2. Vital signs. The presence of fever suggests catheter infection or sepsis, especially if the catheter has been in place longer than 3 days.

  B. Laboratory data

    1. Blood gases. A blood gas sample obtained from the distal port of the catheter can be helpful in determining whether a pulmonary artery catheter is in permanent wedge position. If the catheter is wedged, the oxygen saturation will approximate ar-

terial oxygen saturation, whereas mixed venous saturation is
found in pulmonary artery locations.

2. **Blood cultures.** Should be obtained in the presence of a fever
or elevated white count with an increase in segmented and
banded neutrophils.

C. Radiologic and other studies

1. **Chest x-ray.** A CXR is useful in determining whether the
catheter is kinked or in the correct position. Permanent wedge
may be suggested by a markedly distal location of the catheter
tip. After injection with air, a deflated balloon also points to balloon rupture.

2. **Culture of catheter tip.** If catheter-related sepsis or infection is
suspected, the catheter must be removed and the catheter tip
sent for culture.

V. Plan. For replacement of a pulmonary artery catheter, see Section III, Chapter 12, Pulmonary Artery Catheterization, p 370.

A. **Problems outside the patient.** If simple tapping on the catheter
does not result in a waveform, the cause clearly resides outside the
patient. Transducer, cable, and monitor-related problems should
be addressed first.

B. **Problems inside the patient.** When a good waveform is obtained
by tapping the catheter, the problem most likely resides within the
patient.

1. **Permanent wedge.** This problem is reported much more frequently than actually exists. Often, a well-placed pulmonary
artery catheter is withdrawn when the position is fine.

a. **Inspect the system** thoroughly before you attempt to move
the catheter. The transducer should be evaluated for proper
functioning. The system should be evaluated for leaks, loose
connections, and similar mechanical problems, prior to any
manipulation of the catheter.

b. **Obtain a CXR for positioning of the catheter and evaluation of the balloon.** If the catheter is truly stuck in wedge,
the CXR will show the catheter to be distal in the pulmonary
circulation. Less commonly, the balloon will not deflate
because the catheter is kinked. A CXR is the best tool to
assess this situation.

c. **Check the oxygen saturation.** As mentioned earlier, the
oxygen saturation will be arterial when obtained from a truly
wedged catheter.

d. **Catheter withdrawal.** If the catheter is really wedged and
the waveform cannot be returned to the expected waveform
by manual aspiration or flushing of the catheter, withdraw the
catheter centimeter by centimeter while flushing between
each withdrawal using a pressure-bag flush system. When

an appropriate waveform returns, the balloon should be re-inflated to be certain that the catheter will wedge when desired. The balloon should be inflated with about 1 mL of air to obtain the wedge tracing.

2. **A balloon that will not wedge.** In most cases, the catheter has been pulled back or the balloon is not functioning. The catheter should not be advanced unless a sterile sleeve protects the catheter lying outside the patient. If the balloon is malfunctioning, the catheter should be removed.

3. **Inaccurate or poorly reproducible cardiac outputs.**
   a. **In cases of apparently inappropriate cardiac outputs,** be sure that the constant on the cardiac output computer is correct for the catheter used. The thermodilution technique is not accurate in patients with very low cardiac outputs or significant tricuspid regurgitation. Use the mixed venous oxygen saturation and the Fick oxygen method to confirm a low cardiac output.
   b. **If no cardiac output is obtained,** the catheter may not be properly connected to the computer, or the wire connecting the thermistor to the computer may be fractured. Most computers will flash a code indicating that the catheter is at fault in this circumstance.

4. **Pulmonary artery rupture or erosion.** Treatment depends on the severity of the bleeding. It is prudent to remove the pulmonary artery catheter; if it is crucial for managing the patient, it can be replaced. The new catheter should be directed toward the opposite lung. This procedure requires fluoroscopy. Careful attention to the adequacy of ventilation and blood pressure, serial CXRs, and a low threshold for requesting cardiothoracic surgery consultation are advisable in this situation. This complication can be avoided by always inflating the balloon slowly and carefully, and monitoring the pressure waveform so that the catheter is not overwedged. For replacement of central venous catheters, see Section III, Chapter 6, Central Venous Catheterization, p 350.

REFERENCE

Grossman W, Barry WH: Cardiac catheterization. In: Braunwald E ed. *Heart Disease: A Textbook of Cardiovascular Medicine.* 4th ed. Saunders;1992:180.

56. SEIZURES

I. **Problem.** A 25-year-old woman is found having a seizure 1 day after admission for pyelonephritis.

II. Immediate Questions

A. Has the patient ever had seizures before? A patient with a history of prior seizures is often taking an anticonvulsant. In these patients, a common cause of seizures is failure to take the prescribed medication.

B. Is the patient on any anticonvulsant medications? Find out what medications the patient is supposed to be taking. Is the patient compliant, or receiving all the medications she was on prior to admission? If the patient is to have nothing by mouth (NPO), was an appropriate parenteral form given. Check for interactions with other medications, as some of these can affect the blood levels of anticonvulsants, particularly diphenylhydantoin (Dilantin).

C. Does the patient have a history of alcohol abuse? Alcohol withdrawal seizures commonly occur 6–48 hours after cessation of drinking. They are generalized; one to six will occur over a short period of time (6 hr) and the EEG is normal between seizures. One-third of these patients progress to delirium tremens. (See Section I, Chapter 16, Delirium Tremens, p 85.) Benzodiazepines are an effective treatment for these seizures.

D. Is there a history of barbiturate or sedative hypnotic abuse? Patients addicted to these substances may have a seizure after cessation.

E. Does the patient have a history of diabetes? Hypoglycemia can cause seizures. The most common cause of hypoglycemia is hypoglycemic agents, such as insulin and oral sulfonylureas.

F. Was the seizure generalized or focal in nature? Seizures that begin focally suggest a central nervous system etiology.

G. Are there any electrolyte abnormalities that could be causing the seizure? Recent lab results may reveal the cause of the seizure. Hyponatremia, severe alkalosis, hypernatremia, hypocalcemia, and hypomagnesemia can all cause seizures.

H. Is there any history of renal disease? Uremia can cause generalized seizures.

III. Differential Diagnosis.

Seizures result from abnormal electrical activity in the cerebral cortex. They may result in abnormal motor activity, abnormal behavior, or change in consciousness. Tonic-clonic seizures result in unconsciousness and stiffening of muscles followed by clonic jerking. There may be urinary incontinence, and there is often postictal confusion, lethargy, and headache.

A. Idiopathic epilepsy. The most common etiology of seizures, but must be a diagnosis of exclusion in the acute situation.

B. Tumors. Either primary brain tumors or metastatic lesions. Carcinoma of the breast, lung, or kidney, melanoma, and lymphoma frequently metastasize to the brain.

C. Infection. In adults, intracranial infections such as meningitis, brain abscess, or encephalitis can cause seizures; in children, any infectious process with systemic reaction (fever) can cause seizures (febrile seizures). Rabies, Rocky Mountain spotted fever, Lyme disease, syphilis, toxoplasmosis, Creutzfeldt-Jakob disease and mycotic aneurysm from endocarditis can cause seizures.

D. Trauma. A careful history must be obtained. Are there signs of skull fracture or other trauma?

E. Alcohol/drug withdrawal. Common after hospitalization, resulting in cessation of alcohol or drugs such as barbiturates or benzodiazepines.

F. Chronic renal failure. With uremia.

G. Anoxia. Generalized hypoxemia (post cardiac arrest, carbon monoxide poisoning, bradycardiac rhythms such as third-degree heart block), or focal anoxia (embolism or thrombosis).

H. Electrolyte abnormalities. See II G.

I. Other metabolic disorders. These may include pyridoxine deficiency or thyroid storm in adults; in children, phenylketonuria (PKU), and Tay-Sachs disease (deficiency of hexosaminidase).

J. Collagen-vascular disease. Systemic lupus erythematosus (SLE), vasculitis (polyarteritis), sarcoidosis.

K. Drugs. Seizures may result from cocaine use and amphetamine intoxication.

L. Porphyria. Acute intermittent porphyria.

M. Vascular lesions. Infarction (thrombotic or embolic), hypertensive encephalopathy, carotid sinus disease, subarachnoid hemorrhage.

N. Syncope. Often what is thought to be a seizure is a syncopal attack. Obtain a careful description from both nurses, the patient, and family about the event. See Section I, Chapter 57, Syncope, p 274.

O. Psychogenic seizures or pseudoseizures. May be difficult to distinguish from true tonic-clonic seizures. Often the patient remains conscious, there is no postictal confusion or incontinence, and there is a psychiatric history.

P. Toxemia of pregnancy. Occurs in the third trimester of pregnancy. Hypertension, renal dysfunction (decreased glomerular filtration rate or proteinuria), thrombocytopenia, and coagulopathy may be present.

Q. Hyperventilation. Rapid, shallow breathing, paresthesias, and tremulousness are seen.

R. Inadequate level of prescribed anticonvulsants. This is especially likely with phenytoin (Dilantin), in which the level of effectiveness can be altered by many other medications such as aspirin.

IV. Database
A. Physical examination key points
1. **Vital signs.** Fever suggests an infection. Check blood pressure or palpate pulse to ensure adequate perfusion. A markedly ele-

vated blood pressure suggests a potential cause of the seizure (malignant hypertension); or possibly the result of the source of the seizure (toxemia, cerebral hemorrhage or a thromboembolic stroke). A slow heart rate suggests a bradyarrhythmia.

2. **HEENT.** Nuchal rigidity suggests meningitis or subarachnoid hemorrhage. The tongue may be lacerated from the seizure. Look for evidence of head trauma, including blood behind the tympanic membranes.

3. **Neurologic exam.** Perform a complete neurologic exam including all cranial nerves, full sensory and motor examinations, deep tendon reflexes, Babinski, and mental status examinations. There may be transient deficits after the seizure (the postictal state). Focal findings may suggest a cerebrovascular accident or tumor. Evidence of meningeal irritation, such as pain with flexion of the neck, a positive Kernig's sign (with a hip and knee flexed at 90', pain and resistance is encountered with knee extension), or a positive Brudzinski's sign (flexion of the neck resulting in flexion of the knee and hips) suggests meningitis or a subarachnoid hemorrhage. Evaluate for loss of bladder or bowel control associated with a tonic-clonic or grand mal seizures.

4. **Skin.** Rash may suggest a vasculitis.

B. **Laboratory data**
   1. **Serum electrolytes.** Especially sodium, calcium, and magnesium.
   2. **Serum glucose.** To rule out hypoglycemia or hyperglycemia (hyperosmolar state).
   3. **Arterial blood gases.** To rule out hypoxemia or a severe alkalosis as the cause. A gap-acidosis secondary to lactic acid is often encountered after a tonic-clonic seizure.
   4. **Drug levels of prescribed anticonvulsants.** Perform this evaluation immediately, as a patient seizing with adequate drug levels will need to have new therapy instituted. See Section XVII, Commonly Used Medications, Table 7–13, p 536.
   5. **Drug screen.** Consider to rule out barbiturates or cocaine as the cause.
   6. **Complete blood count with differential.** To rule out infectious causes. Also, a low white blood cell count and anemia may point to a systemic illness such as SLE. In addition, severe thrombocytopenia (< 20,000/mL) can result in cerebral hemorrhage.
   7. **Collagen-vascular workup.** Antinuclear antibodies, sedimentation rate and complement studies, if SLE or vasculitis is suspected.

C. **Radiologic and other studies**
   1. **CT scan or MRI of head.** If this episode represents new-onset seizures and there is no obvious etiology, then an imaging study is indicated. However, this need not be done emergently unless other evidence suggests a space-occupying lesion that may re-

quire emergent treatment, or if the seizures recur without an obvious etiology.

2. **Lumbar puncture.** See Section III, Chapter 10, Lumbar Puncture, p 364. Indicated if meningitis or encephalitis is suspected; it should be done immediately. A CT scan should precede the lumbar puncture if there is papilledema or focal findings on neurologic exam suggesting increased intracranial pressure.

V. Plan. Support life functions (the ABCs of cardiopulmonary resuscitation), and prevent self-inflicted injury during the seizure. Follow with a careful workup to determine the cause and institute appropriate therapy.

   A. Emergency management
   1. Do not interfere if the patient is spontaneously breathing. Specifically, do **not** try to force something into the patient's mouth, such as a tongue depressor. This can lead to injury to the patient or yourself, and is totally unnecessary.
   2. Position the patient in the left lateral decubitus position with a suction device readily available to prevent aspiration if vomiting occurs.
   3. Most seizures will stop within 3 minutes.

   B. Seizure control. See Section VII, Commonly Used Medications, for a discussion of drugs listed here.
   1. A single seizure will usually run its course prior to the onset of action of any intravenous medication, and therefore need not be specifically treated.
   2. Establish intravenous access as soon as possible. If hypoglycemia is the cause of the seizure then give 1 ampoule (50 mL) of D50W. The etiology of the hypoglycemia will need to be determined to assess risk of repeated hypoglycemic episodes. See Section I, Chapter 35, Hypoglycemia, p 178.
   3. To treat a second seizure, or status epilepticus (repeated seizures with no regaining of consciousness between them), diazepam (Valium) IV may be given, usually as 5 mg IV slow push repeated at 10- to 15-minute intervals as needed; or lorazepam (Ativan) 2.5–10 mg IV slow push repeating at 15- to 20-minute intervals as needed to control seizure activity. Lorazepam is replacing diazepam as the treatment of choice in status epilepticus because of its longer half-life.
   4. Phenytoin (Dilantin) intravenously may be used if diazepam or lorazepam fails, or to prevent recurrence of seizures if diazepam or lorazepam has provided temporary control. It must be given slowly, no faster than 50 mg/min intravenously. Hypotension can result if administered too rapidly. Check levels daily after first starting the drug.

5. Phenobarbital may also be used. It is given slowly, usually by IV with a 120–140 mg loading dose. Maintenance doses are given IV, IM, or PO to maintain therapeutic levels.
6. Use of diazepam and phenobarbital (especially when used sequentially) can lead to respiratory depression.
7. Be alert for the complications of aspiration, hyperthermia, and cardiovascular collapse.
8. Long-term anticonvulsant therapy is not indicated for alcohol withdrawal seizures. Benzodiazepines are the treatment of choice. Chlordiazepoxide (Librium) or diazepam (Valium) orally can be used to treat mild to moderate alcohol withdrawal, and alcohol withdrawal seizures. See Section I, Chapter 16, Delirium Tremens, p 85.
9. Refractory seizures that do not respond to the preceding management may require general anesthesia.
10. A neurologist should be consulted in difficult-to-manage patients.
C. **Treating underlying condition.** After the acute seizure episode is controlled, treat the underlying condition. Treat electrolyte abnormalities as outlined in the specific "On Call Problem." Treat CNS lesions as appropriate. Definitive treatment for toxemia is delivery.

REFERENCES

Browning RG, Olsen DW, Steven HA: 50% dextrose: Antidote or toxin. Ann Emerg Med 1990;19:113.
Epilepsy and other seizure disorders. In: Adams RD, Victor M eds. *Principles of Neurology.* 5th ed. McGraw-Hill;1993:273.
French J: The long-term therapeutic management of epilepsy. Ann Intern Med 1994;120:411.
Scheuer ML, Pedley TA: The evaluation and treatment of seizures. N Engl J Med 1990;323:1468.

57. SYNCOPE

I. **Problem.** A patient admitted for palpitations and chest pain loses consciousness while being transported to the ICU.

II. **Immediate Questions**
A. **What was the patient's activity and position immediately prior to the incident?** Syncope in the recumbent position is almost always due to Stokes-Adams attacks (high-grade atrioventricular block). Vasovagal syncope or fainting from orthostatic hypotension requires the patient to have been in the seated or upright position. Exertional syncope is frequently cardiac in origin. Other key activ-

ities to ask about include: turning or twisting the head, coughing, getting up quickly, and micturition.

B. Is the patient still unconscious? Vasovagal syncope rarely lasts more than a few seconds and resolves with recumbency. Persistent unconsciousness suggests a cardiac or neurologic (brain stem stroke or seizure [See Section I, Chapter 56, Seizures, p 269]) cause.

C. What were the vital signs during the episode? What are the vital signs now? Vasovagal syncope is associated with bradycardia during the episode, but frequently a reflex tachycardia is noted after the episode. The blood pressure is usually normal after a vasovagal faint. Orthostatic changes in blood pressure and a tachycardia are frequently evidence of volume depletion or blood loss as the cause. Neurologic causes are generally associated with a normal or elevated blood pressure. Cardiac syncope may occur when arrhythmias result in a pulse < 140 or > 180 BPM.

D. Was there evidence of seizure activity? Some clonic jerking of the limbs may occur with syncope, and in some rare instances, a brief tonic-clonic seizure may occur (convulsive syncope). Fecal and urinary incontinence are more typical of seizures than of other causes of syncope.

E. How quickly was consciousness regained? Was the patient immediately oriented? Vasovagal episodes are brief and usually have an immediate return to full consciousness. Cardiac causes are also associated with a rapid return to full consciousness. Seizures are characterized by postictal confusion and headache.

F. How did the patient feel immediately prior to the loss of consciousness? Vasovagal episodes are normally preceded by a symptom complex consisting of sweating, lightheadedness, and abdominal queasiness. Seizures often have an aura (frequently recurring visual or olfactory sensations). Cardiac and orthostatic syncope is often not preceded by symptoms, or is associated with sensations of the room closing in or going dark.

G. What medical conditions does the patient have? A number of medical conditions predispose to syncope. Diabetics are at risk for hypoglycemia as well as orthostasis secondary to autonomic dysfunction. A history of atherosclerotic vascular disease suggests cardiac causes and arrhythmias as well as cerebrovascular events. Other important illnesses to ask about include: a previous history of a seizure disorder, valvular disorders, and any history of head trauma.

H. What medications is the patient receiving? A variety of medications predispose to orthostatic hypotension, including diuretics, antihypertensives, and tricyclic antidepressants such as amitriptyline (Elavil). Varying degrees of heart block can be induced by verapamil (Calan, Isoptin), diltiazem (Cardizem), digoxin (Lanoxin), and beta-blockers. Many Class I antiarrhythmics can also induce ventricular arrhythmias leading to syncope ("quinidine syncope").

III. Differential Diagnosis

A. Vasovagal syncope. Also called neurocardiogenic syncope. It is by far the most common cause of syncope, and associated with the symptom complex previously described.

B. Sudden decrease in venous return
1. **Micturition syncope**
2. **Cough syncope**
3. **Valsalva maneuver.** Increases vagal tone.

C. Cardiac syncope
1. **Dysrhythmias**
   a. **Tachycardias.** (See Section I, Chapter 58, Tachycardia, p 279.)
      i. **Ventricular tachycardia**
      ii. **Paroxysmal atrial tachycardia**
      iii. **Atrial fibrillation with rapid ventricular response**
      iv. **Atrial flutter**
      v. **Wolff-Parkinson-White (WPW) syndrome.** Look for short PR interval and delta wave.
   b. **Bradycardias.** See Section I, Chapter 8, Bradycardia, p 37.
      i. **Sinus bradycardia**
      ii. **Second- and third-degree atrioventricular block.**
2. **Structural causes**
   a. **Atrial myxoma.** Intermittent obstruction of a valve.
   b. **Aortic stenosis.** Associated with left ventricular outflow obstruction. Syncope is a marker of significant mortality.
   c. **Idiopathic hypertrophic subaortic stenosis.** Same etiology as aortic stenosis.
3. **Pacemaker syncope.** If the patient has a pacemaker, malfunction must be considered as a possible cause of syncope. See Section I, Chapter 51, Pacemaker Troubleshooting, p 250.
4. **Primary pulmonary hypertension.** Caused by decreased pulmonary flow and left-sided return.
5. **Acute myocardial infarction with cardiogenic shock**

D. Orthostatic hypotension
1. **Hypovolemia**
   a. **Dehydration**
   b. **Blood loss**
2. **Medications.** Diuretics, anti-hypertensives, and tricyclic antidepressants such as amitriptyline (Elavil).
3. **Neurologic causes**
   a. **Shy-Drager syndrome.** Idiopathic autonomic dysfunction.
   b. **Diabetes.** Autonomic dysfunction with long-standing diabetes.

E. Cerebrovascular accident. Seldom will a cerebrovascular accident involving the anterior circulation result in syncope unless there is bilateral disruption of the reticular activating system.
1. **Basilar artery insufficiency ("drop attacks")**
2. **Carotid sinus syndrome.** Presents as syncope caused by turning head to one side or too tight a collar.

3. **Subclavian steal syndrome**
4. **Subarachnoid hemorrhage.** May present as brief syncope followed by severe headache.

F. **Miscellaneous causes**
   1. **Hypoxemia**
   2. **Hyperventilation**
   3. **Hypoglycemia.** Often occurs in patients on insulin or oral hypoglycemics who miss a meal or receive the wrong dose.
   4. **Seizures**
   5. **Acute pulmonary embolism**
   6. **Psychogenic causes**

IV. Database

A. Physical examination key points

1. **Vital signs** (see Section II.C). Vitals should be rechecked frequently during the evaluation.
2. **HEENT.** Look for evidence of trauma, and palpate for bony abnormalities. Look for subhyaloid hemorrhages as evidence of subarachnoid hemorrhage. Tongue or cheek lacerations suggest seizure activity. Meningitis and subarachnoid hemorrhage have associated neck stiffness. Carotid bruits suggest diffuse atherosclerosis.
3. **Chest.** Auscultate for crackles and wheezes that may accompany aspiration during the syncopal episode. Palpate for rib injury caused by a fall.
4. **Heart.** Assess rate and rhythm, data which are especially useful during or immediately after episode. Auscultate for new fourth heart sound (S_4), suggestive of acute myocardial infarction and murmur, listening for characteristic changes with position that would differentiate aortic stenosis and idiopathic hypertrophic subaortic stenosis from other systolic murmurs. Assess the jugular venous pulse as an indicator of volume status.
5. **Genitourinary system.** Look for urinary and/or fecal incontinence.
6. **Neurologic exam.** Slow resolution of mental status to normal points to a postictal state. Focal deficits suggest a cerebrovascular event. Persistent mental obtundation suggests hypoglycemia, hypoxemia, or other metabolic derangement.
7. **Reproduction of event.** Perform maneuvers intended to reproduce event. *Caution:* Do this only with appropriate monitoring and resuscitation equipment available (including venous access). Have the patient cough, turn her or his head, and hyperventilate; or perform carotid massage as appropriate.

B. Laboratory data

1. **Hemogram.** Anemia can potentiate cerebral ischemia.

2. **Electrolytes and glucose.** Hypokalemia and hyperkalemia can cause ventricular arrhythmias. Hyponatremia, hypernatremia, hypocalcemia, and hypoglycemia predispose to seizures.

3. **Arterial blood gases.** Look for hypoxemia and hypocarbia. Also, severe alkalosis can cause seizures.

4. **Stool for occult blood.** Evaluate for an acute bleed.

C. **Radiologic and other studies**

1. **Electrocardiogram with a rhythm strip.** Look for tachyarrhythmias or bradyarrhythmias. A short PR interval and delta wave suggest Wolff-Parkinson-White syndrome. Also look for evidence of ischemia or myocardial damage and new conduction abnormalities.

2. **Chest x-ray.** Evaluate the cardiac silhouette for enlargement, possible effusion, or congestive failure. Look for possible causes of hypoxia, such as infiltrates, pneumothoraces, or signs of pulmonary embolism.

3. **Echocardiogram.** Look for valvular lesion, thrombi, new wall motion abnormalities, or myxoma.

4. **Holter monitor.** Useful if an arrhythmia is suspected, particularly in patients with frequent attacks. An event recorder may be more useful if the attacks are infrequent and the evaluation is in the outpatient setting.

5. **CT scan of head.** If seizure or subarachnoid hemorrhage is suspected.

6. **Electroencephalography.** If seizure is suspected.

7. **Tilt-table.** Excellent test for neurocardiogenic syncope.

V. **Plan.** This will be dictated by your initial impression based on the preceding evaluation. The causes of syncope range from a relatively benign vasovagal episode to life-threatening complete heart block. The treatment plan should reflect the severity of the underlying cause. Remember, injuries from a fall secondary to syncope can result in significiant morbidity in many patients, especially the elderly. So a thorough evaluation for injury should be a part of every plan.

A. **Vasovagal syncope**

1. Instruct the patient to assume a recumbent position at the onset of presyncopal symptoms. If unable to lie down, the patient should be seated with their head down.

2. The patient should be made aware of situations that bring on the episodes, such as prolonged standing, and should seek to avoid these situations.

3. For patients with suspected recurrent neurocardiogenic syncope, consider head up tilt-table testing to confirm diagnosis and direct further treatment (beta-blockers, disopyramide).

B. Orthostatic hypotension
1. Assess for signs of volume contraction and correct as indicated. Review patient's medications to eliminate, if possible, those that could cause volume depletion.
2. If gastrointestinal bleeding is diagnosed, see Section I, Chapter 26, Hematemesis, Melena, p 140, and/or Chapter 27, Hematochezia, p 143.
3. Instruct the patient to rise and change positions slowly, with adequate support available.

C. Cardiac syncope
1. Treat any arrhythmias. See Section I, Chapter 8, Bradycardia, p 37, and Chapter 58, Tachycardia, p 286.
2. If arrhythmia is suspected but cannot be confirmed with Holter monitoring, consider electrophysiologic testing, especially if ischemic heart disease is present.
3. If ischemia is the suspected etiology, treat as possible myocardial infarction, and institute a rule-out myocardial infarction protocol.

D. Miscellaneous disorders
1. **Carotid sinus syndrome (carotid sinus hypersensitivity).** Instruct the patient to avoid sudden turning of the head, tight collars, or vigorous rubbing with electric shavers.
2. **Micturition.** Instruct the patient to sit when voiding and to remain seated for several minutes after voiding.
3. **Cough and hyperventilation.** Informing the patient of the cause is frequently the only thing that can be done; however, if hyperventilation is due to anxiety, the anxiety should be addressed and treated appropriately.

REFERENCES

Gruss BP. Differentiation of convulsive syncope and epilepsy with head-up tilt testing. Ann Intern Med 1991;115:871.
Martin JB, Ruskin J. Faintness, syncope, and seizures. In: *Harrison's Principles of Internal Medicine.* 13th ed. Isselbacher et al, eds. McGraw-Hill;1994:90.

58. TACHYCARDIA

I. Problem. You are asked to evaluate an 18-year-old woman presenting to the ER with sudden onset of chest pain, palpitations, and dizziness. Triage evaluation reveals the presence of a rapid, regular, narrow-complex tachycardia at a rate of 180 beats per minute (bpm).

II. Immediate Questions
A. What are the patient's other vital signs? Take particular note of the patient's blood pressure, respiratory rate, and temperature. Hy-

potension accompanying a tachyarrhythmia requires rapid attention. Tachypnea and tachycardia may be present with acute pulmonary embolism (PE); a severe pneumonia; an exacerbation of chronic obstructive pulmonary disease (COPD); or during the presentation of acute pulmonary edema. Tachycardia accompanied by a fever may suggest an infection such as pneumonia, sepsis, or thyrotoxicosis. The presence of pulsus paradoxus (a variation in the systolic blood pressure of more than 10 mm Hg between tidal end inspiration and end expiration) suggests the possibilities of pericardial tamponade or an exacerbation of COPD.

B. **What has been the patient's heart rate previously?** A sudden change in heart rate may signify a change in cardiac rhythm, such as the sudden onset of atrial fibrillation.

C. **Does the patient have any symptoms related to the tachycardia?** Ask about dyspnea, chest pain, dizziness, syncope, agitation, or confusion.

D. **What medication is the patient currently taking?** Drugs that can cause tachyarrhythmias include diuretics, theophylline preparations, sympathomimetic drugs, catecholamine infusions, digoxin, and thyroid supplements. Diuretics can lead to intravascular volume loss as well as hypokalemia and hypomagnesemia that can result in tachyarrhythmias. Theophylline, even in therapeutic doses, may be responsible for a sinus tachycardia; and in toxic doses (serum levels greater than 20 µg/mL) can lead to ventricular tachyarrhythmias.

III. Differential Diagnosis

A. **Sinus tachycardia.** This condition is defined as a sinus node controlled rhythm at a rate greater than 100 bpm. The extensive list of its causes includes: varying states of emotion and pain; fever; anemia; hypoxemia; hemorrhage; infection; thyrotoxicosis; myocardial infarction; pneumothorax; pericarditis; use of drugs or medications that include caffeine, nicotine, and atropine; ingestion or overdoses of amyl nitrite, quinidine, cocaine, antihistamines, decongestants, or tricyclic antidepressants. Sinus tachycardia is typically gradual both in onset and termination. Vagal maneuvers and carotid sinus massage may slow the heart rate temporarily, but the tachycardia will return when these maneuvers are stopped. Sinus tachycardia rarely occurs in quiet patients at rates greater than 140 bpm. Fever can be expected to raise the sinus rate about 10 bpm for every degree above normal core body temperature.

B. **Supraventricular tachyarrhythmias (SVT).** When examining the ECG or rhythm strip of a suspected supraventricular tachyarrhythmia for the first time, check the tracing for the following features:

1. **Regularity.** Atrial fibrillation, multifocal atrial tachycardia, and on occasion atrial flutter are irregular rhythms whereas most other SVTs are regular rhythms.

2. **Baseline.** The baseline is that portion of the ECG between the end of the T wave and the beginning of either the P wave or the next QRS complex. If this section is flat, then the atria are either quiescent or fibrillating, or their activity is hidden in another section of the ECG.

3. **QRS complex.** SVTs generally have QRS complexes with axes and widths that are similar to those found during sinus rhythm, but not always. Wide QRS complexes can result from a rate-related bundle branch block, or antegrade conduction across an accessory atrioventricular pathway.

4. **P waves.** Determine if the P wave morphology and axis during the tachycardia is similar to or different from normal sinus rhythm. If different, then atrial activation is initiated somewhere other than the sinoatrial node.

5. **P wave-QRS complex relationship.** A constant timing relationship between P waves and the QRS complexes is found in most regular SVTs. Atrial flutter may demonstrate a variable relationship depending on the degree of AV conduction. The presence of AV dissociation would indicate a ventricular tachyarrhythmia.

6. After examination of the characteristics of a particular supraventricular tachyarrhythmia, it is then helpful to classify the arrhythmia based on the mechanisms used to sustain it.

    a. **Atrial flutter.** Atrial flutter involves a reentry circuit localized entirely within the atrial myocardium. The atrial rate is typically 250–400 bpm. Coarse, saw-toothed "flutter waves" are usually visible in the inferior leads. The ventricular rate depends on conduction in the AV node and is usually ½ to ⅓ of the atrial rate. If AV conduction is rapid, and the atrial flutter waves are therefore hard to see, carotid sinus massage will transiently decrease AV node conduction and allow a better view of the baseline of the ECG. Atrial flutter can be irregular or regular, depending on whether the conduction through the AV node is variable or constant. Atrial flutter can be seen with rheumatic heart disease; ischemic heart disease; with recent cardiac surgery, as part of the postpericardiotomy syndrome; in cardiomyopathy of various causes; atrial septal defect; acute pulmonary embolism; mitral or tricuspid valve disease; thyrotoxicosis; chronic alcoholism; and pericarditis.

    b. **Atrial fibrillation.** Atrial fibrillation is a rhythm that involves many disorganized atrial electrical circuits leading to chaotic atrial depolarizations. It is characterized by an atrial rate of 350–600 bpm. Distinct P waves are not visible. The ventricular rate is classically described as "irregularly irregular," and is controlled by the rate of conduction of the atrial impulses through the AV node. Ventricular rates are commonly 100–160 bpm in the untreated patient. Carotid sinus massage will temporarily decrease AV node conduction and slow the ventricular rate to allow the baseline to be seen. Predisposing conditions are similar to those for atrial flutter.

c. **Automatic supraventricular tachycardias.** These tachycardias develop because of abnormally enhanced automaticity in the atrial myocardium or bundle of His.

   i. **Paroxysmal atrial tachycardia with block.** This tachycardia is usually related to digitalis toxicity, and therefore occurs in patients with some type of organic heart disease. Enhanced automaticity in the atrial myocardium is the most likely mechanism. Hypokalemia may cause this arrhythmia. There is organized, visible atrial activity, although the P wave axis is different from normal sinus rhythm. The atrial rate is typically 180–240 bpm. Conduction of the rapid atrial discharges through the AV node is partially suppressed by digitalis, resulting in the intermittent AV block.

   ii. **Automatic atrioventricular junctional tachycardia.** The mechanism of this tachycardia is incompletely understood. It is generally attributed to increased automaticity of the pacemaker cells in the AV node. This tachycardia rarely occurs in patients without underlying cardiac disease. It can be seen in patients with digitalis intoxication, acute inferior or posterior myocardial infarctions, following cardiac surgery, or with viral or rheumatic myocarditis. This arrhythmia is usually benign and self-limited. The QRS complex is usually narrow and resembles that of sinus rhythm. The rate rarely exceeds 130 bpm. AV dissociation is commonly visible; P waves are visible between QRS complexes. This arrythmia has a gradual onset and termination.

d. **Reentrant supraventricular tachycardia.** Reentry circuits are the most common mechanism sustaining regular SVTs. Reentry requires myocardium with differing degrees of refractoriness in order to maintain the electrical circuit. These reentry circuits are located within the AV node, the atrial myocardium, or the sinus node; or involve both the atria and ventricles in the case of accessory conduction pathways.

   i. **AV nodal reentry tachycardia.** This is the most common type of reentrant tachycardia, accounting for up to 30% of all SVTs. The reentry circuit usually consists of a slowly conducting antegrade AV nodal pathway and a rapidly conducting retrograde AV nodal pathway. This arrhythmia is characterized by the presence of normal QRS complexes at a regular rate between 150 and 250 bpm. P waves are usually not visible. The onset and termination of the tachycardia are usually abrupt. Carotid sinus massage or vagal maneuvers may result in the abrupt termination of the tachyarrhythmia.

   ii. **Atrioventricular reciprocating tachycardia.** This tachyarrhythmia, also known by the eponym Wolff-Parkinson-White syndrome, involves an accessory conduction pathway between the atria and the ventricles. The QRS complex is usually narrow during tachycardia because antegrade conduction moves through the AV node, and the accessory pathway is conducting the ventricular electrical activity retrograde to the atria. Heart rates may exceed 200 bpm. During sinus rhythm, a "delta" wave, representing ventricular pre-excitation, may be visible as a slurring of the upstroke of the QRS complex. This also results in an abnormally short PR interval (<0.12 secs). This tachyarrhythmia may account for up to 20% of all supraventricular tachycardias. P waves may be visible inside the QRS complex, or in the QT interval. The P waves will have an abnormal axis reflective of the retrograde atrial depolarization.

  e. SVTs of uncertain mechanism. Multifocal atrial tachycardia is an arrhythmia characterized by the presence of multiple foci of atrial depolarization, resulting in more than one P wave morphology. This arrhythmia is found most commonly in patients with chronic pulmonary disease and pulmonary hypertension. The ventricular rhythm is usually irregular as a result of variable conduction through the AV node. The QRS complexes are generally normal. The ventricular rate can range from 100–140 bpm.

C. Ventricular arrhythmias

 1. Accelerated idioventricular rhythm (AIVR). This is a rhythm of ventricular origin with a rate of 50–100 bpm. It can be seen in patients with digitalis intoxication or acute myocardial infarction, as well as in otherwise normal healthy individuals. It is a common arrhythmia seen in patients given reperfusion therapy for acute myocardial infarction, where it is considered an indicator of successful coronary reperfusion. Most AIVRs are benign, except those associated with digitalis intoxication. Onset and termination are gradual. AIVRs do not usually result in hemodynamic collapse. The QRS complexes are wide, consistent with the ventricular origin of the arrhythmia. AIVRs can be recognized by the appearance of a monomorphic ventricular rhythm that appears to overtake a slower sinus rhythm; P waves and fusion beats are frequently visible. No specific therapy is necessary, unless digitalis intoxication is present. If hypotension does result from the AIVR, use of atropine to raise the sinus node rate will usually terminate this arrhythmia and restore hemodynamic stability.

2. **Ventricular tachycardia (VT).** These arrhythmias are characterized by a cardiac rhythm with wide QRS complexes and heart rates of 70–250 bpm. They usually compromise blood pressure and are a common cause of sudden cardiac death. Electrocardiographic criteria suggesting a ventricular arrhythmia, as opposed to a supraventricular arrhythmia, include: 1) a QRS duration >0.14 sec; 2) the presence of fusion and capture beats; 3) identification of P waves in the baseline of the electrocardiogram, suggesting AV dissociation; and 4) a QRS morphology that appears similar to isolated PVCs seen prior to the initiation of sustained VT. A **fusion beat** is a hybrid beat, in which a beat originating in the atrium fuses with one originating in the ventricle. Ventricular tachycardia is invariably associated with organic heart disease, especially coronary artery disease following myocardial infarction, and cardiomyopathies with impaired left ventricular function. The mechanism behind most ventricular tachyarrhythmias involves a reentry circuit located within the ventricular myocardium. There is usually an abnormality of impulse conduction, with a region of normally conducting myocardium located adjacent to a region of slowly conducting myocardium, frequently involving a section of scarred or fibrotic tissue. These areas of slow conduction are the myocardial substrate needed to maintain a reentry electrical circuit. This region of slowly conducting myocardium produces low-amplitude, high-frequency after-depolarizations that help to maintain the reentry circuit. These after-depolarizations are visible on signal-averaged electrocardiograms (SAECG).

3. **Ventricular fibrillation (VF).** This is the most common arrhythmia in cardiac arrest patients. Coronary artery disease is the major underlying etiology. Death is certain unless rapid and immediate electrical defibrillation is instituted. If resuscitation efforts are successful, further investigation is indicated, as recurrence rates are as high as 30% during the first year. Invasive electrophysiologic studies are helpful in finding the patients who are at highest risk for recurrence of VT or VF; these studies have proven to be useful in guiding long-term therapy options.

4. **Torsades de pointes.** This is a distinctive form of polymorphic ventricular tachycardia. This arrhythmia is uniquely characterized by a basic variation in the electrical polarity of the QRS complex, such that the QRS complexes appear to be twisting around an isoelectric baseline. Multiple leads may be necessary to accurately visualize the changes in the electrical polarity. The rate of the tachyarrhythmia can range from 150–280 bpm. Vari-

ation in the R–R interval is commonly seen. Spontaneous termination and recurrences are the rule with this arrhythmia. Torsades de pointes can occasionally progress to a sustained ventricular arrhythmia. The electrocardiographic abnormality that is the hallmark of this tachyarrythmia is a prolonged corrected QT interval during sinus rhythm >0.50 secs. This tachyarrhythmia is seen in quinidine and procainamide toxicity.

IV. Database
A. Physical examination key points
1. **Vital signs.** The blood pressure during the tachycardia is of primary importance, and dictates how rapidly action will be required. Palpation of carotid, brachial, or femoral pulses can give the examiner a rapid estimate of the adequacy of systolic pressure.
2. **Neck.** Distended jugular veins are present with acute decompensation of congestive heart failure, exacerbations of chronic pulmonary disease, pneumothorax, and pericardial tamponade. The presence of cannon "A" waves in the jugular venous pulsations suggests the presence of AV dissociation.
3. **Chest.** Rales and wheezes can be present in many of the associated cardiopulmonary diseases that predispose to tachyarrhythmias.
4. **Heart.** Listen in particular for a third (S_3) or fourth (S_4) heart sound, or a murmur that might suggest mitral valve disease.
5. **Abdomen.** Localized or rebound tenderness may help to indicate a source of infection as the condition responsible for a tachyarrhythmia.
6. **Extremities.** Examine for signs of peripheral perfusion as an assessment of the adequacy of cardiac output.

B. Laboratory data
1. **Serum electrolytes.** Hypokalemia and hypomagnesemia can be responsible for sustained arrhythmias, particularly in patients taking digitalis. Both supraventricular and ventricular arrhythmias can result from potassium and magnesium deficiencies.
2. **Arterial blood gases.** Severe disturbances of acid–base status can be responsible for initiation of tachyarrhythmias.
3. **Hemogram.** An elevated white blood cell count with a left shift suggests the presence of an infection.
4. **Thyroid function studies.** Check in order to exclude hyperthyroidism as a cause of a supraventricular tachyarrhythmia.
5. **Serum drug levels.** In particular, digitalis, theophylline, and antiarrhythmic drug levels should be checked in patients with new onset of a sustained tachyarrhythmia.

C. Electrocardiogram (ECG) and rhythm strip.
A 12-lead ECG is the most important piece of diagnostic information in a patient with acute onset of sustained ventricular tachyarrhythmia. It should be

obtained prior to initiating therapy as long as the patient's condition allows the extra time to perform it. Otherwise you will have to rely on a single lead rhythm strip recorded from the cardiac monitor to direct therapy. Examine the ECG for the presence of visible P waves, fusion or capture beats, and their relationship to the QRS complexes, the rate and regularity of the rhythm, and the width of the QRS complexes. If a baseline ECG is available, look for prolongation of the QT interval.

V. Plan. A discussion of definitive or long-term therapy of tachyarrhythmias is not within the scope of this book. The reader is referred to the reference edited by Horowitz for an in-depth explanation of the use of antiarrhythmic medications, radiofrequency ablative procedures, automatic implantable cardioverter defibrillators, and anti-tachycardia pacemakers. The present discussion will deal primarily with the use of medications for acute treatment of sustained tachyarrhythmias.

   A. Treat any underlying predisposing conditions. Correction of serum electrolyte imbalances is essential. Therefore, treatment with IV potassium and magnesium when appropriate may help prevent further episodes of sustained tachyarrhythmias related to these electrolyte disturbances. Administration of supplemental oxygen may be helpful in the hypoxic patient. If acute digitalis intoxication is responsible for the presence of a life-threatening recurrent tachyarrhythmia, then consider treating the patient with digoxin immune Fab fragments (Digibind). The reader is referred to the Physician's Desk Reference (PDR) for dosage information.

   B. Synchronized electrical cardioversion. If a tachyarrhythmia is responsible for causing an acute unstable episode of congestive heart failure, acute myocardial ischemia, or hemodynamic collapse, the quickest and most appropriate therapy for the termination of the tachyarrhythmia is synchronized electrical cardioversion. If the patient remains conscious during the tachycardia, then it is appropriate to administer an intravenous sedative such as midazolam (Versed) prior to electrical cardioversion. Ventricular fibrillation may result if the electrical shock is not synchronized to the R wave in cases of SVT and VT. Most supraventricular tachyarrhythmias can be terminated using 50–100 joules, and most ventricular tachyarrhythmias respond to 100–200 joules. *Caution:* Electrical cardioversion is contraindicated in cases of digitalis toxicity, and will not be helpful if used for sinus tachycardia.

   C. Carotid sinus massage. This maneuver can be very helpful in establishing the diagnosis of many supraventricular tachycardias, and can result in the termination of some tachycardias, such as AV nodal reentry tachycardia. Carotid sinus massage or other maneuvers that raise vagal tone, like Valsalva's or Mueller's maneuver, should be tried first when you are treating an episode of SVT, as long as the patient's condition will allow this. Vagal maneuvers should be repeated after each pharmacologic agent is administered until the arrhythmia stops. Carotid sinus massage should be done in a monitored setting because of the potential of inducing symptomatic bradycardia or sinus arrest in the case of hypersensitive carotid sinus syndrome.

D. Medications

1. **Adenosine (Adenocard).** The electrophysiologic effects of adenosine include a negative chronotropic action on the sinus node, and a negative dromotropic effect on the AV node. Adenosine is helpful in the management of paroxysmal supraventricular tachycardias caused by a reentry circuit involving the AV node. Adenosine has also been used to diagnose the mechanism of a particular tachycardia, and occasionally to differentiate supraventricular tachycardias with aberrant conduction from ventricular tachycardias. Adenosine (6 mg) is administered as a rapid intravenous dose. The onset of action is 10–30 sec, and its therapeutic effect lasts for only 60–90 sec. If the initial dose does not terminate the tachycardia, then a second bolus of 12 mg is given. Conduction over accessory atrioventricular pathways is not affected. The patient with unstable bronchial asthma should not receive intravenous adenosine. Patients with atrioventricular reciprocating tachycardias (Wolff-Parkinson-White syndrome) should be watched closely, as adenosine may induce atrial fibrillation which could lead to acceleration of the tachyarrhythmia and subsequent cardiac arrest. Dipyridamole, cardiac glycosides, verapamil, and benzodiazepines can potentiate the electrophysiologic effects of adenosine. Therefore, the initial dose should be reduced for patients taking these medications. Aminophylline antagonizes the actions of adenosine, and therefore higher doses may be required.

2. **Digitalis (Digoxin, Lanoxin).** Digitalis is useful in the treatment of many supraventricular tachycardias in order to control the ventricular response. It is an established drug in the treatment of atrial fibrillation or flutter. An initial dose of 0.25–0.50 mg is given IV followed by additional doses of 0.25 mg every 4–6 hr, for a total loading dose of 1.0 mg. Daily maintenance doses of 0.125–0.25 mg are required to sustain adequate serum levels with normal renal function. If digitalis alone does not adequately control the ventricular rate of a SVT, addition of a calcium channel blocker such as verapamil or diltiazem may be helpful.

3. **Verapamil (Calan).** Verapamil IV will convert approximately 90% of episodes of AV nodal reentry tachycardia to sinus rhythm. It is also helpful in the acute management of atrial flutter and fibrillation. An initial bolus of 2.5–10 mg IV is given, then start oral maintenance dose of 80–120 mg tablets Q 8 hr. Verap-

amil is not the drug of choice for patients with congestive heart failure, poor LV function, or acute myocardial infarction; it should *never* be used in the treatment of wide-complex tachyarrhythmias as it will frequently worsen the patient's condition.

4. **Diltiazem (Cardizem, Dilacor).** Diltiazem now comes in an injectable form for the acute management of new-onset atrial fibrillation or flutter, and the treatment of acute episodes of paroxysmal supraventricular tachycardia. The initial dose is 0.25 mg/kg IV administered over 2 minutes (maximum dose 20 mg), to be repeated 0.35 mg/kg in 15 minutes if needed. The patient can then be maintained on an IV infusion of 10 mg/hr, or started on oral maintenance doses of 60–90 mg given Q 6 hr. Precautions are similar to those for verapamil.

5. **Beta-blockers (propranolol, metoprolol, esmolol).** Beta-blockers are helpful in controlling a rapid heart rate in patients with sinus tachycardia, atrial flutter and fibrillation, automatic atrial tachycardia, and supraventricular tachyarrhythmias associated with digitalis intoxication. Beta-blockers should be avoided in patients with impaired left ventricular function or chronic obstructive pulmonary disease. The usual intravenous dose for propranolol (Inderal) is 1–10 mg in divided doses; for metoprolol (Lopressor), 5–15 mg in divided doses; and for esmolol (Brevibloc) 500 μg/kg over 1 minute followed by a continuous infusion of 50 μg/kg/min.

6. **Quinidine sulfate (Quinaglute, Quinidex).** The vagolytic effect of quinidine on the AV node can result in an accelerated ventricular response with atrial fibrillation or flutter. For this reason, treatment with digitalis, calcium channel blockers, or beta-blockers prior to initiating quinidine therapy is recommended.

7. **Lidocaine.** Lidocaine is the initial drug of choice for the treatment of ventricular tachyarrhythmias that are not associated with hemodynamic collapse. A loading dose of 1 mg/kg is given as an IV bolus followed by a continuous infusion of 1–4 mg/min. A second loading dose of 0.5 mg/kg is recommended to be given 5–10 minutes after the initial bolus. Lidocaine may also be helpful in arrhythmias associated with digitalis intoxication.

8. **Procainamide (Pronestyl).** Procainamide is the best drug available to convert ventricular tachyarrhythmias should Lidocaine be unsuccessful. A loading dose of 500–1000 mg is given IV at a rate of 25 mg/min, followed by a continuous infusion of 1–4 mg/min. Hypotension can develop during loading infusions if the drug is administered at rates in excess of 25 mg/min.

   Special Note: Treatment of AV reciprocating tachyarrhythmias, or Wolff-Parkinson-White syndrome, should focus on drugs that prolong the refractory period of the accessory atrioventricular pathway or of the AV node. An acute onset tachyarrhythmia suspicious for an accessory atrioventricular pathway (normal

QRS width, regular R–R interval, rate around 200 bpm, and retrograde P waves visible in ST segment) can be approached with drugs that prolong conduction in the AV node, such as adenosine, verapamil, diltiazem, beta-blockers, or with procainamide. Procainamide is the preferred drug of choice for initial management, as it will prolong the effective refractory period of the accessory bypass pathway and other involved myocardium, and has less chance of accelerating the rate of tachycardia. Procainamide's electrophysiologic properties make this drug an excellent choice for the initial pharmacologic therapy of AV reciprocating tachycardias. Digitalis may shorten the refractory period of the accessory pathway and accelerate ventricular response in some patients with AV reciprocating tachyarrhythmias.

REFERENCES

Horowitz LN ed.: *Current Management of Arrhythmias.* Decker;1991.

Marriott H: *Practical Electrocardiography.* 7th ed. Williams and Wilkins;1983.

Wellens HJJ, Bar FWH, Lie K: The value of the electrocardiogram in the differential diagnosis of tachycardia with widened QRS complex. Am J Med 1978;64:27.

Zipes DP: Specific arrhythmias: Diagnosis and treatment. In: Braunwald E ed. *Heart Disease: A Textbook of Cardiovascular Medicine.* 4th ed. Saunders;1992:667.

59. THROMBOCYTOPENIA

I. **Problem.** You are called to see a 73-year-old patient admitted to the cardiology service with unstable angina. His admission laboratory data reveals a platelet count of 32,000/μL.

II. **Immediate Questions**
   A. **Is the patient bleeding?** The risk of bleeding from trauma increases with a platelet count ≤ 50,000/μL; the risk of spontaneous bleeding increases with a platelet count < 20,000/μL.
   B. **Is there a past history of low platelet count?** Does this appear to be an acute problem such as idiopathic thrombocytopenic purpura (ITP) or is there an underlying disorder contributing to the low platelet count such as cirrhosis with hypersplenism or chronic ITP?
   C. **Is the patient on any medicines that might cause thrombocytopenia?** Drug-induced thrombocytopenia is one of the most common etiologies. A large number of drugs can cause thrombocytopenia. Quinidine and quinine together account for the largest number of cases. Other commonly associated drugs are ethanol, sulfonamides, heparin, gold, thiazide diuretics, cimetidine (Tagamet), and capoten (Captopril).

D. Is there a history of a preceding viral infection? A viral infection days to weeks before the onset of thrombocytopenia suggests a chronic form of ITP or acute interference with normal megakaryocyte maturation.

III. **Differential Diagnosis.** Quantitative platelet disorders can frequently be divided into two categories: decreased production; and peripheral destruction or sequestration.

   A. Pseudothrombocytopenia. Thrombocytopenia may be artifactual, particularly when relying on an automated counter. Platelet autoagglutinins may cause clumping in the presence of EDTA or may cause adherence to neutrophils.

   B. Decreased production

   1. **Infiltrative processes.** Acute and chronic leukemias, carcinomas, and lymphomas crowd normal marrow elements, leading to decreased numbers of megakaryocytes. Granulomatous diseases (eg, tuberculosis) occasionally cause a similar picture.

   2. **Myelodysplasia (preleukemic syndrome).** This condition frequently leads to morphologically abnormal megakaryocytes and results in low platelet levels.

   3. **Drugs.** Some known myelosuppressive drugs are particularly toxic to platelet production; for example, cytosine arabinoside (ARA-C), cyclophosphamide (Cytoxan), busulfan (Myleran), methotrexate (MTX), carboplatin (Paraplatin), and interferon. Thiazide diuretics have been associated with a decreased number of megakaryocytes leading to thrombocytopenia. Thiazides may also induce platelet-directed antibodies that can lead to peripheral destruction. Thrombocytopenia is common in chronic alcoholism. Ethanol has been shown to decrease the number of megakaryocytes.

   4. **Radiation.** Ionizing radiation can affect all marrow elements, frequently megakaryocytes to a lesser extent. Patients who have had therapeutic radiation to large areas of marrow can have transient thrombocytopenia, and recovery to preradiation levels may not occur.

   5. **Nutrition.** Malnutritional states, such as vitamin B_{12} and folate deficiency, and occasionally iron deficiency, can lead to depressed numbers of megakaryocytes.

   6. **Virus infection.** Viral illnesses such as hepatitis B, rubella, and infectious mononucleosis may cause an acute interference with normal megakaryocyte maturation.

   7. **Paroxysmal nocturnal hemoglobinuria.** Can be associated with insufficient platelet production.

   C. Peripheral destruction

   1. **Immune-mediated disorders**

      a. Idiopathic thrombocytopenic purpura (ITP). ITP is an autoimmune disorder, and a frequent cause of thrombocytopenia. The diagnosis can be made definitively if antiplatelet antibodies can be demonstrated; however, this test is not available in all clinical labs. There are two forms of ITP:

   i. **Chronic.** Usually seen in adults.
   ii. **Acute.** Most frequently seen in children; is usually self-limiting.

   b. **Drugs.** May also cause immune destruction; quinidine is the best known. In addition to exerting a toxic effect on mega-karyocytes, quinidine may act as a hapten with antibody complex adhering to the platelet, followed by complement-mediated platelet destruction.

   c. **Systemic lupus erythematosus (SLE).** Can cause autoimmune thrombocytopenia.

   d. **Human immunodeficiency virus (HIV).** An ITP-like syndrome has been associated with HIV. The thrombocytopenia is caused by an IgG antibody; platelets counts may fall below 10,000/μL. The incidence increases with the severity of the disease.

2. **Infection.** Direct platelet toxicity may occur from viruses, gram-positive organisms, or the lipopolysaccharides of gram-negative bacteria. Complement, immunoglobulins, and fibrinogen may also play a role. Disseminated intravascular coagulation (DIC), frequently caused by infection, can lead to a consumptive platelet loss. Thrombocytopenia may also be seen in the absence of DIC in septicemia, as with Rocky Mountain spotted fever and malaria.

3. **Snake bite.** Thrombocytopenia may be related to DIC or direct platelet destruction.

4. **Burns.** Thrombocytopenia may be secondary to sequestration within damaged tissue and can be further aggravated by concomitant sepsis.

5. **Glomerulonephritis.** Thrombocytopenia presumably secondary to immune-mediated mechanisms.

6. **Aortic valvular stenosis.** Occasional cause of thrombocytopenia. Presumed mechanism is direct platelet injury secondary to turbulent flow.

7. **Thrombotic thrombocytopenic purpura (TTP, Moschcowitz's syndrome).** This disease is a pentad of hemolytic anemia with a microangiopathic picture on the peripheral blood smear, thrombocytopenia, fluctuating neurologic findings, fever, and renal dysfunction.

8. **Direct toxins to platelets.** Heparin appears to cause a direct antiplatelet factor causing aggregation (Type II heparin-induced thrombocytopenia) and can induce aggregation in the absence of antibody (Type I heparin-induced thrombocytopenia). The incidence of heparin-induced thrombocytopenia is about 5%. Heparin-induced thrombocytopenia can occur with IV or SC delivery, and with bovine or porcine heparin, but is more com-

mon with bovine. This entity is infrequently associated with thromboembolism.

D. Sequestration. Normally, the spleen may contain 30% of the circulating platelet pool. When the spleen is enlarged and hypersplenism ensues, up to 90% of circulating platelets may be pooled within the spleen.

IV. Database

A. Physical examination key points.
The physical examination should be directed toward evaluation of evidence of bleeding and of peripheral sequestration.

1. **Vital signs.** Fever requires consideration of infectious causes as well as TTP.
2. **Skin and mucous membranes.** Are there petechiae or purpura? The lower extremities frequently reveal petechiae when petechiae may not be easily seen elsewhere. Multiple bruises out of proportion to the degree of trauma may give further evidence of quantitative or qualitative platelet defects. Look for gingival hyperplasia or skin nodules, which suggest leukemia.
3. **Heart.** Severe aortic stenosis can cause thrombocytopenia. A new murmur may indicate bacterial endocarditis.
4. **Abdomen.** Splenomegaly may be associated with thrombocytopenia resulting from sequestration. Chronic alcoholics may have evidence of portal hypertension such as dilated abdominal and chest wall veins, ascites, and splenomegaly. Splenomegaly is also seen with lymphoproliferative and myeloproliferative disorders, as well as infectious causes (eg, infectious mononucleosis and endocarditis). The lack of splenomegaly is also important to note. The presence of palpable splenomegaly makes ITP much less likely.
5. **Neurologic exam.** Fluctuating neurologic findings are frequently seen in TTP.

B. Laboratory data

1. **Peripheral blood smear.** Extremely important to review to rule out pseudothrombocytopenia. Pseudothrombocytopenia can be confirmed by obtaining a normal platelet count from heparin-anticoagulated blood. Large platelets (megathrombocytes) are frequently seen with ITP and may indicate peripheral destruction. Morphology of red blood cells may indicate DIC or TTP with a microangiopathic picture. Look for blasts as a sign of acute leukemia. The presence of left-shifted granulocytes, nucleated red blood cells, and tear drops may indicate marrow infiltration. Left-shifted granulocytes and toxic granulation are consistent with a bacterial infection.
2. **Coagulation studies.** Elevated prothrombin time, partial thromboplastin time, and thrombin time may be seen with DIC and liver disease. They are normal in ITP and TTP.

   3. **Antinuclear antibodies (ANA).** You need to rule out collagen vascular disease as a cause of thrombocytopenia.
   4. **BUN and creatinine.** Renal failure can cause marrow suppression of megakaryocytes and may coexist with other causes such as sepsis, DIC, and TTP.
   5. **Bone marrow** (See Section III, Chapter 5, Bone Marrow Aspiration and Biopsy, p 348). This is essential in the evaluation. The presence of megakaryocytes in adequate or increased numbers implies peripheral destruction. Marrow infiltration or primary marrow disease can be identified with a bone marrow aspirate and biopsy.
   6. **Liver function tests.** Total bilirubin, alkaline phosphatase, and transaminases (AST and ALT) may support viral hepatitis, alcoholic liver disease, or sepsis from a biliary source as the cause.
C. **Radiologic and other studies**
   1. **CT scan of the abdomen.** Demonstrates hepatosplenomegaly or lymphadenopathy in indicated situations.
   2. **Liver/spleen scan.** Demonstrates splenomegaly in questionable cases, and also indicates hepatic dysfunction and findings consistent with portal hypertension.
   3. **Platelet antibodies.** Much variability exists among the techniques for various assays. A negative antiplatelet antibody study does not rule out the presence of antiplatelet antibodies.

V. **Plan**
   A. **Bleeding.** Initially, it is important to determine if there is life-threatening bleeding, in which case platelet transfusion would be indicated. (See Section V, Blood Component Therapy, p 383.) If there is no active bleeding and the thrombocytopenia is immunologic, platelet transfusions are to be avoided. In this situation, the transfusions are frequently ineffective and may actually worsen the thrombocytopenia with further immunologic challenge.
   B. **Immune-mediated destruction.** If this is suspected, all nonessential medicines should be stopped. Do not overlook heparin flush from catheters and Hep-Locks, as well as heparin-banded central venous catheters.
   C. **Treatment of underlying cause.** Of key importance for leukemias, lymphomas, infections, and DIC.
   D. **ITP**
      1. **High-dose steroids** (1–2 mg/kg prednisone) daily is the treatment for ITP. IV immunoglobulins can also be used in steroid-unresponsive ITP or if steroids are contraindicated.
      2. **Splenectomy** may be required in chronic ITP that is unresponsive to steroids or immunoglobulins. If the platelet count is consistently > 50,000/μL, close observation may be best depending on the underlying medical condition(s).
   E. **TTP**
      1. **Plasmapheresis.** Considered standard treatment though the mechanism of action is unknown. May be related to removal of an offending agent or replacement of missing factor(s).

2. **High-dose prednisone.** Frequently used treatment; however, there is no proven benefit.

F. **Prophylactic platelet transfusion.** May be indicated for patients with myeloproliferative disorders or bone marrow suppression from myelotoxic drugs. Frequently, transfusions are given for platelet counts < 20,000/μL. Three units per meter squared, or approximately six units, should give an adequate increment in most adults. Repeated transfusion may cause alloimmunization, with resultant smaller increments after transfusion. Human leukocyte antigen-matched platelets will increase platelet survival, and are indicated in patients receiving multiple platelet transfusions who have a suboptimal response.

REFERENCES

Beutler E: Platelet transfusions: The 20,000/microliter trigger. Blood 1993;81:1411.

George JN: Thrombocytopenia due to diminished or defective platelet production. In: Beutler E, Lichtman MA, Coller BS et al eds. *William's Hematology.* 5th ed. McGraw-Hill, Inc;1995:1281.

George JN. Thrombocytopenia: Pseudothrombocytopenia, hypersplenism, and thrombocytopenia associated with massive transfusion. In: Beutler E, Lichtman MA, Coller BS et al eds. *William's Hematology.* 5th ed. McGraw-Hill, Inc; 1995:1355.

George JN, El-Harake MA: Thrombocytopenia due to enhanced platelet destruction by nonimmunologic mechanisms. In: Beutler E, Lichtman MA, Coller BS et al eds. *William's Hematology.* 5th ed. McGraw-Hill, Inc;1995:1290.

George JN, El-Harake MA, Aster RH: Thrombocytopenia due to enhanced platelet destruction by immunologic mechanisms. In: Beutler E, Lichtman MA, Coller BS et al eds. *William's Hematology.* 5th ed. McGraw-Hill, Inc;1995:1315.

60. TRANSFUSION REACTION

(See also Section V, Blood Component Therapy, p 383.)

I. **Problem.** During a transfusion of packed red blood cells (PRBCs), the patient's temperature rises to 38.5°C (101.3°F).

II. **Immediate Questions.** Fever is a common complication of transfusion and is a sign of transfusion reaction. Transfusion reactions are categorized into broad categories of non-infectious versus infectious complications and may be either mild febrile non-hemolytic transfusion reactions which are self-limited or severe life-threatening hemolytic reactions. Your initial assessment will be directed at differentiating among these.

A. **What are the patient's vital signs?** Presenting signs and symptoms of fever and chills, tachycardia, and tachypnea are nonspecific and will not allow you to differentiate reliably between a self-limited and a life-threatening transfusion reaction.

B. **Does the patient have any complaints?** Fever, frequently accompanied by shaking chills, may be the only clinical symptom of a febrile nonhemolytic transfusion reaction. However, severe acute hemolytic reactions are often accompanied by other symptoms, including nausea, vomiting, headache, and back pain. Often patients will experience bronchospasm and pulmonary edema.

C. **Is there any evidence of generalized bleeding from mucosal membranes, previous venipuncture sites, or the present IV site?** Diffuse bleeding would be consistent with disseminated intravascular coagulation (DIC); it suggests a severe, life-threatening hemolytic reaction.

D. **Has the patient ever been transfused before? If so, has she or he ever reacted to blood products in the past?** Patients who have prior histories of a transfusion are likely to have become alloimmunized to blood group antigens. Patients with a prior history of febrile reactions to transfusion likely have cytotoxic or agglutinating antibodies to HLA antigens present on granulocytes, lymphocytes, and platelets. Although these reactions are troublesome, they are typically self-limited.

E. **Most importantly, does the name on the unit of packed cells match that on the patient's armband?** The majority of fatal acute hemolytic transfusion reactions result from transfusion of ABO incompatible blood. This is frequently the result of human error in patient or specimen identification occurring during situations of high stress.

III. Differential Diagnosis

A. Hemolytic transfusion reaction

1. **Severe sequelae** from a hemolytic transfusion reaction may occur even when a small volume of incompatible blood is transfused. If there is concern that a patient may be experiencing a severe reaction, the transfusion must be stopped immediately. If the label on the transfusion unit of blood does not match that on the patient's arm band, the blood bank should be notified immediately for assistance.

2. **Transfusion of ABO-incompatible blood** results in intravascular hemolysis. The naturally occurring anti-A or anti-B antibodies activate the classical complement pathway resulting in membrane lysis and a liberation of free hemoglobin within the blood stream. Fever, hypotension, shock, and renal failure may result.

B. Self-limiting febrile transfusion reaction. This reaction is not hemolytic. It often occurs in patients who have had numerous transfusions or in multiparous women. While this type of reaction often results in interruption of the transfusion, if no further symptoms develop the transfusion may be restarted.

C. **Transfusion of blood contaminated with microorganisms.** This is an infrequent transfusion reaction. Blood contaminated by cold-growing organisms such as *Pseudomonas* should be considered.

D. **Delayed hemolytic reaction.** Should be suspected if a post-transfusion hemoglobin level cannot be maintained several days after the transfusion. Mild jaundice and fever with or without chills should alert the clinician to the possibility of a delayed hemolytic transfusion reaction. Many of these reactions are not detected because patients have been discharged from the hospital. The serologic findings of a delayed hemolytic transfusion reaction include a positive direct Coombs' test. The previously alloimmunized patient may not have had detectable antibody levels in their routine pre-transfusion antibody screening study. However, after reexposure to the relevant antigen, an amnestic response to the transfused RBCs occurs. IgG antibody alone or IgG with complement may then be detected. A single antibody or multiple antibodies may be involved. The antibodies most often implicated are directed against Rh, Kidd, Duffy, or Kell antigens. Because the antibody titer may again drop to undetectable levels a chart notation or medical alert card may prevent future reactions in patients with known antibodies. Delayed hemolytic transfusion reactions are generally regarded as mild.

IV. **Database**

A. **Physical examination key points**

1. **Vital signs.** If the constellation of hypotension, fever, and tachycardia is present the transfusion reaction must be considered to be a severe hemolytic reaction.

2. **Skin and mucous membranes.** Generalized bleeding may be part of a severe hemolytic reaction.

3. **Chest.** Wheezing or rales are consistent with a life-threatening reaction.

B. **Laboratory data**

1. **Hemogram.** This may point to contaminated blood or show evidence of hemolysis.

2. **Prothrombin time, partial thromboplastin time, thrombin time, fibrinogen, and fibrin split products.** To rule out DIC.

3. **Peripheral smear.** Look for schistocytes as evidence for DIC.

4. **Urine for hemoglobinuria.** If present, it supports the diagnosis of a severe transfusion reaction.

5. **Serum for free hemoglobin.** If positive, indicates hemolysis.

6. **Post-transfusion direct antiglobulin testing.** A negative study in the absence of serum-free hemoglobin is good evidence that an acute hemolytic transfusion has not occurred.

7. **Gram's stain of remaining untransfused blood.** To rule out bacterial contamination of the unit.

V. Plan. The treatment plan depends on the type of reaction.
   A. Severe hemolytic reaction
      1. If a serious transfusion reaction is suspected, the transfusion should be stopped immediately.
      2. **Supportive care** including IV fluids. The patient should be closely monitored for hypotension and decreasing urine output. If oliguria occurs diuretics and mannitol may be required. A renal dose of dopamine (5 mg/kg/min) may be considered as well. If physical signs and laboratory findings indicate DIC, administration of platelets and cryoprecipitate are recommended.
   B. Self-limiting febrile transfusion reactions. The findings of isolated fever and chills in a patient with a previous history of a febrile reaction support the diagnosis of the self-limited febrile transfusion reaction. Antihistamines and antipruritics may be administered. Demerol may be used for patients experiencing severe shaking chills. After premedication, transfusion may be safely resumed. Steps to prevent this type of reaction in the future include decreasing the granulocytes in the transfused unit. Leukofiltration and premedication are indicated for future transfusions.
   C. Transfusion of blood contaminated with microorganisms. Broad-spectrum antibiotics should be instituted if suspected.

REFERENCES

Andreu G, Dewailly J, Leberre C et al: Prevention of HLA immunization with leukocyte-poor packed red cells and platelet concentrates obtained by filtration. Blood 1988;72:964.

Brittingham TE, Chaplin H Jr: Febrile transfusion reaction caused sensitivity to donor leukocytes and platelets. JAMA 1957;165:819.

Brubaker DB: Clinical significance of white cell antibodies in febrile nonhemolytic transfusion reactions. Transfusion 1990;30:733.

Jeter EK, Spivey MA: Noninfectious complications of blood transfusion. Hematol Oncol Clin North Am 1995;9:187.

Sazama K: Reports of 355 transfusion associated deaths: 1976–1985. Transfusion 1990;30:583.

61. WHEEZING

I. Problem. You are cross-covering a patient recently admitted with chest pain who develops respiratory distress and wheezing.

II. Immediate Questions
   A. What are the vital signs? A respiratory rate greater than 30/min may indicate the need for immediate treatment. Associated hypotension may suggest an anaphylactic reaction, an acute myocardial infarction (MI) with pulmonary edema, or a pulmonary em-

bolism. Fever may point to an underlying infection or new pulmonary embolism.

B. Were any diagnostic tests recently performed or medicines administered? A beta-blocker may precipitate an acute attack of bronchospasm when given to a stable or undiagnosed asthmatic. Wheezing after the administration of a drug such as penicillin or radiocontrast dye suggests an anaphylactic reaction.

C. Why was the patient admitted? A patient admitted to rule out MI may have developed acute pulmonary edema. A patient with a gastric ulcer may have gastric outlet obstruction and have aspirated.

D. Is there a history of asthma? Childhood asthma may reactivate at any age, given the right stimuli.

E. Does the patient have any allergies to medications or other substances such as shellfish? It is prudent to inquire about known allergies.

III. Differential Diagnosis

A. Diffuse wheezing

1. **Acute bronchospasm.** May be caused by asthma, exacerbation of chronic obstructive pulmonary disease (COPD), or an anaphylactic reaction.
2. **Aspiration.** May trigger bronchospasm from mucosal irritation or from impacted foreign bodies.
3. **Cardiogenic pulmonary edema.** The primary finding in "cardiac asthma" may be wheezing. Other findings of pulmonary edema should be present, and the chest x-ray will be diagnostic.
4. **Pulmonary embolism (PE).** Mediators may be released that cause not only hypoxemia but also transient bronchospasm.

B. Stridor (upper airway wheezing)

1. **Laryngospasm.** This may be part of an anaphylactic reaction or secondary to aspiration.
2. **Laryngeal or tracheal tumor.** A history of dysphagia, hoarseness, cough, or weight loss and anorexia may be present.
3. **Epiglottitis.** The patient is often unable to speak or to swallow secretions.
4. **Foreign body aspiration**
5. **Vocal cord dysfunction.** Bilaterally paralyzed vocal cords may result in severe stridor and dyspnea. A subgroup of patients has recently been recognized to have "factitious asthma": they voluntarily adduct their vocal cords for psychogenic reasons.

C. Localized wheezing

1. **Tumors.** May obstruct one bronchus, leading to localized wheezing.
2. **Mucous plugging**
3. **Aspirated foreign body**

IV. Database

A. Physical examination key points. Localization of wheezing allows categorization, as outlined in the differential diagnosis.

    1. Vital signs. A fever may indicate an infectious etiology. A pulsus paradoxus greater than 20 mm Hg indicates severe respiratory distress. Hypotension requires immediate assessment and action.

    2. HEENT. Check the mouth carefully. Examine the neck for angioneurotic edema. Palpate the sternocleidomastoid muscles for accessory muscle use. Auscultate over the mouth and larynx in an effort to localize the wheezing.

    3. Chest. Carefully auscultate for localized wheezing. Listen for bibasilar rales, which may be present in pulmonary edema. Rales, increased fremitus, and egophony suggest pneumonia.

    4. Heart. Check carefully for evidence of an S_3 gallop or jugular venous distension, which points to cardiogenic pulmonary edema.

    5. Extremities. Clubbing may indicate underlying lung cancer. Cyanosis indicates underlying hypoxemia. Edema may signify chronic congestive heart failure.

    6. Skin. Urticaria probably indicates an acute allergic reaction. A malar rash points toward acute systemic lupus erythematosus, which can present with acute pneumonitis.

B. Laboratory data

    1. Arterial blood gases. An elevated $PaCO_2$ indicates significant ventilatory failure. Hypoxemia is commonly present during bronchospasm because of $\dot{V}/\dot{Q}$ mismatch. It may worsen after beta-agonist aerosols.

    2. Complete blood count. An increased white blood cell count may indicate an underlying infection; however, an increase in WBCs without a left shift can be seen with an acute MI or PE. Eosinophilia suggests an allergic or asthmatic etiology to the wheezing.

C. Radiologic and other studies

    1. Electrocardiogram. An ECG may show an acute MI or ischemia. Occasionally it will be suggestive of a PE, showing an S wave in lead I, a Q wave in III, T wave inversion in lead III ($S_1Q_3T_3$), new right bundle branch block (RBBB), and right-axis shift. It may also show a change in rhythm.

    2. Chest radiograph. A PE (with infarction) severe enough to cause wheezing may be evident on the chest film. Look for a pleural-based, wedge-shaped lesion (Hampton's hump) or localized oligemia of the pulmonary arteries. Kerley B lines, bilateral pleural effusions, vascular redistribution, and cardiomegaly may suggest congestive heart failure. Look for localized infiltrates or masses suggesting other causes.

V. Plan. Treatment depends on the diagnosis. The preceding differential diagnoses and studies should enable you to form a tentative categorization on which to base initial therapy.

   A. Bronchospasm (asthma, COPD, allergic reaction)
      1. Methylprednisolone (Solu-Medrol) 200 mg IV stat dose.
      2. Nebulized albuterol (Ventolin) 0.5 mL (2.5 mg) or metaproterenol (Alupent) 0.3 mL of 5% solution in 3.0 mL normal saline stat and then every 2–4 hours.

   B. Stridor
      1. Methylprednisolone 200 mg IV stat dose.
      2. Nebulized racemic epinephrine (Micronephrine) 0.5 mL in 3 mL normal saline.
      3. Continuous positive airway pressure (CPAP), 10–15 cm H_2O applied continuously.
      4. Consider intubation or tracheostomy if there is no response to the above measures.

   C. Pulmonary edema
      1. Furosemide (Lasix) 20–80 mg IV.
      2. Nitroglycerin 0.4 mg sublingually, or paste 1/2 in. on skin, or nitroglycerin drip 10–20 mg/min and increase by 5–10 mg every 10 minutes.
      3. Afterload reduction with agents such as intravenous nitroprusside (Nipride), or oral agents such as captopril (Capoten) or enalapril (Vasotec), or any other angiotensin-converting enzyme (ACE) inhibitor.
      4. Intravenous morphine for venodilation and to relieve anxiety. Be prepared to intubate the patient.
      5. Oxygen. Start with 100% O_2 by non-rebreather mask, as long as the patient is not a carbon dioxide (CO_2) retainer.

   D. Miscellaneous disorders. Treatment varies with the disease. Obviously, PE should be treated with anticoagulants. Suspected tumors require additional tests such as bronchoscopy before reasonable treatment can be initiated.

REFERENCES

Aboussouan LS, Stoller JK: Diagnosis and management of upper airway obstruction. Clin Chest Med 1994;15:35.
Leatherman J: Life-threatening asthma. Clin Chest Med 1994;15:453.

II. Laboratory Diagnosis

Notes: The ranges of normal values are given below each test, first in conventional units such as metric (eg, milligrams per liter), and then in international units if there is a difference. Reference ranges for each laboratory may vary from the values given; therefore, you should interpret the results of a patient's laboratory value in light of an individual facility's range.

■ ACTH (ADRENOCORTICOTROPIC HORMONE)
8 am: 20–100 pg/mL or 20–100 ng/L; midnight value: ~50% of am value.
Increased: Addison's disease; ectopic ACTH production (small cell carcinoma, pancreatic islet cell tumors, thymic tumors, renal cell carcinoma).
Decreased: Adrenal adenoma or carcinoma, nodular adrenal hyperplasia, pituitary insufficiency.

■ ACTH STIMULATION TEST
Used to help diagnose adrenal insufficiency. Cosyntropin (Cortrosyn), an ACTH analogue, is given at a dose of 0.25 mg IM or IV. Collect blood at times 0, 30, and 60 minutes for cortisol.
Normal response: Basal cortisol of at least 5 µg/dL, an increase of at least 7 µg/dL, and a final cortisol of 16 µg/dL at 30 minutes or 18 µg/dL at 60 minutes.
Addison's disease (primary adrenal insufficiency) and secondary adrenal insufficiency: Secondary insufficiency is caused by pituitary insufficiency or suppression by exogenous steroids. An ACTH level and pituitary stimulation tests can be used to differentiate primary from secondary adrenal insufficiency.

■ ACID-FAST STAIN
Positive: *Mycobacterium* species (tuberculosis and atypical mycobacteria such as *M avium-intracellulare*), *Nocardia*.

■ ACID PHOSPHATASE
< 3.0 g/mL or 0.11–0.60 U/L.
Radioimmunoassay determination usually specific for the prostate.
Increased: Carcinoma of the prostate (usually metastatic), prostatic surgery or trauma, excessive platelet destruction (immune thrombocytopenic purpura), rarely in bone disease.

■ ALBUMIN, SERUM
3.5–5.0 g/dL or 35–50 g/L.

Decreased: Malnutrition, nephrotic syndrome, cystic fibrosis, multiple myeloma, Hodgkin's disease, leukemia, protein-losing enteropathies, chronic glomerulonephritis, cirrhosis, inflammatory bowel disease, collagen-vascular diseases, hyperthyroidism.

■ ALBUMIN, URINE

Normal < 30 mg/d.

Microalbuminuria 30–200 mg/d (a sign of early renal damage in diabetes mellitus; presence helps identify patients at risk for renal failure, neuropathy, retinopathy and coronary artery disease. Renal function may be preserved with the use of an angiotensin-converting enzyme [ACE] inhibitor).

Note: Microalbuminuria can be seen with prolonged exercise, hematuria, fever or prolonged upright posture.

Nephrotic proteinuria > 3.5 gm/d.

■ ALDOSTERONE

Serum—supine: 3–10 g/dL or 0.083–0.28 nmol/L early am, normal sodium intake; upright: 5–30 g/dL or 0.138–0.83 nmol/L.

Urinary—2–16 µg/24 h or 5.4–44.3 nmol/d.

Increased: Hyperaldosteronism (primary or secondary). Should confirm after oral or IV salt loading.

Decreased: Adrenal insufficiency.

■ ALKALINE PHOSPHATASE

Adult 20–70 U/L.

A γ-glutamyltransferase (GGT) is often useful to differentiate whether an elevated alkaline phosphatase has its origin from bone or liver. A normal GGT suggests bone origin.

Increased: Increased calcium deposition in bone (hyperparathyroidism), Paget's disease, osteoblastic bone tumors, osteomalacia, pregnancy, childhood, liver disease, and hyperthyroidism.

Decreased: Malnutrition, excess vitamin D ingestion.

■ ALPHA-FETOPROTEIN (AFP)

< 30 ng/mL or < 30 µg/L

Increased: Hepatoma, testicular tumor (embryonal carcinoma, malignant teratoma), spina bifida (in mother's serum).

■ ALT (ALANINE AMINOTRANSAMINASE) (SGPT: SERUM GLUTAMIC-PYRUVIC TRANSAMINASE)

8–20 U/L.

Increased: Liver disease–liver metastasis, biliary obstruction, liver congestion, hepatitis (ALT is more elevated than AST in viral hepatitis; AST is more elevated than ALT in alcoholic hepatitis).

■ AMMONIA
Arterial: 15–45 µg/dL or 11–32 µmol N/L.
Increased: Hepatic encephalopathy, Reye's syndrome.

■ AMYLASE
25–125 U/L.
Increased: Acute pancreatitis, pancreatic duct obstruction (stones, stricture, tumor, sphincter spasm secondary to drugs), alcohol ingestion, mumps, parotiditis, renal disease, macroamylasemia, cholecystitis, peptic ulcers, intestinal obstruction, mesenteric thrombosis, after surgery (upper abdominal), ovarian cancer, ruptured ectopic pregnancy, and diabetic ketoacidosis.
Decreased: Pancreatic destruction (pancreatitis, cystic fibrosis), liver disease (hepatitis, cirrhosis).

■ ANION GAP
8–12 mmol/L.
Note: The anion gap is a calculated estimate of unmeasured anions and is used to help differentiate the cause of metabolic acidosis.

$$\text{Anion gap} = (Na^+) - (Cl^- + HCO_3)$$

Increased (High): (> 12 mmol/L): Lactic acidosis, ketoacidosis (diabetic, alcoholic, starvation); uremia; toxins (salicylates, methanol, ethylene glycol, paraldehyde). In addition, dehydration, alkalosis, use of certain penicillins (carbenicillin), and salts of strong acids such as sodium citrate (used as a preservative in packed red cells) can cause a mild increase in the anion gap.
Decreased (Low): (< 8 mmol/L): Seen with bromide ingestion, hypercalcemia, hypermagnesemia, multiple myeloma, and hypoalbuminemia.

■ ANTICARDIOLIPIN ANTIBODIES
See Antiphospholipid Antibodies.

■ ANTI-NEUTROPHIL CYTOPLASMIC ANTIBODIES (ANCAs)
Negative = < 10 EV/mL.
Equivocal = 10–20 EV/mL.
Positive = > 20 EV/mL.

Antibodies to cytoplasmic components of neutrophils, seen in vasculitides. Two types:

1. **C-ANCA (Cytoplasmic-staining ANCA).** Present in ~90% of patients with generalized Wegener's granulomatosis; also seen in rapidly progressive glomerulonephritis and a type of polyarteritis nodosa (microscopic). May be used to follow disease activity; also especially useful in distinguishing active disease from an infectious complication. C-ANCA is not present in other collagen vascular diseases.

2. **P-ANCA (Perinuclear-staining ANCA).** Seen in a variety of collagen vascular diseases such as limited Wegener's granulomatosis, polyarteritis nodosa, Goodpasture's syndrome, and other vasculitides; and also seen in several types of glomerulonephritides.

■ ANTINUCLEAR ANTIBODIES (ANA)

Negative: A useful screening test in patients with symptoms suggesting collagen-vascular disease, especially if titer is $\geq$ 1:160.

Positive: Systemic lupus erythematosus (SLE), drug-induced lupus (procainamide, hydralazine, isoniazid, etc.), scleroderma, mixed connective tissue disease (MCTD), rheumatoid arthritis, polymyositis, juvenile rheumatoid arthritis (JRA) (5–20%). Low titers are also seen in non-collagen-vascular disease.

Specific Immunofluorescent ANA Patterns

1. ANA Patterns

- **Homogenous:** Nonspecific, from antibodies to deoxyribonucleoproteins (DNP) and native double-stranded deoxyribonucleic acid (DNA). Seen in SLE and a variety of other diseases. Antihistone is consistent with drug-induced lupus.
- **Speckled:** Pattern seen in many connective tissue disorders. From antibodies to extractable nuclear antigens (ENA) including antiribonucleoproteins (anti-RNP), anti-Sm, anti-PM-1, and anti-SS. Anti-RNP is positive in MCTD and SLE. Anti-Sm is found in SLE. Anti-SS-A and anti-SS-B are seen in Sjögren's syndrome and subacute cutaneous lupus. The speckled pattern is also seen with scleroderma.
- **Peripheral RIM Pattern:** From antibodies to native double-stranded DNA and DNP. Seen in SLE.
- **Nucleolar Pattern:** From antibodies to nucleolar ribonucleic acid (RNA). Positive in Sjögren's syndrome and scleroderma.

2. Other Autoantibodies

- **Antimitochondrial:** Primary biliary cirrhosis.
- **Anti-Smooth Muscle:** Low titers are seen in a variety of illnesses; high titers ($>$ 1:100) are suggestive of chronic active hepatitis.
- **Antimicrosomal:** Hashimoto's thyroiditis.

■ ANTIPHOSPHOLIPID ANTIBODIES

Note: There are two basic categories of antiphospholipid antibody—anticardiolipin and lupus anticoagulant. Both are associated with recurrent arterial or venous thrombosis or fetal demise.

Anticardiolipin antibody. Two forms: IgG, IgM.

IgG normal $< 23u$.

IgM normal $< 11u$.

Lupus anticoagulant

Negative $=$ normal.

Positive $=$ presence.

Should be suspected with an isolated elevated partial thromboplastin time (PTT) with no other likely cause.

■ AST (ASPARTATE AMINOTRANSAMINASE) (SGOT: SERUM GLUTAMIC-OXALOACETIC TRANSAMINASE)

8–20 U/L.

Generally parallels changes in ALT in liver disease.

Increased: Liver disease, acute myocardial infarction, Reye's syndrome, muscle trauma and injection, pancreatitis, intestinal injury or surgery, factitious increase (erythromycin, opiates), burns, brain damage.

Decreased: Beri-beri, severe diabetes with ketoacidosis, liver disease.

■ B₁₂ (VITAMIN B₁₂)

140–700 pg/mL or 189–516 pmol/L.

Increased: Leukemia, polycythemia vera.

Decreased: Pernicious anemia, bacterial overgrowth, dietary deficiency (rare—humans normally have 2–3 years of stores), malabsorption, pregnancy.

■ BASE EXCESS/DEFICIT

See Table 2–1, p 306. A decrease in base (bicarbonate) is termed **base deficit**; an increase in base is termed **base excess**.

Excess: Metabolic alkalosis (see Section I, Chapter 3, Alkalosis, p 17), respiratory acidosis (see Section I, Chapter 2, Acidosis, p 9).

Deficit: Metabolic acidosis (see Section I, Chapter 2, Acidosis, p 9), respiratory alkalosis (see Section I, Chapter 3, Alkalosis, p 17).

■ BENCE JONES PROTEINS—URINE

Negative: Normal.

Positive: Multiple myeloma, idiopathic Bence Jones proteinuria.

TABLE 2–1. NORMAL BLOOD GAS VALUES.[1]

Measurement	Arterial	Mixed Venous[2]	Venous
pH	7.40	7.36	7.36
(range)	(7.36–7.44)	(7.31–7.41)	(7.31–7.41)
pO_2 (decreases with age)	80–100 mm Hg	35–40 mm Hg	30–50 mm Hg
pCO_2	36–44 mm Hg	41–51 mm Hg	40–52 mm Hg
O_2 saturation (decreases with age)	>95%	60–80%	60–85%
HCO_3^-	22–26 mmol/L	22–26 mmol/L	22–29 mmol/L
Base difference (deficit/excess)	−2 to +2	−2 to +2	−2 to +2

[1] Modified and reproduced with permission from Gomella LG, ed: *Clinician's Pocket Reference.* 7th ed. Appleton & Lange; 1993.
[2] From right atrium.

■ BICARBONATE (SERUM HCO_3^-)

22–29 mmol/L.

See Tables 2–1 and 2–2. Also see Carbon Dioxide, Arterial, for pCO_2 values.

Increased: Metabolic alkalosis, compensation for respiratory acidosis. See Section I, Chapter 2, Acidosis, p 9; and Section I, Chapter 3, Alkalosis, p 17.

Decreased: Metabolic acidosis, compensation for respiratory alkalosis. See Section I, Chapter 2, Acidosis, p 9; and Section I, Chapter 3, Alkalosis, p 17.

■ BILIRUBIN

Total: < 0.2–1.0 mg/dL or 3.4–17.1 µmol/L;
Direct: < 0.2 mg/dL or < 3.4 µmol/L;

TABLE 2–2. ACID BASE DISORDERS WITH APPROPRIATE COMPENSATION.

Disorder	Changes in Normal Values		
	pH	HCO_3^-	pCO_2
Metabolic acidosis	↓	↓↓	↓
Metabolic alkalosis	↑	↑↑	↑
Acute respiratory acidosis	↓	slight↑	↑↑
Chronic respiratory acidosis	slight↓	↑	↑↑
Acute respiratory alkalosis	↑	slight↓	↓↓
Chronic respiratory alkalosis	slight↑	↓	↓↓

Indirect: < 0.8 mg/dL or < 13.7 µmol/L.

Increased Total: Hepatic damage (hepatitis, toxins, cirrhosis), biliary obstruction (gallstone or tumor), hemolysis, fasting.

Increased Direct (Conjugated): Biliary obstruction (gallstone, tumor, stricture), drug-induced cholestasis, Dubin-Johnson syndrome, and Rotor's syndrome.

Increased Indirect (Unconjugated): Hemolytic anemia (transfusion reaction, sickle cell, collagen-vascular disease), Gilbert's disease, Crigler-Najjar syndrome.

■ BLEEDING TIME
Duke, Ivy: < 6 min; Template: < 10 min.

Increased: Thrombocytopenia, thrombocytopenic purpura, von Willebrand's disease, defective platelet function (aspirin, nonsteroidal anti-inflammatory drugs, uremia).

■ BLOOD GAS, ARTERIAL
See Tables 2–1 and 2–2, p 306. For acid-base disorders, see Section I, Chapter 2, Acidosis, p 9; and Chapter 3, Alkalosis, p 17.

■ BLOOD GAS, VENOUS
See Table 2–1, p 306. **Note:** There is little difference between arterial and venous pH and bicarbonate (except with congestive heart failure and shock); therefore, the venous blood gas may be occasionally used to assess acid-base status, but venous oxygen levels are significantly lower than arterial levels.

■ BLOOD UREA NITROGEN (BUN)
7–18 mg/dL or 1.2–3.0 mmol urea/L.

Increased: Renal failure, prerenal azotemia (decreased renal perfusion secondary to congestive heart failure, shock, volume depletion), postrenal obstruction, gastrointestinal bleeding, hypercatabolic states.

Decreased: Starvation, liver failure (hepatitis, drugs), pregnancy, infancy, nephrotic syndrome, overhydration.

■ CBC (COMPLETE BLOOD COUNT, HEMOGRAM)
Note: For normal values, see Table 2–3, p 308. For differential, see specific tests.

■ C-PEPTIDE
Fasting: ≤ 4.0 g/mL or ≤ 4.0 µg/L;

male > 60 years: 1.5–5.0 g/mL or 1.5–5.0 µg/L;
female: 1.4–5.5 g/mL or 1.4–5.5 µg/L.

Decreased: Diabetes (insulin-dependent diabetes mellitus), insulin administration, hypoglycemia.

Increased: Insulinoma. Test is useful to differentiate insulinoma from surreptitious use of insulin as a cause of hypoglycemia.

TABLE 2–3. NORMAL CBC VALUES—ADULTS.[1]

WBC	4800–10,800 cells/µL
RBCs	M: 4.7–6.1 × 10^6 cells/µL
	F: 4.2–5.4 × 10^6 cells/µL
Hemoglobin	M: 14–18 g/dL
	F: 12–16 g/dL
Hematocrit	M: 40–54%
	F: 37–47%
MCV	M: 80–94 fL
	F: 81–99 fL
MCH	27–31 pg
MCHC (%)	33–37%
RDW	11.5–14.5
Platelets	150,000–450,000/µL
■ **Differential**	
Segmented neutrophils	41–71%
Banded (stab) neutrophils	5–10%
Lymphocytes	24–44%
Monocytes	3–7%
Eosinophils	1–3%
Basophils	0–1%

[1] Refer to hospital reference values. Modified and reproduced with permission from Gomella LG, ed: *Clinician's Pocket Reference.* 7th ed. Appleton & Lange; 1993.

■ C-REACTIVE PROTEIN (CRP)

Normal: < 8 mg/L.

An acute phase reactant with a relatively short half-life.

Increased: In infections (increase in bacterial infections > increase in viral infections); tissue injury or necrosis (acute myocardial infarction, malignant disease [especially lung, breast, and gastrointestinal] and organ rejection following transplantation); and inflammatory disorders (rheumatoid arthritis, systemic lupus erythematosus, inflammatory bowel disease, and vasculitides).

■ CALCITONIN

< 100 pg/mL or < 100 g/L.

Increased: Medullary carcinoma of the thyroid, pregnancy, chronic renal insufficiency, Zollinger-Ellison syndrome, pernicious anemia.

■ CALCIUM, SERUM

8.4–10.2 mg/dL (4.2–5.1 mEq/L) or 2.10–2.55 mmol/L;
Ionized: 4.5–4.9 mg/dL (2.2–2.5 mEq/L) or 1.1–1.2 mmol/L.

Note: When interpreting a total calcium value, the albumin must be known. If the albumin is not within normal limits, a corrected calcium can be roughly calculated with the following formula. Values for ionized calcium need no special correction.

$$\text{Corrected total Ca} = 0.8\,(\text{normal albumin} - \text{measured albumin}) + \text{reported Ca}$$

Increased: See Section I, Chapter 30, Hypercalcemia, p 156.
Decreased: See Section I, Chapter 35, Hypocalcemia, p 178.

■ CALCIUM, URINE

Calcium-free diet: < 540 mg or 0.13–1.00 mmol per 24-hour urine; Average calcium diet: 100–300 mg per 24-hour urine

Increased: Hyperparathyroidism, hyperthyroidism, hypervitaminosis D, distal renal tubular acidosis (type I), sarcoidosis, immobilization, osteolytic lesions (bony metastasis, multiple myeloma), Paget's disease, glucocorticoid excess (either endogenous or exogenous), furosemide.

Decreased: Thiazide diuretics, hypothyroidism, renal failure, steatorrhea, rickets, osteomalacia.

■ CARBON DIOXIDE, ARTERIAL (PCO_2)

36–44 mm Hg. See Tables 2–1 and 2–2, p 306.

Increased: Respiratory acidosis, compensation for metabolic alkalosis. See Section I, Chapter 2, Acidosis, p 9; and Chapter 3, Alkalosis, p 17.

Decreased: Respiratory alkalosis, compensation for metabolic acidosis. See Section I, Chapter 2, Acidosis, p 9; and Chapter 3, Alkalosis, p 17.

■ CARBOXYHEMOGLOBIN

Nonsmoker: < 2%;
Smoker: < 6%;
Toxic: > 15%.

Increased: In smokers; cases of smoke inhalation; persons exposed to automobile exhaust inhalation or inadequate ventilation with faulty heating units.

■ CARCINOEMBRYONIC ANTIGEN (CEA)

Nonsmoker: < 3.0 g/mL or < 3.0 µg/L;
Smoker: < 5.0 g/mL or < 5.0 µg/L.

Increased: Carcinoma (colon, pancreas, lung, stomach), smokers, nonneoplastic liver disease, Crohn's disease, and ulcerative colitis. Test used predominantly to monitor patients for recurrence of carcinoma, especially status post resection for colon carcinoma.

■ CATECHOLAMINES, FRACTIONATED

Note: Values are variable and depend on the lab and method of assay used. Normal levels listed in Table 2–4 are based on high-performance liquid chromatography technique.

Increased: Pheochromocytoma, neural crest tumors (neuroblastoma). In extra-adrenal pheochromocytoma, norepinephrine may be markedly elevated compared with epinephrine.

TABLE 2–4. FRACTIONATED CATECHOLAMINES.

Catecholamine	Plasma (Supine)	Urine
Norepinephrine	70–750 pg/mL 414–4435 pmol/L	14–80 µg/24-hr 82.7–473 nmol/d
Epinephrine	0–100 pg/mL 0–546 pmol/L	0.5–20 µg/24-hr 2.73–109 nmol/d
Dopamine	<30 pg/ml <196 pmol/L	65–400 µg/24-hr 424–2612 nmol/d

■ CATECHOLAMINES, URINE, UNCONJUGATED

> 15 years old: < 100 µg/24 h.

Measures free (unconjugated) epinephrine, norepinephrine, and dopamine.

Increased: Pheochromocytoma, neural crest tumors (neuroblastoma).

■ CHLORIDE, SERUM

98–106 mEq/L

Increased: Metabolic non-gap acidosis such as diarrhea, renal tubular acidosis, mineralocorticoid deficiency, hyperalimentation, medications (acetazolamide, ammonium chloride).

Decreased: Vomiting, diabetes mellitus with ketoacidosis, mineralocorticoid excess, renal disease with sodium loss.

■ CHLORIDE, URINE

110–250 mmol per 24-hour urine
See Urinary Electrolytes.

■ CHOLESTEROL (TOTAL)
140–240 mg/dL or 3.63–6.22 mmol/L;
Desired level: < 200 mg/dL or 5.18 mmol/L.
Increased: Primary hypercholesterolemia (types IIA, IIB, III), elevated triglycerides (types I, IV, V), biliary obstruction, nephrosis, hypothyroidism, diabetes, pregnancy.
Decreased: Liver disease (eg, hepatitis), hyperthyroidism, malnutrition (cancer, starvation), chronic anemias, steroid therapy, lipoproteinemias.

High-Density Lipoprotein (HDL) Cholesterol
Fasting male: 30–70 mg/dL or 0.78–1.81 mmol/L;
female: 30–80 mg/dL or 0.78–2.07 mmol/L.
Note: HDL has the best correlation with the development of coronary artery disease; decreased HDL in males leads to an increased risk.
Increased: Estrogen (females), exercise, ethanol.
Decreased: Males, uremia, obesity, diabetes, liver disease, Tangier's disease.

Low-Density Lipoprotein (LDH) Cholesterol
Desired: < 130–160 mg/dL or 3.36–4.14 mmol/L.
Increased: Excess dietary saturated fats, myocardial infarction, hyperlipoproteinemia, biliary cirrhosis, endocrine disease (diabetes, hypothyroidism).
Decreased: Malabsorption, severe liver disease, abetalipoproteinemia.

Triglycerides
See **TRIGLYCERIDES,** p 334.

■ COLD AGGLUTININS
< 1:32: Normal.
Increased: *Mycoplasma* pneumonia; viral infections (especially mononucleosis, measles, mumps); cirrhosis; some parasitic infections.

■ COMPLEMENT C3
80–155 mg/dL or 800–1550 ng/L;
> 60 years: 80–170 mg/dL or 80–1700 ng/L.
Note: Normal values may vary greatly depending on the assay used.
Increased: Rheumatic fever, various neoplasms (gastrointestinal, prostate, others).
Decreased: Systemic lupus erythematosus, glomerulonephritis (poststreptococcal and membranoproliferative), vasculitis, severe hepatic failure.
Variable: Rheumatoid arthritis.

■ COMPLEMENT C4

20–50 mg/dL or 200–500 ng/L.

Increased: Neoplasia (gastrointestinal, lung, others).

Decreased: Systemic lupus erythematosus, chronic active hepatitis, cirrhosis, glomerulonephritis, hereditary angioedema.

Variable: Rheumatoid arthritis.

■ COMPLEMENT CH50 (TOTAL)

33–61 mg/mL or 330–610 ng/L. Tests for complement deficiency in the classical pathway.

Increased: Acute-phase reactants (eg, tissue injury, infections).

Decreased: Hereditary complement deficiencies, any cause of deficiency of individual complement components. See Complement C3 and Complement C4.

■ COOMBS' TEST, DIRECT

Uses patient's erythrocytes; tests for the presence of antibody or complement on the patient's red blood cells.

Positive: Autoimmune hemolytic anemia (leukemia, lymphoma, collagen-vascular diseases, [systemic lupus erythematosus]); hemolytic transfusion reaction; sensitization to some drugs (methyldopa, levodopa, penicillins, cephalosporins).

■ COOMBS' TEST, INDIRECT

More useful for red cell typing. Uses serum that contains antibody from the patient.

Positive: Isoimmunization from previous transfusion, incompatible blood as a result of improper cross-matching.

■ CORTISOL

Serum—8 am: 5.0–23.0 µg/dL or 138–635 nmol/L; 4 pm: 3.0–15.0 µg/dL or 83–414 nmol/L.

Urine (24 hour)—10–100 µg/d or 27.6–276 nmol/d.

Increased: Adrenal adenoma, adrenal carcinoma, Cushing's disease, nonpituitary ACTH-producing tumor, steroid therapy, oral contraceptives.

Decreased: Primary adrenal insufficiency (Addison's disease), Waterhouse-Friderichsen syndrome, ACTH deficiency.

■ CORTROSYN STIMULATION TEST

See ACTH Stimulation Test.

■ COUNTERIMMUNOELECTROPHORESIS (CIE)

Normal = negative.

CIE is an immunologic technique that allows rapid identification of infectious organisms from body fluids, including serum, urine, cerebrospinal fluid, and others. Organisms that can be identified include *Neisseria meningitidis, Streptococcus pneumoniae, Haemophilus influenzae,* and group B streptococcus.

■ CREATINE PHOSPHOKINASE (CPK)
25–145 mU/mL or 25–145 U/L.

Increased: Cardiac muscle (acute myocardial infarction, myocarditis, defibrillation); skeletal muscle (intramuscular injection, hypothyroidism, rhabdomyolysis, polymyositis, muscular dystrophy); cerebral infarction.

CPK isoenzymes MM, MB, BB: MB (normal $< 6\%$) increased in acute myocardial infarction (increases in 4–8 hours, peaks at 24 hours), cardiac surgery; BB not frequently seen or useful.

■ CREATININE CLEARANCE
Male: 100–135 mL/min or 0.963–1.300 mL/s/m²;
Female: 85–125 mL/min or 0.819–1.204 mL/s/m².

A concurrent serum creatinine and a 24-hour urine creatinine are needed. A shorter time interval can be used and corrected for in the formula. A quick formula for estimation is also found in Table 7–15, Aminoglycoside Dosing.

$$\text{Creatinine clearance} = \frac{\text{urine creatinine} \times \text{total urine volume}}{\text{plasma creatinine} \times \text{time in minutes}}$$

To verify if the urine sample is a complete 24-hour collection, determine if the sample contains at least 18–25 mg/kg/24 hr or 125–220 mmol/kg/d creatinine for adult males; or 12–20 mg/kg/24 hr or 106–177 mmol/kg/d for adult females. This test is not a requirement.

Decreased: A decreased creatinine clearance results in an increase in serum creatinine, usually secondary to renal insufficiency. Clearance normally decreases with age. See Creatinine, Serum, Increased.

Increased: Pregnancy, pre-diabetic renal failure.

■ CREATININE, SERUM
Male: 0.7–1.3 mg/dL;
Female: 0.6–1.1 mg/dL.

Increased: Renal failure (prerenal, renal, or postrenal), acromegaly, ingestion of roasted meat, large body mass. Falsely elevated with ketones and certain cephalosporins depending on assay.

■ CREATININE, URINE
Male total creatinine: 14–26 mg/kg/24 h or 124–230 μmol/kg/d;
Female: 11–20 mg/kg/24 h or 97–177 μmol/kg/d. See Creatinine Clearance.

■ CRYOCRIT

≤ 0.4%. (Negative if qualitative.) Cryocrit, a quantitative measure, is preferred over the qualitative method. It should be collected in nonanticoagulated tubes and transported at body temperature. Positive samples can be analyzed for immunoglobulin class, and light chain type on request.

> 0.4%. (Positive if qualitative.) *Monoclonal*—Multiple myeloma, Waldenström's macroglobulinemia, lymphoma, chronic lymphocytic leukemia.

Mixed polyclonal or mixed monoclonal—Infectious diseases (viral, bacterial, parasitic) such as subacute bacterial endocarditis or malaria, systemic lupus erythematosus, rheumatoid arthritis, essential cryoglobulinemia, lymphoproliferative diseases, sarcoidosis, chronic liver disease (cirrhosis).

■ DEXAMETHASONE SUPPRESSION TEST

Used in the differential diagnosis of Cushing's syndrome.

Overnight Dexamethasone Suppression Test

In the rapid version of this test, the patient takes 1 mg of dexamethasone PO at 11 pm; a fasting 8 am plasma cortisol is obtained. Normally, the cortisol level should be < 5 µg/dL or < 138 nmol/L. A value > 5 µg/dL or > 138 nmol/L suggests the diagnosis of Cushing's syndrome; however, suppression may not occur with obesity, alcoholism, or depression. In these patients, the best screening test is a 24-hour urine for free cortisol.

Low-Dose Dexamethasone Suppression Test

After collection of baseline serum cortisol and 24-hour urine free cortisol levels, dexamethasone 0.5 mg PO is administered Q 6 hr for eight doses. Serum cortisol and 24-hour urine for free cortisol are repeated on the second day. Failure to suppress to a serum cortisol of < 5 µg/dL (138 nmol/L) and a urine free cortisol < 30 µg/dL (82 nmol/L) confirms the diagnosis of Cushing's syndrome.

High-Dose Dexamethasone Suppression Test

If the low-dose test is positive, dexamethasone 2 mg PO Q 6 hr for eight doses is administered. A fall in urinary free cortisol to 50% of the baseline value occurs in patients with Cushing's disease, but not in patients with adrenal tumors or ectopic ACTH production.

■ ERYTHROPOIETIN (EPO)

Normal = 5–30 mU/mL.

There is an inverse relationship between erythropoietin and hematocrit.

Decreased or normal levels: Myelodysplastic syndrome, polycythemia vera, chronic renal disease, early pregnancy, and in pre-term infants.

Increased: AZT-treated HIV infection, normocytic anemias, and with a microcytic anemia.

RIA measurement detects erythropoietin in both the active and inactive forms while the mouse bioassay assesses functional hormones.

■ ETHANOL LEVEL

See Drug Levels, Table 7–13, p 536.

■ FERRITIN

Male: 15–200 ng/mL or 15–220 µg/L;
Female: 12–150 ng/mL or 12–150 µg/L.
Decreased: Iron deficiency, severe liver disease.
Increased: Hemochromatosis, hemosiderosis, sideroblastic anemia, any inflammatory process (acute-phase reactant).

■ FIBRIN DEGRADATION PRODUCTS (FDP)

< 10 µg/mL.
Increased: Any thromboembolic condition (deep venous thrombosis, myocardial infarction, pulmonary embolus); disseminated intravascular co-agulation; hepatic dysfunction.

■ FIBRINOGEN

150–450 mg/dL or 150–450 g/L.
Decreased: Congenital; disseminated intravascular coagulation (sepsis, amniotic fluid embolism, abruptio placentae, prostatic or cardiac surgery); burns; neoplastic and hematologic malignancies; acute severe bleeding; snake bite.
Increased: Inflammatory processes (acute-phase reactant).

■ FOLATE RED BLOOD CELL

160–640 ng or 360–1450 nmol/mL RBC.
More sensitive for detecting folate deficiency from malnourishment if the patient has started proper nutrition before the serum folate is measured (even one well-balanced hospital meal).
Increased: See Folic Acid.
Decreased: See Folic Acid.

■ FOLIC ACID (SERUM FOLATE)

2–14 ng/mL or 4.5–31.7 nmol/L.
Increased: Folic acid administration.
Decreased: Malnutrition, malabsorption, massive cellular growth (cancer), hemolytic anemia, pregnancy.

■ FTA-ABS (FLUORESCENT TREPONEMAL ANTIBODY ABSORBED)

Nonreactive.

Positive: Syphilis (test of choice to confirm diagnosis). May be negative in early primary syphilis; may remain positive after adequate treatment.

■ FUNGAL SEROLOGIES

Negative ($< 1:8$). This is a complement-fixation fungal antibody screen that usually detects antibodies to *Histoplasma, Blastomyces, Aspergillus,* and *Coccidioides.*

■ GASTRIN

Male: < 100 pg/mL or < 100 ng/L;

Female: < 75 pg/mL or < 100 ng/L.

Increased: Zollinger-Ellison syndrome, pyloric stenosis, pernicious anemia, atrophic gastritis, ulcerative colitis, renal insufficiency, steroid and calcium administration.

■ GLUCOSE

Fasting: 70–105 mg/dL or 3.89–5.83 nmol/L:

2 hours postprandial: 70–120 mg/dL or 3.89–6.67 mmol/L.

Increased: See Section I, Chapter 31, Hyperglycemia, p 161.

Decreased: See Section I, Chapter 36, Hypoglycemia, p 181.

■ GAMMA-GLUTAMYLTRANSFERASE (GGT)

Male: 9–50 U/L;

Female: 8–40 U/L. Generally parallels changes in serum alkaline phosphatase and 5′-nucleotidase in liver disease.

Increased: Liver disease (hepatitis, cirrhosis, obstructive jaundice); pancreatitis.

■ GLYCOHEMOGLOBIN (HEMOGLOBIN A$_{1C}$)

4.6–7.1%.

Increased: Poorly controlled diabetes mellitus.

■ GRAM'S STAIN

Rapid Technique

Spread a thin layer of specimen onto glass slide and allow to dry. Fix with heat. Apply Gentian violet (15–20 seconds); follow with iodine (15–20 seconds), then alcohol (just a few seconds until effluent is barely decolorized).

Rinse with water and counterstain with safranin (15–20 seconds). Examine under oil immersion lens: gram-positive organisms are dark blue and gram-negatives are red.

Gram-Positive Cocci: *Staphylococcus, Streptococcus, Enterococcus, Micrococcus, Peptococcus* (anaerobic), and *Peptostreptococcus* (anaerobic) species.

Gram-Positive Rods: *Clostridium* (anaerobic), *Corynebacterium, Listeria, Bacillus,* and *Bacteroides* (anaerobic) species.

Gram-Negative Cocci: *Neisseria, Branhamella, Moraxella, Acinetobacter* species.

Gram-Negative Coccoid Rods: *Haemophilus, Pasteurella, Brucella, Francisella, Yersinia,* and *Bordetella* species.

Gram-Negative Straight Rods: *Acinetobacter (Mima, Herellea), Aeromonas, Bacteroides* (anaerobic), *Campylobacter* (comma-shaped) species, *Eikenella, Enterobacter, Escherichia, Fusobacterium* (anaerobic), *Helicobacter, Klebsiella, Legionella* (small, pleomorphic; take weakly staining), *Proteus, Providencia, Pseudomonas, Salmonella, Serratia, Shigella, Vibrio, Yersinia.*

■ HAPTOGLOBIN

26–185 mg/mL.

Increased: Obstructive liver disease; any inflammatory process.

Decreased: Hemolysis (eg, transfusion reaction); severe liver disease.

■ HELICOBACTER ANTIBODIES

Normal = negative.

Serological test to detect antibodies to *Helicobacter pylori* in patients with peptic ulcer disease. High titers of IgG to *Helicobacter* almost universally with *H pylori* infection (sensitivity > 95% and specificity > 95%). More sensitive than biopsy for detecting presence of *H pylori*. It may take 6 months or longer for antibodies to decline appreciably after treatment.

■ HEMATOCRIT

See Table 2–3, p 308 , for normal values.

Increased: See Section I, Chapter 54, Polycythemia, p 260.

Decreased: See Section I, Chapter 5, Anemia, p 25.

■ HEMOGLOBIN

See Table 2–3, p 308, for normal values.

Increased: See Section I, Chapter 54, Polycythemia, p 260.

Decreased: See Section I, Chapter 5, Anemia, p 25.

■ HEPATITIS TESTS

See Table 2–5, p 319.

- **HBsAg:** Hepatitis B surface antigen (formerly Australia antigen). Indicates either chronic or acute infection with hepatitis B. Used by blood banks to screen donors.
- **Total Anti-HBc:** IgG and IgM antibody to hepatitis B core antigen. Confirms either previous exposure to hepatitis B virus (HBV) or ongoing infection. Used by blood banks to screen donors.
- **Anti-HBc IgM:** IgM antibody to hepatitis B core antigen. Early and best indicator of acute infection with hepatitis B.
- **HBeAg:** Hepatitis B$_e$ antigen. When present, indicates high degree of infectiousness. Order *only* when evaluating a patient with *chronic* HBV infection.
- **Anti-HBe:** Antibody to hepatitis B antigen. Order with HbeAg. Presence is associated with resolution of active inflammation; but often means virus is integrated into host DNA, especially if host remains HBsAg positive.
- **Anti-HBs:** Antibody to hepatitis B surface antigen. Typically indicates immunity associated with clinical recovery from an HBV infection or previous immunization with hepatitis B vaccine. Order *only* to assess effectiveness of vaccine.
- **HBV-DNA:** Detects presence of viral DNA in serum (pg/mL) quantitatively to confirm infection and assess therapy. Very expensive assay.
- **Anti-HAV:** Total antibody to hepatitis A virus. Confirms previous exposure to hepatitis A virus.
- **Anti-HAV IgM:** IgM antibody to hepatitis A virus. Indicates recent acute infection with hepatitis A virus.
- **Anti-HDV:** Total antibody to delta-agent hepatitis. Confirms previous exposure. Order *only* in patients with known chronic HBV infection.
- **Anti-HDV IgM:** IgM antibody to delta-agent hepatitis. Indicates recent infection. Order *only* in patients with known chronic HBV infection.
- **Anti-HCV:** Antibody against hepatitis C (formerly known as non-A non-B hepatitis). Order to evaluate both acute and chronic hepatitis. Has a low false positive rate. Used by blood banks to screen donors.
- **Anti-HCV RIBA:** Measures antibody to 4 separate HCV antigens. Used to confirm positive anti-HCV test.
- **HCV-RNA:** Detects presence of virus by either sensitive RT-PCR or quantitatively by branched DNA. Confirms infection or response to therapy. Very expensive assay.

■ HUMAN CHORIONIC GONADOTROPIN, SERUM (HCG BETA SUBUNIT)

< 3.0 mIU/mL;

7–10 days postconception: > 3 mIU/mL; 30 days: 100–5000 mIU/mL;

TABLE 2–5. HEPATITIS PANEL TESTING.

Profile Name	Tests	Purpose
■ Screening		
Admission: High-risk patients (homosexuals, IV drug users, dialysis patients)	HBsAg Anti-HCV	To screen for chronic or active infection.
All pregnant women	HBsAg	To screen for chronic or active infection.
Percutaneous inoculation	HBsAg Anti-HCV	Test serum of patient (if known) for possible infectivity. Start Hep B vaccination if health care worker not previously immunized.
	Anti-HBs	Determine if vaccinated health care worker is immune and protected.
Pre-HBV vaccine in high-risk patients	HBsAg Anti-HBc	To determine if an individual is infected or already has antibodies and is immune.
■ Diagnosis		
Differential diagnosis of acute hepatitis	Anti-HAV IgM HBsAg Anti-HBc IgM Anti-HCV	To differentiate between hepatitis A, hepatitis B and hepatitis C (Anti-HCV may take 4–8 weeks to become positive)
Differential diagnosis of chronic hepatitis (Abnormal Liver Function Tests [LFTs])	HBsAg Anti-HCV (and RIBA or HCV RNA if Anti-HCV is positive)	To rule out chronic hepatitis B or C as a cause of chronically elevated LFTs.
■ Monitoring		
Chronic hepatitis B	LFTs HBsAg HBeAg/Anti-HBe Anti-HDV IgM α-fetoprotein HBV DNA	To test for activity, late seroconversion or disease latency in known hepatitis B carrier, superinfection with HDV, development of hepatoma, or resolution of infection after therapy or spontaneously.
Chronic hepatitis C	LFTs HCV RNA α-fetoprotein	To test for activity of hepatitis, likelihood of response to interferon or development of hepatoma
Postvaccination screening	Anti-HBs	To ensure immunity after vaccination
Sexual contact	HBsAg	To monitor sexual partners with acute or chronic hepatitis B

10 weeks: 50,000–140,000 mIU/mL; > 16 weeks: 10,000–50,000 mIU/mL; thereafter: levels slowly decline.

Increased: Pregnancy, testicular tumors, trophoblastic disease (hydatidiform mole, choriocarcinoma levels usually > 100,000 mIU/mL).

■ 5-HIAA (5-HYDROXYINDOLEACETIC ACID)

2–8 mg or 10.4–41.6 μmol/24-h urine collection. 5-HIAA is a serotonin metabolite.

Increased: Carcinoid tumors; certain foods (banana, pineapple, tomato).

■ HUMAN IMMUNODEFICIENCY VIRUS (HIV) ANTIBODY TEST

Negative: Used in the diagnosis of acquired immunodeficiency syndrome (AIDS) and HIV infection, and to screen blood for use in transfusion. May be negative in early HIV infection.

ELISA (Enzyme-Linked Immunoabsorbent Assay)

Used to detect HIV antibody. A positive test is usually repeated and then confirmed by Western blot analysis.

Positive: AIDS, asymptomatic HIV infection, false-positive test.

Western Blot

The technique used as the reference procedure for confirming the presence or absence of HIV antibody, usually after a positive HIV antibody by ELISA determination.

Positive: AIDS, asymptomatic HIV infection.

Note: In the future, polymerase chain reaction will become a viable tool for detection of the HIV virus. It will be especially useful in very early infection, when antibody may not be present.

■ INTERNATIONAL NORMALIZED RATIO (INR)

See also Prothrombin Time, p 329.

Normal = 1.0

The INR is used to standardize prothrombin results in patients taking anticoagulants.

- **INR 2–3:** Therapeutic range for most indications, including atrial fibrillation, deep vein thrombosis, pulmonary embolus, and transient ischemic attacks.
- **INR 3.0–4.5:** Prevention of arterial thrombo-embolism with mechanical valves. This range may also be required in hypercoagulable states, or in recurrent arterial or venous thromboembolic disease.

■ IRON
Males: 65–175 µg/dL or 11.64–31.33 µmol/L;
Females: 50–170 µg/dL or 8.95–30.43 µmol/L.
Increased: Hemochromatosis, hemosiderosis caused by excessive iron intake, excess destruction or decreased production of erythrocytes, liver necrosis.
Decreased: Iron deficiency anemia, nephrosis (loss of iron-binding proteins), anemia of chronic disease.

■ IRON BINDING CAPACITY, TOTAL (TIBC)
250–450 µg/dL or 44.75–80.55 µmol/L.
The normal iron/TIBC ratio is 20–50%; < 15% is characteristic of iron deficiency anemia. An increased ratio is seen with hemochromatosis.
Increased: Acute and chronic blood loss, iron deficiency anemia, hepatitis, oral contraceptives.
Decreased: Anemia of chronic disease, cirrhosis, nephrosis, hemochromatosis.

■ 17-KETOGENIC STEROIDS (17-KGS)
Males: 5–23 mg or 17–80 µmol/24-h urine;
Females: 3–15 mg or 10–52 µmol/24-h urine.
Increased: Adrenal hyperplasia.
Decreased: Panhypopituitarism, Addison's disease, acute steroid withdrawal.

■ 17-KETOSTEROIDS (17-KS)
Males: 9–22 mg or 31–76 µmol/24-h urine;
Females: 6–15 mg or 21–52 µmol/24-h urine.
Increased: Cushing's syndrome, 11- and 21-hydroxylase deficiency, severe stress, exogenous steroids, excess ACTH or androgens.
Decreased: Addison's disease, anorexia nervosa, panhypopituitarism.

■ KOH PREP
Negative: Normal.
Positive: Superficial mycoses (*Candida, Trichophyton, Microsporum, Epidermophyton, Keratinomyces*).

■ LACTATE DEHYDROGENASE (LDH)
45–100 U/L.
Increased: Acute myocardial infarction, cardiac surgery, hepatitis, pernicious anemia, malignant tumors, pulmonary embolus, hemolysis, renal infarction.

LDH Isoenzymes (LDH 1–LDH 5): Normally, the ratio LDH 1/LDH 2 is < 0.6–0.7. If the ratio becomes > 1 or approaches 1, suspect a recent myocardial infarction. With an acute myocardial infarction, the LDH begins to rise at 10–12 hours, peaks at 48–72 hours, and remains elevated for 7–10 days. LDH 5 is increased in hepatitis.

■ LACTIC ACID (LACTATE)

4.5–19.8 mg/dL or 0.5–2.2 mmol/L.

Increased: Lactic acidosis resulting from hypoxia, hemorrhage, circulatory collapse, sepsis, cirrhosis, exercise.

■ LEUKOCYTE ALKALINE PHOSPHATASE SCORE (LAP SCORE)

70–140.

Increased: Leukemoid reaction, Hodgkin's disease, polycythemia vera, myeloproliferative disorders, pregnancy, liver disease, acute inflammation.

Decreased: Chronic myelogenous leukemia, pernicious anemia, paroxysmal nocturnal hemoglobinuria, nephrotic syndrome.

■ LIPASE

Variable depending on the method; 10–150 U/L by turbidimetric method.

Increased: Acute pancreatitis; pancreatic duct obstruction (stone, stricture, tumor, drug-induced spasm); fat emboli. Usually normal in mumps.

■ LUPUS ANTICOAGULANT

See Antiphospholipid Antibody, p 305.

■ LYMPHOCYTES, TOTAL

1800–3000/mL.

Often used to assess nutritional status. Calculated by multiplying the white cell count by the percentage of lymphocytes: < 900, severe; 900–1400, moderate; 1400–1800, minimal nutritional deficit. Lymphopenia is also seen with certain viral infections. including human immunodeficiency virus.

■ MAGNESIUM

1.6–2.4 mg/dL or 0.80–1.20 mmol/L.

Increased: Renal failure, hypothyroidism, magnesium-containing antacids, Addison's disease, severe dehydration.

Decreased: See Section I, Chapter 38, Hypomagnesemia, p 190.

■ MAGNESIUM, URINE

6.0–10.0 mEq/d or 3.00–5.00 mmol/d.

Increased: Hypermagnesemia, diuretics, hypercalcemia, metabolic acidosis, hypophosphatemia.

Decreased: Hypomagnesemia, hypocalcemia, hypoparathyroidism, metabolic alkalosis.

■ METANEPHRINES, URINE

Total: < 1.0 mg or 0.574 mmol/24-h urine;

Fractionated metanephrines-normetanephrines: < 0.9 mg or 0.517 mmol/24-h urine;

Fractionated metanephrines: < 0.4 mg or 0.230 mg/24-h urine.

Increased: Pheochromocytoma, neural crest tumors (neuroblastoma), false positives with drugs (phenobarbital, hydrocortisone, others).

■ MONOSPOT

Negative: Normal.
Positive: Mononucleosis.

■ MYOGLOBIN, URINE

Qualitative negative.

Positive: Disorders affecting skeletal muscle (crush injury, rhabdomyolysis, electrical burns, delirium tremens, surgical procedures), acute myocardial infarction.

■ NITROGEN BALANCE

+4 to +20 g/d or +275 to +1400 mmol/d;

Urinary nitrogen: 12–24 g/24-h urine or 850–1700 mmol/24-h urine.

Most often used in the assessment of patients receiving hyperalimentation. A positive nitrogen balance is usually the goal. The following equation may be used to compute the nitrogen balance:

$$\text{Nitrogen Balance} = \frac{\text{24-hr protein intake (g)}}{6.25} - (\text{24-hr urine nitrogen} + 4)$$

■ 5'-NUCLEOTIDASE

2–15 U/L.

Increased: Obstructive liver disease.

■ OSMOLALITY, SERUM

275–295 mOsm/kg.

A rough estimation of osmolality is $[2(Na) + BUN/2.8 + glucose/18])$. The calculation will not be accurate if foreign substances that increase the osmolality (eg, mannitol) are present. If foreign substances are suspected, osmolality should be measured directly.

Increased: Hyperglycemia; alcohol ingestion; increased sodium resulting from water loss (diabetes insipidus, hypercalcemia, diuresis); ethylene glycol ingestion; mannitol.

Decreased: Low serum sodium, diuretics, Addison's disease, hypothyroidism, syndrome of inappropriate antidiuretic hormone (SIADH), iatrogenic causes (poor fluid balance).

■ OSMOLALITY, URINE

Spot 50–1400 mOsm/kg; > 850 mOsm/kg after 12 hours of fluid restriction.

The loss of the ability to concentrate urine, especially during fluid restriction, is an early indicator of impaired renal function.

■ OXYGEN, ARTERIAL (pO$_2$)

See Table 2–1, p 387; see also Section VI, Ventilator Management, p 387.
Decreased:

- **Ventilation-perfusion ($\dot{V}/\dot{Q}$) abnormalities:** COPD, asthma, atelectasis, pneumonia, pulmonary embolus, adult respiratory distress syndrome, pneumothorax, cystic fibrosis, obstructed airway.
- **Alveolar hypoventilation:** Skeletal abnormalities, neuromuscular disorders, Pickwickian syndrome.
- **Decreased pulmonary diffusing capacity:** Pneumoconiosis, pulmonary edema, pulmonary fibrosis.
- **Right-to-left shunt:** Congenital heart disease (tetralogy of Fallot, transposition, others).

■ pH, ARTERIAL

See Tables 2–1 and 2–2, p 306.
Increased: Metabolic and respiratory alkalosis. See Section I, Chapter 3, Alkalosis, p 17.
Decreased: Metabolic and respiratory acidosis. See Section I, Chapter 2, Acidosis, p 9.

■ PARATHYROID HORMONE (PTH)

Normal based on relationship to serum calcium, usually provided on the lab report. Also, reference values will vary depending on the laboratory and whether N-terminal, C-terminal, or midmolecule is measured.

PTH midmolecule: 0.29–0.85 ng/mL or 29–85 pmol/L with calcium 8.4–10.2 mg/dL or 2.1–2.55 mmol/L.

Increased: Primary hyperparathyroidism, secondary hyperparathyroidism (hypocalcemic states such as chronic renal failure, others).

Decreased: Hypoparathyroidism and hypercalcemia not resulting from hyperparathyroidism, hypoparathyroidism.

■ PARTIAL THROMBOPLASTIN TIME (PTT)

27–38 seconds.

Prolonged: Heparin and any defect in the intrinsic clotting mechanism, such as severe liver disease or disseminated intravascular coagulation (includes factors I, II, V, VIII, IX, X, XI, and XII); prolonged use of a tourniquet before drawing a blood sample; hemophilia A and B; lupus anticoagulant; liver disease. See Section I, Chapter 12, Coagulopathy, p 64.

■ PHOSPHORUS

2.7–4.5 mg/dL or 0.87–1.45 mmol/L.

Increased: Hypoparathyroidism, pseudohypoparathyroidism, excess vitamin D, secondary hypoparathyroidism, acute and chronic renal failure, acromegaly, tumor lysis (lymphoma or leukemia treated with chemotherapy), alkalosis, factitious increase (hemolysis of specimen).

Decreased: See Section I, Chapter 40, Hypophosphatemia, p 199.

■ PLATELETS

See Table 2–3, p 308.

Platelet counts may be normal in number, but abnormal in function (eg, aspirin therapy); platelet function with a normal platelet count can be assessed by measuring bleeding time.

Increased: Primary thrombocytosis (idiopathic myelofibrosis, agnogenic myeloid metaplasia, polycythemia vera, primary thrombocythemia, chronic myelogenous leukemia). Secondary thrombocytosis (collagen-vascular diseases, chronic infection [osteomyelitis, tuberculosis], sarcoidosis, hemolytic anemia, iron deficiency anemia, recovery from B$_{12}$ deficiency or iron deficiency, solid tumors and lymphomas; after surgery, especially postsplenectomy; response to drugs such as epinephrine or withdrawal of myelosuppressive drugs).

Decreased: See Section I, Chapter 59, Thrombocytopenia, p 289.

■ POTASSIUM, SERUM

3.5–5.1 mmol/L.

Increased: See Section I, Chapter 32, Hyperkalemia, p 166.

Decreased: See Section I, Chapter 37, Hypokalemia, p 185.

■ POTASSIUM, URINE

25–125 mmol/24-hr urine; varies with diet. See Urine Electrolytes, p 337.

■ PROLACTIN

Females: 1–25 ng/mL;
Males: 1–20 ng/mL.

Increased: Pregnancy, nursing after pregnancy, prolactinoma, hypothalamic tumors, sarcoidosis or granulomatous disease of the hypothalamus, hypothyroidism, renal failure, Addison's disease, phenothiazines, butyrophenones (eg, haloperidol [Haldol]).

Decreased: Sheehan's syndrome.

■ PROSTATIC-SPECIFIC ANTIGEN (PSA)

< 4 ng/dL.

Most useful as a measure of response to therapy for prostate cancer. Values > 8.0 ng/dL are associated with carcinoma at the 90% confidence level.

Increased: Prostate cancer, some cases of benign prostatic hypertrophy, prostatic infarction.

Decreased: Total prostatectomy, response to therapy for prostatic carcinoma.

■ PROTEIN ELECTROPHORESIS, SERUM AND URINE (SERUM PROTEIN ELECTROPHORESIS [SPEP]; URINE PROTEIN ELECTROPHORESIS [UPEP])

Quantitative analysis of the serum proteins is often used in the workup of hypoglobulinemia, macroglobulinemia, α_1-antitrypsin deficiency, collagen disease, liver disease, myeloma, and occasionally in nutritional assessment. Serum electrophoresis yields five different bands (see Figure 2–1, p 327; and Table 2–6, p 328). If a monoclonal gammopathy or a low globulin fraction is detected, quantitative immunoglobulins should be checked.

Urine protein electrophoresis can be used to evaluate proteinuria and can detect Bence Jones (light-chain) protein that is associated with myeloma, Waldenström's macroglobulinemia, and Fanconi's syndrome.

■ PROTEIN, SERUM

6.0–7.8 g/dL or 60–78 g/L.

Increased: Multiple myeloma, Waldenström's macroglobulinemia, benign monoclonal gammopathy, lymphoma, sarcoidosis, chronic inflammatory disease.

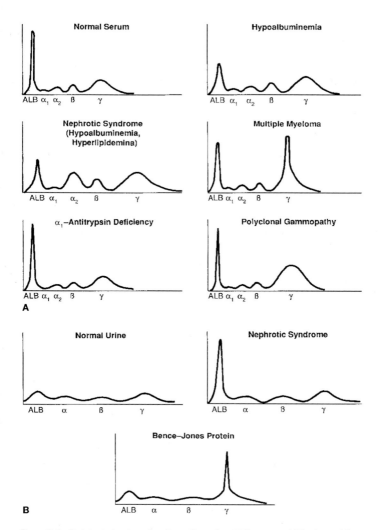

Figure 2–1. Protein electrophoresis patterns. Examples of **(A)** serum and **(B)** urine protein electrophoresis patterns.

TABLE 2–6. NORMAL SERUM PROTEIN COMPONENTS AND FRACTIONS AS DETERMINED BY ELECTROPHORESIS ALONG WITH ASSOCIATED CONDITIONS.[1]

Protein Fraction	Percentage of Total Protein	Constituents	Increased	Decreased
Albumin	52–68	Albumin	Dehydration (only known cause)	Nephrosis, malnutrition, chronic liver disease
α$_1$-Globulin	2.4–4.4	Thyroxine-binding globulin, antitrypsin, lipoproteins, glycoprotein, transcortin	Inflammation, neoplasia	Nephrosis, α$_1$-antitrypsin deficiency (emphysema-related)
α$_2$-Globulin	6.1–10.1	Haptoglobin, glycoprotein, macroglobulin, ceruloplasmin	Inflammation, infection, neoplasia, cirrhosis	Severe liver disease, acute hemolytic anemia
β-Globulin	8.5–14.5	Transferrin, glycoprotein, lipoprotein	Cirrhosis, obstructive jaundice	Nephrosis
γ-Globulins (immunoglobulins)	10–21	IgA, IgG, IgM, IgD, IgE	Infections, collagen-vascular diseases, leukemia, myeloma	Agammaglobulinemia, hypogammaglobulinemia, nephrosis

[1] Reproduced with permission from Gomella LG, ed: *Clinician's Pocket Reference*. 7th ed.: Appleton & Lange; 1993.

Decreased: Any cause of decreased albumin or any cause of hypogammaglobulinemia such as common variable hypogammaglobulinemia.

■ PROTEIN, URINE

See also Albumin, Urine
< 100 mg/24-hr urine;
Spot: < 10 mg/dL (< 20 mg/dL if early-morning collection);
Dipstick: negative.

Increased: Nephrotic syndrome, glomerulonephritis, lupus nephritis, amyloidosis, venous congestion of kidney (renal vein thrombosis, severe congestive heart failure), multiple myeloma, pre-eclampsia, postural proteinuria, polycystic kidney disease, diabetic nephropathy, radiation nephritis, malignant hypertension.

False positive: Gross hematuria, very concentrated urine, pyridium, very alkaline urine.

■ PROTEIN C PLASMA

Normal = 60–130%

Decreased: Hypercoagulable states resulting in recurrent venous thrombosis; chronic liver disease; disseminated intravascular coagulation (DIC); post-operatively; neoplastic disease and autosomal recessive deficiency.

■ PROTEIN S PLASMA

Normal = 60–140%

Decreased: See Protein C. Protein S is a cofactor of protein C; should be ordered along with protein C.

■ PROTHROMBIN TIME (PT)

See International Normalized Ratio (INR), p 320.
11.5–13.5 seconds.
Evaluates extrinsic clotting mechanism (factors I, II, V, VII, and X).

Prolonged: Drugs such as sodium warfarin (Coumadin), decreased vitamin K, fat malabsorption, liver disease, prolonged use of a tourniquet before drawing a blood sample, disseminated intravascular coagulation (DIC), lupus anticoagulant (usually selectively increased PTT). See Section I, Chapter 12, Coagulopathy, p 64.

■ QUANTITATIVE IMMUNOGLOBULINS

IgG: 650–1500 mg/dL or 6.5–15 g/L;
IgM: 40–345 mg/dL or 0.4–3.45 g/L;

IgA: 76–390 mg/dL or 0.76–3.90 g/L;
IgE: 0–380 IU/mL or KIU/L;
IgD: 0–8 mg/dL or 0–80 mg/L.

Increased: Multiple myeloma (myeloma immunoglobulin increased, other immunoglobulins decreased), Waldenström's macroglobulinemia (IgM increased, others decreased), lymphoma, carcinoma, bacterial infection, liver disease, sarcoidosis, amyloidosis, myeloproliferative disorders.

Decreased: Hereditary immunodeficiency, leukemia, lymphoma, nephrotic syndrome, protein-losing enteropathy, malnutrition.

■ RED BLOOD CELL COUNT (RBC)

See Table 2–3, p 308. Also see Hematocrit.

■ RED BLOOD CELL INDICES

See Table 2–3, p 308.

MCV (Mean Cell Volume)

Increased: Megaloblastic anemia (B_{12}, folate deficiency), reticulocytosis, chronic liver disease, alcoholism, hypothyroidism, aplastic anemia.

Decreased: Iron deficiency, sideroblastic anemia, thalassemia, some cases of lead poisoning, hereditary spherocytosis.

MCH (Mean Cellular Hemoglobin)

Increased: Macrocytosis (megaloblastic anemias, high reticulocyte counts).

Decreased: Microcytosis (iron deficiency).

MCHC (Mean Cellular Hemoglobin Concentration)

Increased: Very severe, prolonged dehydration; spherocytosis.

Decreased: Iron deficiency anemia, overhydration, thalassemia, sideroblastic anemia.

RDW (Red Cell Distribution Width)

Measure of the degree of anisocytosis.

Increased: Combination of a macrocytic and microcytic anemia or recovery from iron deficiency anemia.

■ RED BLOOD CELL MORPHOLOGY

Poikilocytosis: Irregular RBC shape (sickle, burr).
Anisocytosis: Irregular RBC size (microcytes, macrocytes).
Basophilic stippling: Lead, heavy metal poisoning, thalassemia.
Howell-Jolly bodies: Seen after a splenectomy and in some severe anemias.
Sickling: Sickle cell disease and trait.

Nucleated RBCs: Severe bone marrow stress (hemorrhage, hemolysis), marrow replacement by tumor, extramedullary hematopoiesis.

Target cells: Thalassemia, hemoglobinopathies (sickle cell disease), obstructive jaundice, any hypochromic anemia, after splenectomy.

Spherocytes: Hereditary spherocytosis, immune or microangiopathic hemolysis.

Helmet cells (Schistocytes). Microangiopathic hemolysis, hemolytic transfusion reaction, other hemolytic anemias.

Burr cells (Acanthocytes): Severe liver disease; high levels of bile, fatty acids, or toxins.

Polychromasia: Appearance of a bluish-gray red cell on routine Wright's stain suggests reticulocytes.

■ RETICULOCYTE COUNT

0.5–1.5%.

If the patient's hematocrit is abnormal, a corrected reticulocyte count should be calculated as follows:

$$\text{Corrected reticulocyte count} = \% \text{ reticulocytes} \times \frac{\text{patient's hematocrit}}{45\%}$$

Increased: Hemolysis, acute hemorrhage, therapeutic response to treatment for iron, vitamin B_{12}, or folate deficiency.

Decreased: Infiltration of bone marrow by carcinoma, lymphoma or leukemia, marrow aplasia, chronic infections such as osteomyelitis, toxins, drugs ($>$ 100 reported), many anemias.

■ RETINOL BINDING PROTEIN (RBP)

3–6 mg/dL.

Increased: Chronic renal disease.

Decreased: Malnutrition states, vitamin A deficiency, intestinal malabsorption of fats, chronic liver disease.

■ RHEUMATOID FACTOR (RA LATEX TEST)

$<$ 15 IU by microscan kit or $<$ 1:40.

Increased: Rheumatoid arthritis, systemic lupus erythematosus, Sjögren's syndrome, scleroderma, dermatomyositis, polymyositis, syphilis, chronic inflammation, subacute bacterial endocarditis, hepatitis, sarcoidosis, interstitial pulmonary fibrosis.

■ SCHLICHTER TEST

Bactericidal $\geq$ 1:8 dilution.

Used most frequently to ensure adequate antimicrobial levels in patients with osteomyelitis or bacterial endocarditis.

■ SEDIMENTATION RATE (ESR)

- **Wintrobe Scale:** Males: 0–9 mm/h;
Females: 0–20 mm/h.
- **ZETA Scale:** 40–54%, normal; 55–59%, mildly elevated; 60–64%, moderately elevated; > 65%, markedly elevated.
- **Westergren Scale:** Males < 50 years: 15 mm/h; males > 50 years: 20 mm/h;
- Females < 50 years, 25 mm/h; females > 50 years: 30 mm/h.
- This is a very nonspecific test. The ZETA method is not affected by anemia. The Westergren scale remains the preferred method.

Increased: Any type of infection, inflammation, rheumatic fever, endocarditis, neoplasm, acute myocardial infarction.

■ SGGT (SERUM GAMMA-GLUTAMYLTRANSFERASE)

See Gamma-Glutamyltransferase (GGT).

■ SGOT (SERUM GLUTAMIC-OXALOACETIC TRANSAMINASE) OR AST (SERUM ASPARTATE AMINOTRANSAMINASE)

See AST.

■ SGPT (SERUM GLUTAMIC-PYRUVIC TRANSAMINASE) OR ALT (SERUM ALANINE AMINOTRANSAMINASE)

See ALT.

■ SODIUM, SERUM

136–145 mmol/L.
Increased: See Section I, Chapter 33, Hypernatremia, p 170.
Decreased: See Section I, Chapter 39, Hyponatremia, p 193.

■ SODIUM, URINE

40–210 mmol/24-h urine. See Urinary Electrolytes, p 337.

■ STOOL FOR OCCULT BLOOD (HEMOCCULT TEST)

Negative: Normal.
Positive: Swallowed blood; ingestion of red meat; any gastrointestinal tract lesion (ulcer, carcinoma, polyp); large doses of vitamin C (> 500 mg/d). See also Section I, Chapter 27, Hematochezia, p 143, and Chapter 26, Hematemesis, Melena, p 140.

■ STOOL FOR WBC
Occasional WBCs, usually PMNs.
Increased: *Shigella, Salmonella,* enteropathogenic *Escherichia coli,* pseudomembranous colitis (*Clostridium difficile*), ulcerative colitis.

■ T₃ (TRIIODOTHYRONINE) RADIOIMMUNOASSAY
120–195 ng/dL or 1.85–3.00 nmol/L.
Increased: Hyperthyroidism, T_3 thyrotoxicosis, exogenous T_4, any cause of increased thyroid-binding globulin such as oral estrogens, pregnancy, or hepatitis.
Decreased: Hypothyroidism, euthyroid sick state, any cause of decreased thyroid-binding globulin (eg, malnutrition).

■ T₃ RU (RESIN UPTAKE)
24–34%.
Increased: Hyperthyroidism; medications (phenytoin [Dilantin], steroids, heparin, aspirin, others); nephrotic syndrome.
Decreased: Hypothyroidism, pregnancy, medications (estrogens, iodine, propylthiouracil, others).

■ T₄ TOTAL (THYROXINE)
5–12 µg/dL or 65–155 nmol/L;
Males: 5–10 µg/dL: 5–10 µg/dL or 65–129 nmol;
Females: 5.5–10.5 µg/dL or 71–135 nmol/L.
Increased: Hyperthyroidism; exogenous thyroid hormone; any cause of increased thyroid-binding globulin (eg, estrogens, pregnancy, or hepatitis) euthyroid sick state.
Decreased: Hypothyroidism, euthyroid sick state, any cause of decreased thyroid-binding globulin (eg, malnutrition).

■ THROMBIN TIME
10–14 seconds.
Increased: Heparin, disseminated intravascular coagulation, elevated fibrin degradation products, fibrinogen deficiency, congenitally abnormal fibrinogen molecules. See Section I, Chapter 12, Coagulopathy, p 64.

■ THYROGLOBULIN
0–60 ng/mL or < 60 µg/L.
Used primarily to detect recurrence in patients who undergo surgical resection for nonmedullary thyroid carcinoma.
Increased: Differentiated thyroid carcinomas (papillary, follicular), thyroid adenoma, Graves' disease, toxic goiter, nontoxic goiter, thyroiditis.
Decreased: Hypothyroidism, testosterone, steroids, phenytoin.

■ THYROID-BINDING GLOBULIN (TBG)

1.5–3.4 mg/dL or 15–34 mg/L.

Increased: Hypothyroidism, pregnancy, oral contraceptives, estrogens, hepatitis, acute porphyria, familial.

Decreased: Hyperthyroidism, androgens, anabolic steroids, corticosteroids, nephrotic syndrome, severe illness, phenytoin, liver failure, malnutrition.

■ THYROID-STIMULATING HORMONE (TSH)

0.7–5.3 mU/mL.

Newer sensitive assays are excellent screening tests for hyperthyroidism as well as hypothyroidism; they allow you to distinguish between a low normal and a decreased TSH.

Increased: Hypothyroidism.

Decreased: Hyperthyroidism. Fewer than 1% of cases of hypothyroidism are from pituitary or hypothalamic disease resulting in a decreased TSH.

■ TRANSFERRIN

220–400 mg/dL or 2.20–4.00 g/L.

Increased: Acute and chronic blood loss, iron deficiency anemia, hepatitis, oral contraceptives.

Decreased: Anemia of chronic disease, cirrhosis, nephrosis, hemochromatosis.

■ TRIGLYCERIDES

Males: 40–160 mg/dL or 0.45–1.81 mmol/L;

Females: 35–135 mg/dL or 0.40–1.53 mmol/L; may vary with age.

Increased: Hyperlipoproteinemias (types I, IIb, III, IV, V), hypothyroidism, liver diseases, diabetes mellitus, alcoholism, pancreatitis, acute myocardial infarction, nephrotic syndrome.

Decreased: Malnutrition, congenital abetalipoproteinemia.

■ URIC ACID

Males: 4.5–8.2 mg/dL or 0.27–0.48 mmol/L;

Females: 3.0–6.5 mg/dL or 0.18–0.38 mmol/L.

Increased: Gout; renal failure; destruction of massive amounts of nucleoproteins (tumor lysis after chemotherapy, leukemia or lymphoma); toxemia of pregnancy; drugs (especially diuretics); hypothyroidism; polycystic kidney disease; parathyroid diseases.

Decreased: Uricosuric drugs (salicylates, probenecid, allopurinol), Wilson's disease, Fanconi's syndrome, pregnancy.

■ URINALYSIS, ROUTINE

Appearance

- **Normal:** Yellow, clear, straw-colored
- **Pink/red:** Blood, hemoglobin, myoglobin, food coloring, beets
- **Orange:** Pyridium, bile pigments
- **Brown/black:** Myoglobin, bile pigments, melanin, cascara bark, iron, nitrofurantoin, metronidazole, sickle cell crisis
- **Blue:** Methylene blue, *Pseudomonas* urinary tract infection (rare), hereditary tryptophan metabolic disorders
- **Cloudy:** Urinary tract infection (pyuria), blood, myoglobin, chyluria, mucus (normal in ileal loop specimens), phosphate salts (normal in alkaline urine), urates (normal in acidic urine), hyperoxaluria
- **Foamy:** Proteinuria, bile salts

pH
(4.6–8.0)

Acidic: High-protein diet; methenamine mandelate; acidosis; ketoacidosis (starvation, diabetic); diarrhea; dehydration.

Basic: Urinary tract infection, especially involving Proteus; renal tubular acidosis; diet (high vegetable, milk, immediately postprandial); sodium bicarbonate or acetazolamide therapy; vomiting; metabolic alkalosis; chronic renal failure.

Specific Gravity
Normal: 1.001–1.035.

Increased: Volume depletion, congestive heart failure (CHF), adrenal insufficiency, diabetes mellitus, syndrome of inappropriate antidiuretic hormone (SIADH), increased proteins (nephrosis). If markedly increased (1.040–1.050), suspect artifact, excretion of radiographic contrast medium, or some other osmotic agent.

Decreased: Diabetes insipidus, pyelonephritis, glomerulonephritis, water load with normal renal function.

Bilirubin
Negative dipstick.

Positive: Obstructive jaundice, hepatitis, cirrhosis, CHF with hepatic congestion, congenital hyperbilirubinemia (Dubin-Johnson syndrome).

Blood (Hemoglobin)
Negative dipstick.

Positive: Hematuria (See Section I, Chapter 28, Hematuria, p 147); free hemoglobin (from trauma, transfusion reaction, or lysis of red cells); or myoglobin (crush injury, burn, or tissue ischemia).

Glucose
Negative dipstick.

Positive: Diabetes mellitus; other endocrine disorders (pheochromocytoma, hyperthyroidism, Cushing's syndrome, hyperadrenalism); stress states (sepsis, burns); pancreatitis; renal tubular disease; iatrogenic (steroids, thiazides, birth control pills); false positive with vitamin C ingestion.

Ketones
Negative dipstick.
Positive: Starvation, high-fat diet, alcoholic and diabetic ketoacidosis, vomiting, diarrhea, hyperthyroidism, pregnancy, febrile states.

Leukocyte Esterase
Negative dipstick.
Positive: Infection (test detects 5 or more WBC/HPF or lysed WBCs).

Microscopy
Note: Many laboratories will no longer perform urine microscopy on a routine basis when the dipstick is negative and the gross appearance is normal.

- **RBCs:** (Normal: 0–3/HPF). Trauma, urinary tract infection, prostatic hypertrophy, genitourinary tuberculosis, stones, malignant and benign tumors, glomerulonephritis, and any cause of blood on dipstick (see earlier).
- **WBCs:** (Normal: 0–4/HPF). Infection anywhere in the urinary tract, genitourinary tuberculosis, renal tumors, acute glomerulonephritis, radiation damage, interstitial nephritis (analgesic abuse). (Glitter cells represent WBCs lysed in hypotonic solution.)
- **Epithelial cells:** (Normal: occasional). Acute tubular necrosis, necrotizing papillitis.
- **Parasites:** (Normal: none). *Trichomonas vaginalis, Schistosoma haematobium.*
- **Yeast:** (Normal: none). *Candida albicans* (especially in diabetics and immunosuppressed patients, or if a vaginal infection is present).
- **Spermatozoa:** (Normal: after intercourse or nocturnal emission).
- **Crystals:** Normal:

  Acid urine: Calcium oxalate (small square crystals with a central cross), uric acid.
  Alkaline urine: Calcium carbonate, triple phosphate (resemble coffin lids).
  Abnormal: Cystine, sulfonamide, leucine, tyrosine, cholesterol, or excessive amounts of the crystals noted earlier.

- **Contaminants:** Cotton threads, hair, wood fibers, amorphous substances (all usually unimportant).
- **Mucus:** (Normal: small amounts.) Large amounts suggest urethral disease. Ileal loop urine normally has large amounts.

- **Hyaline cast:** (Normal: occasional.) Benign hypertension, nephrotic syndrome.
- **RBC cast:** (Normal: none.) Acute glomerulonephritis, lupus nephritis, subacute bacterial endocarditis, Goodpasture's disease, vasculitis, malignant hypertension.
- **WBC cast:** (Normal: none.) Pyelonephritis.
- **Epithelial cast:** (Normal: occasional.) Tubular damage, nephrotoxin, viral infections.
- **Granular cast:** (Normal: none.) Results from breakdown of cellular casts, leads to waxy casts.
- **Waxy cast:** (Normal: none.) End stage of a granular cast; evidence of severe chronic renal disease, amyloidosis.
- **Fatty cast:** (Normal: none.) Nephrotic syndrome, diabetes mellitus, damaged renal tubular epithelial cells.
- **Broad cast:** (Normal: none.) Chronic renal disease.

Nitrite
Negative dipstick.
Positive: Infection (a negative test does not rule out infection).

Protein
See also Albumin, Urine, p 302.
Negative dipstick.
Positive: See Protein, Urine, p 329.

Reducing Substance
Negative dipstick.
Positive: Glucose, fructose, galactose.
False positives: Vitamin C, antibiotics.

Urobilinogen
Negative dipstick.
Positive: Bile duct obstruction, suppression of gut flora with antibiotics.

■ URINARY ELECTROLYTES
These "spot urines" are of limited value because of large variations in daily fluid and salt intake. Results are usually indeterminate if a diuretic has been given. Sodium is most useful in the differentiation of volume depletion, oliguria, or hyponatremia. Chloride is useful in the diagnosis and treatment of metabolic alkalosis. Urinary potassium levels are often used in the evaluation of hypokalemia.

- **Chloride < 10 mmol/L:** Chloride-sensitive metabolic alkalosis. See Section I, Chapter 3, Alkalosis, p 17.
- **Chloride > 20 mmol/L:** Chloride-resistant metabolic alkalosis. See Section I, Chapter 3, Alkalosis, p 17.

- **Potassium < 10 mmol/L:** Hypokalemia, from extrarenal losses.
- **Potassium > 10 mmol/L:** Renal potassium wasting (diuretics, brisk urinary output).
- **Sodium < 20 mmol/L:** Volume depletion, hyponatremic states, prerenal azotemia (CHF, shock, others), hepatorenal syndrome, edematous states.
- **Sodium > 40 mmol/L:** Acute tubular necrosis, adrenal insufficiency, renal salt wasting, syndrome of inappropriate antidiuretic hormone (SIADH).
- **Sodium > 20–40 mmol/L:** Indeterminate.

■ URINARY INDICES

See Table 2–7. These are used in determining the etiology of oliguria. See Section I, Chapter 50, Oliguria/Anuria, p 244.

TABLE 2–7. URINARY INDICES IN ACUTE RENAL FAILURE ACCOMPANIED BY OLIGURIA: DIFFERENTIAL DIAGNOSIS OF OLIGURIA.[1]

Index	Prerenal	Renal (ATN)
Urine osmolality	> 500	< 350
Urinary sodium	< 10–20	> 30–40
Urine/serum creatinine	> 40	< 20
Fractional excreted sodium[2]	< 1	> 1
Renal failure index[3]	< 1	> 1

[1] Modified and reproduced with permission from Gomella LG, ed.: *Clinician's Pocket Reference.* 7th ed. Appleton & Lange; 1993.

[2] Fractional excreted sodium $= \dfrac{\text{(urine/serum sodium)}}{\text{(urine/serum creatinine)}} \times 100.$

[3] Renal failure index $= \dfrac{\text{(urine sodium} \times \text{serum creatinine)}}{\text{(urine creatinine)}}.$

■ VANILLYLMANDELIC ACID (VMA), URINE

2–7 mg/dL or 10.1–35.4 mmol/d.

VMA is urinary metabolite of both epinephrine and norepinephrine.

Increased: Pheochromocytoma; neural crest tumors (neuroblastoma, ganglioneuroma). False positive with methyldopa, chocolate, vanilla, others.

■ VDRL TEST (VENEREAL DISEASE RESEARCH LABORATORY) OR RAPID PLASMA REAGIN (RPR)

Normal: Nonreactive.

Good for screening syphilis. Almost always positive in secondary syphilis, but frequently becomes negative in late syphilis. Also, in some patients with HIV infection, the VDRL can be negative in primary and secondary syphilis.

Positive (reactive): Syphilis, systemic lupus erythematosus, pregnancy and drug addiction. If reactive, confirm with FTA-ABS (false positives may occur with bacterial or viral illnesses).

■ WHITE BLOOD CELL COUNT

See Table 2–3, p 308.

Increased: See Section I, Chapter 47, Leukocytosis, p 229.

Decreased: See Section 1, Chapter 48, Leukopenia, p 234.

■ WHITE BLOOD CELL DIFFERENTIAL

See Table 2–3, p 308. Many hospitals are now performing differentials on automated machines. The newer automated differentials can differentiate neutrophils, lymphocytes, monocytes, eosinophils and basophils. A manual differential must be done to differentiate segmented and banded neutrophils.

Neutrophils

40–70% segmented neutrophils, 5–10% banded neutrophils.

Increased: Exercise, pain, stress, infection, burns, drugs, thyrotoxicosis, steroids, malignancy, chronic inflammatory disease (vasculitis, collagen-vascular disease, colitis), lithium, epinephrine, asplenia, idiopathic.

Decreased: Congenital, immune-mediated, drug-induced, infectious (viral, rickettsial, parasitic).

Lymphocytes

Normal: 24–44%.

Increased: Measles; German measles (rubeola); mumps, whooping cough (*Bordetella pertussis*); smallpox; chicken pox (varicella); influenza; viral hepatitis; infectious mononucleosis (Epstein-Barr virus); virtually any viral infection; acute and chronic lymphocytic leukemias.

Decreased: Following stress, burns, trauma; normal finding in 22% of population; uremia; some viral infections (including human immunodeficiency virus).

Lymphocytes, Atypical

Normal: 0–3%.

> 20%: Infectious mononucleosis (Epstein-Barr virus), cytomegalovirus infection, viral hepatitis, toxoplasmosis.

> 3%, < 20%: Viral infections (mumps, rubeola, varicella), rickettsial infections, tuberculosis.

Monocytes
Normal: 3–7%.

Increased: Subacute bacterial endocarditis, brucellosis (*Brucella*), typhoid fever (*Salmonella typhi*), kala-azar (visceral leishmaniasis [*Leishmania*]), trypanosomiasis (*Trypanosoma*), rickettsial infection, ulcerative colitis, sarcoidosis, Hodgkin's disease, monocytic leukemias, collagen-vascular diseases.

Decreased: Myelodysplasia, aplastic anemia, hairy cell leukemia, cyclic neutropenia, thermal injuries, collagen-vascular diseases.

Eosinophils
Normal: 0–3%.

Increased: Allergies, parasites, skin diseases, malignancy, drugs, asthma, Addison's disease, collagen-vascular diseases. (A handy mnemonic is **NAACP: N**eoplasm, **A**llergy, **A**ddison's disease, **C**ollagen-vascular diseases, **P**arasites).

Decreased: After steroids; ACTH; after stress (infection, trauma, burns); Cushing's syndrome.

Basophils
Normal: 0–1%.

Increased: Chronic myeloid leukemia; rarely, in recovery from infection and from hypothyroidism.

Decreased: Acute rheumatic fever, lobar pneumonia, after steroid therapy, thyrotoxicosis, stress.

■ WHITE BLOOD CELL MORPHOLOGY
- **Auer rod:** Acute myelogenous leukemias.
- **Döhle bodies:** Severe infection, burns, malignancy, pregnancy.
- **Hypersegmentation:** Megaloblastic anemias, iron deficiency, myeloproliferative disorders, drug induced.
- **Toxic granulation:** Severe illness (sepsis, burns, high temperature).

■ ZINC
60–130 µg/dL or 9–20 µmol/L.

Increased: Atherosclerosis, coronary artery disease.

Decreased: Inadequate dietary intake (parenteral nutrition, alcoholism); malabsorption; increased needs such as pregnancy or wound healing; acrodermatitis enteropathica.

REFERENCE

Burtis CA, Ashwood ER: *Tietz's Textbook of Clinical Chemistry.* 2nd ed. Saunders;1994.

III. Procedures

1. ARTERIAL LINE PLACEMENT

(See also Section I, Chapter 6, Arterial Line Problems, p 31.)

Indications. Frequent sampling of arterial blood; hemodynamic monitoring when continuous blood pressure readings are needed, such as a patient with malignant hypertension or a patient in shock, where indirect cuff pressures may be inaccurate.

Contraindications. Poor collateral circulation. Avoid the femoral artery if severe aortoiliac atherosclerosis is present. Coagulopathy is a relative contraindication. See Section I, Chapter 12, Coagulopathy, p 64.

Materials. 20-gauge (or smaller) 1.5- to 2-in. catheter-over-needle assembly (Angiocath), arterial line setup per ICU routine (transducer, tubing, and pressure bag with heparinized saline), armboard, sterile dressing, lidocaine.

Procedure

1. The radial artery is most frequently used; this approach is described here. Other sites, in decreasing order of preference, are the dorsalis pedis, femoral, brachial, and axillary arteries. Axillary arteries are infrequently used; catheters in these arteries should be placed by an intensivist or anesthesiologist.
2. Verify the patency of the collateral circulation between the radial and ulnar arteries using the **Allen test** See Section III, Chapter 2, Arterial Puncture, p 342.
3. Place the extremity on an armboard with a roll of gauze behind the wrist to hyperextend the joint. Prep with povidone-iodine and drape with sterile towels. The operator should wear gloves and a mask.
4. Raise a very small skin wheal at the puncture site with 1% lidocaine using a 25-gauge needle. Carefully palpate the artery and choose the puncture site where it appears most superficial.
5. While palpating the path of the artery with your nondominant hand, advance the 20-gauge catheter-over-needle assembly into the artery at a 30-degree angle to the skin with the needle bevel up. Once a "flash" of blood is seen in the hub, hold the needle steady and advance the entire unit 1–2 mm so that the needle and catheter are in the artery. Advance the catheter over the needle into the artery. Remove the needle whip briefly, occluding the artery with manual pressure and connect the pressure tubing.
6. Suture in place with 3-0 silk and apply a sterile dressing.
7. Splint the dorsum of the wrist to limit mobility and provide catheter stability.

8. Kits are available with a needle and guide wire that allow the Seldinger technique to be used, especially useful for femoral artery cannulation.
9. Arterial lines should be replaced using a different site every 4 days to decrease risk of infection.

Complications. Thrombosis, hematoma, arterial embolism, arterial spasm, infection, hemorrhage, pseudoaneurysm formation.

2. ARTERIAL PUNCTURE

Indications. Blood gas determination; need for arterial blood in chemistry determinations such as ammonia levels.

Contraindications. Systemic fibrinolytic states, such as following thrombolytic therapy, are relative contraindications to arterial puncture.

Materials. Blood gas sampling kit *or* 3– to 5–mL syringe, 23– to 25–gauge needle (20–22 gauge for femoral artery), 1 mL heparin (1000 U/mL), alcohol or povidone/iodine swabs, and a cup of ice.

Procedure

1. Use a heparinized syringe for blood gas and a nonheparinized syringe for chemistry determinations. Obtain a blood gas kit (contains a preheparinized syringe), or a small syringe (3–5 mL) with a small–gauge needle (23–25 gauge for radial artery, 20–22 gauge acceptable for femoral artery). Heparinize the syringe (if not preheparinized), by drawing up about 0.5–1 mL of heparin, pulling the plunger all the way back, and discarding the heparin.
2. Arteries, in the order of preference, are radial, femoral, and brachial. If using the radial artery, perform the **Allen test** to verify collateral flow from the ulnar artery. Have the patient make a tight fist. Occlude both the radial and ulnar arteries at the wrist and have the patient make a fist and release several times. Then have the patient open her or his hand. The hand should appear pale. While maintaining pressure on the radial artery, release the ulnar artery. If the ulnar-brachial arterial arch is patent, the entire hand should flush red within 10 seconds. If the Allen test is positive (the radial distribution will remain white beyond 10 seconds), the artery should not be used.
3. Hyperextension of the wrist joint or elbow will often bring the radial and brachial arteries closer to the surface.
4. If using the femoral artery, the mnemonic NAVEL will aid in locating the important structures in the groin. Palpate the femoral artery just two fingerbreadths below the inguinal ligament. From lateral to medial, the structures are **n**erve, **a**rtery, **v**ein, **e**mpty space, **l**ymphatic. You may wish to inject 1% lidocaine subcutaneously for anesthesia. Palpate the artery proximally and distally with two fingers, or trap the artery between two fingers placed on either side of the vessel.

5. Prep the area with either a povidone-iodine solution or an alcohol swab. Hold the syringe like a pencil with the needle bevel up and enter the skin at a 60–90-degree angle. Maintain slight negative pressure on the syringe.
6. Obtain blood on the downstroke or on slow withdrawal. Aspirate very slowly. A good arterial sample should require only minimal back pressure. If a glass or blood-gas syringe is used, the barrel will usually rise spontaneously. You should obtain 2–3 mL.
7. If the vessel cannot be located, redirect the needle without coming out of the skin.
8. Withdraw the needle quickly and apply *firm* pressure at the site for at least 5–10 minutes, even if the sample was not obtained, to avoid a hematoma.
9. If the sample is for a blood gas, expel any air from the syringe, mix the contents thoroughly by twirling the syringe between your fingers, and make the syringe airtight with a cap. Place the syringe on ice before the sample is processed.

Complications. Localized bleeding; thrombosis of the artery, which may lead to arterial insufficiency; infection.

3. ARTHROCENTESIS (DIAGNOSTIC AND THERAPEUTIC)

Indications:

Diagnostic: Arthrocentesis is helpful in the diagnosis of new-onset arthritis, and to rule out infection in acute or chronic unremitting joint effusion.

Therapeutic: The procedure is used to instill steroids and maintain drainage of septic arthritis.

Contraindications: None. Care must be taken, however, not to cause excessive trauma if a coagulopathy or thrombocytopenia is present or if the patient is taking anticoagulant medications.

Materials: Betadine, alcohol swabs, sterile gloves, lidocaine or ethyl chloride spray, an 18- or 20-gauge needle (a smaller-gauge needle if aspirating finger or toe joints), a large syringe (size depends on the amount of fluid present), a 3-mL syringe with a 25-gauge needle, and two heparinized tubes for cell count and crystal examination.

Discuss with your microbiology laboratory their preference for transporting fluid for bacterial, fungal, and acid-fast bacillus (AFB) cultures, and Gram's stain. A Thayer-Martin plate is needed if you suspect *Neisseria gonorrhoeae* (GC). A small syringe containing a long-acting corticosteroid such as Depo-Medrol or triamcinolone is optional for therapeutic arthrocentesis.

Procedure

General

1. Obtain consent. Describe the procedure and complications.
2. Determine the optimal site for aspiration and mark with indelible ink. Alternately, make an indentation in the skin with the retracted tip of a ball-point pen.
3. Wear gloves (universal precautions) to protect yourself against hepatitis and HIV. When aspiration is to be followed by corticosteroid injection, maintaining a sterile field with sterile implements minimizes the risk of infection to the patient.
4. Clean the area with betadine, and dry and wipe over the aspiration site with alcohol. Betadine can render cultures negative. Let the alcohol dry before beginning the procedure.
5. Anesthetize the area with lidocaine using a 25–gauge needle, taking care not to inject the solution into the joint space. Lidocaine is bactericidal. Avoid preparations containing epinephrine, especially in a small digit. Alternately, spray the area with ethyl chloride just prior to needle aspiration.
6. Insert the aspirating needle, applying a small amount of vacuum to the syringe. Remove as much fluid as possible, repositioning the syringe if necessary.
7. If a corticosteroid is to be injected, remove the aspirating syringe from the needle, which is still in the joint space. It is helpful to ensure that the syringe can easily be removed from the needle before undertaking Step 6. Attach the syringe containing the corticosteroid, pull back on the plunger to ensure that the needle is not in a vein, and inject contents. ***Caution:*** *Never inject steroids when there is a possibility that the joint is infected.* Remove the needle and syringe, and apply pressure to the area. Generally, the equivalent of 40 mg of methylprednisolone is injected into large joints such as the knee and 20 mg into medium-sized joints such as the ankle or wrist. Preparations of intra-articular steroids are equivalent in potency. Injections of 0.5 cc into the knee or shoulder and 0.25 cc into the ankle or wrist are recommended dosages.
8. Joint fluid is sent for cell count and differential, crystal exam, Gram's stain, and cultures for bacteria, fungi, and AFB as indicated. See Section I, Chapter 46, Joint Swelling, p 224.

Arthrocentesis of the Knee

1. The knee should be fully extended with the patient supine. Wait until the patient's quadriceps muscle has relaxed, as its contraction plants the patella against the femur, making aspiration painful.
2. Insert the needle posterior to the *medial* portion of the patella into the patellar-femoral groove. Direct the advancing needle slightly posteriorly and inferiorly. (See Figure 3–1.)

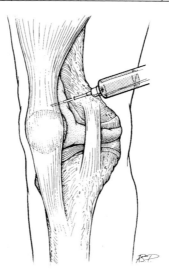

Figure 3–1. Arthrocentesis of the knee.

Arthrocentesis of the Wrist: The easiest site for aspiration lies between the navicular bone and radius on the dorsal wrist.

1. Locate the distal radius between the tendons of the extensor pollicus longus and the extensor carpi radialis longus of the second finger. This site is just ulnar to the anatomic snuff box.
2. Direct the needle perpendicular to the mark. (See Figure 3–2.)

Arthrocentesis of the Ankle

1. The most accessible site lies between the tibia and the talus. The angle of the foot to leg is positioned at 90 degrees. Make a mark lateral and anterior to the medial malleolus and medial and posterior to the tibialis anterior tendon. Direct the advancing needle posteriorly toward the heel.
2. The subtalar ankle joint does not communicate with the ankle joint and is difficult to aspirate even by an expert. Keep in mind that "ankle pain" may originate in the subtalar joint rather than in the ankle. (See Figure 3–3.)

Complications: Infection, bleeding, pain. Postinjection flareups of joint pain and swelling can occur after steroid injection and can persist up to 48

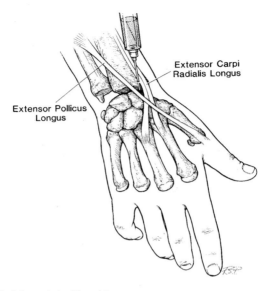

Figure 3–2. Arthrocentesis of the wrist.

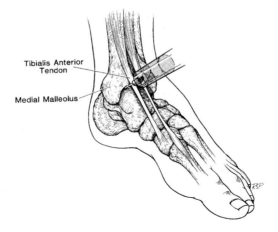

Figure 3–3. Arthrocentesis of the ankle.

hours. This complication is thought to be a crystal-induced synovitis resulting from the crystalline suspension used in long-acting steroids.

4. BLADDER CATHETERIZATION

(See also Section I, Chapter 23, Foley Catheter Problems, p 125.)

Indications: Relieve urinary retention; collect an uncontaminated urine sample; monitor urinary output in critically ill patients; perform bladder tests (cystogram, cystometrogram, determination of postvoid residual urine quantity).

Contraindications: Urethral disruption associated with pelvic fracture, acute prostatitis (relative).

Materials. Prepackaged Foley catheter tray (may need to add a catheter), catheter of choice (16- to 20-French Foley in adults).

Procedure

1. Have the patient in a well-lit area in a supine position. With females, knees should be flexed wide and heels placed together to adequately expose the meatus.
2. Open the kit and put on the gloves. Prepare all the materials before you attempt to insert the catheter. Open the prep solution and soak the cotton balls; apply the sterile drapes.
3. Inflate and deflate the balloon of the Foley catheter with 5–10 mL of sterile water to ensure proper functioning. Coat the end of the catheter with lubricant jelly.
4. In females, use one gloved hand to prep the urethral meatus in a pubis-toward-anus direction; hold the labia apart with the other gloved hand. With uncircumcised males, retract the foreskin to prep the glands; use a gloved hand to hold the penis still.
5. The hand used to hold the penis or labia should not touch the catheter while you are inserting it. You can use disposable forceps in the kit to insert the catheter, or use the forceps to prep; you can then insert the catheter with your gloved hand.
6. In males, stretch the penis upward perpendicular to the body to eliminate any folds in the urethra that might lead to a false passage. Use *gentle* pressure to slowly advance the catheter. Any significant resistance that is encountered may represent a stricture and requires urologic consultation. In males with benign prostatic hypertrophy (BPH), a Coude-tip catheter may facilitate passage. Other means to facilitate catheter passage are ensuring that the penis is well stretched; and instilling 30–50 mL of sterile surgical lubricant into the urethra with a catheter-tipped syringe.
7. In both males and females, insert the catheter to the hilt of the drainage end. Compress the penis toward the pubis. These maneu-

vers ensure that the balloon will be inflated in the bladder and not in the urethra. Inflate the balloon with 5–10 mL of sterile water. After inflation, pull the catheter back so that the balloon will come to rest against the bladder neck. There should be good urine return when the catheter is in place. **Caution:** *any male who is uncircumcised should have the foreskin repositioned to prevent massive edema of the glans after the catheter is inserted.*

8. If no urine returns, attempt to irrigate with 25–50 mL of sterile saline via a catheter-tipped syringe. **Note:** *A catheter that will not irrigate is in the urethra, not the bladder.*
9. Catheters in females can be taped to the leg. In males, the catheter should be taped to the abdominal wall to decrease urethral stricture formation (avoids catheter damage to urethra at penoscrotal junction).

Complications: Infection, bleeding, false passage.

5. BONE MARROW ASPIRATION AND BIOPSY

Indications: Evaluation of anemia, thrombocytopenia, leukopenia, leukocytosis, thrombocytosis, malignancy primary to the marrow (leukemia, myeloma) or metastatic to the marrow (lung cancer, breast cancer); evaluation of iron stores; evaluation for possible disseminated infection (tuberculosis, fungal disease).

Contraindications: Infection near the puncture site. Relative contraindications include severe coagulopathy or thrombocytopenia uncorrected by transfusion of cryoprecipitate fresh frozen plasma or platelets.

Materials: Commercial kits containing all necessary materials are presently available. If you do not have such a kit, you will need the following items: bone marrow biopsy needle (Jamshidi, Westerman, or similar type); sterile gloves and surgical drapes; iodine prep solution and alcohol; 22– and 26–gauge needles; at least two 10–mL syringes; 1% lidocaine solution; No. 11 scalpel blade, 4 × 4 gauze pads; and several microscope slides for staining.

Procedure

1. You must explain the procedure in detail to the patient or legally responsible individual and obtain their informed consent.
2. Local anesthesia is usually all that is required; however, it is reasonable to premedicate extremely anxious patients with an anxiolytic or sedative such as diazepam (Valium) or lorazepam (Ativan), or with an analgesic.
3. Bone marrow can be obtained from numerous sites, the most common being the sternum, the anterior iliac crest, and the posterior iliac crest. The posterior iliac crest is the safest and is the method de-

scribed here. The patient may be positioned on either the abdomen or on the side opposite the biopsy site.

4. Identify the posterior iliac crest with palpation and mark the desired biopsy site with indelible ink.

5. Use sterile gloves and follow strict aseptic technique for the remainder of the procedure.

6. Prep the biopsy site with sterile iodine solution and allow the skin to dry. Then wipe the site free of iodine with sterile alcohol. Next, cover the surrounding areas with surgical drapes.

7. Using a 26-gauge needle, administer 1% lidocaine solution subcutaneously to raise a skin wheal. Then, with the 22-gauge needle, infiltrate the deeper tissues with lidocaine until you reach the periosteum. At this point, you should advance the needle just through the periosteum and infiltrate lidocaine subperiosteally. An area approximately 2 cm in diameter should be infiltrated, using repeated periosteal punctures.

8. Once local anesthesia has been obtained, use a No. 11 scalpel blade to make a 2- to 3-mm skin incision over the biopsy site.

9. Insert the bone marrow biopsy needle through the skin incision; then advance it with a rotating motion that alternates between clockwise and counterclockwise rotation and gentle pressure until you reach the periosteum. Once the needle is firmly seated on the periosteum, advance it through the outer table of bone into the marrow cavity with the same rotating motion and gentle pressure. Generally, a slight change in the resistance to needle advancement signals entry into the marrow cavity. At this point, you should advance the needle 2–3 mm.

10. Remove the stylet from the biopsy needle and attach a 10-mL syringe to the hub of the biopsy needle. Withdraw the plunger on the syringe briskly and aspirate 1–2 mL of marrow into the syringe. The patient may experience severe, instantaneous pain. Slow withdrawal of the plunger or collection of more than 1–2 mL of marrow with each aspiration will result in excessive contamination of the specimen with peripheral blood.

11. The marrow aspiration specimen can be used to prepare coverslips for viewing under the microscope, and for special studies such as cytogenetics and cell markers or for culture. Repeat aspirations may be required to obtain enough marrow to perform all of the preceding tests. Also note that certain studies may require heparin or EDTA for collection. You should contact the appropriate laboratory prior to the procedure to be sure that you collect the specimens in the appropriate solution.

12. If a biopsy is to be obtained, replace the stylet and withdraw the needle. Reinsert the needle at a slightly different angle and location, still within the area of periosteum previously anesthetized. Once you have reentered the marrow cavity, remove the stylet again. Advance the needle 5–10 mm using the same alternating rotating motion with gentle pressure. Withdraw the needle several millimeters (but not

outside of the marrow cavity) and redirect it at a slightly different angle; then advance it again. Repeat this maneuver several times. 2–3 cm of core material should enter the needle. Rotate the needle rapidly on its long axis in a clockwise and then counterclockwise direction. This will sever the biopsy specimen from the marrow cavity. Withdraw the needle completely without replacing the stylet. Some operators prefer to hold their thumb over the open end of the needle to create a negative pressure in the needle as it is withdrawn. This may help to prevent loss of the core biopsy.

13. Remove the core biopsy from the needle by inserting a probe (provided with the biopsy needle) into the distal end of the needle and then gently pushing the specimen the full length of the needle and finally out the hub end. The direction is important, as an attempt to push the specimen out the distal end may damage the biopsy. Most biopsy needles are tapered at this end, presumably allowing the specimen to expand inside the needle and to prevent specimen loss when the needle is withdrawn from the patient.

14. The core biopsy is usually collected in formalin solution. Again, plans for special studies should be made prior to the procedure to allow for any special handling of the biopsy material.

15. Observe the biopsy site for excess bleeding and apply local pressure for several minutes. Clean the area thoroughly with alcohol and apply an adhesive strip or gauze patch. Instruct the patient to assume a supine position, and place a pressure pack between the bed or table and the biopsy site for 10–15 minutes. This is not an absolute requirement in patients without an underlying coagulopathy or thrombocytopenia, but will still serve to decrease local hematoma formation. Patients with an underlying tendency to bleed should maintain pressure for 20–25 minutes. A patient who is stable at this point may resume normal activities.

Complications: Local bleeding and hematoma, pain, possible infection.

6. CENTRAL VENOUS CATHETERIZATION

(See also Section I, Chapter 10, Central Venous Line Problems, p 51.)

Indications. Administration of fluids and medications when peripheral administration is impossible, inappropriate, or unreliable; hemodynamic monitoring; transvenous pacemaker placement.

Contraindications. A coagulopathy dictates the use of the femoral or median basilic vein approach to avoid bleeding complications.

Materials. Generally, two approaches are used to place central venous lines. One of these involves puncturing the vein with a relatively small needle through which a thin guide wire is placed in the vein. After the needle has been withdrawn, the intravascular appliance or a sheath through which a smaller catheter will be placed is introduced into the vein over the guide wire. The other technique involves puncturing the vein with a larger-bore needle through which the intravascular catheter will fit. There are commercially available disposable trays that provide all necessary needles, wires, sheaths, dilators, suture materials, and topical anesthetics. Some hospitals insist that these materials be assembled when central line placement becomes necessary. If needles, guide wires, and sheaths are collected from different places, it is very important to make sure that the needle will accept the guide wire, that the sheath and dilator will pass over the guide wire, and that the appliance to be passed through the sheath will indeed fit the inside lumen of the sheath. Supplies should include the following items:

1. Small needle (16–18 gauge)
2. Guide wire
3. 5- to 10-mL syringe
4. Scalpel
5. Intravascular appliance (triple-lumen catheter or a sheath through which a Swan-Ganz pulmonary artery catheter could be placed)
6. Heparinized flush solution: 1 mL of 1:100 U heparin in 10 mL of normal saline (to be used to fill all lumens prior to placement, to prevent clotting of the catheter during placement)
7. Lidocaine 1% with or without epinephrine
8. Povidone-iodine (Betadine) prep solution
9. Alcohol pads
10. Sterile towels
11. 4 × 4 gauze sponges
12. 21-gauge needle to draw up the lidocaine.

Also, sterile procedure is highly recommended (mask, sterile gown, and gloves).

Note: If the catheter is introduced through a large-bore needle, an appropriately-sized large-bore needle is required (12–14 gauge); a smaller needle and guide wire are not required. There seems to be little rationale for placement of a single-lumen catheter when multiple lumens can be installed for potential use at virtually the same risk. For these reasons, the ensuing discussion focuses on the over-the-guide wire technique and placement of either a triple-lumen catheter or a sheath through which a smaller catheter will eventually be placed.

Right Internal Jugular Vein Approach

Actually, three different sites are described and used in accessing the right internal jugular vein: (1) anterior (medial to the sternocleidomastoid muscle belly); (2) middle (between the two heads of the sternocleidomastoid muscle belly); and (3) posterior (lateral to the sternocleidomastoid muscle belly). The middle approach is most commonly used and has the advantage of well-defined landmarks.

Procedure

1. Sterilize the site with povidone-iodine and drape with sterile towels.
2. Administer local anesthesia with lidocaine in the area to be explored.
3. Place the patient in Trendelenburg (head down) position.
4. Use a small-bore thin-walled needle with syringe attached to locate the internal jugular vein. It may be helpful to have a small amount of anesthetic in the syringe to inject during exploration for the vein, if the patient notes some discomfort.
5. The internal diameter of the needle used to locate the internal jugular vein should be large enough to accommodate the passage of the guide wire.
6. Percutaneous entry should be made at the apex of the triangle formed by the two heads of the sternocleidomastoid muscle and the clavicle.
7. The needle should be directed slightly laterally toward the ipsilateral breast and kept as superficial as possible.
8. Often a notch can be palpated on the posterior surface of the clavicle. This actually can help locate the vein in the lateral/medial plane, as the vein lies deep to this shallow notch.
9. Successful puncture of the vein is accomplished at an unnerving depth of needle insertion, and is heralded by sudden aspiration of nonpulsatile venous blood.
10. After the needle is detached from the syringe, the guide wire should pass with ease all the way to the right atrium. Once the wire is passed, remove the needle.
11. Leave enough wire outside the patient to accommodate the length of the intravascular catheter, sheath, etc., **with an adequate amount to allow control over the distal end of the guide wire at all times.**
12. Nick the skin with a No. 11 scalpel blade.
13. The catheter or sheath should be introduced over the guide wire while the depth of the guide wire is kept relatively constant, to avoid irritation of the right atrium or ventricle and possible ventricular ectopy.
14. When the sheath or catheter is placed over the guide wire, the proximal end of the guide wire should be held until the catheter or sheath completely passes over the distal end of the guide wire.
15. Then the distal end of the guide wire is controlled while the catheter or sheath is advanced through the incised skin and into the vein.
16. Once the catheter or sheath is in place, the guide wire is removed.
17. An occlusive sterile dressing should be applied.
18. A chest x-ray should be obtained to verify position of the line as well as to identify complications such as a pneumothorax.

Complications

1. Remarkably safe; the literature describes literally thousands of attempts uncomplicated by pneumothorax.
2. It is likely that errant attempts at internal jugular puncture will end up in the mediastinum. It is possible to perforate endotracheal tube cuffs by this approach. This is usually not a subtle event and generally requires prompt replacement of the now faulty endotracheal tube before safe deep line placement can proceed.
3. The other procedural miscue is inadvertent puncture of the carotid artery. This commonly occurs if the needle is inserted medial to where it should be on the middle approach; it is also common with the anterior approach. With arterial puncture, the syringe fills without negative pressure because of arterial pressure, and bright red blood pulsates from the needle after the syringe is removed. The needle should be removed and manual pressure applied for 10–15 minutes to ensure adequate hemostasis.
4. A chest x-ray should always be obtained after the procedure to check for positioning of the catheter and to rule out pneumothorax.

Advantages. Central venous access from this site allows virtually every potential use of the deep line, including hemodynamic assessment (both central venous pressure and pulmonary artery measurements are easily done), temporary pacemaker placement, endomyocardial biopsy, as well as administration of fluids, drugs, and parenteral nutrition.

Disadvantages

1. The major disadvantage of this site is patient discomfort. The site is difficult to dress, and is uncomfortable for patients who have the capacity to turn their heads.
2. The risk of infectious contamination for this line is intermediate between that for femoral lines and that for subclavian lines, and is probably related to the difficulty in keeping the site occlusively dressed.

Left Internal Jugular Vein Approach

The left internal jugular vein is not commonly used for central line placement. Better options exist and should be exhausted before resorting to this approach.

Procedure. Similar to right internal jugular vein approach.

Complications. In addition to the usual procedural complications common to central lines, this approach has some unique complications.

1. There are case reports of inadvertent left brachiocephalic vein and superior vena cava puncture with intravascular wires, catheters, and sheaths.
2. Laceration of the thoracic duct.

Advantages. None over right internal jugular vein approach.

Disadvantages. See complications for right internal jugular vein approach. Laceration of the thoracic duct and puncture of the left brachiocephalic vein and superior vena cava are also possible.

Subclavian Approach (Left or Right)

Procedure

1. A small rolled-up towel placed between the shoulder blades facilitates this approach.
2. Place the patient in the Trendelenburg position.
3. Use sterile preparation and appropriate draping.
4. Anesthetize the skin with local anesthetic.
5. Percutaneous entry is then made at the distal third of the clavicle.
6. A small amount of topical anesthetic in the syringe can be used to anesthetize periosteal surfaces while the vein is located, but hopefully only one puncture will be needed.
7. The guide wire should fit inside the lumen of the needle used to find the vein.
8. Direct the needle under the clavicle, above the first rib and toward the jugular notch. (See Figure 3–4.)
9. Apply constant negative pressure while the needle is advanced.
10. Successful entry is marked by free flow of nonpulsatile venous blood.

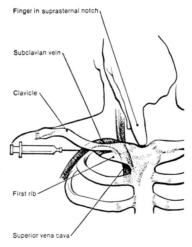

Figure 3–4. Technique for catheterization of the subclavian vein. (Reproduced, with permission, from Gomella, LG, ed. *Clinician's Pocket Reference.* 7th ed. Appleton & Lange; 1993:211.)

11. The patient's head should be directed to face the operator while the guide wire is inserted. This facilitates guide wire placement down the superior vena cava as opposed to up the internal jugular vein.
12. Remove the syringe.
13. Advance the guide wire through the needle.
14. The guide wire should slide easily through the needle, essentially to the hub of the needle.
15. If there is resistance to passage of the guide wire, it is important to reattach the syringe and reposition the needle so that the blood flows freely.
16. If the resistance is more distal than the tip of the needle, the guide wire is likely coursing cephalad at the internal jugular vein (an awake patient may remark that the ipsilateral ear hurts). Another pass of the guide wire with the entry needle pulled back slightly is appropriate. Placing the guide wire in the internal jugular vein from the subclavian approach accomplishes nothing. The catheter placed over the guide wire will also end up in the internal jugular vein.
17. Once the guide wire is passed, remove the needle.
18. Follow steps 11 through 18 for placement via the right internal jugular vein.

Complications

1. Arterial puncture is usually obvious, as bright red blood spurts from the needle when the syringe is detached or the syringe spontaneously fills without negative pressure. The needle is then withdrawn and manual pressure applied to stop arterial bleeding. Significant bleeding deep to the clavicle may occur and is heavily dependent on the patient's coagulation system and the size of the puncture. This underscores the importance of knowing the patient's coagulation profile before making the decision of central line placement.
2. Pneumothorax can be detected when a sudden gush of air is aspirated instead of blood. A postprocedure chest x-ray should always be done to rule out pneumothorax and check for line placement. A pneumothorax requires chest tube placement in virtually all cases, especially when the patient is being supported on a ventilator. The left-sided approach is associated with higher risk for pneumothorax because of the higher dome of the left pleura compared with the right.
3. Hemothorax.
4. Air embolus.

Advantages

1. The left subclavian approach affords a gentle, sweeping curve to the apex of the right ventricle, and is the preferred entry site for placement of a temporary transvenous pacemaker without fluoroscopic assistance.

2. Hemodynamic measurements are often easier to record from the left subclavian approach.
3. From the left subclavian vein approach, the catheters do not have to negotiate an acute angle as is commonly the case at the junction of the right subclavian with the right brachiocephalic vein en route to the superior vena cava. This is also a common site for kinking of the deep line.
4. Lowest risk of infection of various central line sites.

Disadvantages. Risk of pneumothorax.

Femoral Vein Approach

The femoral line is an option probably underutilized in critical care settings.

Procedure

1. Place the patient in the supine position.
2. Use sterile preparation and appropriate draping. Administer local anesthesia in the area to be explored.
3. Palpate the femoral artery.
4. Guard the artery with the fingers of one hand.
5. Explore for the vein just medial to the operator's fingers with a needle and syringe.
6. It may be helpful to have a small amount of anesthetic in the syringe to inject with exploration.
7. The needle is directed cephalad at about a 30-degree angle and should be inserted below the femoral crease.
8. Puncture is heralded by the return of venous, nonpulsatile blood on application of negative pressure to the syringe.
9. Advance the guide wire through the needle.
10. The guide wire should pass with ease into the vein to a depth at which the distal tip of the guide wire is always under the operator's control. The operator should maintain control of the guide wire at its entry point through the skin while passing the sheath/dilator or catheter over the distal end of the wire.
11. Remove the needle once the guide wire has advanced into the femoral vein.
12. If the catheter is 6-French or larger, a skin incision with a scalpel blade is generally needed. The catheter can then be advanced along with the guide wire in unison into the femoral vein. **Be sure always to control the distal end of the guide wire.**
13. Follow steps 14 through 17 for the right internal jugular vein approach.

Complications

1. The femoral deep line has the highest incidence of contamination and sepsis. If an occlusive dressing can remain in place and remain free from contamination, this is a safe option.

2. Deep vein thrombosis (DVT) has occurred from femoral vein catheterization as well as with other sites. The risk for DVT increases if the catheter remains in place for prolonged periods.

Advantages

1. The procedure is safe, in that arterial and venous sites are compressible. This route or the median basilic vein approach is preferred in the presence of a coagulopathy or severe lung disease.
2. It is impossible to cause pneumothorax from this site.
3. Placement can be accomplished without interrupting cardiopulmonary resuscitation.
4. This site can be used to place a variety of intravascular appliances, including temporary pacemakers, pulmonary artery catheters (expertise with fluoroscopy is needed), and triple-lumen catheters.

Disadvantages

1. This approach has the highest rate of infection.
2. Fluoroscopy is required for placement of pulmonary artery catheters or transvenous pacemakers.

Median Basilic Vein Approach

It is possible in some patients, particularly men with well-developed upper extremities, to place an 8-French-sized introducer into the median basilic vein. The median basilic vein is directed medially at the antecubital fossa. The cephalic vein runs laterally at the antecubital fossa and should not be relied on to pass a deep line because the line will commonly hang up at the origin of the axillary vein. Passage to the central circulation may occur via the cephalic vein, but should be tested using a long, thin guide wire and fluoroscopy before this approach is counted on for central access.

Procedure

1. Use sterile preparation with appropriate draping.
2. Administer local anesthesia with lidocaine.
3. Place an intracath needle into the vein through which the guide wire will pass.
4. Advance the guide wire through the intracath.
5. Once the guide wire has passed into the median vein, remove the intracath.
6. Incise the skin with a No. 11 scalpel. Advance the sheath/dilator system or triple-lumen catheter over the wire and into the vein **while controlling either the proximal or distal end of the guide wire at all times.**
7. Follow steps 14 through 17 for the right internal jugular vein approach.

Complications. Thrombophlebitis (line should be removed in 48–72 hours).

Advantages

1. Noncompressible bleeding is avoided. This route or the femoral route is preferred in the presence of coagulopathy or severe lung disease.
2. No risk of pneumothorax.

Disadvantages

1. Cannot be used in all patients.
2. Fluoroscopy is required for placement of pulmonary artery catheters or temporary pacemakers.
3. Uncomfortable and immobilizing.

7. ENDOTRACHEAL INTUBATION

(See also Section VI, Ventilator Management, p 387.)

Indications. Airway management during cardiopulmonary resuscitation; any indication for using mechanical ventilation, such as coma or respiratory failure.

Contraindications. (Relative) massive maxillofacial trauma; fractured larynx; suspected cervical spinal cord injury. Nasotracheal intubation is contraindicated in suspected basilar skull fractures. Fiberoptic intubation or tracheostomy may be indicated in those instances.

Materials. Endotracheal tube (ETT), usually 7.0–9.0 mm internal diameter for most adults; laryngoscope handle and blade (No. 3 straight or curved); 10-mL syringe; adhesive tape; suction equipment; malleable stylet (optional).

Procedure

1. Orotracheal intubation is most commonly used and is described here. The use of orotracheal intubation should be strongly discouraged in the case of suspected cervical spine injuries; nasotracheal intubation is preferred.
2. Any patient who is hypoxic or apneic must be ventilated with 100% oxygen using a bag and mask prior to attempting endotracheal intubation. Remember to avoid prolonged periods without ventilation if the intubation is difficult.
3. Extend the laryngoscope blade to 90 degrees to verify that the light is working and check the balloon on the tube for leaks.
4. Place the patient's head in the so-called "sniffing position" (neck flexed anteriorly and head extended posteriorly). Use suction to clear the upper airway if needed.

5. Hold the laryngoscope in the left hand, hold the mouth open with the right hand, insert blade in the right side of the mouth and use the blade to push the tongue to the patient's left making certain the tongue remains anterior to the blade. Advance carefully toward the midline until the epiglottis is seen.

6. With the *straight laryngoscope blade* pass the blade under the epiglottis, and lift the blade upward; the vocal cords or arytenoid cartilage should be visualized. If they are not visualized, first slowly back out the laryngoscope and watch for the vocal cords to "pop" into view. Secondly, ask an assistant to press down on the thyroid cartilage ("apply cricoid pressure"). When using a *curved* blade, place it anterior to the epiglottis and gently lift anteriorly. The handle should not be used to pry the epiglottis open, but rather should be gently lifted in both cases. (See Figure 3–5.) Thrust the left arm upward at a 45-degree angle so as to avoid back pressure on the teeth.

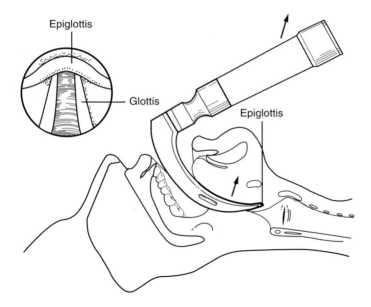

Figure 3–5. Endotracheal intubation. Advance blade to groove between base of tongue and epiglottis. (Reproduced, with permission, from Vander Salm TJ, ed. *Atlas of Bedside Procedures.* 2nd ed. Little, Brown;1988:21.)

7. While maintaining visualization of the cords, grasp the ETT in the right hand and pass it through the cords. With more difficult intubations, a malleable stylet can be used to direct the tube.
8. Gently inflate the balloon with air from a 10-mL syringe until there is an adequate seal (about 5 mL). Ventilate the patient while auscultating in the axillary areas and visualizing both sides of the chest to verify positioning. If the left side does not seem to be ventilating, it may signify that the tube has been advanced down the right mainstem bronchus. Withdraw the tube 1–2 cm and recheck the breath sounds. Confirm positioning with a stat chest x-ray.
9. Tape the tube in position and insert an oropharyngeal airway to prevent the patient from biting the ETT.

Complications. Bleeding; oral or pharyngeal trauma; improper tube positioning (esophageal or right mainstream bronchus intubation); aspiration; obstruction of the ETT or kinking.

REFERENCE

Einarsson O, Rochester CL, Rosenbaum SH: Airway management in respiratory emergencies. Clin Chest Med 1994;15:13.

8. GASTROINTESTINAL TUBES

Indications: Gastrointestinal (GI) decompression (paralytic ileus, obstruction, postoperatively); lavage of the stomach for GI bleeding or drug overdose; prevention of aspiration in obtunded patient (you should protect the airway by endotracheal intubation first); feeding a patient who is unable to swallow.

Contraindications: Nasal fractures, basilar skull fracture.

Materials: Gastrointestinal tube of choice, lubricant jelly, catheter tip syringe, glass of water with straw, stethoscope.

1. **Nasogastric tubes**
   a. **Levine:** Single-lumen tube that must be placed on intermittent suction to evacuate gastric contents.
   b. **Salem sump:** The best tube for continuous suction. The Salem sump is a double-lumen tube, with the smaller tube acting as an air intake vent. Use 14- to 18-French size in adults.
   c. **Ewald:** Large (18–36 French) double-lumen tube, especially suited for gastric lavage of drug overdoses; more often inserted by the orogastric route.
2. **Feeding tubes.** Although any small-bore nasogastric tube can be used as a feeding tube, certain weighted tubes are designed to pass into the duodenum and decrease the risk of aspiration of gastric contents.
   a. **Dobhoff, Entriflex, Keogh:** These have a weighted mercury tip with stylet.

      b. Vivonex: Tungsten-tipped.
3. **Sengsten-Blakemore tube:** A triple-lumen tube used exclusively for tamponade of esophageal varices to control bleeding. One lumen is for aspiration, one is for the gastric balloon, and the third is for the esophageal balloon.

Procedure

1. Inform the patient of the nature of the procedure and encourage them to cooperate. Choose the nasal passage that appears most patent by occluding one nostril and having the patient sniff.
2. Lubricate the distal 3–4 in. of the tube with a water-soluble jelly (K-Y Jelly or viscous 2% lidocaine) and insert the tube gently along the floor of the nasal passageway. Maintain gentle pressure that will allow the tube to pass into the nasopharynx. Running the tube under warm water prior to lubrication makes it more pliable and may help facilitate its placement. Flexing the head also helps facilitate passage of the tube.
3. When the patient can feel the tube in the back of the throat, ask him or her to swallow small amounts of water through a straw as you advance the tube 2–3 in. at a time.
4. To be sure that the tube is in the stomach, aspirate gastric contents or blow air into the tube and listen over the stomach with your stethoscope for a "pop" or "gurgle."
5. Attach sump tubes (Salem sump) to "continuous low wall suction" and the single-lumen tube (Levine) to "intermittent suction".
6. Feeding tubes are more difficult to insert because they are more flexible. You can use a stylet or guide wire, or attach the smaller tube to a larger, stiffer tube by wedging both into a gelatin capsule. Pass the tube in the usual fashion and allow it to remain in the stomach for 10–15 minutes. After this time, the capsule will dissolve and the larger tube can be removed.
7. Always verify the position of feeding tubes by chest x-ray before beginning feedings.
8. Tape the tube securely in place but do not allow it to apply pressure to the nasal ala. Patients have been disfigured by ischemic necrosis of the nose caused by a poorly positioned tube.

Complications: Inadvertent passage into the trachea; coiling of the tube in the mouth or pharynx; bleeding from the nose, pharynx, or stomach.

9. INTRAVENOUS TECHNIQUES

    Indications. To establish intravenous access for the administration of fluids, blood, or medications.
    Materials. Intravenous fluid, connecting tubing, tourniquet, alcohol swab, intravenous cannulas (a catheter over a needle, such as Intracath,

Angiocath, and Jelco or a butterfly needle), antiseptic ointment, dressing, and tape. You will find it helpful to rip the tape into strips and to flush the air out of the tubing with the intravenous fluid before you begin the procedure.

Procedure

1. An upper, nondominant extremity is the site of choice for an IV. Choose a distal vein so that if the vein is damaged, you can reposition the IV more proximally. Avoid veins that cross a joint space. Also avoid the leg, as there is a high incidence of superficial thrombophlebitis. If no extremity vein can be found, try the external jugular vein. If all these fail, the only alternative is a central line or a cutdown.

2. Apply a tourniquet above the proposed IV site. Techniques to help expose difficult-to-locate veins include (1) wrapping the extremity in a warm towel; (2) leaving the arm in a dependent position for a few minutes after the tourniquet is applied; or (3) using a blood pressure cuff as a tourniquet, inflated so that the arterial flow is still maintained. Carefully clean the site with an alcohol or povidone-iodine swab. If a large-bore IV is to be used (16 or 14 French), local anesthesia with 1% lidocaine may be helpful.

3. Stabilize the vein distally with the thumb of your free hand. Using the catheter-over-needle assembly (Intracath or Angiocath), enter the skin alongside the vein first, and then stick the vein along the side at about a 20-degree angle. Once the vein is punctured, blood should appear in the "flash" chamber. Advance 4–5 mm to be sure that BOTH the needle AND the tip of the catheter have entered the vein. Carefully withdraw the needle as you advance the catheter into the vein. (See Figure 3–6.) *Never withdraw the catheter over the needle as this procedure can shear off the plastic tip and cause a catheter embolus.* Apply pressure with your thumb over the vein just proximal to the site, to prevent significant blood loss while you connect the IV line to the catheter.

4. Observe the site with the IV fluid running, for signs of induration or swelling that indicate improper placement or damage to the vein.

5. Tape the IV securely in place; apply a drop of povidone-iodine or antibiotic ointment and a sterile dressing at the puncture site over the needle. Ideally, the dressing should be changed every 24–48 hours to help reduce infections. Armboards are also useful to help maintain an IV site, especially near a joint.

6. If the veins are deep and difficult to locate, a small 3- to 5-mL syringe can be mounted on the catheter assembly. Proper position inside the vein is determined by aspiration of blood.

7. If venous access is limited, a "butterfly" needle can be used (see Figure 3–7); or the external jugular vein may be considered as an alternative site.

8. All intravenous lines should be changed every 72 hours to decrease the risk of infection.

Complications. Thrombophlebitis; localized infection or sepsis.

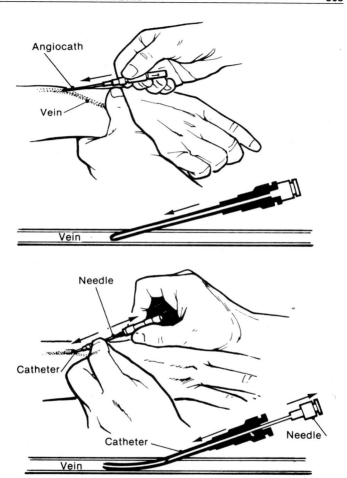

Figure 3–6. To insert a catheter-over-needle assembly into a vein, stabilize the skin and vein with gentle traction. Enter the vein and advance the catheter while holding the needle steady; then remove the needle. (Reproduced, with permission, from Gomella, LG, ed. *Clinician's Pocket Reference.* 7th ed. Appleton & Lange;1993:234.)

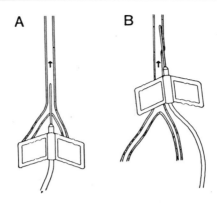

Figure 3–7. Two techniques for entering the vein for intravenous access: **(A)** direct puncture; and **(B)** side entry. (Reproduced, with permission, from Gomella TL ed. *Neonatology: Management, Procedures, On-Call Problems, Diseases and Drugs.* Appleton & Lange;1994;165.)

10. LUMBAR PUNCTURE

Indications. Diagnostic purposes; measurement of cerebrospinal fluid pressure; injection of various agents (contrast media, chemotherapy).

Contraindications. Increased intracranial pressure (papilledema, mass lesion); infection near the puncture site; planned myelography or pneumoencephalography; coagulopathy (see Section I, Chapter 12, Coagulopathy, p 64).

Materials. A sterile, disposable lumbar puncture (LP) kit or minor procedure tray, spinal needles (21-gauge), sterile specimen tubes.

Procedure
1. Examine the optic disc for evidence of papilledema, and review the CT (computed tomographic) scan of the head if available. Remember, a CT scan must be done prior to a lumbar puncture if there is papilledema or any focal neurologic findings.
2. Place the patient in the lateral decubitus position close to the edge of the bed or table. The patient (held by an assistant, if possible) should be positioned with knees pulled up toward the stomach and head flexed on the chest. This enhances flexion of the vertebral spine and widens the interspaces between the spinous processes. Try to position the patient so that the hips and shoulders are perpendicular to the bed. Place a pillow beneath the patient's side between the iliac crest and inferior costal margin, to prevent sagging

and ensure alignment of the spinal column. In an obese patient, or a patient with arthritis or scoliosis, the sitting position, leaning forward, may be preferred.

3. Draw an imaginary line between the iliac crests. This should cross the spine at the L4 vertebral body and assist in locating the L4–L5 interspace. You may want to make a mark in the skin with your fingernail in the middle of the L4–L5 interspace prior to sterilizing the area for easier identification later.

4. Open the kit, put on sterile gloves, and prep the area with povidone-iodine solution in a circular fashion, starting at the center and covering several interspaces. This step will need to be repeated twice. Next, drape the patient.

5. With a 25-gauge needle and 1% lidocaine, raise a skin wheal over the L4–L5 interspace. Anesthetize the deeper structures with a 22-gauge needle.

6. Examine the spinal needle and stylet for defects; and then insert the 20-gauge needle with stylet into the skin wheal and into the spinous ligament. Use an 18-gauge needle in arthritic or obese patients, in that landmarks are easier to feel with a larger needle. Hold the needle between the index fingers of both hands, with your thumbs holding the hub of the needle and stylet, and guiding the needle. Direct the needle perpendicular to the long axis of the spine and parallel to the bed. Aim the needle toward the umbilicus. (See Figure 3–8.)

7. Advance the needle through the major structures and "pop" into the subarachnoid space through the dura. An experienced operator can feel these layers, but an inexperienced one may need to remove the stylet periodically every 2–3 mm to look for return of fluid. Direct the bevel of the needle parallel to the long axis of the body so that the dural fibers are separated rather than sheared. This method helps to minimize "spinal headaches."

8. If no fluid returns, it is sometimes helpful to rotate the needle slightly. If there is still no fluid, and you think that you are in the subarachnoid space, 1 mL of air can be injected as it is not uncommon for a piece of tissue to clog the needle. **NEVER** inject saline or distilled water. If spinal fluid cannot be aspirated, the bevel of the needle probably lies in the epidural space; advance it with the stylet in place.

9. If unsuccessful in the L4–L5 interspace, attempt the procedure one interspace above or below the current location.

10. When fluid returns, attach a manometer and stopcock, and measure the pressure. Normal opening pressure is 70–180 mm water. Increased pressure may result from congestive heart failure (CHF), ascites, subarachnoid hemorrhage, infection, or a space-occupying lesion. Decreased pressure may result from needle position, obstructed flow, or severe volume depletion.

11. Collect 0.5- to 2.0-mL samples in serial, labeled containers. Send them to the lab in this order:

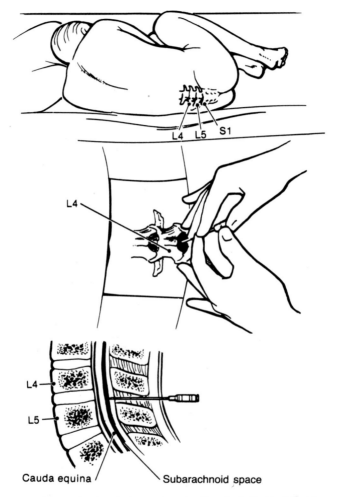

Figure 3–8. When performing a lumbar puncture, place the patient in the lateral decubitus position and locate the L4–L5 interspace. Control the spinal needle with two hands and enter the subarachnoid space. (Reproduced, with permission, from Gomella LG, ed. *Clinician's Pocket Reference.* 7th ed. Appleton & Lange;1993:239.)

- Tube 1 for cell count and differential;
- Tube 2 for glucose and protein;
- Tube 3 for bacterial culture and gram stain;
- Tube 4 for cell count and differential and special studies: VDRL, AFB, and fungal smear and culture; cryptococcal antigen; and counterimmune electrophoresis (CIE) or latex agglutination for *Streptococcus pneumoniae, Haemophilus influenzae, Neisseria meningitidis*, as well as two less commonly found organisms, beta-hemolytic streptococci and *Staphylococcus aureus*.

Obtaining cell counts from tubes 1 and 4 permits better differentiation between a subarachnoid hemorrhage and a traumatic tap. In a traumatic tap, the number of red blood cells in the first tube should be much higher than that in the last tube. In a subarachnoid hemorrhage, the cell counts should be similar. Xanthochromia indicates the presence of old blood, and suggests subarachnoid hemorrhage rather than a traumatic tap.

12. Withdraw the needle and place a sterile dressing over the site.
13. Instruct the patient to remain recumbent for 12–24 hours, and encourage an increased fluid intake to help prevent "spinal headaches." Interpret the results based on Table 3–1.

Complications. Spinal headache (the most common complication, seen about 20% of the time) typically is improved by recumbency and aggravated by upright posture. Its onset usually occurs within 24–48 hours of the procedure, but may occur up to 1 week after the procedure. To help prevent spinal headaches, keep the patient recumbent for 12–24 hours, encourage the intake of fluids, use the smallest needle possible, and keep the bevel of the needle parallel to the long axis of the body to help prevent a persistent cerebrospinal fluid leak. If the headache is persistent and resistant to usual measures, consult an anesthesiologist, as a "blood patch" should be considered. Other complications include trauma to nerve roots, herniation of either the cerebellum or the medulla, and meningitis.

TABLE 3-1. DIFFERENTIAL DIAGNOSIS OF CEREBROSPINAL FLUID.[1]

Condition	Color	Opening Pressure (mm H$_2$O)	Protein (mg/100 mL)	Glucose (mg/100 mL)	Cells (per mL)
Adult (normal)	Clear	70–180	15–45	45–80	0–5 lymphs
Viral infection	Clear or opalescent	Normal or slightly increased	Normal or slightly increased	Normal	10–500 lymphs (polys early)
Bacterial infection	Opalescent or yellow, may clot	Increased	50–1500	Decreased, usually <20	25–10,000 polys
Granulomatous (TB, fungal)	Clear or opalescent	Often increased	Increased but usually <500	Decreased, usually 20–40	10–500 lymphs
Subarachnoid hemorrhage	Bloody or usually xanthochromic after 2–8 hours	Usually increased	Increased	Normal	WBC/RBC ratio of CSF same as blood Cell count tube 1 equals tube 4

WBC = white blood cell; RBC = red blood cell; lymphs = lymphocytes; polys = polymorphonuclear leukocytes; TB = tuberculosis.
[1] Modified and reproduced with permission from Gomella LG, ed: *Clinician's Pocket Reference.* 7th ed.: Appleton & Lange; 1993.

11. PARACENTESIS

Indications: Determination of the cause of ascites; ruling out bacterial peritonitis; therapeutic removal of fluid in patients with tense ascites for symptomatic relief (early satiety, abdominal discomfort, dyspnea).

Contraindications. Coagulopathy (relative); multiple prior abdominal operations; uncooperative patient.

Materials: Minor procedure tray; Angiocath or Jelco assembly (18- to 20-gauge with a 1-1/2-in. needle); 20–60-mL syringe; sterile specimen containers.

Procedure

1. Obtain informed consent. The patient's bladder needs to be empty.
2. If there is any doubt about the presence of ascites, confirmation should be made by abdominal ultrasound. If the amount of ascites is small, ultrasound can be used to help locate the fluid during the procedure.
3. The entry site is usually the midline, 3–4 cm below the umbilicus. Avoid old surgical scars since bowel may adhere to the abdominal wall. Alternately, you can locate an entry site in the left or right lower quadrant midway between the umbilicus and the anterior superior iliac spine (lateral to the rectus sheath).
4. Prep the patient's skin with povidone-iodine solution and drape him or her. Raise a skin wheal with 1% lidocaine over the proposed entry site.
5. With the Angiocath mounted on the syringe, advance the needle into the anesthetized area carefully while gently aspirating. You will meet some resistance as you enter the fascia. When you get free return of fluid, leave the catheter in place, remove the needle, reattach the syringe, and aspirate. Sometimes it is necessary to reposition the catheter because of abutting bowel or bowel wall.
6. Aspirate the amount of fluid needed for tests (30–50 mL). Bedside inoculation of blood culture bottles with ascitic fluid increases the sensitivity of cultures. For a therapeutic tap, a 16–18-gauge needle can be connected to vacuum bottles with phlebotomy tubing. Large-volume paracentesis (up to 5 liters) can be safely performed in patients with tense ascites if the fluid is removed over a period of 60–90 minutes.
7. Remove the needle quickly, apply a sterile 4 × 4 gauze, and apply pressure to the site with tape.
8. Depending on the patient's clinical picture, send samples for albumin, total protein, glucose,lactate dehydrogenase, amylase, cell count and differential, Gram's stain, bacterial culture, acid-fast bacillus and fungal smears, and cultures and cytology. See Table 3–2 for differential diagnosis of the fluid obtained.

TABLE 3–2. TESTING OF ASCITIC FLUID.

1) Albumin gradient
   $ALB_{serum} - ALB_{ascites} = X$
      If X > 1.1 g/dL, then portal hypertension
      If X < 1.1 g/dL, then no portal hypertension
2) Total Protein < 1.0 g/dL, high risk for spontaneous bacterial peritonitis
3) Cell Count—absolute neutrophil count > 250/μL, presume infected
4) Bacterial Culture: Blood culture bottles 85% sensitivity
                      Routine cultures 50% sensitivity
5) Bacterial Peritonitis—Spontaneous versus secondary
      Secondary: A) polymicrobial, B) total protein > 1.0 g/dL; C) LDH > normal serum
         value; D) glucose < 50 mg/dL
6) Food fibers: Found in most causes of perforated viscus
7) Cytology: Bizarre cells with large nuclei may represent reactive mesothelial cells and *not* a
   malignancy. Malignant cells suggest a tumor.

Complications: Peritonitis; perforated bowel; intra-abdominal hemorrhage; perforated bladder.

REFERENCES

Runyon BA: Care of patients with ascites. N Engl J Med 1994;330:337.
Runyon BA, Montano AA, Akriviadis EA et al: The serum-ascites albumin gradient is superior to the exudate-transudate concept in the differential diagnosis of ascites. Ann Intern Med 1992;117:215.

12. PULMONARY ARTERY CATHETERIZATION

(See also Section I, Chapter 55, Pulmonary Artery Catheter Problems, p 265.)

Indications: Pulmonary artery catheterization is generally undertaken in acutely ill patients when a question exists regarding the patient's volume status or cardiac output. Some specific examples include (1) differentiating the etiology of pulmonary infiltrates between congestive heart failure and acute respiratory distress syndrome (ARDS) or pneumonia; (2) determining whether poor urine output is due to volume depletion, acute renal failure, or poor forward cardiac output; and (3) determining whether a patient with acute myocardial infarction and tachycardia has volume depletion, stress, or left ventricular failure.

Contraindications: If a pulmonary artery catheter is needed to manage a patient in a critical care setting, there are no absolute contraindications. As with all indwelling catheters that involve frequent manipulation, pulmonary artery catheters should be changed every 3 to 4 days to avoid the increased likelihood of an infection.

Materials: In most institutions, a single brand of a flow-directed balloon-tipped pulmonary artery catheter (often called a Swan-Ganz catheter) is available. Use an insertion kit that provides the catheter as well as a sheath and the various syringes, needles, preparation material, local anesthetic, and other items that will be used to insert the catheter.

The pulmonary artery catheter has four or five ports: air inflation port, thermistor, distal port, right atrial port, and (in some) a port for fluid or medication administration. (See Figure 3–9.) The air inflation port is used to inflate the balloon to facilitate passage of the catheter from the right cardiac chambers to the pulmonary artery. The thermistor can be used to measure cardiac outputs by thermal dilution when connected to a cardiac output computer. The distal port is used to measure pulmonary artery pressure and pulmonary capillary wedge pressure (PCWP) with the catheter in the pulmonary artery. The right atrial port is used to administer fluids, to measure right atrial pressure, or to inject fluid to measure cardiac output in conjunction with the thermistor and the cardiac output computer. (See Figure 3–9.) The catheter is often marked so that the clinician can determine how

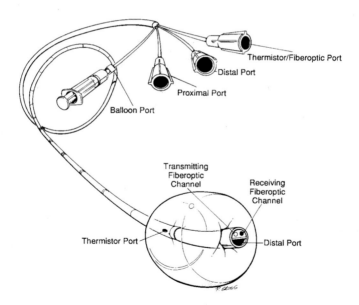

Figure 3–9. An example of a pulmonary artery catheter. This one features an oximetric measuring feature. (Reproduced, with permission, from Gomella, LG ed., *Clinician's Pocket Reference.* 7th ed. Appleton & Lange;1993:362.)

far the distal tip lies from the entry site. This information may help in catheter placement without fluoroscopy.

Procedure

1. The patient's informed consent is usually required.
2. Choose the site of operation; prep and drape the area. The choice of site is dictated by patient variables and operator experience. The easiest sites to place a pulmonary artery catheter without fluoroscopic guidance are the right internal jugular vein and the left subclavian vein. In a patient receiving thrombolytic therapy, femoral and median basilic veins are preferable routes.
3. In general, use a strict sterile approach with gown, gloves, and mask.
4. Prepare the pulmonary artery catheter by flushing the lumens with heparinized saline solution (1 mL of 1:100 U heparin in 10 mL of normal saline). Check the balloon function, and tap the catheter to be sure that an appropriate waveform is present. You should set the pressure transducer level to the middle of the patient's chest.
5. Cannulate the central vein. (See Section III, Chapter 6, Central Venous Catheterization, p 350, for details.) In general, *never* push a guide wire when there is resistance; *always* keep one hand on the guide wire.
6. Once the sheath is in place, you can advance the prepared catheter into the sheath. Once it has been advanced approximately 15 cm, the balloon will have cleared the tip of the sheath. You can then gently inflate the balloon with 1.0–1.5 cm^3 of air. The maximum amount of air for use with smaller catheters (5 French) is 1.0 cm^3. If there is resistance to full inflation, check to see that the balloon has cleared the sheath or that it is not in an extravascular location via fluoroscopy.
7. Once the balloon is inflated, advance the catheter to the level of the right atrium under the guidance of the pressure waveform and the electrocardiogram. Monitor the waveform and electrocardiogram at all times while advancing the balloon catheter. Advance the catheter with the balloon inflated and withdraw it with the balloon deflated. Pulmonary artery catheters usually come with a preformed curve on the tip. You should insert the catheter with its tip pointing anteriorly and to the left. Positioning in the right atrium is probably best determined by watching for the characteristic waveform. The right atrium is generally located approximately 20 cm from the right internal jugular or subclavian vein insertion site and approximately 25–30 cm from the left subclavian vein insertion site. The catheter should be advanced steadily. An abrupt change in the pressure tracing will occur as the catheter enters the right ventricle. There is generally little ectopy on entry into the right ventricle; however, as you advance the catheter into the right ventricular outflow tract, premature ventricular contractions (PVCs) may occur. Keep advancing the catheter until the ectopy disappears and the pulmonary artery tracing is obtained. If this does not occur, deflate the balloon, withdraw the catheter, and try again with the balloon inflated after slightly ro-

tating the catheter. The PCWP will then be obtained by advancing the catheter another 10–15 cm. The catheter's final position should be such that the PCWP is obtained with full balloon inflation and the pulmonary artery pressure (PAP) tracing is present with the balloon deflated. In the "ideal position," transition from PAP to PCWP (and vice versa) will occur within three or fewer heartbeats. ***Caution:*** *Never* withdraw the catheter with the balloon inflated. See Figure 3–10 for normal waveforms. See Table 3–3 for normal pulmonary artery catheter measurements.

8. Suture the catheter in place and dress the site according to each institution's practice. A chest x-ray should be obtained to document the catheter's present position as well as to rule out a pneumothorax or other complication from central venous catheterization.

9. Common problems: Catheter placement is much more difficult if severe pulmonary artery hypertension is present. If there is significant cardiac enlargement, particularly dilation of the right heart structures, the catheter may have a propensity to coil and get lost in its path to the right ventricular outflow tract. Fluoroscopy may be required to get the catheter into the correct position; moreover, it will hold this position poorly. Placement of the catheter in the pulmonary artery may also be difficult in the setting of a low cardiac output as the balloon-tipped catheter is dependent on blood flow to carry it through the right heart chambers.

10. Cardiac output can be measured by thermal dilution. First, connect the thermistor to the cardiac output computer. Then rapidly inject fluid (usually 10 mL of normal saline) through the right atrial port. Have someone set the computer as you inject the bolus. The computer will display the cardiac output. Repeat this procedure two more times. If all these values are approximately the same, then average the readings and record. For normal cardiac output and index, consult Table 3–3.

11. You can often differentiate various clinical entities by measuring the blood pressure, PCWP, and cardiac output, and calculating the systemic vascular resistance. (See Table 3–4.) Abnormalities in various pressures obtained from pulmonary artery catheterization can often help diagnose various disease states. (See Table 3–5.)

Complications

1. Most complications that occur in the course of pulmonary artery catheterization are related to central vein cannulation and include arterial puncture and pneumothorax.

2. Arrhythmias are another common complication. The most common of these are transient PVCs that occur when the catheter is advanced into the right ventricular outflow tract. If a patient with a pulmonary artery catheter suddenly develops frequent premature ventricular complexes, displacement of the catheter should be suspected.

3. Ventricular tachycardia (VT) and ventricular fibrillation (VF) are rare occurrences.

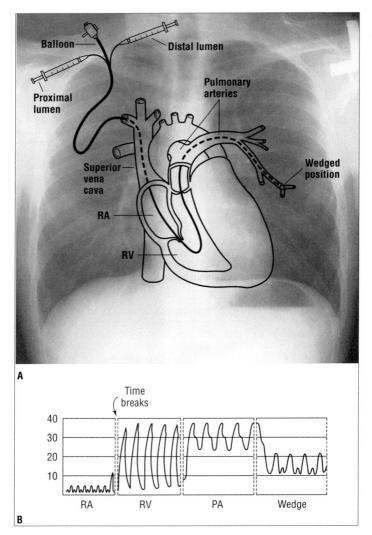

Figure 3–10. **(A)** Positioning and **(B)** pressure waveforms seen as the pulmonary artery catheter is advanced. (Reproduced, with permission, from Stillman RM, ed. *Surgery Diagnosis and Therapy.* Appleton & Lange;1989.)

TABLE 3–3. NORMAL PULMONARY ARTERY CATHETER MEASUREMENTS.

Parameter	Range
Right atrial pressure (RAP)	1–7 mm Hg
Right ventricular systolic pressure	15–25 mm Hg
Right ventricular diastolic pressure	0–8 mm Hg
Pulmonary artery systolic pressure	15–25 mm Hg
Pulmonary artery diastolic pressure	8–15 mm Hg
Pulmonary artery mean pressure	10–20 mm Hg
Pulmonary capillary wedge pressure (wedge)	6–12 mm Hg
Cardiac output (CO)	3.5–5.5 L/min
Cardiac index	2.8–3.2 L/min/m^2
Mixed venous O_2 saturation	>60%
Systemic vascular resistance (SVR)	900–12 dynes/sec/cm^5

$$SVR = \frac{(\text{mean arterial pressure} - \text{central venous pressure (or RAP)})}{CO} \times 80$$

4. Transient right bundle branch block (RBBB) occurs occasionally as the catheter passes through the right ventricular outflow tract. In a patient with preexisting left bundle branch block, this can result in complete heart block. In this setting, some form of backup pacing should be readily available. Complete heart block has been reported but is a rare occurrence.
5. Significant pulmonary infarcts and pulmonary artery rupture are serious but infrequent complications of pulmonary artery catheters secondary to permanent wedge or peripheral placement of the catheter.

TABLE 3–4. COMMONLY ENCOUNTERED HEMODYNAMIC SUBSETS.

	BP	PCWP	CO	SVR
Volume depletion	Decreased	Decreased	Decreased or normal	Increased
Volume overload (Normal left ventricular function)	Normal or increased	Increased	Increased	Normal or decreased
Sepsis, early	Normal or decreased	Normal or decreased	Increased	Decreased
Sepsis, late	Decreased	Decreased	Decreased	Decreased
Cardiogenic shock	Decreased	Increased	Decreased	Increased

$$SVR = \frac{80 \, (\text{aortic mean pressure} - \text{right atrial mean pressure})}{\text{cardiac output}}$$

BP = Blood pressure; PCWP = pulmonary capillary wedge pressure; CO = cardiac output; SVR = systemic vascular resistance.

TABLE 3–5. DIFFERENTIAL DIAGNOSIS OF COMMON PULMONARY ARTERY CATHETER READINGS.[1]

Low right atrial pressure	Volume depletion
High right atrial pressure	Volume overload; congestive heart failure; cardiogenic shock; increased pulmonary vascular resistance (hypoxia, ventilator effect of PEEP, pulmonary disease, primary pulmonary hypertension)
Low right ventricular pressure	Volume depletion
High right ventricular pressure	Volume overload; congestive heart failure; cardiogenic shock; increased pulmonary vascular resistance (hypoxia, ventilator effect of PEEP, pulmonary disease, primary pulmonary hypertension)
High pulmonary artery pressure	Congestive heart failure; increased pulmonary vascular resistance (hypoxia, ventilator effect of PEEP, pulmonary disease, primary pulmonary hypertension); cardiac tamponade
Low wedge pressure	Volume depletion
High wedge pressure	Cardiogenic shock, left ventricular failure, ventricular septal defect, mitral regurgitation and stenosis, volume overload, cardiac tamponade

PEEP = positive end-expiratory pressure.
[1] Modified and reproduced with permission from Gomella LG, Lefor AT, eds: *Surgery On Call Reference,* 2nd ed.: Appleton & Lange; 1996.

6. Most complications and problems tend to increase with the length of time the catheter is in place. There is a significant risk of bacteremia and subacute bacterial endocarditis in chronically instrumented, severely ill patients. In the setting of unexplained fever, the catheter and sheath should always be removed and cultured. The catheter and sheath should be replaced at a different site if use of a pulmonary catheter is still indicated.

13. SKIN BIOPSY

Indications. Any skin lesion or eruption for which the diagnosis is unclear; any skin condition that has been unresponsive to therapy.

Contraindications. Any skin lesion that is suspected to be a malignancy should be referred to a dermatologist or plastic surgeon for excisional biopsy rather than a punch biopsy.

Materials. A 2-, 3-, 4-, or 5-mm skin punch; 3 mL lidocaine 1% solution; 3-mL syringe; 26-gauge needle; sterile gloves; 4 × 4 gauze pads; 70% alcohol solution; pair of curved iris scissors and fine-tooth forceps (ordinary forceps may distort a small biopsy specimen and should not be used);

specimen bottle containing 10% formalin; suturing materials for 3- to 5-mm skin punch biopsies; skin marking pen.

Procedure

1. If more than one lesion is present, choose one that is well developed and representative of the dermatosis. For patients with vesiculobullous disease, an early edematous lesion should be chosen rather than a vesicle. Avoid lesions that are excoriated or infected.

2. Mark the area to be biopsied with a skin marking pen. Inject the lidocaine to form a skin wheal over the site of the biopsy.

3. After putting on sterile gloves and preparing a sterile field, perform the punch biopsy. First, immobilize the skin with the fingers of one hand, applying pressure perpendicular to the skin wrinkle lines with the skin punch. Core out a cylinder of skin by twirling the punch between the fingers of the other hand. As the punch enters into the subcutaneous fat, resistance will lessen. At this point, the punch should be removed. The core of tissue usually pops up slightly and can be cut at the level of the subcutaneous fat with curved iris scissors, without the use of forceps. If tissue core does not rise, it may be elevated by use of a hypodermic needle or fine-tooth forceps. Be sure to include a portion of the subcutaneous fat in the specimen.

4. Place the specimen in the specimen container.

5. Hemostasis can be achieved by pressure with the gauze pad.

6. Defects from 1.5- and 2-mm punches usually do not require suturing, and will heal with very minimal scarring. Punch defects that are 2–4 mm can generally be closed with a single suture.

7. A dry dressing should be applied and removed the following day.

8. Sutures can be removed as early as 3 days post procedure from the face, and 7–10 days from other areas.

Complications. Infection (unusual); hemorrhage (usually controlled by simple application of pressure); keloid formation, especially in a patient with a prior history of keloid formation.

14. THORACENTESIS

Indications. Diagnosis of pleural effusion; therapeutic removal of pleural fluid; instillation of sclerosing compounds to obliterate the pleural space.

Contraindications. Pneumothorax, hemothorax, or respiratory impairment on the contralateral side; coagulopathy (relative); a patient receiving positive pressure ventilation (relative).

Materials. Prepackaged thoracentesis kit; or minor procedure tray plus 20- to 60-mL syringe, 20- or 22-gauge 1.5-in needle, three-way stopcock, specimen containers.

Procedure

1. It takes at least 300 mL of fluid to visualize a pleural effusion on a standard posteroanterior chest x-ray.
2. Discuss the procedure with the patient and obtain informed consent. Teach the patient the Valsalva maneuver; or make sure the patient can hum (to increase intrathoracic pressure at a later point in the procedure).
3. The usual site for a thoracentesis is the posterolateral back above the diaphragm but under the fluid level. Percuss out the fluid level; or use the chest x-ray and count ribs. The site will be above the rib to avoid the neurovascular bundle that travels below the rib.
4. Prep the area with povidone-iodine and drape. The patient should be sitting up comfortably; leaning too far forward causes the effusion to move anteriorly away from the thoracentesis site. The bed stand is helpful in order to keep the patient upright and leaning slightly forward.
5. Make a skin wheal over the proposed site with a 25-gauge needle and lidocaine. Change to a 22-gauge 1.5-in needle, and infiltrate up and over the rib; try to anesthetize the deeper structures and the pleura. During this time, you should be aspirating. (See Figure 3–11.) Once fluid returns, note the depth of the needle and mark it with a hemostat. This gives you the approximate depth before you enter the pleural space. Remove the needle.

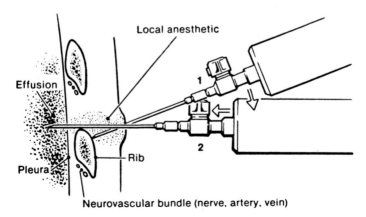

Figure 3–11. In a thoracentesis, the needle is passed over the top of the rib to avoid the neurovascular bundle. (Reproduced, with permission, from Gomella LG, ed. *Clinician's Pocket Reference.* 7th ed. Appleton & Lange;1993:258.)

6. Measure the 16- to 18-gauge thoracentesis needle with a hemostat to the same depth as the first needle. Penetrate through the anesthetized area with the thoracentesis needle. Always go over the top of the rib to avoid the neuromuscular bundle that runs below the rib. (See Figure 3–11.) Never pull the catheter back over the needle, as this can shear the tip of the catheter. Attach the three-way stopcock and tubing, and aspirate the amount of fluid needed. Turn the stopcock and evacuate the fluid through the tubing. *Never remove more than 1000–1500 mL per tap!* If you use a prepackaged catheter-over-needle kit (Arrow brand and others), an 0.5 cm horizontal skin incision must be made to allow passage of the catheter. Once fluid is withdrawn through the needle, advance the catheter into the pleural space and remove the needle.

7. Have the patient hum or do the Valsalva maneuver as you withdraw the needle. These actions increase intrathoracic pressure and decrease the chance of a pneumothorax. Bandage the site.

8. Obtain a chest x-ray to evaluate the fluid level and to rule out a pneumothorax. An expiratory film is best because a small pneumothorax is more likely to be visualized.

9. Send samples of pleural fluid for the following studies: pH, specific gravity, protein, LDH, glucose, cell count and differential, Gram's stain and bacterial cultures. Optional lab studies are: cytology, fungal, and AFB smears and cultures; amylase if you suspect an effusion secondary to pancreatitis (usually on the left); and a Sudan stain and triglycerides if a chylothorax is suspected. See Table 3–6 for the differential diagnosis.

Complications. Pneumothorax, hemothorax, infection, pulmonary laceration, hypoxemia, vasovagal attack.

REFERENCE

Light RW: *Pleural Diseases.* 3rd ed. Williams and Wilkins;1995.

TABLE 3–6. DIFFERENTIAL DIAGNOSIS OF PLEURAL FLUID.[1]

Transudate: Nephrosis, congestive heart failure, cirrhosis.
Exudate: Infection (pneumonia, tuberculosis, malignancy, empyema, peritoneal dialysis, pancreatitis, chylothorax).

Lab Value	Transudate	Exudate
Specific gravity	<1.016	>1.016
Protein (pleural fluid)	<2.5 g/100 mL	>3 g/100 mL
Protein ratio (pleural fluid-to-serum ratio)	<0.5	>0.6
LDH ratio (pleural fluid-to-serum ratio)	<0.5	>0.6
Pleural fluid LDH	<200 IU	>200 IU
Fibrinogen (clot)	No	Yes
Cell count and differential	Low WBC count	WBC count > 2500/mL; suspect an inflammatory exudate (early polys, later monos)

Grossly bloody tap: trauma, pulmonary infarction, tumor, and iatrogenic causes.
pH: The pH of pleural fluid is usually > 7.3. If between 7.2 and 7.3, suspect tuberculosis or malignancy or both. If < 7.2, suspect an empyema.
Glucose: Normal pleural fluid glucose is two-thirds serum glucose. If the pleural fluid glucose is *much, much* lower than the serum glucose, then consider empyema or rheumatoid arthritis (0–16 mg/100 mL) as the cause of the effusion.
Triglycerides and positive Sudan stain: Chylothorax.

LDH = lactic dehydrogenase; WBC = white blood cells; polys = polymorphonuclear leukocytes; monos = monocytes.
[1] Modified and reproduced with permission from Gomella LG, Lefor AT, eds: *Surgery On Call Reference,* 2nd ed.: Appleton & Lange; 1996.

IV. Fluids and Electrolytes

Daily maintenance requirements for the average 70-kg male are as follows:

Fluid	2000–2500	mL
Dextrose	100–200	g
Sodium	60–100	mEq
Potassium	40–60	mEq

These requirements can be met with an infusion of D5¼ NS with 20–30 mEq of potassium chloride per liter infused at 100 mL/h. The preceding combination of fluid and electrolytes may differ depending on other clinical parameters such as congestive heart failure, cirrhosis, hyponatremia, hypernatremia, hyperkalemia, and renal insufficiency. Maintenance fluids should be used for only 48–72 hours, at which time more effective measures of nutritional support (enteral tube feedings) should be instituted. For patients with severe volume depletion, normal saline can be administered as rapidly as 500–1000 mL/h until the patient is stabilized. For patients undergoing nasogastric suction, measured losses can be replaced every 4 hours with an equal volume of normal saline. Additional potassium may have to be added to the maintenance fluids to replace that lost with gastric suction. (See Tables 4–1 and 4–2.)

TABLE 4–1. COMPOSITION OF COMMONLY USED CRYSTALLOID SOLUTIONS.[1]

Fluid	Glucose (g/L)	Na	Cl	K (mEq/L)	Ca	HCO₃	kcal/L
D5W (5% dextrose in water)	50	—	—	—	—	—	170
D10W (10% dextrose in water)	100	—	—	—	—	—	340
D20W (20% dextrose in water)	200	—	—	—	—	—	680
D50W (50% dextrose in water)	500	—	—	—	—	—	1700
½ NS (0.45% NaCl)	—	77	77	—	—	—	—
NS (0.9% NaCl)	—	154	154	—	—	—	—
3% NS	—	513	513	—	—	—	—
D5 ¼ NS	50	38	38	—	—	—	170
D5 ½ NS (0.45% NaCl)	50	77	77	—	—	—	170
D 5% NS (0.9% NaCl)	50	154	154	—	—	—	170
D5LR (5% dextrose in lactated Ringer's)	50	130	110	4	3	27	180
Lactated Ringer's	—	130	110	4	3	27	<10

NS = normal saline.
[1] Modified and reproduced with permission from Gomella LG, ed: *Clinician's Pocket Reference.* 7th ed.: Appleton & Lange; 1993.

TABLE 4–2. COMPOSITION AND DAILY PRODUCTION OF BODY FLUIDS.[1]

Fluid	Electrolytes (mEq/L)				Average Daily Production (mL)
	Na	Cl	K	HCO₃	
Sweat	50	40	5	0	Varies
Saliva	100	15	26	50	1500
Gastric juice	60–100	100	10	0	1500–2000
Duodenum	130	90	5	0–10	300–2000
Bile	145	100	5	15–35	100–800
Pancreatic juice	140	75	5	70–115	100–800
Ileum	140	100	5	15–30	2000–3000
Diarrhea	50	40	35	45	—

[1] Modified and reproduced with permission from Gomella LG, ed: *Clinician's Pocket Reference.* 7th ed.: Appleton & Lange; 1993.

V. Blood Component Therapy

■ RED CELL TRANSFUSIONS

Prior to transfusion of any red cell products, two things must be considered: (1) the absolute level of hemoglobin (HGB) or hematocrit (HCT) and (2) the patient's symptoms. Transfusion should not be undertaken strictly to achieve a specific HCT.

GENERAL GUIDELINES

1. Hemoglobin > 10 g/dL: No transfusion.
2. Hemoglobin 8–10 g/dL: Avoid transfusion unless a therapeutic trial shows a marked improvement in symptoms.
3. Hemoglobin 6–8 g/dL: Try to avoid transfusion by reducing activity and treating the underlying disease.
4. Hemoglobin < 6 g/dL: Transfusion almost always indicated.

ANEMIA

(See also Section I, Chapter 5, Anemia, p 25.)

When confronted with a chronic anemia, the clinician must consider whether the HGB and HCT accurately reflect the red blood cell (RBC) mass. The RBC mass is more important with respect to oxygen transport than the measured HCT or HGB; however, a low HGB or HCT usually reflects a low RBC mass. An increased plasma volume may result in a dilutional change in the hemoglobin and make an anemia appear more severe. Increased plasma volume may occur in congestive heart failure (CHF), pregnancy, and paraproteinemia.

Acute Blood Loss. In the setting of acute blood loss and hypotension, restoration of blood volume and tissue perfusion as well as improvement of oxygen-carrying capacity must be accomplished. You should use electrolyte solutions or colloids initially. Blood losses of 500–1000 mL in an adult do not usually require blood transfusion unless there is an underlying anemia or there are other medical conditions that require added oxygen-carrying capacity.

RBC Products—Availability and Indications

1. **Whole blood.** There are few indications for transfusion of whole blood today, except for transfusion of the massively bleeding patient when volume and oxygen-carrying capacity can be supplied in one product. Stored whole blood is not adequate replacement for platelets or labile coagulation factors.

2. **Packed RBCs.** Basically a unit of whole blood with two-thirds of the plasma removed. This has become the standard red cell product for most transfusions.

3. **Leukocyte-poor RBCs.** In this product, 70–90% of the leukocytes have been removed by a variety of techniques. Leukocyte-poor red cells are used in patients with a history of repeated febrile reactions to standard packed RBC transfusions. These reactions are usually due to leukocyte antigens. Leukocyte-poor RBCs are indicated for patients expected to require extensive blood product support. These products will decrease the risk of anti-allo platelet antibody formation.

4. **Washed RBCs.** Virtually all plasma and nonerythrocyte cellular elements are removed. Washed cells are indicated in patients with febrile reactions to leukocyte-poor RBCs, in patients with allergic reactions to plasma components (IgA deficiency), and in patients with paroxysmal nocturnal hemoglobinuria when exposure to complement may exacerbate the hemolytic process.

5. **Frozen stored RBCs.** Used primarily for autologous transfusion for elective surgery and to maintain availability of units for patients with alloantibodies to high-incidence blood group antigens.

6. **Cytomegalovirus (CMV)-negative products.** Patients undergoing organ and bone marrow transplantation require aggressive immunosuppressive therapy to ensure engraftment and avoid graft rejection. If these patients or candidates for organ or bone marrow transplantation are CMV-negative prior to their transplant, CMV-negative blood products will minimize the risk of CMV infection complicating their transplantation course.

Complications: See Section I, Chapter 60, Transfusion Reaction, p 294.

■ PLATELET TRANSFUSIONS

(See also Section I, Chapter 59, Thrombocytopenia, p 289.)

Indications: Platelet transfusions are indicated for any patient with a major bleeding event having a qualitative or quantitative platelet disorder. Prophylactic platelet transfusions are most commonly indicated with radiation- or chemotherapy-induced bone marrow suppression. Studies of leukemic patients have shown that spontaneous major bleeding increases dramatically with platelet counts < 5000 mL. Minor bleeding increases as the platelet count falls below 10,000. The threshold for prophylactic platelet transfusion varies with the clinical setting and with the institution. Most centers transfuse prophylactically for platelet counts < 20,000. Patients with lifelong quantitative or qualitative platelet disorders should not be transfused prophylactically solely on the basis of platelet count, bleeding time, or other platelet function studies. Overutilization of platelets increases the risk of alloimmunization and subsequent inadequate response to platelet transfusions. Likewise, patients with idiopathic thrombocytopenic purpura (ITP) should not be prophylactically transfused.

Complications

1. **Transmission of viral infections**
2. **Reactions to plasma components, RBCs, and WBCs.** Reactions to RBC antigens rarely cause a hemolytic transfusion reaction. They can cause alloimmunity and a potential for problems such as the use of Rh-positive platelets in an Rh-negative female. The patient should receive intravenous anti-D globulin (RhoGAM) if she is of childbearing age.
3. **Possible transmission of bacterial infections.** A potential problem because of the storage time and storage temperature of platelet concentrates.
4. **Development of alloimmunization.** This problem eventually develops in two-thirds of patients receiving multiple transfusions of platelets. May necessitate the use of HLA-matched platelets to achieve adequate posttransfusion counts.

■ PLASMA COMPONENT THERAPY

The following is a list of commonly available plasma products and selected remarks about indications and complications.

Fresh-Frozen Plasma

1. Contains all factors, but titers of factors VIII and V decline with long-term storage. Can be used for replacement of other factor deficiencies, but problems include long turnaround time because of the need for thawing, and the potential volume of plasma needed to correct certain factor deficiencies.
2. Other side effects include urticaria, fever, nausea, headaches, and pruritus. These can usually be treated or prevented with antihistamines and antipyretics.
3. Transmission of viral infections is less likely than with the factor concentrates.

Cryoprecipitate

1. Contains high levels of factor VIII, von Willebrand factor, and fibrinogen. Useful in factor VIII deficiency, von Willebrand's disease, fibrinogen disorders, and uremic bleeding.
2. Risk of transfusion-associated hepatitis is high.

Factor VIII Concentrate

1. Various preparations are available. Only genetically engineered preparations should be used so as to avoid transmitting human immunodeficiency virus (HIV) and viral hepatitis.
2. Use is limited to patients with factor VIII deficiency.

Vitamin K-Dependent Factor Concentrates (Konyne, Proplex)

1. Contains factors II, VII, IX, and X; protein C; and protein S. Useful in these specific factor deficiencies and in patients with factor VIII inhibitors.
2. Risk of hepatitis and thromboembolic disease exists because of the presence of activated factors in some preparations.

Single-Donor Plasma

1. Collected from one donor unit of whole blood. Levels of factors V and VIII decline appreciably with storage; single-donor plasma should not be used to replace these factors.
2. Risk of hepatitis and other infections is equivalent to the risk associated with transfusing a unit of whole blood.

Gamma Globulin. There are many different forms of intravenous and intramuscular gamma globulins available with a wide variety of indications and reactions.

1. **Indications**
   a. Nonspecific immunoglobulin for non-B hepatitis prophylaxis. Hepatitis B immunoglobulin is used for prophylaxis for hepatitis B. Specific immunoglobulins can also be used for postexposure prophylaxis for varicella and rabies.
   b. Prophylactic or therapeutic intravenous use in patients with inherited or acquired humoral immune deficiencies.
   c. Treatment of acute and chronic immune thrombocytopenic purpura (ITP).
2. **Reactions.** The following are adverse effects that might result from the administration of gamma globulin.
   a. **Anaphylactoid reaction.** An immediate reaction attributed to complement activation. Symptoms and signs may include flushing, chest tightness, dyspnea, fever, chills, nausea, vomiting, hypotension, and back pain. These are uncommon reactions with the currently available preparations but can occur with both intravenous and intramuscular administration. Therapy consists of discontinuation of the infusion and use of diphenhydramine (Benadryl), steroids, epinephrine, and vasopressors if necessary.
   b. **Inflammatory reaction.** This is characteristically a delayed reaction. Signs and symptoms may include headache, malaise, fever, chills, and nausea. The reaction disappears with discontinuation of gamma globulin therapy.

REFERENCES

McCullough J: Transfusion medicine. In: Handin RI, Lux SE, Stossel TP eds: *Blood: Principles and Practice of Hematology.* Lippincott;1995:1947.

Mollison PL, Engelfriet CP, Contreras M: The transfusion of platelets, leucocytes, and plasma components. In: *Blood Transfusion in Clinical Medicine.* 9th ed. Blackwell Scientific Publications;1993:638.

Mollison PL, Engelfriet CP, Contreras M: The transfusion of red cells. In: *Blood Transfusion in Clinical Medicine.* 9th ed. Blackwell Scientific Publications;1993:377.

VI. Ventilator Management

1. INDICATIONS AND SETUP

I. Indications

  A. Ventilatory failure. This condition is judged by the degree of hypercarbia. A $PaCO_2 > 50$ Torr indicates ventilatory failure; however, many patients will have chronic ventilatory failure with renal compensation (retaining HCO_3^-) to adjust the pH toward normal. Thus, absolute pH is often a better guide to determine the need for ventilatory assistance than $PaCO_2$. A respiratory acidosis with a rapidly falling pH or an absolute pH < 7.24 is an indication for ventilatory support.

  The prototype of pure ventilatory failure is the drug overdose patient in whom there is a sudden loss of central respiratory drive with uncontrolled hypercarbia. Patients with sepsis, neuromuscular disease, and chronic obstructive pulmonary disease (COPD) may also have hypercarbic ventilatory failure.

  B. Hypoxemic respiratory failure. Inability to oxygenate is an important indication for ventilatory support. A $PaO_2 < 60$ Torr on $\geq$ 50% inspired fraction of oxygen (FiO_2) constitutes hypoxemic respiratory failure. Although these patients can sometimes be managed with higher FiO_2 delivery systems, such as partial or nonrebreather masks, or continuous positive airway pressure (CPAP) delivered by mask, they are at high risk for respiratory arrest. They should be closely monitored in an intensive care unit (ICU) if they are not intubated. Worsening of the respiratory status necessitates prompt intubation and ventilatory support.

  The prototype disease for hypoxemic respiratory failure is adult respiratory distress syndrome (ARDS), in which the high shunt fraction leads to refractory hypoxemia.

  C. Mixed respiratory failure. In actuality, most patients have failure of both ventilation and oxygenation. The indications for ventilatory support remain the same as listed earlier.

  An example of mixed respiratory failure is COPD with acute bronchitis. Bronchospasm alters the ventilation-perfusion ratio ($\dot{V}/\dot{Q}$) relationships, leading to worsening hypoxemia. Bronchospasm and accumulated secretions lead to a high work of breathing and consequent hypercarbia.

  D. Neuromuscular failure. This is actually not a category of ventilatory failure but deserves separate mention because of differing management. Hypercarbia occurs just before arrest; thus criteria other than arterial blood gases (ABGs) are needed.

  1. In progressive tachypnea, respiratory rates > 24/min are an early sign of respiratory failure. A progressive rise in the respiratory rate, or sustained respiratory rates > 35/min, are indications for ventilatory support.

2. Abdominal paradox indicates dyssynergy of chest wall muscles and diaphragms and impending respiratory failure. It is manifested by inward movement of the abdominal wall during inspiration rather than the normal outward motion.

3. A vital capacity < 15 mL/kg (1000 mL for a person with a normal-size body) is associated with acute respiratory arrest as well as an inability to clear secretions. Similarly, a negative inspiratory force less than −25 cm H_2O implies impending respiratory arrest.

   Guillain-Barré syndrome is the prototype of a neuromuscular disease in which the preceding criteria require strict attention. A patient with Guillain-Barré syndrome should be closely observed and followed with frequent vital capacity (VC) measurements. A rapidly falling VC, or VC < 1000 mL, requires respirator support.

II. Partial Ventilatory Assistance

A. CPAP (continuous positive airway pressure) may be administered by full face mask or nasal mask. Pressures of 5–15 cm H_2O may be used to recruit alveoli and improve oxygenation for refractory hypoxemia.

B. BIPAP (bidirectional positive airway pressure) may provide significant ventilatory assistance in patients with chronic neuromuscular diseases, COPD, or pneumonia; or for patients in whom intubation is not an option. Initial settings would be IPAP (inspiratory pressure) 12 cm; EPAP (expiratory pressure) 4 cm; Patient Assist Mode, backup rate 12 breaths per minute. IPAP can then be titrated upward to increase the effective tidal volume.

C. CPAP or BIPAP requires intensive respiratory therapy support for titration of O_2 and pressure as well as adjustments of the mask since leaks are common. Necrosis of the bridge of the nose may occur. Contraindications include: rapidly progressive respiratory failure, pneumothorax, and gastric distension. Partial ventilatory support should be administered only in an ICU or stepdown unit.

III. Tracheal Intubation
See Section III, Chapter 7, Endotracheal Intubation. Endotracheal intubation is actually the most difficult and complication-ridden part of ventilator initiation. Skill and experience on the clinician's part are required for correct placement. Aspiration, esophageal intubation, and right mainstem bronchus intubation are common complications. Bilateral breath sounds always need to be confirmed by chest auscultation in each axilla. An immediate postintubation portable chest x-ray (CXR) should be obtained. An inline CO_2

sensor can be used for rapid confirmation of tracheal intubation. Intubation can be accomplished by three routes:

A. Nasotracheal intubation. This can be accomplished blindly and in an awake patient. Intubation requires experience and adequate local anesthesia. Complications include intubation of the esophagus, nosebleeds, kinking of the endotracheal tube (ETT), and postobstructive sinusitis. A smaller ETT is usually required for nasotracheal versus orotracheal intubation; this leads to a higher work of breathing because of increased resistance, difficulties with adequate suctioning, and higher ventilation pressures. Nasotracheal ETTs are more comfortable than orotracheal ETTs; they are less damaging to the larynx because they are better stabilized in the airway. This type of intubation should be avoided in the presence of facial trauma if possible.

B. Orotracheal intubation. Placement of orotracheal tubes requires normal neck mobility to allow hyperextension of the neck for direct visualization of the vocal cords. Larger ETTs can be placed via this route. Adequate local anesthesia or sedation is necessary for safe placement without aspiration.

C. Tracheostomy. Tracheostomy is a surgical procedure most often done acutely for upper airway obstruction; however, in patients who require more than 14–21 days of ventilatory support, a tracheostomy is recommended. Tracheostomy tubes facilitate the weaning process by decreasing tube resistance, as the tube is shorter and has a wider radius. Patients can eat with a tracheostomy, and find the tubes more comfortable than those used for tracheal intubation.

IV. Ventilator Setup

A. The ventilator. All contemporary ventilators are time- and volume-cycled. Newer models also have pressure-targeted modes (pressure control or pressure support). Elaborate alarm systems are present to alert personnel to inadequate ventilation, high pressure, disconnection of the ETT, and so forth.

Effective ventilation is measured by changes in $PaCO_2$. Minute ventilation (V_e) can be calculated by tidal volume $\times$ breath rate. Thus, ventilation may be adjusted by changing the breath rate, the tidal volume, or both. Tidal volumes > 10 mL/kg may cause overdistension of alveoli and increase the risk of pneumothorax. Most initial tidal volumes are therefore set at 8–10 mL/kg ideal body weight.

Oxygenation is adjusted by changing FiO_2. Prolonged $FiO_2 > 60\%$ may cause pulmonary fibrosis. Thus, down-adjustment to "safe levels" sufficient to maintain O_2 saturation $> 90\%$ should be attempted as indicated by ABGs. If an O_2 saturation $> 90\%$ cannot be maintained when decreasing the $FiO_2 < 60\%$, other means to increase oxygenation such as positive end-expiratory pressure (PEEP) should be used.

The mode of ventilation should be specified:

1. **Control mode** delivers a set rate and tidal volume without regard to patient efforts.
2. **Assist control (AC) mode** allows the patient to trigger machine breaths once a threshold of inspiratory flow or effort is made. AC mode also supplies a backup rate in cases of apnea or paralysis.
3. **Intermittent mandatory ventilation (IMV)** provides a set number of machine breaths per minute and allows the patient to make spontaneous breaths as well. Synchronized intermittent mandatory ventilation (SIMV) allows synchronization of the IMV breaths with patient efforts. As the rate is turned down, the patient assumes more and more of the work of breathing.
4. **Continuous positive airway pressure (CPAP)** allows completely spontaneous respirations while the patient is still connected to the ventilator. A set amount of continuous pressure may be applied as well (from 0–30 cm H_2O).
5. **Pressure support.** Pressure support is an early inspiratory boost given to augment spontaneous respiratory efforts. Thus, in CPAP mode, pressure support can be used to overcome the work of breathing imposed by the ventilatory system (endotracheal tube, tubing, demand valves). Typically, a 8–10 cm pressure boost is used. Pressure support can also be used at higher levels during ventilator weaning (see Section VI, Chapter 4, Weaning, p 402).
6. **Pressure control.** Recent-model ventilators may be set to operate in a pressure-limited mode rather than volume-targeted. A set pressure boost is maintained for a measured time period in this mode. The goal is the limitation of peak airway pressures below 40 cm H_2O and thus minimization of barotrauma or overstretching of the lung. Pressure control is primarily used in ARDS. Often inverse ratio ventilation (increasing inspiratory time) is done simultaneously. Because this stimulates a breath holding maneuver, it feels unnatural to patients, and they usually require deep sedation and/or paralysis in this mode. ***Caution:*** Pressure control should be used *only under supervision of ICU-trained faculty or fellows.*
7. **Initial ventilator settings** should be dictated by the underlying condition as well as by previous blood gas results. An example of settings for a 70 kg patient after respiratory arrest would be:

   - FiO_2 1.0 (100%)
   - Assist control mode
   - Rate 14
   - Tidal volume 700 mL

An attempt should be made to supply the patient with at least as much minute ventilation as was required prior to intubation. Thus, a patient with pulmonary edema, ARDS, or neuromuscular disease may require a minute ventilation rate of 14–22 L/min. The AC mode will generally be more comfortable and will alleviate the work of breathing to a large extent. Sample settings might be:

- FiO_2 1.0
- Assist control mode
- Rate 18
- Tidal volume 700 mL

The patient with COPD, on the other hand, should not be overventilated initially. Such patients may have a chronically high bicarbonate because of renal compensation, and overventilation may cause a severe alkalosis. Sample settings might be:

- FiO_2 0.5 (50%)
- SIMV mode
- Pressure support 10 cm
- Rate 12
- Tidal volume 700 mL

B. Additional setup requirements
   1. **Restrain the patient's hands,** in that their natural reaction to the ETT upon awakening is to pull it out.
   2. **Place a nasogastric tube** to decompress the stomach or to continue essential oral medications.
   3. **Obtain a stat portable CXR** to confirm ETT placement and to reassess any underlying pulmonary disease. The tip of the ETT should be 3–4 cm above the carina.
   4. **Treat any underlying pulmonary disease** (maximize bronchodilators in status asthmaticus or vasodilators and diuretics in pulmonary edema).
   5. **Consider prophylactic measures.** Heparin 5000 U SC Q 12 hr may reduce the incidence of pulmonary embolism while the patient is at bed rest. Stress ulceration bleeding can be prevented by the use of any of the following: antacids; H_2 antagonists (cimetidine, ranitidine); sucralfate (Carafate); or tube feedings (enteral nutrition).
   6. **Order other medications as needed** such as morphine for pain and lorazepam (Ativan) for agitation.

2. ROUTINE MODIFICATION OF SETTINGS

Arterial blood gases (ABGs) should be monitored and adjusted to a normal pH (7.37–7.44) and a $PaO_2 > 60$ Torr on less than 60% O_2. Tachypnea should be investigated for adequacy of ventilation or for any new cause (eg, fever) prior to sedating the patient.

I. Adjusting PaO$_2$

  A. To decrease: FiO$_2$ should be decreased in increments of 10–20% every 30 minutes. The "rule of sevens" states that there will be a 7-Torr fall in PaO$_2$ for each 1% decrease in FiO$_2$.

  B. To increase

    1. Ventilation has some effect on PaO$_2$ (as shown by the alveolar air equation); therefore, correction of the respiratory acidosis will improve oxygenation.

    2. Positive end-expiratory pressure (PEEP) can be added in increments of 2–4 cm H$_2$O. PEEP recruits previously collapsed alveoli, holds them open, and restores functional residual capacity (FRC) to a better physiologic level. It counteracts pulmonary shunts and will raise PaO$_2$. PEEP increases intrathoracic pressure and may thus impede venous return and decrease cardiac output. This is particularly true in the presence of volume depletion and shock. If PEEP levels > 12–14 cm H$_2$O are needed, the placement of a Swan-Ganz catheter is recommended to monitor mixed venous oxygen levels and cardiac output.

II. Adjusting PaCO$_2$

  A. To decrease

    1. Increase the rate or tidal volume.

    2. Check for leaks in the system.

  B. To increase

    1. Decrease the rate.

    2. You may have to switch from AC mode to SIMV mode to eliminate patient-driven central hyperventilation.

    3. An old (but tried and true!) method is to place increased exhalation tubing to increase deadspace. The patient is then rebreathing his or her CO$_2$.

3. TROUBLESHOOTING

AGITATION

  I. Problem. The ventilator patient becomes agitated, struggles constantly, tries to pull out all tubes, and actively fights the respirator.

  II. Immediate Questions

    A. Is the patient still properly connected? Hypoxemia or hypercarbia resulting from disconnection of the respirator may result in agitation.

   B. What were the most recent ABGs? Again, hypoxemia or hypercarbia can cause agitation. Adjusting the settings can correct either problem.

   C. What does the CXR show? Atelectasis from mucous plugging or pneumothorax, which can occur spontaneously in asthmatics or as a result of barotrauma, can result in hypoxemia or hypercarbia.

   D. What is the underlying diagnosis? What are the current medications and IV fluids? Agitation may be related to the underlying diagnosis or to a medication, and unrelated to the patient's respiratory status. Cimetidine (Tagamet) and narcotics can cause confusion, especially in the elderly. Multiple metabolic disturbances (eg, hyponatremia and hypernatremia) can lead to confusion and possibly agitation. See Section 1, Chapter 13, Coma, Acute Mental Status Changes, p 69.

   E. What are the ventilator settings? The ventilator setting may have been set incorrectly, resulting in hypoxemia or hypercarbia. Barotrauma resulting in pneumothorax is associated with high PEEP settings, high tidal volumes, and peak inspiratory pressures > 45 cm.

III. Differential Diagnosis

   A. Causes of respiratory decompensation

      1. Worsening of underlying pulmonary disease

      2. Pneumothorax

      3. Endotracheal tube displacement. The tube may be outside the trachea, high in the glottis, or down the right mainstem bronchus.

      4. Mucous plugs. May result in atelectasis and hypoxemia.

      5. Ventilator malfunction

      6. Pulmonary embolism. Immobilization is a major risk for PE.

      7. Aspiration

      8. Inadequate oxygenation or respiratory muscle fatigue

   B. Sepsis

   C. ICU psychosis

   D. Medications. Multiple medications such as digoxin (Lanoxin), lidocaine, theophylline, imipenem-cilastatin (Primaxin), diazepam (Valium) and other benzodiazepines, meperidine and other narcotics, and cimetidine may cause psychosis, especially in high doses or with decreased clearance states.

   E. Electrolyte imbalance. Hyponatremia, hypernatremia, hypercalcemia, hypocalcemia, and hypophosphatemia can cause confusion which can lead to agitation.

IV. Database

   A. Physical examination key points

1. **Endotracheal tube.** Carefully check the patency, position, and function of the endotracheal tube (ETT).
2. **Vital signs.** Tachypnea may suggest hypoxemia. Tachycardia and hypertension can result from agitation or be associated with respiratory failure or an underlying problem such as myocardial infarction (MI). Hypotension implies sepsis, cardiogenic shock, or possibly tension pneumothorax or massive PE. An elevated temperature suggests sepsis or possibly a pulmonary infection. Tachycardia, tachypnea, and fever may be associated with PE or MI. A pulsus paradoxus > 20 mm Hg implies severe respiratory distress or pericardial tamponade.
3. **HEENT.** Check for distended neck veins suggesting pericardial tamponade or congestive heart failure (CHF). Tracheal deviation may be caused by a tension pneumothorax.
4. **Chest.** Auscultate for bilateral breath sounds. Absent breath sounds on one side suggest pneumothorax or an improperly placed ETT. Bilaterally absent breath sounds can be secondary to either bilateral pneumothoraces or severe respiratory failure.
5. **Extremities.** Check for cyanosis.
6. **Skin.** Palpate for subcutaneous emphysema, which can result from a very high PEEP or may be seen in asthmatics.

B. **Laboratory data**
1. **ABGs.** To rule out hypoxemia and hypercarbia as well as a severe acidosis and alkalosis.
2. **Electrolyte panel.** Including calcium and phosphorus.

C. **Radiologic and other studies.** A CXR to rule out atelectasis and pneumothorax and to evaluate underlying pulmonary pathology.

V. **Plan**
A. **Emergency management**
1. **Examine the patient** as outlined earlier. Carefully check the ETT function, ventilator connections, and chart.
2. **Suction the patient vigorously.** This confirms tube patency and clears out any mucous plugs.
3. **Bag the patient manually** to check for ease of ventilation. Marked difficulty can be seen with tension pneumothorax.
4. **Obtain ABGs, electrolyte panel, and stat CXR.**
5. **If the patient appears cyanotic** or "air hungry," turn the inspired fraction of oxygen (FiO_2) to 1.0 and the ventilator mode to "Assist Control" (AC).
6. **If hypotension and unilaterally absent breath sounds** are found concomitantly, consider chest tube insertion for tension pneumothorax. Patients on ventilators can rapidly die of tension pneumothoraces.
7. **If you suspect ICU psychosis,** reassure the patient. Have a family member help reorient the patient. Often a familiar voice

will work wonders! Ask the nurses to move the patient to a room with a window; this environmental feature has been shown to reduce ICU psychosis.
8. **Check the ventilator settings.** Perhaps too much effort is required to open the valves or to initiate a breath.
9. **If everything else is stable** and the patient is endangering himself or herself, sedate them. Haloperidol (Haldol) 0.5–2.0 mg IM or IV and lorazepam (Ativan) 0.5–2.0 mg IV are the currently recommended agents.

4. HYPOXEMIA

I. **Problem.** The respirator patient requires $\geq 60\%$ FiO_2 to maintain a $PaO_2 > 60$ Torr.

II. **Immediate Questions**
   A. **What is the sequence of ABGs?** In other words, is this an acute or a slowly developing change? A rapid deterioration implies an immediate life-threatening process such as a tension pneumothorax or a massive pulmonary embolism (PE).
   B. **What is the underlying diagnosis?** A patient with long-bone fractures may develop fat embolus syndrome, a patient with sepsis may develop adult respiratory distress syndrome (ARDS), or a patient with head injury might develop neurogenic pulmonary edema.
   C. **What are the ventilator settings? Has a change been made recently?** An error may have been made with the ventilator settings; or recent changes may have been made too aggressively in an attempt to wean the patient from the ventilator.

III. **Differential Diagnosis**
   A. **Shunts secondary to alveolar filling or by obstructed bronchi with consequent collapse**
      1. **Pneumonia**
      2. **Pulmonary contusion**
      3. **Atelectasis.** The ETT may be placed too far in the right mainstem bronchus, or there may be mucous plugs.
      4. **ARDS or cardiogenic pulmonary edema**
   B. **Cardiac level shunt.** An acute ventricular septal defect, especially in the setting of an acute myocardial infarction (MI), may develop. Sudden pulmonary hypertension may occasionally lead to a patent foramen ovale and physiologic shunt at the atrial level. A tip-off to this development is a worsening shunt and PaO_2 as positive end-expiratory pressure (PEEP) is increased.
   C. **Shunts secondary to pneumothorax**
   D. **Ventilation/perfusion ($\dot{V}/\dot{Q}$) mismatch**
      1. **Bronchospasm**

      2. **Pulmonary embolism**
      3. **Aspiration.** Still possible, even when an ETT is in place.
  E. Inadequate ventilation
      1. **Ventilator disconnection or malfunction**
      2. **Incorrect settings.** Has the patient recently been changed to IMV which has resulted in hypoventilation?
      3. **Sedatives.** These can result in hypoxemia secondary to hypoventilation. Sedatives should be used cautiously, especially during weaning.
      4. **Neuromuscular disease.** Hypophosphatemia or aminoglycosides can cause neuromuscular weakness, which can cause hypoxemia secondary to hypoventilation and lack of sighing.

IV. Database
  A. Physical examination key points
      1. **Endotracheal tube.** Confirm proper ETT position and listen for any leaks.
      2. **Vital signs.** Tachypnea implies worsening of the respiratory status. Tachycardia can be associated with a variety of conditions including PE, sepsis, MI, and worsening of underlying pulmonary pathology. Fever can be seen with PE, MI, or an infection.
      3. **Neck.** Stridor suggests upper airway obstruction.
      4. **Chest.** Check for bilateral breath sounds, signs of consolidation, or new onset of wheezing. Unilateral breath sounds suggest a pneumothorax or possibly displacement of the ETT in one of the mainstem bronchi. Palpate the chest for new subcutaneous emphysema, which can occur in asthmatics or as a result of high PEEP.
      5. **Heart.** New murmurs or a new third heart sound (S_3) or fourth heart sound (S_4) may be seen with an MI.
      6. **Extremities.** Check nailbeds for cyanosis from worsening of pulmonary status. Also check legs for unilateral edema or other signs of phlebitis which point to PE.
      7. **Skin.** Check for new rashes which may suggest a drug or anaphylactic reaction.
  B. Laboratory data
      1. **Repeat ABGs or check oximetry** to assess accuracy of initial ABGs and progression of deterioration.
      2. **Sputum appearance and Gram's stain** may direct antibiotic therapy if pneumonia is present.
      3. **A Swan-Ganz catheter** will have to be in place to measure mixed venous oxygen saturation ($\dot{V}O_2$). $\dot{V}O_2$ is a direct reflection of oxygen delivery to the tissues and extraction of oxygen. It can be used to determine the presence of an intracardiac shunt.

C. **Radiologic and other studies**
1. **Stat CXR.** To rule out atelectasis and pneumothorax, and to evaluate underlying pulmonary disease.
2. **Electrocardiogram.** An evolving MI may be evident. New right-axis deviation, right bundle branch block, P pulmonale, or an S wave in lead I, a Q wave in lead III, and a T wave in lead III ($S_1Q_3T_3$) imply PE; however, these characteristic findings are often absent. Sinus tachycardia is the most common electrocardiographic finding with PE.
3. **V/Q scan.** To be obtained if clinical suspicion is high for PE.
4. **Swan-Ganz catheter.** To measure PaO_2 and to exclude a cardiac shunt as well as to measure cardiac output and maximum O_2 consumption.

V. **Plan**
A. **Suction.** Vigorously suction the patient to prove patency of the ETT and dislodge mucous plugs.
B. **Correct anemia.** Oxygen delivery to tissue depends on the hemoglobin as well as the cardiac output and PaO_2.
C. **Treat underlying disorders**
1. **Insert chest tube** for pneumothorax.
2. **Reassess choice of antibiotic agents.** A pneumonia secondary to *Legionella* requires erythromycin (1 g IV Q 6 hr).
3. **Consider more vigorous chest physical therapy** or even bronchoscopy for recalcitrant mucous plugging or atelectasis.
4. **Maximize bronchodilators** if bronchospasm is the problem. Corticosteroids such as hydrocortisone 125 mg or methylprednisolone 60 mg should be added and given Q 6 hr. Aerosolized albuterol (Ventolin) or metaproterenol (Alupent) should be given at least Q 4 hr.
5. **Cardiogenic pulmonary edema** should be vigorously treated with afterload reduction and diuresis.
D. **Optimize ventilator settings**
1. **Correct any hypoventilation.** This may mean giving up on weaning, and using the AC mode with the patient essentially controlled on a high minute ventilation.
2. **Increase FiO_2 to 100%.** Your first priority is to prevent anoxic brain or cardiac damage. You may then reduce the FiO_2 as other maneuvers further improve the pO_2.
3. **PEEP will recruit unused, collapsed, or partially collapsed alveoli to overcome pulmonary shunts.** It should be added in 2- to 4-cm of H_2O increments while monitoring cardiac output and blood pressure.
4. **Oxygen consumption ($\dot{V}O_2$)** can be markedly reduced by administering a neuromuscular blocking agent as a last resort. Remember to provide adequate analgesia and sedation as well. Nerve stimulation studies should be done routinely to monitor

the neuromuscular blockade; otherwise these agents should be used for < 24 hours.

E. Optimize hemodynamics
1. **Consider Swan-Ganz placement** when high levels of PEEP are in use, when shock of unclear cause is present, when a cardiac shunt is suspected, or when volume status is unclear.
2. **Correct volume excess** because it will obviously worsen CHF and ARDS.
3. **Volume depletion** will likewise alter both cardiac output and V/Q ratios and may adversely affect oxygen delivery. A drop in blood pressure with the addition of PEEP almost always results from volume depletion.
4. **Correct anemia** so as to maximize O_2 delivery. If ARDS is present, red blood cell transfusions should either be washed or administered through leukocyte removal filters to prevent an exacerbation of the ARDS secondary to the transfusion.
5. **Correct low cardiac output** to maximize O_2 delivery. Inotropic agents (eg, dobutamine) and agents for afterload reduction (eg, IV nitroglycerin or nitroprusside) can be used.

5. HYPERCARBIA

I. Problem. The patient's $PaCO_2$ remains > 40 Torr. $PaCO_2$ is a direct reflection of both CO_2 production and alveolar ventilation. $PaCO_2$ increases when ventilation/perfusion (V/Q) mismatch worsens or dead-space increases.

II. Immediate Questions
  A. What is the sequence of arterial blood gases? In other words, is this an acute or a slowly developing change? Rapid deterioration implies an immediate life-threatening process such as a tension pneumothorax or a massive pulmonary embolism.
  B. What is the underlying diagnosis? Worsening of underlying pulmonary disease (pneumonia, atelectasis, or bronchospasm) can cause hypoventilation. Congestive heart failure (CHF) can cause V/Q mismatch and CO_2 retention.

III. Differential Diagnosis
  A. Inadequate minute ventilation ($\dot{V}_e$)
1. **Too low a rate, inadequate tidal volume, or both**
2. **Patient tiring during synchronized intermittent mandatory ventilation or weaning**
3. **ETT leak**
4. **Worsening bronchospasm**
5. **Pulmonary embolism (PE).** Keep in mind that immobilization is a major risk factor.

B. **Increased CO_2 production**
   1. **High-carbohydrate feedings**
   2. **Increased metabolism.** Causes include hyperthyroidism, fever, sepsis, and high work of breathing as well as rewarming after surgical procedures (a common but frequently overlooked cause of CO_2 production).
C. **Oversedation.** Decreases central ventilatory drive.

IV. **Database**
   A. **Physical examination key points**
      1. **Endotracheal tube.** Check ETT position and look for a leak.
      2. **Vital signs.** Tachycardia can be associated with fever, sepsis, worsening bronchospasm, PE, and hyperthyroidism. Tachypnea can be seen with PE, worsening bronchospasm, or sepsis. Fever suggests infection but can also be seen with hyperthyroidism and PE.
      3. **Chest.** Auscultate looking for onset of new wheezes or a change in the equality of breath sounds.
      4. **Heart.** Listen for a new loud P_2 which suggests a PE.
      5. **Extremities.** Check patient's legs for unilateral edema or other signs of thrombophlebitis.
      6. **Musculoskeletal exam.** Check for signs of respiratory fatigue: abdominal paradox or accessory muscle is seen with severe respiratory failure.
   B. **Laboratory data**
      1. **Arterial blood gases.** Repeat ABGs or check oximetry to assess accuracy of initial ABGs and progression of deterioration.
      2. **Complete blood count (CBC) with differential.** An increased white count with an increase in banded neutrophils suggests an infection or sepsis.
   C. **Radiologic and other studies.** With a CXR, proper ETT position can be ensured and new pulmonary infiltrates can be ruled out.

V. **Plan**
   A. **Check position and functioning of ETT.** If there is a persistent leak, replace the tube.
   B. **Verify proper ventilator function.** Check with particular care for leaky connections.
   C. **Drugs.** Verify that the ordered sedatives are the drugs that were actually given and note time of last dose. If the patient is oversedated, you can either increase the minute ventilation ($\dot{V}_e$); or reverse sedation with naloxone (Narcan) 0.4 mg IV for narcotics or flumazenil (Mazicon) 0.2 mg IV over 15 seconds for benzodiazepines. Flumazenil dosing may be repeated Q 1 min up to a total dose of 1 mg.

    D. Look for a source of sepsis. Adjust antibiotics as indicated. Lower $\dot{V}O_2$ by treating fever with Tylenol or a cooling blanket.

    E. Review ventilator settings. If the tidal volume is too low, dead-space ventilation will be present. Correct this condition by increasing the tidal volume. If the patient is tiring on a low SIMV rate, switch to either a higher rate or change to "Assist Control" (AC) mode.

    F. Review the patient's nutrition regimen. If the patient is critically ill with bronchospasm or ARDS, you may be forced to reduce CO_2 production by decreasing the percentage of carbohydrates in tube feedings or IV hyperalimentation fluid.

6. HIGH PEAK PRESSURES

  I. Problem. The ventilator peak pressures remain consistently above 50 cm H_2O.

II. Immediate Questions

    A. Is this a new problem or has it developed progressively? The answer to this question will be readily available on the respiratory therapy bedside flow sheet.

    B. What is the underlying diagnosis? Severe status asthmaticus or acute respiratory distress syndrome (ARDS) can cause high ventilatory peak pressures.

    C. What are the most recent ABGs? A decrease in the pO_2 or an increase in the pCO_2 may point to a worsening of the underlying pulmonary disease.

    D. Has ETT function or position changed? Is it possible to suction the patient? The tube could be kinked or plugged by secretions.

III. Differential Diagnosis

    A. ETT

        1. **Too small or obstructed** by secretions.

        2. **Kinked**, especially if placed nasotracheally.

        3. **Migration** down the right mainstem so that the entire tidal volume flows into one lung. This condition also increases coughing and anxiety.

    B. Incorrect ventilator settings

        1. **High tidal volume.** Tidal volumes > 10 mL/kg may increase distension pressure tremendously.

        2. **High positive end-expiratory pressure.** PEEP should always be used at the lowest possible level.

        3. **High minute ventilation.** A high minute ventilation may lead to the phenomenon of "auto PEEP," in which the patient has inadequate time to exhale, leading to "stacked breaths." Auto PEEP

may cause hypotension because of high intrathoracic pressure decreasing venous return.
  C. **Worsening lung disease.** All of these conditions show concomitant falls in lung compliance:
    1. **Severe status asthmaticus**
    2. **Adult respiratory distress syndrome (ARDS)**
    3. **Cardiogenic pulmonary edema**
    4. **Interstitial lung disease**
  D. **Uncooperative or agitated patient**
    1. **Biting the ETT**
    2. **Fighting the ventilator**
    3. **Coughing**
  E. **Abdominal distension**
  F. **Tension pneumothorax.** It is always imperative to exclude this as a cause of new onset of high peak pressures because death can occur quickly.

IV. **Database**
  A. **Physical examination key points**
    1. **ETT.** Check position to rule out migration down the right mainstem bronchus; check patency of the ETT.
    2. **Vital signs.** Tachycardia and tachypnea can occur with worsening of the underlying pulmonary disease and with agitation. Hypotension and tachycardia are seen with tension pneumothorax.
    3. **HEENT.** An increase in jugular venous distension (JVD) implies CHF. Tracheal deviation can be seen with tension pneumothorax.
    4. **Chest.** Absent breath sounds, especially with hypotension, and unilateral hyperresonance to percussion point to tension pneumothorax. Rales suggest CHF.
    5. **Heart.** A third heart sound (S_3) over the apex implies left ventricular dysfunction/congestive heart failure.
    6. **Abdomen.** Examine for tenderness and distension.
    7. **Extremities.** New cyanosis is consistent with worsening of underlying pulmonary disease. Edema will be seen with biventricular or right-sided heart failure.
    8. **Skin.** Check for subcutaneous emphysema which can be associated with barotrauma or with severe asthma.
  B. **Laboratory data**
    1. **Arterial blood gases.** Repeat ABGs or check oximetry to assess accuracy of initial ABGs and progression of deterioration.
    2. **Complete blood count (CBC) with differential.** An increased white count with an increase in banded neutrophils suggests an infection or sepsis.

   C. **Radiologic and other studies.** Use a stat portable CXR to check
      ETT position, rule out kinking, rule out pneumothorax, and assess
      any change in underlying pulmonary disease.
   D. **Ventilator**
      1. Ask the respiratory therapist to measure "Auto PEEP" or check
         for it via the wave forms.
      2. **View the peak airway pressure pattern.** A rapid rise and fall
         suggest a kinked or obstructed ETT.

V. **Plan**
   A. **Try to suction the patient.** If they are biting down, insert an oral
      airway or sedate them. If the patient is not biting down on the ETT
      but the suction tube will not go down, the tube is kinked or blocked,
      possibly by a mucus plug, and must be replaced.
   B. **Ambu bag the patient and confirm equal breath sounds.** Un-
      equal breath sounds may result from a tension pneumothorax or
      from improper positioning of the ETT. Reposition the ETT if nec-
      essary. On an average-sized person, an oral ETT should not be in
      farther than 24 cm at the lip; however, there is considerable vari-
      ability among patients and the CXR should always be reviewed. If
      there is considerable resistance to bagging, a tension pneumotho-
      rax, auto PEEP, or a mucus plug may be present.
   C. **Place a chest tube** if a pneumothorax is present.
   D. **Adjust the ventilator.** Try to reduce the PEEP to the minimum
      needed for adequate oxygenation. Try reducing high tidal volumes
      to 8 mL/kg body weight. Increase FiO_2 as needed to ensure
      adequate oxygenation.
   E. **Sedation** may have to be increased.
   F. **Adjustment of alarms.** If all possibilities have been evaluated,
      alarms may be increased to higher levels; however, the risk of an
      acute tension pneumothorax will increase with higher peak pres-
      sures.

7. WEANING

   I. **Requirements.** Once the underlying cause of respiratory failure has
      been corrected, it is time for the most arduous task of all: weaning the
      patient from the respirator.
      A. **Stabilization.** The underlying disease is under optimum control.
      B. **Initiation of weaning.** The process is begun in the early morning.
         Patients prefer to rest at night rather than work at breathing.
         1. **$PaO_2 \geq 60$ Torr on no PEEP; and $FiO_2 \leq 0.5$.**
         2. **Minute ventilation < 10 L/min.**
         3. **Negative inspiratory force more negative than -20 cm H_2O.**

4. **Vital capacity > 800 mL.**
5. **Tidal volume > 300 mL.**

II. Weaning Techniques

A. **T-Piece (or T-tube bypass).** The patient is taken off the respirator for a limited period of time, and the ETT is connected to a constant flow of O_2 (usually 40%). If the patient tolerates breathing independently, the length of time off the respirator is progressively increased. This is a tried and true method. It is particularly easy to use in patients with no underlying lung disease (eg, a patient recovering from a drug overdose).

This technique, however, has several drawbacks. No alarms are available as the patient is totally disconnected from the ventilator. It is time-consuming for the respiratory therapists and nurses. Perhaps most importantly, it is much more work for the patient than breathing spontaneously without an ETT. This is due to the relatively small diameter of the tube. Remember that resistance increases by the fourth power of the radius of a tube.

B. **Synchronized intermittent mandatory ventilation.** In this method, fewer and fewer machine breaths are given as the patient begins taking spontaneous breaths in the intervals. For example, a patient breathing at a rate of 14 in AC mode is switched to SIMV mode, rate 14. The rate is then decreased to 10, to 6, to 4, and then to 0. Most physicians either place the patient on continuous positive airway pressure mode at this juncture or observe the patient briefly on a T-piece.

This method has several theoretical advantages over T-piece weaning. Backup alarms, including automatic rates in case of apnea, are in place. A graded assumption of work is done allowing respiratory muscle "retraining"; however, this method has never been proven clearly superior to T-piece weaning. Moreover, there is still a high work of breathing because of the ETT resistance as well as the inherent resistance of the SIMV circuit valves.

One way to decrease the work of breathing with the SIMV weaning technique is to add pressure support (PS) to the system. Pressure support is a positive pressure boost that is initiated when a certain liter flow rate during inspiration is sensed by the respirator. It then supplies a set amount of positive pressure (and by Boyle's law, it also supplies some tidal volume). A PS level of 8–12 cm will overcome the increased work caused by the ETT resistance.

C. **Continuous positive airway pressure and pressure support.** In this method, the patient is switched to the spontaneous breathing mode, which in modern ventilators is the CPAP mode. In current usage, CPAP is equivalent to PEEP, except that it is used exclusively in spontaneously breathing mode. Anywhere from 0–30 cm pressure may be used, but generally the lowest level possible (usually 0–5 cm) is preferred. Pressure support may be used concomitantly to augment the patient's spontaneous breaths. It can then be progressively decreased as the patient increases tidal volumes. For example, PS levels of 25, then 20, then 15, and finally 10 can be used while monitoring the patient's breath rate, tidal volumes, and ABGs.

This method requires an alert, cooperative patient who is breathing spontaneously; if those conditions do not pertain, why wean anyway? Machine backup functions remain in place in case of apnea or other inadequate parameters.

III. Timing. Deciding when to extubate the patient is part of the art of medicine. Still, the fulfillment of certain criteria ensures success. The following weaning parameters (as discussed earlier) are acceptable:

    A. Respiratory rate is < 30/min.
    B. ABGs show a pH > 7.35 and adequate oxygenation or ≤ 50 FiO_2.
    C. The patient is awake and alert.
    D. A normal gag reflex is present.
    E. The stomach is not distended.

IV. Postextubation care. After extubation, it is important to encourage the patient to cough frequently and forcefully. Respiratory therapy treatments should be continued. Incentive spirometry should be used several times an hour while the patient is awake to encourage deep breathing. The patient must be carefully observed for stridor, respiratory muscle fatigue, or other signs of failure. Oxygen should be given at the same level or at a level slightly higher than was given via the respirator prior to intubation. The ABGs should be checked 2–4 hours after extubation to confirm adequate ventilation and oxygenation.

REFERENCES

Glauser FL, Polatty C, Sessler CN: Worsening oxygenation in the mechanically ventilated patient: Causes, mechanisms and early detection. Am Rev Respir Dis 1988;138:458.

Luce JM et al: Intermittent mandatory ventilation. Chest 1981;79:678.

MacIntyre NR: Weaning from mechanical ventilatory support: Volume-assisting intermittent breaths versus pressure-assisting every breath. Respir Care 1988; 33:121.

Marcy TW, Marini JJ: Respiratory distress in the ventilated patient. Clin Chest Med 1994;15:55.

Slutsky AS: ACCP consensus conference—Mechanical ventilation. Chest 1993; 104:1833.

Tobin MJ: Mechanical ventilation. N Engl J Med 1994;330:1056.

VII. Commonly Used Medications

This section is designed to serve as a quick reference to commonly used medications. You should be familiar with all of the indications, contraindications, side effects, and drug interactions of any medications that you prescribe. Such detailed information is beyond the scope of this manual and can be found in the package insert, *Physicians Desk Reference (PDR)*, or the American Hospital Formulary Service.

Drugs in this section are listed in alphabetical order by generic names. Some of the more common trade names are listed for each medication.

Drugs under the control of the Drug Enforcement Agency (Schedule II-V controlled substances) are indicated by the symbol [C].

GENERIC DRUGS: GENERAL CLASSIFICATION

Analgesic/Anti-Inflammatory/Antipyretic Agents

Acetaminophen
Acetaminophen with butalbital and
  caffeine
Acetaminophen with codeine
Aspirin
Aspirin with butalbital and caffeine
Aspirin with codeine
Buprenorphine
Butorphanol
Codeine
Dezocine
Diclofenac sodium
Diflunisal
Etodolac
Fenoprofen
Fentanyl transdermal system
Flurbiprofen
Hydromorphone
Ibuprofen

Indomethacin
Ketoprofen
Ketorolac
Levorphanol
Meperidine
Methadone
Morphine sulfate
Nabumetone
Nalbuphine
Naproxen
Oxaprozin
Oxycodone
Pentazocine
Piroxicam
Propoxyphene
Sulindac
Tolmetin
Tramadol

405

Antacids/Antigas

Aluminum carbonate
Aluminum hydroxide
Aluminum hydroxide with magnesium hydroxide
Aluminum hydroxide with magnesium hydroxide and simethicone
Aluminum hydroxide with magnesium trisilicate and alginic acid

Calcium carbonate
Dihydroxyaluminum sodium carbonate
Magaldrate
Simethicone

Antianxiety Agents

Alprazolam
Buspirone
Chlordiazepoxide
Clorazepate
Diazepam

Doxepin
Hydroxyzine
Lorazepam
Oxazepam

Antiarrhythmics

Adenosine
Amiodarone
Bretylium
Digoxin
Diltiazem
Disopyramide
Esmolol
Lidocaine

Mexiletine
Procainamide
Propafenone
Quinidine
Sotalol
Tocainide
Verapamil

Antibiotics

Amikacin
Amoxicillin
Amoxicillin/potassium clavulanate
Ampicillin
Ampicillin/sulbactam
Atovaquone
Azithromycin
Aztreonam
Cefaclor
Cefadroxil
Cefamandole
Cefazolin
Cefixime
Cefmetazole
Cefonicid
Cefoperazone
Cefotaxime

Cefotetan
Cefoxitin
Cefpodoxime
Cefprozil
Ceftazidime
Ceftizoxime
Ceftriaxone
Cefuroxime
Cephalexin
Cephalothin
Cephapirin
Cephradine
Chloramphenicol
Ciprofloxacin
Clarithromycin
Clindamycin
Clofazimine

Cloxacillin
Cortisporin, otic
Dapsone
Demeclocycline
Dicloxacillin
Dirithromycin
Doxycycline
Erythromycin
Ethambutol
Gentamicin
Imipenem/cilastatin
Isoniazid
Lomefloxacin
Loracarbef
Metronidazole
Mezlocillin
Nafcillin
Neomycin sulfate
Nitrofurantoin
Norfloxacin
Ofloxacin

Oxacillin
Penicillin G aqueous
Penicillin G benzathine
Penicillin G procaine
Penicillin V
Pentamidine
Piperacillin
Piperacillin/tazobactam
Pyrazinamide
Rifabutin
Rifampin
Silver sulfadiazine
Streptomycin
Tetracycline
Ticarcillin
Ticarcillin/potassium clavulanate
Tobramycin
Trimethoprim
Trimethoprim/sulfamethoxazole
Trimetrexate
Vancomycin

Anticoagulant/Thrombolytic and Related Agents

Abciximab
Alteplase, recombinant (TPA)
Aminocaproic acid
Anistreplase
Antihemophilic Factor VIII
Aprotinin
Desmopressin (DDAVP)
Dipyridamole

Enoxaparin
Heparin
Pentoxifylline
Protamine Sulfate
Streptokinase
Ticlopidine
Urokinase
Warfarin

Anticonvulsants

Carbamazepine
Clonazepam
Diazepam
Ethosuximide
Gabapentin
Lamotrigine

Lorazepam
Pentobarbital
Phenobarbital
Phenytoin
Valproic acid

Antidepressants

Amitriptyline
Bupropion
Desipramine
Doxepin
Fluoxetine

Imipramine
Lithium carbonate
Maprotiline
Nefazodone
Nortriptyline

Paroxetine
Sertraline
Trazodone

Trimipramine
Venlafaxine

Antidiabetic Agents

Acarbose
Acetohexamide
Chlorpropamide
Glipizide
Glyburide

Insulin
Metformin
Tolazamide
Tolbutamide

Antidiarrheal Agents

Bismuth subsalicylate
Diphenoxylate with atropine
Kaolin/Pectin

Lactobacillus
Loperamide
Octreotide

Antidotes

Acetylcysteine
Charcoal
Digoxin immune Fab
Flumazenil
Ipecac syrup

Mesna
Naloxone
Sodium polystyrene sulfonate
Succimer

Antiemetics

Chlorpromazine
Dimenhydrinate
Dronabinol
Droperidol
Granisetron
Meclizine
Metoclopramide

Ondansetron
Prochlorperazine
Promethazine
Scopolamine
Thiethylperazine
Trimethobenzamide

Antifungal Agents

Amphotericin B
Clotrimazole
Fluconazole
Flucytosine
Itraconazole

Ketoconazole
Miconazole
Nystatin
Terconazole
Tioconazole

Antigout Agents

Allopurinol
Colchicine

Probenecid
Sulfinpyrazone

Antihistamines

Astemizole
Chlorpheniramine
Clemastine fumarate
Cyproheptadine
Diphenhydramine
Hydroxyzine
Loratadine
Terfenadine

Antihyperlipidemics

Cholestyramine
Colestipol
Fluvastatin
Gemfibrozil
Lovastatin
Niacin
Pravastatin
Simvastatin

Antihypertensives

Acebutolol
Amlodipine
Atenolol
Benazepril
Betaxolol
Bisoprolol
Captopril
Carteolol
Carvedilol
Clonidine
Diltiazem
Doxazosin
Enalapril
Felodipine
Fosinopril
Guanabenz
Guanadrel
Guanethidine
Guanfacine
Hydralazine
Isradipine
Labetalol
Lisinopril
Losartan
Methyldopa
Metoprolol
Minoxidil
Moexipril
Nadolol
Nicardipine
Nifedipine
Nitroglycerin
Nitroprusside
Penbutolol
Pindolol
Prazosin
Propranolol
Quinapril
Ramipril
Terazosin
Timolol
Verapamil

Antineoplastic Agents

Aldesleukin (IL-2)
Altretamine
Asparaginase
Bleomycin
Busulfan
Carboplatin
Chlorambucil
Cisplatin
Cladribine
Cyclophosphamide
Cytarabine
Dacarbazine
Dactinomycin
Daunorubicin
Diethylstilbestrol
Doxorubicin
Etoposide
Fludarabine phosphate

Fluorouracil
Flutamide
Goserelin
Hydroxyurea
Idarubicin
Ifosfamide
Leuprolide
Megestrol acetate
Melphalan
Mercaptopurine

Methotrexate
Mitomycin
Mitoxantrone
Paclitaxel
Plicamycin
Tamoxifen citrate
Teniposide
Thiotepa
Vinblastine
Vincristine

Antiparkinsonism Agents

Amantadine
Benztropine
Bromocriptine
Carbidopa/levodopa

Pergolide
Selegiline
Trihexyphenidyl

Antipsychotic Agents

Chlorpromazine
Clozapine
Fluphenazine
Haloperidol
Lithium carbonate
Mesoridazine

Perphenazine
Prochlorperazine
Risperidone
Thioridazine
Thiothixene
Trifluoperazine

Antitussive, Decongestant, Expectorant, and Mucolytic Agents

Acetylcysteine
Benzonatate
Codeine
Dextromethorphan

Guaifenesin
Phenylephrine
Pseudoephedrine

Antiviral Agents

Acyclovir
Amantadine
Didanosine
Famciclovir
Foscarnet
Ganciclovir

Rimantadine
Stavudine
Valacyclovir
Zalcitabine
Zidovudine

Bronchodilators

Albuterol
Aminophylline
Bitolterol
Metaproterenol

Pirbuterol
Salmeterol
Terbutaline
Theophylline

Cardiovascular Agents

Acebutolol
Atenolol
Atropine
Bepridil
Digoxin
Diltiazem
Dobutamine
Dopamine
Ephedrine
Epinephrine
Esmolol
Hydralazine
Isoproterenol
Isosorbide dinitrate
Isosorbide mononitrate
Labetalol

Metoprolol
Milrinone
Nadolol
Nicardipine
Nifedipine
Nitroglycerin
Nitroprusside
Norepinephrine
Penbutolol
Phenylephrine
Pindolol
Propranolol
Sodium polystyrene sulfonate
Timolol
Verapamil

Cathartics/Laxatives

Bisacodyl
Docusate calcium
Docusate potassium
Docusate sodium
Glycerin suppositories
Lactulose
Magnesium citrate

Magnesium hydroxide
Mineral oil
Polyethylene glycol-electrolyte
   solution
Psyllium
Sorbitol

Diuretics

Acetazolamide
Amiloride
Bumetanide
Chlorothiazide
Chlorthalidone
Ethacrynic acid
Furosemide
Hydrochlorothiazide
Hydrochlorothiazide and amiloride

Hydrochlorothiazide and
   spironolactone
Hydrochlorothiazide and
   triamterene
Indapamide
Mannitol
Metolazone
Spironolactone
Torsemide

Estrogens

Esterified estrogens
Estradiol topical
Estradiol transdermal

Estrogen, conjugated
Ethinyl estradiol

Gastrointestinal Agents

Cimetidine
Cisapride
Dicyclomine
Famotidine
Lactulose
Lansoprazole
Mesalamine enema
Metoclopramide
Misoprostol
Nizatidine

Octreotide
Olsalazine
Omeprazole
Pancreatin
Pancrelipase
Propantheline
Ranitidine
Sulfasalazine
Sucralfate
Vasopressin

Hormones/Synthetic Substitutes
Also see **Estrogens** and **Thyroid/Antithyroid**

Betamethasone
Cortisone
Desmopressin
Dexamethasone
Epoetin alfa (Erythropoietin)
Fligrastim (G-CSF)
Fludrocortisone acetate
Glucagon
Gonadorelin
Hydrocortisone
Insulin
Interferon alfa
Interferon beta-1b

Interferon gamma-1b
Levonorgestrel Implants
Medroxyprogesterone
Methylprednisolone
Metyrapone
Oxytocin
Pancreatin
Pancrelipase
Prednisolone
Prednisone
Sargramostim (GM-CSF)
Steroids
Vasopressin

Immunosuppressive Agents

Antithymocyte globulin (ATG)
Azathioprine
Cyclosporine
Methotrexate

Muromonab-CD3 (OKT-3)
Mycophenolate mofetil
Tacrolimus (FK-506)

Local Anesthetic Agents

Anusol

Lidocaine

Muscle Relaxants

Atracurium
Baclofen
Carisoprodol
Chlorzoxazone
Cyclobenzaprine
Dantrolene

Diazepam
Methocarbamol
Pancuronium
Succinylcholine
Vecuronium

Ophthalmic Agents

Apraclonidine
Betaxolol
Chloramphenicol
Ciprofloxacin
Cortisporin
Dipivefrin
Erythromycin

Gentamicin
Levobunolol
Metipranolol
Sulfacetamide
Timolol
Tobramycin

Plasma Volume Expanders

Albumin
Hetastarch

Plasma protein fraction

Respiratory and Nasal Inhalants
Also see Bronchodilators

Beclomethasone
Budesonide
Cromolyn sodium
Dornase alfa
Flunisolide

Ipratropium
Nedocromil
SSKI
Triamcinolone

Sedatives/Hypnotics

Diphenhydramine
Estazolam
Flurazepam
Hydroxyzine
Midazolam

Secobarbital
Temazepam
Triazolam
Zolpidem

Supplements

Calcium salts
Cholecalciferol
Cyanocobalamin (B_{12})
Ferrous sulfate
Folic acid
Iron dextran
Leucovorin

Magnesium oxide
Magnesium sulfate
Phytonadione (vitamin K)
Potassium supplements
Pyridoxine (B_6)
Sodium bicarbonate
Thiamine (B_1)

Thyroid/Antithyroid

Levothyroxine
Liothyronine
Methimazole

Propylthiouracil
SSKI

Toxoids/Vaccines/Serums

Hepatitis A vaccine
Hepatitis B immune globulin
Hepatitis B vaccine
Immune globulin, intravenous

Pneumococcal vaccine, polyvalent
Tetanus immune globulin
Tetanus toxoid
Varicella vaccine

Urinary Tract Agents

Belladonna and opium
  suppositories
Bethanechol
Finasteride
Flavoxate

Mesna
Oxybutynin
Phenazopyridine
Terazosin

Miscellaneous

α-protease inhibitor
Demeclocycline
Diazoxide
Disulfiram
Edrophonium
Gallium nitrate
Lindane (γ benzene hexachloride)

Pamidronate
Permethrin
Physostigmine
Propofol
Sumatriptan
Tacrine

GENERIC DRUGS: INDICATIONS AND DOSAGE

■ Abciximab (ReoPro)

Indications: Prevention of acute ischemic complications in patients undergoing PTCA.

Action: Inhibits platelet aggregation.

Dosage: 0.25 mg/kg administered 10–60 minutes prior to PTCA, then 10 mcg/min continuous infusion for 12 hr.

Supplied: Injection 2 mg/mL.

Notes: Used concomitantly with heparin; may cause allergic reactions.

■ Acarbose (Precose)

Indications: Treatment of non-insulin-dependent diabetes mellitus (NIDDM).

Action: Inhibits alpha-glucosidase enzymes in the small intestine. This action slows the digestion of ingested carbohydrates which reduces the peaks in blood glucose that occur postprandially.

Dosage: Initial dose is 25 mg TID (break 50 mg tablet in half). Adjust dose upward to 50 mg TID after 4 to 8 weeks based on tolerability and one-hour postprandial blood glucose concentrations. Maintenance dose ranges from 50 to 100 mg TID.

Supplied: Tablets (scored): 50 mg, 100 mg.

Notes: Patients should swallow their dose with the first bite of each main meal. Adverse effects include abdominal pain, flatulence, and diarrhea. Should not be used in patients with inflammatory bowel disease, colonic ulceration, partial intestinal obstruction, or other chronic intestinal disease. May be used in combination with a sulfonylurea to improve glycemic control.

■ Acebutolol (Sectral) [See Table 7–6, p 529]

■ Acetaminophen (Tylenol, Others)
Indications: Mild pain, headache, fever.
Actions: Non-narcotic analgesic, antipyretic.
Dosage: 650 mg PO or PR Q 4–6 hr or 1000 mg PO Q 6 hr.
Supplied: Tablets 325 mg, 500 mg; elixir 120 mg/5 mL; drops 80 mg/0.8 mL.
Notes: Decrease dose with alcohol use; overdose causes hepatotoxicity which is treated with N-acetylcysteine; has no anti-inflammatory or platelet-inhibiting action.

■ Acetaminophen With Butalbital and Caffeine (Fioricet)
Indications: Mild pain, headache especially associated with stress.
Actions: Non-narcotic analgesic
Dosage: 1–2 tablets or capsules PO Q 4–6 hr PRN
Supplied: Each tablet or capsule contains 325 mg acetaminophen, 40 mg caffeine, and 50 mg butalbital.
Notes: May be habit-forming.

■ Acetaminophen With Codeine (Tylenol #1, #2, #3, #4) [C]
Indications: #1, #2, #3 for relief of mild to moderate pain; #4 for relief of moderate to severe pain.
Actions: Combined effects of acetaminophen and a narcotic analgesic.
Dosage: 1–2 tablets Q 3–4 hr PRN.
Supplied: Tablets; capsules; elixir per 5 mL: acetaminophen 120 mg and codeine 12 mg.
Notes: Codeine in #1 = 7.5 mg, #2 = 15 mg, #3 = 30 mg, #4 = 60 mg.

■ Acetazolamide (Diamox)
Indications: Diuresis, glaucoma, alkalinization of urine, refractory epilepsy.

Actions: Carbonic anhydrase inhibitor.
Dosage: *Diuretic:* 250–375 mg IV or PO Q 24 hr in divided doses.
Glaucoma: 250 mg–1000 mg PO Q day in divided doses.
Supplied: Tablets 125 mg, 250 mg; capsule SR 500 mg, injection 500 mg/vial.
Notes: Contraindicated in renal failure, sulfa hypersensitivity; follow Na^+ and K^+; watch for metabolic acidosis.

■ Acetohexamide (Dymelor) [See Table 7–12, p 535]

■ Acetylcysteine (Mucomyst)
Indications: Mucolytic agent as adjuvant therapy of chronic bronchopulmonary diseases and cystic fibrosis; as antidote to acetaminophen hepatotoxicity, most effective if given within 24 hours of ingestion.
Actions: Splits disulfide linkages between mucoprotein molecular complexes; protects liver by restoring glutathione levels in acetaminophen overdose.
Dosage: *Nebulizer:* 3–5 mL of 20% solution diluted with equal volume of water or normal saline administered TID–QID.
Antidote: PO or NG: 140 mg/kg diluted 1:4 in carbonated beverage as loading dose, then 70 mg/kg Q 4 hr for 17 doses.
Supplied: Solution 10%, 20%.
Notes: Watch for bronchospasm when used by inhalation in asthmatics; activated charcoal will adsorb acetylcysteine when given at the same time for acute acetaminophen ingestion.

■ Acyclovir (Zovirax)
Indications: Treatment of herpes simplex and herpes zoster viral infections.
Actions: Interferes with viral DNA synthesis.
Dosage: *Oral:*

- Initial genital herpes: 200 mg PO Q 4 hr while awake, for a total of 5 capsules/day for 10 days.
- Chronic suppression: 400 mg PO BID–TID.
- Intermittent therapy: same as for initial treatment, except treat for 5 days initiated at the earliest prodrome.
- Herpes zoster: 800 mg PO 5 times per day for 7 days.

Intravenous: 5–10 mg/kg/dose IV Q 8 hr.
Supplied: Capsules 200 mg; tablets 400mg, 800 mg; suspension 200 mg/5 mL; injection 500 mg/vial.
Notes: Adjust dose in renal insufficiency.

■ Adenosine (Adenocard)
Indications: Paroxysmal supraventricular tachycardia, including that associated with Wolff-Parkinson-White syndrome.

Actions: Class IV antiarrhythmic, slows conduction time through the AV node.

Dosage: 6 mg rapid IV bolus over 1 to 3 seconds followed by 20 mL saline flush; if no response in 1 to 2 minutes, then give 12 mg dose.

Supplied: Injection 6 mg/2 mL.

Notes: Doses > 12mg are not recommended; caffeine and theophylline antagonize the effects of adenosine, persantine may enhance the effect.

■ Albumin (Albuminar, Buminate, Albutein, others)

Indications: Plasma volume expansion for shock resulting from burns, surgery, hemorrhage, or other trauma.

Actions: Maintenance of plasma colloid oncotic pressure.

Dosage: 25 gm IV initially; subsequent infusions should depend upon clinical situation and response.

Supplied: Solution 5%, 25%.

Note: Contains 130–160 mEq Na^+/L.

■ Albuterol (Proventil, Ventolin)

Indications: Treatment of bronchospasm in reversible obstructive airway disease, prevention of exercise-induced bronchospasm.

Actions: Beta-adrenergic sympathomimetic bronchodilator; little effect on alpha receptors.

Dosage: 2–4 inhalations Q 4–6 hr; 1 Rotocap inhaled Q 4–6 hr; 2–4 mg PO TID–QID; nebulized treatment, 0.25–0.5 mL of a 2.5 mg/mL solution in 3 mL of normal saline.

Supplied: Tablets 2 mg, 4 mg; tablets, extended release 4 mg; syrup 2 mg/5 mL; metered dose inhaler; Rotocap 200 µg; solution for nebulization 0.083%, 0.5%.

■ Aldesleukin [IL-2] (Proleukin)

Indications: Treatment of metastatic renal cell carcinoma, melanoma, and colorectal cancer.

Actions: Human recombinant interleukin-2. Promotes proliferation, differentiation, and recruitment of T and B cells, natural killer cells and thymocytes. It can also stimulate lymphokine-activated killer (LAK) cells and tumor-infiltrating lymphocyte (TIL) cells.

Dosage: 600,000 IU/kg (0.037 mg/kg) administered every 8 hours by a 15-min infusion for 14 doses. Following 9 days of rest, repeat schedule for another 14 doses, for a maximum of 28 doses per cycle.

Supplied: Injection 18 million IU per mL.

Notes and Caution: Administer *only* in a hospital with an ICU and specialist available; may cause severe hypotension and capillary leaking, resulting in reduced organ perfusion.

■ Allopurinol (Zyloprim, Lopurin, Others)

Indications: Gout, treatment of hyperuricemia of malignancy, uric acid urolithiasis.

Actions: Xanthine oxidase inhibitor.

Dosage: Initial 100 mg PO Q day; usual 300 mg PO Q day.

Supplied: Tablets 100 mg, 300 mg.

Notes: Aggravates acute gouty attacks; do *not* administer until acute attack resolves.

■ Alpha-Protease Inhibitor (Prolastin)

Indications: Panacinar emphysema for α_1-antitrypsin deficiency.

Actions: Replacement of human α_1-protease inhibitor.

Dosage: 60 mg/kg IV once weekly.

Supplied: Injection $\geq$ 20 mg/mL.

Notes: May cause delayed fever up to 12 hours after administration. Fever typically resolves over 24 hours.

■ Alprazolam (Xanax) [C]

Indications: Management of anxiety and panic disorders, and anxiety associated with depression.

Actions: Benzodiazepine; CNS depressant.

Dosage: 0.25–2 mg PO TID.

Supplied: Tablets 0.25 mg, 0.5 mg, 1.0 mg, 2.0 mg.

Notes: Reduce dose in elderly and debilitated patients.

■ Alteplase, Recombinant [t-PA] (Activase)

Indications: Treatment of acute MI and pulmonary embolism.

Actions: A tissue plasminogen activator used as a thrombolytic agent.

Dosage: Front loading protocol: 15 mg IV bolus, then 50 mg over 30 minutes, then 35 mg over 60 minutes.

Notes: May cause bleeding; heparin should be given following alteplase to prevent reocclusion.

■ Altretamine (Hexalen)

Indications: Palliative treatment of ovarian cancer.

Actions: Unknown; may use liver enzyme system to activate cytotoxic properties.

Dosage: 260 mg/m^2/day PO divided Q 6 hr, for 14–21 consecutive days of a 28-day cycle.

Supplied: Capsules 50 mg.

Notes: May cause neurologic and hematologic toxicity.

■ Aluminum Carbonate (Basaljel)

Indications: Hyperacidity (peptic ulcer, hiatal hernia, etc.), supplement to management of hyperphosphatemia.

Actions: Neutralizes gastric acid; binds phosphate.

Dosage: 2 capsules or tablets, or 10 mL (in water) Q 2 hr PRN.

Supplied: Tablets, capsules, suspension.

■ Aluminum Hydroxide (Amphojel, Alternagel)

Indications: Hyperacidity (peptic ulcer, hiatal hernia, etc.), supplement to the management of hyperphosphatemia.

Actions: Neutralizes gastric acid; binds phosphate.

Dosage: 10–30 mL or 2 tablets PO Q 4–6 hr.

Supplied: Tablets 300 mg, 600 mg; chewable tablets 500 mg; suspension 320 mg/5mL, 600 mg/5 mL.

Notes: Can be used in renal failure; may cause constipation.

■ Aluminum Hydroxide With Magnesium Hydroxide (Maalox)

Indications: Hyperacidity (peptic ulcer, hiatal hernia, etc.).

Actions: Neutralizes gastric acid.

Dosage: 10–60 mL or 2–4 tablets PO QID or PRN.

Supplied: Tablets, suspension.

Notes: Doses QID are best given after meals and at bedtime; may cause hypermagnesemia in renal insufficiency.

■ Aluminum Hydroxide With Magnesium Hydroxide and Simethicone (Mylanta, Mylanta II, Maalox Plus)

Indications: Hyperacidity with bloating.

Actions: Neutralizes gastric acid.

Dosage: 10–60 mL or 2–4 tablets PO QID or PRN.

Supplied: Tablets, suspension.

Notes: May cause hypermagnesemia in renal insufficiency; Mylanta II contains twice the amount of aluminum and magnesium hydroxide as Mylanta.

■ Aluminum Hydroxide, Magnesium Trisilicate, and Alginic Acid (Gaviscon)

Indications: Symptomatic relief of heartburn; hiatal hernia.

Actions: Neutralizes gastric acid.

Dosage: 2–4 tablets or 15–30 mL PO QID followed by water.

Supplied: Tablets, suspension.

Notes: May cause hypermagnesemia in renal insufficiency.

■ Amantadine (Symmetrel)

Indications: Treatment or prophylaxis of Influenza A viral infections; parkinsonism.

Actions: Prevents release of infectious viral nucleic acid into the host cell; releases dopamine from intact dopaminergic terminals.

Dosage: *Influenza A:* 200 mg PO QD or 100 mg PO BID.
　　　　　 Parkinsonism: 100 mg PO QD–BID.

Supplied: Capsules 100 mg; syrup 50 mg/5 mL.

Notes: Reduce dose in renal insufficiency.

■ Amikacin (Amikin)

Indications: Treatment of serious infections caused by gram-negative bacteria.

Actions: Aminoglycoside antibiotic, inhibits protein synthesis.

Dosage: 5–7.5 mg loading dose; followed by 5 mg/kg/24 hr divided Q 8–24 hr based on renal function; refer to aminoglycoside dosing in Table 7–15, p 537.

Supplied: Injection 100 mg/2 mL, 500 mg/2 mL.

Notes: May be effective against gram-negative bacteria resistant to gentamicin and tobramycin; monitor renal function carefully for dosage adjustments; monitor serum levels (Table 7–14, p 536).

■ Amiloride (Midamor)

Indications: Hypertension and congestive heart failure.

Actions: Potassium-sparing diuretic.

Dosage: 5–10 mg PO Q day.

Supplied: Tablets 5mg.

Notes: Hyperkalemia may occur; monitor serum potassium levels.

■ Aminocaproic Acid (Amicar)

Indications: Treatment of excessive bleeding resulting from systemic hyperfibrinolysis and urinary fibrinolysis.

Actions: Inhibits fibrinolysis via inhibition of plasminogen activator substances.

Dosage: 100 mg/kg IV, then 1 gm/m^2/hr to maximum of 18 gm/m^2/day or 100 mg/kg/dose Q 8 hr.

Supplied: Tablets 500 mg; syrup 250 mg/mL; injection 250 mg/mL.

Notes and Caution: Administer for 8 hr or until bleeding is controlled; Contraindicated in disseminated intravascular coagulation; *not for upper urinary tract bleeding.*

■ Aminophylline

Indications: Asthma and bronchospasm.

Actions: Relaxes the smooth muscle of the bronchi and pulmonary blood vessels.

Dosage: *Acute asthma:* Load 6 mg/kg IV, then 0.4–0.9 mg/kg/hr IV continuous infusion.

Supplied: Tablets 100 mg, 200 mg; solution 105 mg/5 mL; suppositories 250 mg, 500 mg; injection 25 mg/mL.

Notes: Individualize dosage; signs of toxicity include nausea, vomiting, irritability, tachycardia, ventricular arrhythmias, and seizures; follow serum levels carefully (Table 7–13, p 536); aminophylline is about 85% theophylline; erratic absorption with rectal doses.

■ Amiodarone (Cordarone)

Indications: Treatment of recurrent ventricular fibrillation or hemodynamically unstable ventricular tachycardia.

Actions: Class III antiarrhythmic.

Dosage: *Oral:*

- Loading dose: 800–1600 mg/day PO for 1–3 weeks
- Maintenance: 600–800 mg/day PO for 1 month, then 200–400 mg/day.

Intravenous: 15 mg/min for 10 min, followed by 1 mg/min for 6 hr, followed by a maintenance infusion of 0.5 mg/min.

Supplied: Tablets 200 mg; injection 150 mg/3 mL.

Notes: Average half-life is 53 days; potentially toxic effects leading to pulmonary fibrosis, liver failure, ocular opacities, as well as exacerbation of arrhythmias. Response requires 1 month as a rule; IV concentrations > 2 mg/mL should be administered via a central catheter.

■ Amitriptyline (Elavil, Others)

Indications: Depression, peripheral neuropathy, chronic pain, cluster and migraine headaches.

Actions: Tricyclic antidepressant.

Dosage: Initial dose 50–100 mg PO Q HS, may be increased to 300 mg Q HS.

Supplied: Tablets 10 mg, 25 mg, 50 mg, 75 mg, 100 mg, 150 mg; injection 10 mg/mL.

Notes: Strong anticholinergic side effects; may cause urine retention and sedation.

■ Amlodipine (Norvasc)

Indications: Treatment of hypertension, chronic stable angina, and vasospastic angina.

Actions: Calcium channel blocking agent

Dosage: 2.5–10 mg PO Q day

Supplied: Tablets 2.5 mg, 5 mg, 10 mg.

Notes: May be taken without regard to meals

■ Amoxicillin (Amoxil, Larotid, Polymox, Others)

Indications: Treatment of susceptible gram-positive bacteria (streptococci), and gram-negative bacteria (*Haemophilus influenzae, Escherichia coli, Proteus mirabilis*).

Actions: Inhibits cell wall synthesis.

Dosage: 250–500 mg PO TID.

Supplied: Capsules 250 mg, 500 mg; suspension 50 mg/5mL, 125 mg/5 mL, 250 mg/5mL.

Notes: Cross-hypersensitivity with penicillin; may cause diarrhea; skin rash is common; many hospital strains of *E coli* are resistant.

■ Amoxicillin/Potassium Clavulanate (Augmentin)

Indications: Treatment of infections caused by beta-lactamase producing strains of *H influenzae, S aureus,* and *E coli.*

Actions: Combines a beta-lactamase antibiotic and a beta-lactamase inhibitor.

Dosage: 250–500 mg as amoxicillin PO Q 8 hr.

Supplied: (amoxicillin/potassium clavulanate) Tablets 250/125 mg, 500/125 mg; chewable tablets 125/31.25 mg, 250/62.5 mg; suspension 125/31.25 mg per 5 mL, 250/62.5 mg per 5 mL.

Note: *Do not substitute* two 250 mg tablets for one 500 mg tablet or an overdose of clavulanic acid will occur; may cause diarrhea and GI intolerance.

■ Amphotericin B (Fungizone)

Indications: Severe systemic fungal infections.

Actions: Binds to the sterols in the fungal membrane, altering membrane permeability.

Dosage: Test dose of 1 mg, then 0.25–1.5 mg/kg/24 hr IV over 4–6 hours. Doses often range from 25–50 mg Q day or every other day; total dose varies with indication.

Supplied: Powder for injection 50 mg/vial.

Notes: Monitor renal function; hypokalemia and hypomagnesemia may be seen from renal wasting; pretreatment with acetaminophen and antihistamines (diphenhydramine) to help minimize adverse affects associated with IV infusion.

■ Ampicillin (Amcil, Omnipen, Others)

Indications: Treatment of susceptible gram-negative (*Shigella, Salmonella, E coli, H influenzae, P mirabilis*) and gram-positive (streptococci) bacteria.

Actions: Beta-lactam antibiotic, inhibits cell wall synthesis.

Dosage: 500 mg–2 gm PO, IM, or IV Q 6 hr.

Supplied: Capsules 250 mg, 500 mg; suspension 100 mg/mL, 125 mg/5 mL, 250 mg/5 mL, 500 mg/5 mL; powder for injection 125 mg, 250 mg, 500 mg, 1 gm, 2 gm, 10 gm vials.

Notes: Cross-hypersensitivity with penicillin; can cause diarrhea and skin rash; many hospital strains of *E coli* are now resistant.

■ Ampicillin/Sulbactam (Unasyn)

Indications: Treatment of infections caused by beta-lactamase producing organisms of *S aureus, Enterococcus, H influenzae, P mirabilis,* and *Bacteroides* species.

Actions: Combines a beta-lactam antibiotic and a beta-lactamase inhibitor.

Dosage: 1.5–3.0 gm IM or IV Q 6 hr.

Supplied: Powder for injection 1.5 gm, 3.0 gm vials.

Notes: 2:1 ratio of ampicillin:sulbactam; adjust dosage in renal failure; monitor patient for hypersensitivity reactions.

■ Anistreplase (Eminase)

Indications: Treatment of acute myocardial infarction.

Actions: Thrombolytic agent.

Dosage: 30 U IV over 2–5 min.

Supplied: Vials containing 30 U.

Notes: May not be effective if readministered > 5 days after previous dose of anistreplase, streptokinase, or a streptococcal infection due to production of antistreptokinase antibody.

■ Antihemophilic Factor [Factor VIII] (Monoclate)

Indications: Treatment of classical hemophilia A.

Actions: Provides Factor VIII needed to convert prothrombin to thrombin.

Dosage: 1 AHF unit/kg increases Factor VIII concentration in the body by ~2%. Units required = (kg) (desired Factor VIII increase as % normal) × (0.5).

- Prophylaxis of spontaneous hemorrhage = 5% normal.
- Hemostasis following trauma or surgery = 30% normal.
- Head injuries, major surgery or bleeding = 80–100% normal.

The patient's percentage of normal level of Factor VIII concentration must be ascertained prior to dosing for these calculations.

Supplied: Check each vial for the number of units it contains.

Note: AHF is not effective in controlling bleeding of patients with von Willebrand's disease.

■ Antithymocyte Globulin [ATG] (Atgam)

Indications: Management of allograft rejection in renal transplant patients.

Actions: Reduces the number of circulating, thymus-dependent lymphocytes.

Dosage: 10–30 mg/kg/day.

Supplied: Injection 50 mg/mL.

Notes and Caution: Do *not* administer to a patient with prior history of severe systemic reaction to any other equine gamma globulin preparation; discontinue treatment if severe unremitting thrombocytopenia or leukopenia occurs.

■ Anusol, Anusol-HC

Indications: Symptomatic relief of pain from external and internal hemorrhoids and anorectal surgery.

Actions: Local anesthetic.

Dosage: One suppository Q AM, HS, and following each bowel movement; apply cream or ointment freely to anal area Q 6–12 hr.

Supplied: Suppository, cream, ointment.

Note: Anusol-HC also contains hydrocortisone for anti-inflammatory effect.

■ Apraclonidine (Iodipine) [See Table 7–11, pp 533 & 534]

■ Aprotinin (Trasylol)

Indications: Reduction or prevention of blood loss in patients undergoing CABG

Actions: Protease inhibitor, antifibrinolytic

Dosage: *High dose:* 2 million KIU load, 2 million KIU for the pump-priming dose, followed by 500,000 KIU/hr until surgery is completed.

Low dose: 1 million KIU load, 1 million KIU for pump-priming dose, followed by 250,000 KIU/hr until surgery is completed.

Maximum total dose = 7 million KIU.

Supplied: Injection 1.4 mg/mL

Notes: 1 KIU = 0.14 mg of aprotinin.

■ Asparaginase (Elspar)

Indications: Treatment of leukemia

Actions: Hydrolyzes serum asparagine to nonfunctional aspartic acid, depriving the tumor cell of the needed amino acid.

Dosage: Varies with individual protocols.

Supplied: Injection 10,000 IU

Notes: May cause anaphylaxis and sudden death.

■ Aspirin (Bayer, St. Joseph, Others)

Indications: Mild pain, headache, fever, inflammation, prevention of emboli, and prevention of myocardial infarction.

Actions: Inhibits prostaglandins.

Dosage:

- Pain, fever: 325–650 mg Q 4–6 hr PO or PR.
- Rheumatoid arthritis: 3–6 gm/day PO in divided doses.
- Platelet inhibitory action: 325 mg PO Q day.
- Prevention of MI: 325 mg PO Q day.

Supplied: Tablets 325 mg, 500 mg; chewable tablets 80 mg; enteric-coated tablets 325 mg, 500 mg, 650 mg, 975 mg; tablets SR 650 mg, 800 mg; suppositories 60 mg, 120 mg, 125 mg, 130 mg, 195 mg, 200 mg, 300 mg, 325 mg, 600 mg, 650 mg, 1.2 gm.

Notes: GI upset and erosion are common adverse reactions; discontinue use 1 week prior to surgery to avoid post-operative bleeding complications. See drug levels for salicylates (Table 7–13, p 536).

■ Aspirin With Butalbital and Caffeine (Fiorinal) [C]

Indications: Mild pain, headache especially when associated with stress.

Actions: Non-narcotic analgesic.

Dosage: 1–2 tablets (capsules) PO Q 4–6 hr PRN.

Supplied: Each capsule or tablet contains 325 mg aspirin, 40 mg caffeine, and 50 mg butalbital.

Notes: This compound is also available with codeine: #1 = 7.5 mg; #2 = 15 mg; #3 = 30 mg; significant drowsiness associated with use.

■ Aspirin With Codeine (Empirin #1, #2, #3, #4) [C]

Indications: Relief of mild to moderate pain.

Actions: Combined analgesic effects of aspirin and codeine.

Dosage: 1–2 tablets PO Q 3–4 hr PRN.

Supplied: Tablets 325 mg aspirin, with codeine as specified below.

Notes: Codeine in #1 = 7.5 mg, #2 = 15 mg, #3 = 30 mg, #4 = 60 mg.

■ Astemizole (Hismanal)

Indications: Allergic rhinitis.

Actions: Antihistamine.

Dosage: 10 mg PO daily.

Supplied: Tablet 10 mg.

Notes: Astemizole is nonsedating and should be taken on an empty stomach (1 hr before or 2 hrs after meal); may affect allergy skin testing for weeks after one dose. It may also cause ventricular arrhythmias when used concurrently with the macrolide antibiotics, itraconazole or ketoconazole, or the selective serotonin reuptake inhibitor antidepressants (fluoxetine, paroxetine and sertraline).

■ Atenolol (Tenormin) [See Table 7–6, p 529]

■ Atovaquone (Mepron)
Indications: Treatment of mild to moderate *Pneumocystis carinii* pneumonia.
Actions: Inhibits nucleic acid and ATP synthesis.
Dosage: 750 mg PO TID for 21 days.
Supplied: Suspension 750 mg/5 mL.
Notes: Should be taken with meals.

■ Atracurium (Tracrium)
Indications: Adjunct to anesthesia to facilitate endotracheal intubation.
Actions: Nondepolarizing neuromuscular blocker; skeletal muscle relaxant.
Dosage: 0.4–0.5 mg/kg IV bolus, then 0.08–0.1 mg/kg every 20–45 min PRN.
Supplied: Injection 10 mg/mL.
Notes: Patient must be intubated and on controlled ventilation; use adequate amounts of sedation and analgesia.

■ Atropine
Indications: Preanesthesia, symptomatic bradycardia, asystole.
Actions: Atropine is an anticholinergic and antimuscarinic agent.
Dosage: Emergency cardiac care, bradycardia: 0.5 mg IV Q 5 min up to 2.0 mg total; asystole 1.0 mg IV, repeat in 5 min.
        Preanesthetic: 0.3–0.6 mg IM.
Supplied: Tablets 0.3 mg, 0.4 mg, 0.6 mg; injection 0.05 mg/mL, 0.1 mg/mL, 0.3 mg/mL, 0.4 mg/mL, 0.5 mg/mL, 0.8 mg/mL, 1.0 mg/mL.
Notes: Can cause blurred vision, urinary retention, dried mucous membranes.

■ Azathioprine (Imuran)
Indications: Adjunct for the prevention of rejection following organ transplantation; rheumatoid arthritis; systemic lupus erythematosus (SLE).
Actions: Immunosuppressive agent.
Dosage: 1–3 mg/kg IV or PO daily.
Supplied: Tablets 50 mg; injection 100 mg/20 mL.
Notes: May cause GI intolerance; injection should be handled with cytotoxic precautions.

■ Azithromycin (Zithromax)

Indications: Treatment of mild to moderate upper and lower respiratory tract infections, and nongonococcal urethritis.

Actions: Macrolide antibiotic.

Dosage: Respiratory tract: 500 mg on Day 1 of treatment cycle, followed by 250 mg PO Q day for 4 more days.

  Non-gonococcal urethritis: 1 gm as a single dose.

Supplied: Capsule 250 mg; suspension 100 mg/5 mL, 200 mg/5 mL, 1 gm single-dose packet.

Notes: Should be taken on an empty stomach. Avoid use of astemizole and terfenadine within 10 days of initiation of treatment with azithromycin.

■ Aztreonam (Azactam)

Indications: Treatment of infections caused by aerobic gram-negative bacteria including *Pseudomonas aeruginosa*.

Actions: Monobactam antibiotic, inhibits cell wall synthesis.

Dosage: 1–2 gm IV/IM Q 6–12 hr.

Supplied: Injection 500 mg, 1 gm, 2 gm.

Notes: Not effective against gram-positive or anaerobic bacteria; may be given to penicillin-allergic patients.

■ Baclofen (Lioresal)

Indications: Management of spasticity secondary to severe chronic disorders such as multiple sclerosis (MS) or spinal cord lesions.

Actions: Centrally acting skeletal muscle relaxant.

Dosage: 5 mg PO TID initially, increase every 3 days to maximum effect; maximum 80 mg/day.

Supplied: Tablets 10 mg, 20 mg.

Notes: Use caution in epileptic and neuropsychiatric disturbances.

■ Beclomethasone (Beconase, Vancenase Nasal Inhalers)

Indications: Allergic rhinitis refractory to conventional therapy with antihistamines and decongestants.

Actions: Inhaled corticosteroid; anti-inflammatory agent.

Dosage: 1 spray intranasally BID–QID.

Supplied: Nasal metered-dose inhaler.

Notes: Nasal spray delivers 42 µg/dose.

■ Beclomethasone (Beclovent Inhaler, Vanceril Inhaler)

Indications: Chronic asthma.

Actions: Inhaled corticosteroid.

Dosage: 2–4 inhalations TID–QID (max 20/day).

Supplied: Oral metered-dose inhaler.
Notes: Not effective for acute asthmatic attacks; may cause oral candidiasis. Rinse mouth after use to prevent candidiasis.

■ Belladonna and Opium Suppositories (B & O Supprettes) [C]

Indications: Treatment of bladder spasms; moderate to severe pain.
Actions: Antispasmodic.
Dosage: One suppository PR Q 4–6 hr PRN.

- 15A = 30 mg powdered opium; 16.2 mg belladonna extract.
- 16A = 60 mg powdered opium; 16.2 mg belladonna extract.

Supplied: Suppositories 15A, 16A.
Notes: Anticholinergic side effects; advise patients about sedation, urinary retention, constipation.

■ Benazepril (Lotensin) [See Table 7–3, p 527]

■ Benzonatate (Tessalon Perles)

Indications: Symptomatic relief of nonproductive cough.
Actions: Anesthetizes the stretch receptors in the respiratory passages.
Dosage: 100 mg PO TID.
Supplied: Capsules 100 mg.
Notes: May cause sedation. **Caution:** Instruct patient *not* to chew or puncture capsule; it must be swallowed whole.

■ Benztropine (Cogentin)

Indications: Treatment of parkinsonism and drug-induced extrapyramidal disorders.
Actions: Antimuscarinic agent.
Dosage: 1–6 mg PO, IM, or IV in divided doses.
Supplied: Tablets 0.5 mg, 1.0 mg, 2.0 mg; injection 1 mg/mL.
Note: Anticholinergic side effects.

■ Bepridil (Vascor)

Indications: Treatment of chronic stable angina.
Actions: Calcium channel blocking agent.
Dosage: 200–400 mg PO daily.
Supplied: Tablets 200 mg, 300 mg, 400 mg.
Notes: May cause agranulocytosis and serious ventricular arrhythmias, including torsade de pointes.

■ Betamethasone (Celestone) [See Table 7–2, p 526]

■ Betaxolol, Ophthalmic (Betoptic) [See Table 7–11, pp 533 & 534]

■ Betaxolol (Kerlone) [See Table 7–6, p 529]

■ Bethanechol (Urecholine, Duvoid, Others)
Indications: Neurogenic atony of the bladder with urinary retention, acute postoperative and postpartum functional (nonobstructive) urinary retention.
Actions: Parasympathomimetic stimulant.
Dosage: 10–50 mg PO TID–QID or 5 mg SC TID–QID and PRN.
Supplied: Tablets 5 mg, 10 mg, 25 mg, 50 mg; injection 5 mg/mL.
Notes and Caution: Contraindicated in bladder outlet obstruction, asthma, coronary artery disease; *do not* administer IM or IV.

■ Bisacodyl (Dulcolax)
Indications: Constipation, bowel prep.
Actions: Stimulant laxative.
Dosage: 5–10 mg PO or 10 mg PR PRN.
Supplied: Enteric-coated tablets 5 mg; suppository 10 mg.
Notes and Cautions: do not use with an acute abdomen or bowel obstruction; instruct patient *not* to chew tablets; *do not* administer within 1 hour of giving antacids or milk.

■ Bismuth Subsalicylate (Pepto-Bismol)
Indications: Indigestion, nausea, and diarrhea.
Actions: Antisecretory and anti-inflammatory effects.
Dosage: Two tablets or 30 mL PO PRN.
Supplied: Tablets, chewable 262 mg; liquid 262 mg/15 mL, 524 mg/15 mL.

■ Bisoprolol (Zebeta) [See Table 7–6, p 529]

■ Bitolterol (Tornalate)
Indications: Prophylaxis and treatment of asthma and reversible bronchospasm.
Actions: Sympathomimetic bronchodilator.
Dosage: Two inhalations Q 8 hr.
Supplied: Aerosol 0.8%.

■ Bleomycin (Blenoxane)

Indications: Treatment of cervical, ovarian, squamous cell, testicular cancer, and lymphoma.

Actions: Antibiotic, antineoplastic agent.

Dosage: 0.25–0.5 U/kg/dose IV, IM, or SC once or twice weekly.

Supplied: Injection 15 U.

Notes: Pulmonary toxicity is increased with total doses of > 400 U.

■ Bretylium (Bretylol)

Indications: Acute treatment of ventricular fibrillation or tachycardia unresponsive to conventional therapy.

Actions: Class III antiarrhythmic.

Dosage: 5 mg/kg IV rapid injection (1 minute); may repeat Q 15–30 min with 10 mg/kg (max 30 mg/kg); maintenance, 1–2 mg/min IV infusion.

Supplied: Injection 50 mg/mL.

Notes: Nausea and vomiting are associated with rapid IV bolus; should gradually reduce dose and discontinue in 3–5 days; effects are seen within first 10–15 min; transient rise in BP seen initially; hypotension most frequent adverse effect and occurs within the first hour of treatment.

■ Bromocriptine (Parlodel)

Indications: Hyperprolactinemia and Parkinson's syndrome.

Actions: Acts directly on the striatal dopamine receptors.

Dosage: *Hyperprolactinemia:* 5–7.5 mg daily.
        Parkinsonism: 1.25 mg PO BID initially, titrated to effect.

Supplied: Tablets 2.5 mg; capsules 5 mg.

Notes: Nausea and vertigo are common side effects.

■ Budesonide (Rhinocort)

Indications: Management of allergic and non-allergic rhinitis.

Actions: Intranasal steroid.

Dosage: Two sprays in each nostril BID.

Supplied: Nasal inhaler.

■ Bumetanide (Bumex)

Indications: Edema from congestive heart failure, hepatic cirrhosis, and renal disease.

Actions: Loop diuretic.

Dosage: 0.5–2.0 mg PO daily; 0.5–1.0 mg IV Q 8–24 hr.

Supplied: Tablets 0.5 mg, 1 mg; injection 0.25 mg/mL.

Notes: Monitor patient's fluid and electrolyte status during treatment.

■ Buprenorphine (Buprenex)
Indications: Relief of moderate to severe pain.
Actions: CNS agent; narcotic agonist-antagonist.
Dosage: 0.3 mg IM or slow IV push Q 6 hr PRN.
Supplied: Injection 0.324 mg/mL (= 0.3 mg of buprenorphine).
Notes: May induce withdrawal syndrome in opioid-dependent subjects.

■ Bupropion (Wellbutrin)
Indications: Treatment of depression.
Actions: Weak inhibition of neuronal uptake of serotonin and norepinephrine; also inhibition of the neuronal reuptake of dopamine.
Dosage: 200–450 mg Q day divided BID–TID.
Supplied: Tablets 75 mg, 100 mg.
Notes: Has been associated with seizures; avoid use of alcohol and other CNS depressants.

■ Buspirone (BuSpar)
Indications: Short-term relief of anxiety.
Actions: Antianxiety agent with agonist effects on presynaptic dopamine receptors.
Dosage: 5–10 mg PO TID.
Supplied: Tablets 5 mg, 10 mg.
Notes: Minimal potential for abuse, or for physical or psychological dependence.

■ Busulfan (Myleran)
Indications: Treatment of leukemia.
Actions: Alkylating agent.
Dosage: Induction with 4–8 mg/day, then maintenance therapy with 1–3 mg/day.
Supplied: Tablets 2 mg.

■ Butorphanol (Stadol)
Indications: Analgesic for moderate to severe pain.
Actions: Narcotic agonist-antagonist.
Dosage: 2 mg IM or IV Q 3–4 hr PRN.
Supplied: Injection 1 mg/mL, 2 mg/mL.
Notes: May induce withdrawal syndrome in opioid-dependent patients.

■ Calcium Carbonate (Tums, Alka-mints)
Indications: Hyperacidity associated with peptic ulcer disease, hiatal hernia, etc.

Actions: Neutralizes gastric acid.
Dosage: 500 mg–1.5 gm PO PRN.
Supplied: Chewable tablets 350 mg, 420 mg, 500 mg, 550 mg, 750 mg, 850 mg; suspension.
Notes: Calcium carbonate contains 40% elemental calcium (20 mEq calcium/g).

■ Calcium Salts

Indications: Electromechanical dissociation secondary to hypocalcemia or calcium channel blocker toxicity, life-threatening hypercalcemia, symptomatic hypocalcemia.
Actions: Dietary supplement; increased myocardial contractility, binding phosphate.
Dosage: *Replacement:* 1–2 gm PO Q day.
    Cardiac emergencies: Calcium chloride 0.5–1.0 gm IV Q 10 min or calcium gluconate 1–2 gm IV Q 10 min.
    Hyperphosphatemia in end-stage renal disease: 2 tablets with each meal.
Supplied: Oral: Tablets 500 mg, 650 mg, 975 mg, 1 g; Calcium chloride injection 10% (100 mg/mL); calcium gluconate injection 10% (100 mg/mL).
Notes: Calcium chloride contains 270 mg (13.6 mEq) elemental calcium per gram, and calcium gluconate contains 90 mg (4.5 mEq) elemental calcium per gram.

■ Captopril (Capoten) [See Table 7–3, p 527]

Indications: Diabetic nephropathy, congestive heart failure, hypertension, and following myocardial infarction.
Actions: Angiotensin-converting enzyme inhibitor.
Dosage: 25–50 mg PO TID.
Supplied: Tablets 12.5 mg, 25 mg, 50 mg, 100 mg.
Notes: Use with caution in renal failure. Give 1 hour before meals; can cause rash, proteinuria, and nonproductive cough. For first dose, give 6.25 mg; then increase dose.

■ Carbamazepine (Tegretol)

Indications: Epilepsy; trigeminal neuralgia.
Actions: Anticonvulsant.
Dosage: 200 mg PO BID initially; increase by 200 mg/day; usual dosage is 800–1200 mg/day.
Supplied: Tablets 200 mg; chewable tablets 100 mg; suspension 100 mg/5 mL.
Notes and Caution: Can cause severe hematologic side effects; monitor CBC; monitor serum drug levels, consult Table 7–13, p 536. Generic products are *not* interchangeable with Tegretol (trade name).

■ Carbidopa/Levodopa (Sinemet)
Indications: Parkinson's disease.
Actions: Increases CNS dopamine levels.
Dosage: Start at 10/100 (mg carbidopa/mg levodopa) PO BID–TID; titrate as needed.
Supplied: Tablets 10/100, 25/100, 25/250.
Notes: May cause psychiatric disturbances, orthostatic hypotension, dyskinesia, and cardiac arrhythmias.

■ Carboplatin (Paraplatin)
Indications: Treatment of cervical, ovarian, and lung cancer.
Actions: Alkylating agent.
Dosage: 300-360 mg/m^2 on Day 1 of treatment schedule every 4 weeks.
Supplied: Injection 50 mg, 150 mg, 450 mg
Notes: May cause bone marrow suppression, vomiting, and anaphylaxis.

■ Carisoprodol (Soma)
Indications: Adjunct to sleep and physical therapy for the relief of painful musculoskeletal conditions.
Actions: Centrally acting muscle relaxant.
Dosage: 350 mg PO QID.
Supplied: Tablets 350 mg.
Notes: Avoid alcohol and other CNS depressants.

■ Carteolol (Cartrol) [See Table 7–6, p 529]

■ Carvedilol (Coreg) [See Table 7–6, p 529]

■ Cefaclor (Ceclor) [See Table 7–8, p 530]

■ Cefadroxil (Duricef, Ultracef) [See Table 7–7, p 530]

■ Cefamandole (Mandol) [See Table 7–8, p 530]

■ Cefazolin (Ancef, Kefzol) [See Table 7–7, p 530]

■ Cefixime (Suprax) [See Table 7–9, p 531]

■ **Cefmetazole (Zefazone) [See Table 7–8, p 530]**

■ **Cefonicid (Monocid) [See Table 7–8, p 530]**

■ **Cefoperazone (Cefobid) [See Table 7–9, p 531]**

■ **Cefotaxime (Claforan) [See Table 7–9, p 531]**

■ **Cefotetan (Cefotan) [See Table 7–8, p 530]**

■ **Cefoxitin (Mefoxin) [See Table 7–8, p 530]**

■ **Cefpodoxime (Vantin) [See Table 7–9, p 531]**

■ **Cefprozil (Cefzil) [See Table 7–8, p 530]**

■ **Ceftazidime (Fortaz, Ceptaz, Tazidime, Tazicef) [See Table 7–9, p 531]**

■ **Ceftizoxime (Cefizox) [See Table 7–9, p 531]**

■ **Ceftriaxone (Rocephen) [See Table 7–9, p 531]**

■ **Cefuroxime (Ceftin, Zinacef) [See Table 7–8, p 530]**

■ **Cephalexin (Keflex, Keftab) [See Table 7–7, p 530]**

■ **Cephalothin (Keflin) [See Table 7–7, p 530]**

■ **Cephapirin (Cefadyl) [See Table 7–7, p 530]**

■ **Cephradine (Velosef) [See Table 7–7, p 530]**

■ **Charcoal, Activated (Superchar, Actidose, Liqui-Char)**
Indications: Emergency treatment in poisoning by most drugs and chemicals.
Actions: Adsorbent detoxicant.
Dosage: *Acute intoxication:* 30–100 gm/dose.
  Gastrointestinal dialysis: 25–50 gm Q 4–6 hr.
Supplied: Powder, liquid.
Notes: Administer with a cathartic; some liquid dosage forms are in sorbitol base. Protect airway in lethargic or comatose patient.

■ **Chlorambucil (Leukeran)**
Indications: Treatment of ovarian cancer, leukemia, and lymphoma.
Actions: Alkylating agent.
Dosage: Initially 0.1–0.2 mg/kg/day for 3–6 wk, then maintenance therapy with no more than 0.1 mg/kg/day.
Supplied: Tablets 2 mg.

■ **Chloramphenicol (Chloromycetin)**
Indications: Serious infections caused by gram-positive and gram-negative aerobic and anaerobic bacteria. Can be used to treat *Enterococcus* resistant to ampicillin and vancomycin.
Action: Interferes with protein synthesis.
Dosage: 50–100 mg/kg/day IV in four divided doses.
Supplied: Powder for injection.
Notes and Caution: Aplastic anemia has been associated with the use of this drug; monitor hematology labs closely. Reduce dosage with hepatic impairment. *Pseudomonas aeruginosa* is almost universally resistant.

■ **Chloramphenicol, Ophthalmic (Chloromycetin Ophthalmic) [See Table 7–11, pp 533 & 534]**

■ **Chlordiazepoxide (Librium) [C]**
Indications: Anxiety, tension, alcohol withdrawal.
Actions: Benzodiazepine.
Dosage: *Mild anxiety, tension:* 5–10 mg PO TID–QID or PRN.

Severe anxiety, tension: 25–50 mg IM or IV TID–QID or PRN.
Alcohol withdrawal: 50–100 mg IM or IV; repeat in 2–4 hr if needed, up to 300 mg in 24 hr; gradually taper daily dosage.

Supplied: Tablets and capsules 5 mg, 10 mg, 25 mg; injection 100 mg/vial.

Notes: Reduce dose in the elderly; absorption of IM doses can be erratic.

■ Chlorothiazide (Diuril)

Indications: Hypertension, edema, congestive heart failure.

Actions: Thiazide diuretic.

Dosage: 500 mg–1.0 gm PO or IV Q day–BID.

Supplied: Tablets 250 mg, 500 mg; suspension 250 mg/5 mL; injection 500 mg/vial.

Notes: Contraindicated in anuria.

■ Chlorpheniramine (Chlor-Trimeton, Others)

Indications: Allergic reactions.

Actions: Antihistamine.

Dosage: 4 mg PO or IV Q 4–6 hr or 8–12 mg PO BID of sustained release.

Supplied: Tablets 4 mg; chewable tablets 2 mg; tablets SR 8 mg, 12 mg; syrup 2 mg/5 mL; injection 10 mg/mL, 100 mg/mL.

Notes: Anticholinergic side effects and sedation are common.

■ Chlorpromazine (Thorazine)

Indications: Psychotic disorders, apprehension, intractable hiccups, control of nausea and vomiting.

Actions: Phenothiazine antipsychotic, antiemetic.

Dosage: *Acute anxiety, agitation:* 10–25 mg PO or PR BID–TID.
Severe symptoms: 25 mg IM, can repeat in 1 hour; then 25–50 mg PO or PR TID.
Hiccups: 25–50 mg PO BID–TID.

Supplied: Tablets 10 mg, 25 mg, 50 mg, 100 mg, 200 mg; capsules sustained-release 30 mg, 75 mg, 150 mg, 200 mg, 300 mg; syrup 10 mg/5 mL; concentrate 30 mg/mL, 100 mg/mL; suppositories 25 mg, 100 mg; injection 25 mg/mL.

Notes: Beware of extrapyramidal side effects, and sedation; drug has alpha-adrenergic blocking properties.

■ Chlorpropamide (Diabinese) [See Table 7–12, p 535]

■ Chlorthalidone (Hygroton, Others)
Indications: Hypertension, edema associated with congestive heart failure, steroid and estrogen therapy.
Actions: Thiazide diuretic.
Dosage: 50–100 mg PO Q day.
Supplied: Tablets 25 mg, 50 mg, 100 mg.
Notes: Contraindicated in anuric patients.

■ Chlorzoxazone (Paraflex, Parafon Forte DSC)
Indications: Adjunct to rest and physical therapy for the relief of discomfort associated with acute, painful musculoskeletal conditions.
Actions: Centrally acting skeletal muscle relaxant.
Dosage: 250–500 mg PO TID–QID.
Supplied: Tablets 250 mg, caplets 500 mg.

■ Cholecalciferol [Vitamin D_3] (Delta D)
Indications: Dietary supplement for treatment of vitamin D deficiency.
Actions: Enhances intestinal calcium absorption.
Dosage: 400–1000 IU PO daily.
Supplied: Tablets 400 IU, 1000 IU.
Notes: 1 mg cholecalciferol = 40,000 IU of vitamin D activity.

■ Cholestyramine (Questran)
Indications: Adjunctive therapy for the reduction of serum cholesterol in patients with primary hypercholesterolemia; relief of pruritus associated with partial biliary obstruction.
Actions: Binds bile acids in the intestine to form insoluble complexes.
Dosage: Individualize dose to 4 gm 1–6 times a day.
Supplied: 4 gm cholestyramine resin/9 gm of powder.
Notes: Administer by mixing 4 gm cholestyramine in 2–6 oz. of non-carbonated beverage; give before meals.

■ Cimetidine (Tagamet)
Indications: Duodenal ulcer, ulcer prophylaxis in hypersecretory states such as trauma, burns, surgery, Zollinger-Ellison syndrome, etc., gastro-esophageal reflux disease (GERD).
Actions: Histamine-2 receptor antagonist.
Dosage: Active ulcer: 2,400 mg/day IV continuous infusion or 300 mg IV Q 6–4 hr; 400 mg PO BID or 800 mg Q HS. *Maintenance therapy:* 400 mg PO Q HS.
GERD: 800 mg PO BID, maintenance 800 mg po Q HS.
Supplied: Tablets 200mg, 300 mg, 400 mg, 800 mg; liquid 300 mg/5 mL; injection 300 mg/2 mL.

Notes: Extend dosing interval with renal insufficiency; decrease dose in the elderly; has many drug interactions.

■ Ciprofloxacin, Ophthalmic (Ciloxan) [See Table 7–11, pp 533 & 534]

■ Ciprofloxacin (Cipro)
Indications: Broad spectrum activity against a variety of gram-positive and gram-negative aerobic bacteria.
Actions: Quinolone antibiotic.
Dosage: 250–750 mg PO Q 12 hr or 200–400 mg IV Q 12 hr.
Supplied: Tablets 250 mg, 500 mg, 750 mg; injection 200 mg, 400 mg.
Notes and Caution: Little activity against streptococci; drug interactions with theophylline, caffeine, sucralfate, and antacids; nausea, vomiting and abdominal discomfort are common side effects; *contraindicated in pregnancy.*

■ Cisapride (Propulsid)
Indications: Gastroesophageal reflux.
Actions: Gastrointestinal prokinetic agent.
Dosage: 10–20 mg PO QID.
Supplied: Tablets 10 mg, 20 mg.
Notes: Should be administered 15 min before meals. Concomitant administration with ketoconazole, itraconazole and miconazole is contraindicated due to potential QT interval prolongation and the development of ventricular arrhythmias.

■ Cisplatin (Platinol)
Indications: Treatment of cervical, ovarian, testicular, and other solid tumors.
Actions: Alkylating agent.
Dosage: 20-70 mg/m² IV. Dosage and duration of therapy is dependent on individual treatment protocols.
Supplied: Injection 1 mg/mL.
Notes: Agent is nephrotoxic; hydrate patients with 1–2 liters of fluid prior to infusion.

■ Cladribine (Leustatin)
Indications: For the treatment of hairy cell leukemia, lymphoma, and AML.
Actions: Antineoplastic agent.
Dosage: 0.09 mg/kg/day IV continuous infusion for 7 consecutive days.

Supplied: Injection 1 mg/mL.
Notes: May cause bone marrow suppression and irreversible neuro-toxicity.

■ Clarithromycin (Biaxin)
Indications: Treatment of upper and lower respiratory tract infections, skin and skin structure infections, and infections caused by non-tuberculosis *Mycobacterium* .
Actions: Antibacterial: macrolide antibiotic.
Dosage: 250–500 mg PO BID.
  Mycobacterium: 500–1000 mg PO BID.
Supplied: Tablets 250 mg, 500 mg; suspension 125 mg/5 mL, 250 mg/5 mL.
Notes: Increases theophylline and carbamazepine levels; avoid concurrent use with astemizole and terfenadine. May produce metallic taste.

■ Clemastine Fumarate (Tavist)
Indications: Allergic rhinitis.
Actions: Antihistamine.
Dosage: 1.34 mg BID to 2.68 mg TID, maximum 8.04 mg/day.
Supplied: Tablets 1.34 mg, 2.68 mg; syrup 0.67 mg/5 mL.

■ Clindamycin (Cleocin)
Indications: Susceptible strains of streptococci, pneumococci, staphylococci, and gram-positive and gram-negative anaerobes; no activity against gram-negative aerobes.
Actions: Bacteriostatic, interferes with protein synthesis.
Dosage: 150–450 mg PO QID; 300–600 mg IV Q 6 hr or 900 mg IV Q 8 hr.
Supplied: Capsules 75 mg, 150 mg, 300 mg; suspension 75 mg/5 mL; injection 300 mg/2 mL.
Notes: Beware of diarrhea that may represent pseudomembranous colitis caused by *C difficile* following clindamycin use.

■ Clofazimine (Lamprene)
Indications: Treatment of leprosy, and as part of combination therapy for *Mycobacterium avium* complex in HIV patients.
Actions: Bactericidal, inhibits DNA synthesis.
Dosage: 100–300 mg PO Q day.
Supplied: Capsules 50 mg, 100 mg.
Notes: To be taken with meals. May change skin pigmentation to pink or brownish–black; may cause skin dryness and GI intolerance.

■ Clonazepam (Klonopin) [C]

Indications: Lennox-Gastaut syndrome, akinetic and myoclonic seizures, absence seizures.

Actions: Benzodiazepine anticonvulsant.

Dosage: 1.5 mg/day PO in 3 divided doses; increase by 0.5–1.0 mg/day every 3 days PRN up to 20 mg/day.

Supplied: Tablets 0.5 mg, 1.0 mg, 2.0 mg.

Notes: CNS side effects including sedation.

■ Clonidine (Catapres)

Indications: Hypertension; opioid, alcohol and tobacco withdrawal.

Actions: Centrally acting alpha-adrenergic stimulant.

Dosage: 0.1 mg PO BID adjusted daily by 0.1–0.2 mg increments (maximum 2.4 mg/day).

Supplied: Tablets 0.1 mg, 0.2 mg, 0.3 mg.

Notes: Dry mouth, drowsiness, sedation occur frequently. More effective for hypertension when combined with diuretics; rebound hypertension can occur with abrupt cessation of doses above 0.2 mg BID.

■ Clonidine Transdermal (Catapres TTS)

Indications: Hypertension.

Actions: Centrally acting alpha-adrenergic stimulant.

Dosage: Apply one patch every 7 days to a hairless area on the upper arm or torso; titrate according to individual therapeutic requirements.

Supplied: TTS-1, TTS-2, TTS-3 (programmed to deliver 0.1, 0.2, 0.3 mg respectively of clonidine per day, for one week).

Notes: Doses > two TTS-3 are usually not associated with increased efficacy.

■ Clorazepate (Tranxene) [C]

Indications: Acute anxiety disorders, acute alcohol withdrawal symptoms, adjunctive therapy in partial seizures.

Actions: Benzodiazepine.

Dosage: 15–60 mg/day PO in single or divided doses.

Supplied: Capsules and tablets 3.75 mg, 7.5 mg, 15 mg.

Notes: Monitor patients with renal and hepatic impairment since drug may accumulate in the body; drug also has CNS depressant effects.

■ Clotrimazole (Lotrimin, Mycelex)

Indications: Treatment of candidiasis and tinea infections.

Actions: Antifungal agent.

Dosage: *Oral:* One troche dissolved slowly in mouth 5 times a day for 14 days.

Vaginal:
- Cream: one applicatorful Q HS for 7–14 days.
- Tablets: 100 mg vaginally Q HS for 7 days; or 200 mg (2 tabs) vaginally Q HS for 3 days; or 500 mg tab vaginally HS X 1.

Topical: Apply 3–4 times daily for 10–14 days.
Supplied: Cream 1%; solution 1%; lotion 1%; troche 10 mg; vaginal tablets 100 mg, 500 mg; vaginal cream 1%.
Note: Oral prophylaxis commonly used in immunosuppressed patients.

■ Cloxacillin (Cloxapen, Tegopen) [See Table 7–4, p 527]

■ Clozapine (Clozaril)
Indications: Severe schizophrenia that does not respond to standard therapy.
Actions: Tricyclic "atypical" antipsychotic agent.
Dosage: Initial 25 mg Q day–BID, increase dose to 300–450 mg/day over 2 weeks. Maintain patient at lowest dose possible.
Supplied: Tablets 25 mg, 100 mg.
Notes: Monitor blood counts frequently due to the risk of agranulocytosis. May also cause drowsiness and seizures.

■ Codeine [C]
Indications: Mild to moderate pain; symptomatic relief of cough.
Actions: Narcotic analgesic, depresses the cough reflex.
Dosage: *Analgesic:* 15–60 mg PO, SC, or IM QID PRN.
Antitussive: 5–15 mg PO or SC Q 4 hr PRN.
Supplied: Tablets 15 mg, 30 mg, 60 mg; injection 30 mg/mL, 60 mg/mL.
Notes: Most often used in combination with acetaminophen for pain or with other agents as an antitussive; 120 mg IM equivalent to 10 mg morphine IM.

■ Colchicine
Indications: Acute gout.
Actions: Inhibits migration of leukocytes; reduces production of lactic acid by leukocytes.
Dosage: Initially 0.5–1.2 mg PO or IV, then 0.5–1.2 mg Q 1–2 hr until GI side effects develop (maximum of 8 mg/day PO; no more than 4 mg/day if given IV).
Supplied: Tablets 0.5 mg, 0.6 mg; injection 1 mg/2 mL.
Notes: Use with caution in elderly and patients with renal impairment. Colchicine 1–2 mg IV within 24–48 hours of an acute attack can be diag-

nostic and therapeutic in a monarticular arthritis. Extravasation with IV use can lead to severe local irritation and tissue damage.

■ Colestipol (Colestid)

Indications: Adjunctive therapy for the reduction of serum cholesterol in patients with primary hypercholesterolemia.

Actions: Binds bile acids in the intestine to form an insoluble complex.

Dosage: 15-30 gm Q day divided into 2–4 doses.

Supplied: Tablets 1 mg, granules.

Notes: Instruct patient not to use dry powder by itself; mix with beverages, soups, cereals, etc.

■ Cortisone (Cortone) [See Table 7–2, p 526]

■ Cortisporin Ophthalmic [See Table 7–11, p 533 & 534]

■ Cortisporin Otic

Indications: Treatment of superficial bacterial infections of the external auditory canal by organisms sensitive to neomycin or polymyxin; suspension may also be used in the treatment of infections in the mastoid and fenestrated cavities.

Actions: Topical antibiotic combination.

Dosage: 4 drops instilled into external auditory canal 3–4 times daily.

Supplied: Otic solution, otic suspension.

Notes: Use suspension in cases of ruptured ear drum.

■ Cromolyn Sodium (Intal, Nasalcrom, Opticrom)

Indications: Adjunct to the treatment of asthma; prevention of exercise-induced asthma; allergic rhinitis; ophthalmic allergic manifestations.

Actions: Antiasthmatic; mast cell stabilizer.

Dosage: *Inhalation:* 20 mg (as powder in capsule) inhaled QID or metered-dose inhaler 2 puffs QID.

　　　　　　　　Nasal instillation: Spray once in each nostril 2–6 times daily.

　　　　　　　　Ophthalmic: 1–2 drops in each eye 4–6 times daily.

Supplied: Capsules for inhalation 20 mg; solution for nebulization 20 mg/2 mL; metered dose inhaler; nasal solution 40 mg/mL; ophthalmic solution 4%.

Notes: Inhalation of dry powder can cause cough and bronchospasm; patient may need to switch to metered dose inhaler. Drug may require 2–4 weeks for maximal effect in perennial allergic disorders.

■ Cyanocobalamin/Vitamin B₁₂

Indications: Pernicious anemia and other vitamin B_{12} deficiency states.
Actions: Dietary supplement of vitamin B_{12}.
Dosage: 100 µg, IM or SC Q day for 5–10 days; then 100 µg IM twice a week for 1 month, then 100 µg IM monthly.
Supplied: Tablets 25 µg, 50 µg, 100 µg, 250 µg, 500 µg, 1000 µg; injection 30 g/mL, 100 g/mL, 1000 g/mL.
Notes: Oral absorption highly erratic, altered by many drugs and not recommended; may be used with hyperalimentation.

■ Cyclobenzaprine (Flexeril)

Indications: Adjunct to rest and physical therapy for the relief of muscle spasm associated with acute painful musculoskeletal conditions.
Actions: Centrally acting skeletal muscle relaxant.
Dosage: 10 mg PO TID.
Supplied: Tablets 10 mg.
Notes: Do not use longer than 2–3 weeks; has sedative and anticholinergic properties.

■ Cyclophosphamide (Cytoxan)

Indications: Treatment of breast, ovarian, and soft tissue sarcoma, leukemia, and lymphoma.
Actions: Alkylating agent.
Dosage: *IV:* Initial dose 40–50 mg/kg IV divided over 2–5 days; or 10–15 mg/kg IV Q 7–10 days; or 3–5 mg/kg IV twice weekly.
  Oral: 1–5 mg/kg/day.
Supplied: Tablets 25 mg, 50 mg; powder for injection.
Notes: May cause bone marrow suppression and hemorrhagic cystitis; SIADH has occurred with doses > 50 mg/kg.

■ Cyclosporine (Sandimmune, Neoral)

Indications: Prophylaxis of organ rejection in kidney, liver, heart, and bone marrow transplants in conjunction with adrenal corticosteroids.
Actions: Immunosuppressant, reversible inhibition of immunocompetent lymphocytes.
Dosage: *Oral:* 15 mg/kg/day beginning 12 hr prior to transplant; after 2 weeks, taper dose by 5 mg per week to 5–10 mg/kg/day.
  IV: If patient cannot take drug PO, give 1/3 oral dose IV.
Supplied: Capsules 25 mg, 100 mg; oral solution 100 mg/mL; injection 50 mg/mL.
Notes and Caution: May elevate BUN and Cr, which may be confused with renal transplant rejection. Drug should be administered in glass containers; has many drug interactions. **Caution:** The trade names Neoral and Sandimmune are *not* interchangeable.

■ Cyproheptadine (Periactin)

Indications: Allergic reactions; especially good for itching.
Actions: Phenothiazine antihistamine; antipruritic.
Dosage: 4 mg PO TID, maximum of 0.5 mg/kg/day.
Supplied: Tablets 4 mg; syrup 2 mg/5 mL.
Notes: Anticholinergic side effects and drowsiness common; may stimulate appetite in some patients.

■ Cytarabine (Cytosar-U)

Indications: Leukemia.
Actions: Antimetabolite; antineoplastic.
Dosage: 100 mg/m^2/day IV by continuous infusion on days 1–7, or 100 mg/m^2 IV Q 12 hr on days 1–7.

- Refractory leukemia: 3 gm/m^2 IV Q 12 hr for 4–12 doses.
- Intrathecal use: 5–75 mg/m^2 once daily for 4 days or once every 4 days.

Supplied: Powder for injection.
Notes: Patients can tolerate higher total doses when the drug is given by rapid IV injection as compared to slower infusions.

■ Dacarbazine (DTIC-Dome)

Indications: Treatment of soft tissue and uterine sarcoma, melanoma, and Hodgkin's disease.
Actions: Antineoplastic agent.
Dosage: Dependent on individual protocol.
Supplied: Injection 5 mg/mL, 10 mg/mL.
Notes: May cause myelosuppression.

■ Dactinomycin (Cosmegen)

Indications: Treatment of Wilms' tumor, rhabdomyosarcoma, choriocarcinoma, testicular carcinoma, Ewing's sarcoma, and sarcoma botryoides.
Actions: Antibiotic, antineoplastic.
Dosage: 0.5 mg/day IV for 5 days.
Supplied: Injection 0.5 mg.
Notes: Severe soft tissue damage may occur with extravasation.

■ Dantrolene Sodium (Dantrium)

Indications: Treatment of clinical spasticity resulting from upper motor neuron disorders such as spinal cord injuries, strokes, cerebral palsy, or multiple sclerosis; treatment of malignant hyperthermic crisis.
Actions: Skeletal muscle relaxant.
Dosage: *Spasticity:* Initially 25 mg PO Q day, titrate to effect by 25 mg up to maximum dose of 100 mg PO QID PRN.

Malignant hyperthermia:

- Treatment: Continuous rapid IV push beginning at 1 mg/kg until symptoms subside or 10 mg/kg is reached.
- Postcrisis follow-up: 4–8 mg/kg/day in 3–4 divided doses for 1–3 days to prevent recurrence.

Supplied: Capsules 25 mg, 50 mg, 100 mg; powder for injection 20 mg/vial.
Note: Monitor patient's ALT and AST closely.

■ Dapsone
Indications: Leprosy, *Pneumocystis carinii* pneumonia.
Actions: Unknown; bactericidal.
Dosage: 50–100 mg PO Q day.
Supplied: Tablets 50 mg, 100 mg.

■ Daunorubicin (Cerubidine)
Indications: Leukemia.
Actions: Antibiotic, antineoplastic.
Dosage: Varies with individual protocol.
Supplied: Injection 20 mg.
Notes: Drug causes severe tissue necrosis if extravasation occurs.

■ Demeclocycline (Declomycin)
Indications: Treatment of SIADH (syndrome of inappropriate antidiuretic hormone) secretion; chlamydial and bacterial infections (drug is an antimicrobial of the tetracycline family).
Actions: Antagonizes action of ADH on renal tubules; bacteriostatic, inhibits protein synthesis.
Dosage: *SIADH:* 300–600 mg PO Q 12 hr.
        Antimicrobial: 150–300 mg PO Q 12 hr.
Supplied: Capsules 150 mg; tablets 150 mg, 300 mg.
Notes: Reduce dose in renal failure; drug may cause diabetes insipidus.

■ Desipramine (Norpramine)
Indications: Endogenous depression.
Actions: Tricyclic antidepressant.
Dosage: 25–200 mg/day in single or divided doses; usually as a single dose HS.
Supplied: Tablets 25 mg, 50 mg, 75 mg, 100 mg, 150 mg; capsules 25 mg, 50 mg.
Notes: Many anticholinergic side effects including blurred vision, urinary retention, and dry mouth.

■ Desmopressin (DDAVP, Stimate)

Indications: Diabetes insipidus (intranasal and parenteral administration); bleeding due to hemophilia A and Type I von Willebrand's disease (parenteral administration).

Actions: Synthetic analogue of vasopressin, a naturally occurring human antidiuretic hormone; increases factor VIII.

Dosage: Diabetes insipidus:

- Intranasal 0.1–0.4 mL (10-40 µg) daily in 2–3 divided doses.
- Parenteral 0.5–1 mL (2-4 µg) daily in 2 divided doses. When converting from intranasal to parenteral dosing, use 1/10th of intranasal dose.

   Hemophilia A and von Willebrand's disease (Type I): 0.3 µg/kg diluted to 50 mL with NSS infused slowly over 15–30 min.

Supplied: Injection 4 g/mL; nasal solution 0.1 g/mL.

Note: In very young and old patients, adjust fluid intake to avoid water intoxication and hyponatremia.

■ Dexamethasone (Decadron) [See Table 7–2, p 526]

■ Dextromethorphan (Mediquell, Benylin DM)

Indications: Control of nonproductive cough.

Actions: Depresses the cough center in the medulla.

Dosage: 10–20 mg PO Q 4 hr PRN.

Supplied: Chewy squares 15 mg; lozenges 5 mg; syrup 5 mg/5 mL, 7.5 mg/5 mL, 10 mg/5 mL, 15 mg/5 mL; liquid, sustained-action 30 mg/5 mL.

Notes: May be found in combination products with guaifenesin.

■ Dezocine (Dalgan)

Indications: Pain management.

Actions: Narcotic agonist-antagonist.

Dosage: 5–20 mg IM or 2.5–10 mg IV Q 2–4 hr PRN.

Supplied: Injection 5 mg/mL, 10 mg/mL, 15 mg/mL.

Notes: May cause withdrawal in patients dependent on narcotics.

■ Diazepam (Valium) [C]

Indications: Anxiety, alcohol withdrawal, muscle spasm, status epilepticus, and preoperative sedation.

Actions: Benzodiazepine.

Dosage:

- Status epilepticus: 0.2–0.5 mg/kg/dose IV Q 15–30 min to maximum dose of 30 mg.
- Anxiety, muscle spasm: 2–10 mg PO or IM Q 3–4 hr PRN.
- Preoperative: 5–10 mg PO or IM 20–30 min before procedure; can be given IV just prior to procedure.

- Alcohol withdrawal: Initial dose 2–5 mg IV; then 5–10 mg Q 5–10 min, not to exceed 100 mg in 1 hr. May require up to 1000 mg in 24-hour period for severe withdrawal symptoms. Titrate to agitation; avoid excessive sedation, which may lead to aspiration or respiratory arrest.

Supplied: SR capsules 15 mg; tablets 2 mg, 5 mg, 10 mg; solution 1 mg/mL, 5 mg/mL; injection 5 mg/mL.

Notes: Do not exceed 5 mg/min IV as respiratory arrest can occur; absorption of IM dose may be erratic.

■ Diazoxide (Hyperstat, Proglycem)
Indications: Management of hypoglycemia due to hyperinsulinism.
Actions: Relaxes smooth muscle in the peripheral arterioles; inhibits pancreatic insulin release.
Dosage: 3–8 mg/kg/24 hr PO divided Q 8–12 hr.
Supplied: Injection 300 mg/20 mL; capsules 50 mg; oral suspension 50 mg/mL.
Notes: Sodium retention and hyperglycemia frequently occur; possible thiazide diuretic cross-hypersensitivity; cannot be titrated.

■ Diclofenac (Cataflam, Voltaren) [See Table 7–10, p 532]

■ Dicloxacillin (Dynapen, Dycill) [See Table 7–4, p 527]

■ Dicyclomine (Bentyl, Others)
Indications: Treatment of functional irritable bowel syndromes.
Actions: Smooth muscle relaxant.
Dosage: 20 mg PO QID titrated to a maximum dose of 160 mg/day or 20 mg IM Q 6 hr.
Supplied: Capsules 10 mg, 20 mg; tablets 20 mg, syrup 10 mg/5 mL, injection 10 mg/mL.
Notes: Anticholinergic side effects may limit dose.

■ Didanosine [ddl] (Videx)
Indications: Treatment of HIV infection in patients who are zidovudine-intolerant.
Actions: Antiviral agent.
Dosage: Adults:

- ≥ 60 kg: 200 mg PO BID.
- < 60 kg: 125 mg PO BID.

Supplied: Chewable tablets 25 mg, 50 mg, 100 mg, 150 mg; powder packets 100 mg, 167mg, 250 mg, 375 mg; powder for solution 2 gm, 4 gm.

Notes: Reconstitute powder with water; instruct patient to take on empty stomach. Side effects include pancreatitis, peripheral neuropathy, diarrhea and headache.

■ Diethylstilbestrol (DES)
Indications: Treatment of breast and prostate cancer.
Actions: Hormone; antineoplastic.
Dosage: 50 mg PO TID; may be increased to 200 mg PO TID depending on patient tolerance.
Supplied: Tablets 50 mg.

■ Diflunisal (Dolobid)
Indication: Mild to moderate pain; osteoarthritis.
Actions: Nonsteroidal anti-inflammatory agent, salicylic acid.
Dosage: *Pain:* 500 mg PO BID.
          Osteoarthritis: 500–1500 mg PO in 2–3 divided doses.
Supplied: 250 and 500 mg tablets.
Notes: May prolong prothrombin time.

■ Digoxin (Lanoxin, Lanoxicaps)
Indications: CHF, atrial fibrillation and flutter, paroxysmal atrial tachycardia.
Actions: Positive inotrope, increases refractory period of AV node.
Dosage: *PO digitalization:* 0.50–0.75 mg PO; then 0.25 mg PO Q 6–8 hr until total dose is between 1.0 to 1.5 mg.
          IV digitalization: 0.25–0.50 mg or IV; then 0.25 mg Q 4–6 hr until total dose of ~1 mg.
          Daily maintenance: 0.125–0.500 mg PO, or IV Q day (average daily dose 0.125–0.250 mg).
Supplied: Capsules 0.05 mg, 0.1 mg, 0.2 mg; tablets 0.125 mg, 0.25mg, 0.5 mg; elixir 0.05 mg/mL; injection 0.1 mg/mL, 0.25 mg/mL.
Notes: Can cause heart block; low potassium can potentiate toxicity; reduce dose in renal failure. Symptoms of toxicity include nausea, vomiting, headache, fatigue, visual disturbances (yellow–green halos around lights), cardiac arrhythmias (Drug Levels, Table 7–13, p 536); IM injection can be painful, has erratic absorption, and should not be used. Therapeutic levels: 0.5–2.0 ng/mL.

■ Digoxin Immune Fab (Digibind)
Indications: Treatment of life-threatening digoxin intoxication.
Actions: Antigen-binding fragments bind digoxin, inactivating it prior to elimination through the urine.
Dosage: Based on serum level and patient's weight; see dosing charts provided with the drug.

Supplied: Injection 40 mg/vial.
Notes: Each vial will bind approximately 0.6 mg of digoxin; in renal failure redosing may be required after several days due to breakdown of the immune complex.

■ Dihydroxyaluminum Sodium Carbonate (Rolaids)
Indications: Heartburn, gastroesophageal reflux, and acid ingestion.
Actions: Neutralizes gastric acid.
Dosage: 1–2 tablets PRN.
Supplied: Chewable tablets, 334 mg.

■ Diltiazem (Cardizem, Dilacor)
Indications: Treatment of angina pectoris, prevention of reinfarction, hypertension; atrial fibrillation or flutter, and paroxysmal SVT.
Actions: Calcium channel blocking agent.
Dosage: *Oral:* 30 mg PO QID initially; titrate to 180–360 mg/day in 3–4 divided doses as needed.

- Sustained-release: 60–120 mg PO BID; titrate to effect, maximum dose 360 mg/day.
- Continuous dose: 180–300 mg PO Q day.

IV: 0.25 mg/kg IV bolus over 2 min; may repeat dose in 15 min 0.35 mg/kg. May begin continuous infusion of 5–15 mg/hr.
Supplied: Tablets 30 mg, 60 mg, 90 mg, 120 mg; capsules SR 60 mg, 90 mg, 120 mg; capsules CD or XR 120 mg, 180 mg, 240 mg, 300 mg (CD only); injection 5 mg/mL.
Notes: Contraindicated in sick sinus syndrome, AV block, and hypotension. Cardizem CD and Dilacor XR are *not* interchangeable.

■ Dimenhydrinate (Dramamine)
Indications: Prevention and treatment of nausea, vomiting, dizziness or vertigo of motion sickness.
Actions: Antiemetic.
Dosage: 50–100 mg PO Q 4–6 hr, maximum of 400 mg/day; 50 mg IM/IV PRN.
Supplied: Tablets 50 mg; chewable tablets 50 mg; capsules 50 mg; liquid 12.5 mg/4 mL; injection 50 mg/mL.
Notes: Anticholinergic side effects.

■ Diphenhydramine (Benadryl, Others)
Indications: Allergic reactions, motion sickness, potentiate narcotics, sedation, cough suppression, treatment of extrapyramidal reactions.
Actions: Antihistamine, antiemetic.
Dosage: 25–50 mg PO, IV or IM BID–TID.

Supplied: Tablets and capsules, 25 mg, 50 mg; elixir 12.5 mg/5mL; syrup 12.5 mg/5mL; injection 10 mg/mL, 50 mg/mL.

Notes: Anticholinergic side effects, including dry mouth, urinary retention; causes sedation; increase dosing interval in moderate to severe renal failure.

■ Diphenoxylate With Atropine (Lomotil) [C]

Indications: Diarrhea.

Actions: A constipating meperidine congener, reduces GI motility.

Dosage: Initially 5 mg PO TID–QID until under control; then 2.5–5.0 mg PO BID.

Supplied: Tablets 2.5 mg diphenoxylate/0.025 mg atropine; liquid 2.5 mg diphenoxylate/0.025 mg atropine per 5 mL.

Notes: Atropine-type side effects (headache, drowsiness).

■ Dipivefrin (Propine) [See Table 7–11, p 533 and 534]

■ Dipyridamole (Persantin)

Indications: Prevention of postoperative thromboembolic disorders.

Actions: Antiplatelet activity.

Dosage: 75–100 mg PO TID–QID.

Supplied: Tablets 25 mg, 50 mg, 75 mg.

Notes: Aspirin potentiates the antiplatelet effects. Drug may cause nausea and vomiting.

■ Dirithromycin (Dynabac)

Indication: Bronchitis (caused by *S pneumoniae* and *M catarrhalis*); community-acquired pneumonia (caused by *S pneumoniae, L pneumophila* and *M pneumoniae*); pharyngitis (caused by group A streptococci); and skin and soft tissue infections (caused by *S aureus*).

Actions: Macrolide antibiotic.

Dosage: 500 mg Q day for 7 days.

Supplied: 250 mg tablets.

■ Disopyramide (Norpace, Napamide)

Indications: Suppression and prevention of premature ventricular contractions.

Actions: Class 1a antiarrhythmic.

Dosage: 400–800 mg/day divided Q 6 hr for regular-release products and Q 12 hr for sustained-release products.

Supplied: Capsules 100 mg, 150 mg; SR Capsules 100 mg, 150 mg.

Notes: Has anticholinergic side effects (urinary retention); negative inotropic properties may induce CHF; decrease dose in impaired hepatic function.

■ Disulfiram (Antabuse)

Indications: Alcohol consumption deterrent.

Actions: Blocks oxidation of alcohol to produce unpleasant reaction when alcohol is consumed.

Dosage: 500 mg PO Q day for 1–2 weeks, then 250 mg PO Q day.

Supplied: Tablets 250 mg, 500 mg.

Notes: Instruct patients to avoid all hidden forms of alcohol (cough syrup, mouthwashes, sauces etc.); CBC and LFTs should be checked periodically.

■ Dobutamine (Dobutrex)

Indications: Short-term use in patients with cardiac decompensation secondary to depressed contractility.

Actions: Positive inotropic agent.

Dosage: Continuous IV infusion of 2.5–15 µg/kg/min; rarely 40 µg/kg/min may be required; titrate according to response.

Supplied: Injection 250 mg/20 mL.

Notes: Monitor ECG for increase in heart rate, blood pressure, and increased ectopic activity; monitor pulmonary wedge pressure and cardiac output if possible.

■ Docusate Calcium (Surfak, Others) [See Docusate Sodium]

■ Docusate Potassium (Dialose) [See Docusate Sodium]

■ Docusate Sodium (DOSS, Colace, Others)

Indications: Constipation-prone patient; adjunct to painful anorectal conditions (hemorrhoids).

Actions: Softens stools.

Dosage: 50–500 mg PO Q day.

Supplied: *Calcium*: Capsules 50 mg, 240 mg.

Potassium: Capsules 100 mg, 240 mg.

Sodium: Capsules 100 mg, 240 mg, 250 mg, 300 mg; syrup 50 mg/15 mL, 60 mg/15 mL; liquid 150 mg/15 mL; solution 50 mg/mL.

Notes: No significant side effects; no laxative action.

■ Dopamine (Intropin, Dopastat)

Indications: Short-term use in patients with cardiac decompensation secondary to decreased contractility; drug increases organ perfusion.

Actions: Positive inotropic agent.

Dosage: 5 µg/kg/min by continuous infusion, titrated by increments of 5 µg/kg/min to maximum of 20 µg/kg/min based on effect.

Supplied: Injection 40 mg/mL, 80 mg/mL, 160 mg/mL.

Notes: Dosage > 10 µg/kg/min may decrease renal perfusion; monitor urinary output; monitor ECG for increase in heart rate, blood pressure, and increased ectopic activity; monitor PCWP and CO if possible.

■ Dornase Alpha (Pulmozyme)

Indications: To reduce the frequency of respiratory infections in patients with cystic fibrosis.

Actions: An enzyme that selectively cleaves DNA.

Dosage: 2.5 mg inhaled once daily.

Supplied: Solution for inhalation, 1 mg/mL.

Notes: To be used with recommended nebulizer.

■ Doxazosin (Cardura)

Indications: Treatment of hypertension and benign prostatic hyperplasia.

Actions: Alpha-1-adrenergic blocker

Dosage: Initial dose 1 mg PO Q day, may be increased to 16 mg PO Q day.

Supplied: Tablets 1 mg, 2 mg, 4 mg, 8 mg.

Notes: Doses > 4 mg increase the likelihood of excessive postural hypotension.

■ Doxepin (Sinequan, Adapin)

Indications: Depression or anxiety.

Actions: Tricyclic antidepressant.

Dosage: 50–150 mg PO Q day, usually Q HS but can be taken in divided doses.

Supplied: Capsules 10 mg, 25 mg, 50 mg, 75 mg, 100 mg, 150 mg; oral concentrate 10 mg/mL.

Notes: Anticholinergic, CNS and cardiovascular side effects.

■ Doxorubicin (Adriamycin)

Indications: Treatment of breast, endometrial, and ovarian cancer, and leukemia.

Actions: Antibiotic, antineoplastic.

Dosage: 60–75 mg/m^2 IV as a single dose, at 21-day intervals.

Supplied: Powder for injection: lyophilized: 10 mg, 20 mg, 50 mg, 100 mg; lyophilized, rapid dissolution: 10 mg, 20 mg, 50 mg, 150 mg.

Formula: aqueous injection: 2 mg/mL (5, 10, 25 mL); preservative-free: 2 mg/mL (5, 10, 25, 100 mL).
Notes: May cause myelosuppression and cardiotoxicity.

■ Doxycycline (Vibramycin)
Indications: Broad-spectrum antibiotic including activity against *Rickettsiae, Chlamydia,* and *M pneumoniae.*
Actions: Similar to tetracycline; interferes with protein synthesis.
Dosage: 100 mg PO Q 12 hr on day 1, then 100 mg PO Q day or BID; or 100 mg IV Q 12 hr.
Supplied: Tablets 50 mg, 100 mg; capsules 50 mg, 100 mg; syrup 50 mg/5mL; powder for oral suspension 25 mg/5mL; powder for injection 100 mg, 200 mg per vial.
Notes: Useful for chronic bronchitis; tetracycline of choice for patients with renal impairment.

■ Dronabinol (Marinol) [C]
Indications: Nausea and vomiting associated with cancer chemotherapy; appetite stimulation.
Actions: Antiemetic.
Dosage: *Antiemetic:* 5–15 mg/m^2/dose Q 4–6 hr PRN.
Appetite stimulant: 2.5 mg PO before lunch and supper.
Supplied: Capsules 2.5 mg, 5 mg, 10 mg.
Notes: Principal psychoactive substance present in marijuana; many CNS side effects.

■ Droperidol (Inapsine)
Indications: Nausea and vomiting; premedication for anesthesia.
Actions: Tranquilization, sedation, and antiemetic.
Dosage: *Nausea:* 1.25–2.5 mg IV PRN.
Premedication: 2.5–10 mg IV.
Supplied: Injection 2.5 mg/mL.
Notes: May cause drowsiness, moderate hypotension and occasionally tachycardia.

■ Edrophonium (Tensilon)
Indications: Diagnosis of myasthenia gravis; acute myasthenic crisis; curare antagonist.
Actions: Anticholinesterase.
Dosage: *Test for myasthenia gravis:* 2 mg IV in one min; if tolerated, give 8 mg IV; a positive test is a brief increase in strength.
Supplied: Injection 10 mg/mL.
Notes: Can cause severe cholinergic effects; keep atropine available.

■ Enalapril (Vasotec) [See Table 7–3, p 527]

■ Enoxaparin (Lovenox)

Indications: Prevention of DVT.
Actions: Low molecular weight heparin.
Dosage: 30 mg SC BID or 40 mg once a day.
Supplied: Injection 30 mg/0.3 mL.
Notes: Does not significantly affect bleeding time, platelet function, PT or APTT.

■ Ephedrine

Indications: Treatment of hypotension.
Actions: Sympathomimetic that stimulates both alpha and beta receptors.
Dosage: 25–50 mg IM or IV Q 10 min to maximum 150 mg/day or 25–50 mg PO Q 3–4 hr PRN.
Supplied: Injection 25 mg/mL, 50 mg/mL.

■ Epinephrine (Adrenalin, Sus-Phrine, Others)

Indications: Cardiac arrest, anaphylactic reactions, acute asthma.
Actions: Beta-adrenergic agonist with some alpha effects.
Dosage: Emergency cardiac care: 0.5–1.0 mg (5–10 mL of 1:10,000) IV Q 5 min to response.
Anaphylaxis: 0.3–0.5 mL of 1:1000 dilution SC; may repeat Q 10–15 min to maximum of 1 mg/dose and 5 mg/day.
Asthma: 0.3–0.5 mL of 1:1000 dilution SC repeated at 20 min–4 hr intervals; OR 1 inhalation (metered dose) repeated in 1–2 min; OR suspension 0.1–0.3 mL SC for extended effect.
Supplied: Injection 1:1000, 1:10,000, 1:100,000; suspension for injection 1:200.
Notes: Sus-Phrine offers sustained action; in acute cardiac settings can be given via endotracheal tube if a central line is not available.

■ Epoetin Alfa (Epogen, Procrit)

Indications: Treatment of anemia associated with chronic renal failure, zidovudine treatment in HIV-infected patients, and patients receiving cancer chemotherapy.
Actions: Erythropoietin supplementation.
Dosage: 50–150 U/kg 3 times weekly; adjust dose Q 4–6 weeks as needed.
Supplied: Injection 2000 U, 3000 U, 4000 U, 10,000 U.
Notes: May cause hypertension, headache, tachycardia, nausea and vomiting.

■ Erythromycin (E-Mycin, Ilosone, Erythrocin, Eryc, Others)

Indications: Infections caused by Group A streptococci (*S pyrogenes*), alpha-hemolytic streptococci and *N gonorrhoeae* infections in penicillin-allergic patients; *S pneumoniae; Mycoplasma pneumoniae;* and Legionnaire's disease.

Actions: Bacteriostatic, interferes with protein synthesis.

Dosage: Oral dose variable depending on formulation, usually 250–500 mg PO QID or 500 mg–1 gm IV QID.

Supplied:

- *Powder for injection as lactobionate and gluceptate salts:* 250 mg, 500 mg, 1 gm.
- *Base:* Tablets 250 mg, 333 mg, 500 mg; capsules 125 mg, 250 mg.
- *Estolate:* Chewable tablets 125 mg, 250 mg; capsules 125 mg, 250 mg; drops 100 mg/mL; suspension 125 mg/5mL, 250 mg/5mL.
- *Stearate* Tablets 250 mg, 500 mg.
- *Ethylsuccinate:* Chewable tablets 200 mg; tablets 400 mg; suspension 200 mg/5mL, 400 mg/5mL.

Notes: Frequent mild GI disturbances; estolate salt is associated with cholestatic jaundice; erythromycin base not well absorbed from the GI tract; some forms such as Eryc are better tolerated with respect to GI irritation. Avoid concurrent use of astemizole and terfenadine.

■ Erythromycin, Ophthalmic (Ilotycin) [See Table 7–11, pp 533 & 534]

■ Esmolol (Brevibloc)

Indications: Supraventricular tachycardia, noncompensatory sinus tachycardia.

Actions: Beta-adrenergic blocking agent.

Dosage: Initiate treatment with 500 µg/kg load over 1 min, then 50 µg/kg/min for 4 min; if inadequate response, repeat loading dose and follow with maintenance infusion of 100 µg/kg/min for 4 min; continue titration process by repeating loading dose followed by incremental increases in the maintenance dose of 50 µg/kg/min for 4 min until desired heart rate is reached or a decrease in blood pressure occurs; average dose is 100 µg/kg/min.

Supplied: Injection 10 mg/mL, 250 mg/mL.

Notes: Monitor closely for hypotension; decreasing or discontinuing infusion will reverse hypotension in about a minute.

■ Estazolam (ProSom) [C]

Indications: Insomnia.

Actions: Benzodiazepine, sedative-hypnotic.
Dosage: 1–2 mg PO Q HS PRN.
Supplied: Tablets 1 mg, 2 mg.

■ Esterified Estrogens (Estratab, Menest)

Indications: Vasomotor symptoms, atrophic vaginitis, or kraurosis vulvae associated with menopause, female hypogonadism.
Actions: Estrogen supplementation.
Dosage: *Menopause:* 0.3–1.25 mg Q day.
  Hypogonadism: 2.5 mg PO Q day–TID.
Supplied: Tablets 0.3 mg, 0.625 mg, 1.25 mg, 2.5 mg.

■ Estradiol Topical (Estrace)

Indications: Atrophic vaginitis and kraurosis vulvae associated with menopause.
Actions: Estrogen supplementation.
Dosage: 2–4 gm Q day for 2 weeks, then 1 gm 1–3 times a week.
Supplied: Vaginal cream.

■ Estradiol Transdermal (Estraderm)

Indications: Severe vasomotor symptoms associated with menopause; female hypogonadism.
Actions: Hormonal replacement.
Dosage: 0.05 system twice weekly; adjust dose as necessary to control symptoms.
Supplied: Transdermal patches 0.05 mg, 0.1 mg (delivers 0.05 mg or 0.1 mg per 24 hr).

■ Estrogens, Conjugated (Premarin)

Indications: Moderate to severe vasomotor symptoms associated with menopause; atrophic vaginitis; palliative therapy of advanced prostatic carcinoma; prevention of estrogen deficiency-induced osteoporosis.
Actions: Hormonal replacement.
Dosage: 0.3–1.25 mg/day PO cyclically; prostatic carcinoma requires 1.25–2.5mg PO TID.
Supplied: Tablets 0.3 mg, 0.625 mg, 0.9 mg, 1.25 mg, 2.5 mg; injection 25 mg/mL.
Notes and Caution: Do not use during pregnancy; associated with an increased risk of endometrial carcinoma if progesterone is not also given, gallbladder disease, and thromboembolism and possibly breast cancer. Generic products are *not* equivalent.

■ Ethacrynic Acid (Edecrin)

Indications: Edema, CHF, ascites, any situation in which rapid diuresis is desired.

Actions: Loop diuretic.
Dosage: 50–200 mg PO Q day or 50 mg IV PRN.
Supplied: Tablets 25 mg, 50 mg; powder for injection 50 mg.
Notes: Contraindicated in anuria; many severe side effects.

■ Ethambutol (Myambutol)
Indications: Pulmonary tuberculosis, and other mycobacterial infections.
Actions: Inhibits cellular metabolism.
Dosage: 15–25 mg/kg PO Q day as single dose.
Supplied: Tablets 100 mg, 400 mg.
Notes: May cause vision changes and GI upset.

■ Ethinyl Estradiol (Estinyl, Feminone)
Indications: Vasomotor symptoms associated with menopause, female hypogonadism.
Actions: Estrogen supplementation.
Dosage: 0.02–1.5 mg/day divided Q day–TID.
Supplied: Tablets 0.02 mg, 0.05 mg, 0.5 mg.

■ Ethosuximide (Zarontin)
Indications: Absence seizures.
Actions: Anticonvulsant.
Dosage: 500 mg Q day PO initially; increase by 250 mg/day every 4–7 days as needed.
Supplied: Capsules 250 mg; syrup 250 mg/5mL.
Notes: Blood dyscrasias, CNS and GI side effects may occur; caution in patients with renal or hepatic impairment. See Drug Levels, Table 7–13, p 536.

■ Etodolac (Lodine) [See Table 7–10, p 532]

■ Etoposide (VePesid)
Indications: Treatment of gestational trophoblastic disease, ovarian, testicular, and lung cancer.
Actions: Mitotic inhibitor.
Dosage: 35–100 mg/m²/day IV. Number of doses and duration of therapy is dependent on individual protocols.
Supplied: Capsules 50 mg; injection 20 mg/mL.
Notes: May cause severe bone marrow suppression; has low stability in concentrated solutions.

■ Famciclovir (Famvir)
Indications: Management of acute herpes zoster (shingles).

Actions: Inhibits viral DNA synthesis.
Dosage: 500 mg PO Q 8 hr for 7 days.
Supplied: Tablets 500 mg.

■ Famotidine (Pepcid)

Indications: Short-term treatment of active duodenal ulcer and benign gastric ulcer, maintenance therapy for duodenal ulcer; hypersecretory conditions, and gastroesophageal reflux disease (GERD).
Actions: H_2-antagonist.
Dosage: *Ulcer:* 20–40 mg PO HS or 20 mg IV Q 12 hr.
       Hypersecretory: 20–160 mg PO Q 6 hr.
       GERD: 20 mg PO BID, maintenance 20 mg PO Q HS
Supplied: Tablets 10 mg, 20 mg, 40 mg; suspension 40 mg/5mL; injection 10 mg/mL.
Notes: Decrease dose in severe renal failure.

■ Felodipine (Plendil)

Indications: Treatment of hypertension.
Actions: Calcium channel blocking agent.
Dosage: 5–20 mg PO Q day.
Supplied: Extended-release tablets 5 mg, 10 mg.
Notes: Closely monitor blood pressure in elderly patients and patients with impaired hepatic function; doses > 10 mg should not be used in these patients. Bioavailability is increased when administered with grapefruit juice.

■ Fenoprofen (Nalfon) [Table 7–10, p 532]

■ Fentanyl Transdermal System (Duragesic) [C]

Indications: Management of chronic pain.
Actions: Narcotic.
Dosage: Apply patch to upper torso every 72 hours; dose is calculated from the narcotic requirements for the previous 24 hours.
Supplied: Transdermal patches that deliver 25 µg/hr, 50 µg/hr, 75 µg/hr, 100 µg/hr.
Notes: 0.1 mg of fentanyl is equivalent to 10 mg of morphine IM.

■ Ferrous Sulfate

Indications: Iron deficiency anemia; iron supplementation.
Actions: Dietary supplementation.

Dosage: 100–200 mg/day of elemental iron divided TID–QID.
Supplied: Tablets 195 mg, 300 mg, 325 mg; SR capsules 150 mg, 250 mg; drops 75 mg/0.6 mL, 125 mg/mL; elixir 220 mg/5mL; syrup 90 mg/5mL.
Notes: May turn stools and urine dark; can cause GI upset, constipation; Vitamin C taken with ferrous sulfate will increase the absorption of iron especially in patients with atrophic gastritis. Ferrous sulfate contains 20% elemental iron.

■ Filgrastim [G-CSF] (Neupogen)
Indications: To decrease the incidence of infection in febrile neutropenic patients.
Actions: Recombinant granulocyte colony stimulating factor.
Dosage: 5 µg/kg/day SC or IV as a single daily dose; administer until the patient is no longer neutropenic.
Supplied: Injection 300 µg/mL.
Notes: May cause bone pain.

■ Finasteride (Proscar)
Indications: Treatment of benign prostatic hyperplasia.
Actions: Inhibits 5 alpha-reductase.
Dosage: 5 mg PO Q day.
Supplied: Tablets 5 mg.

■ Flavoxate (Urispas)
Indications: Symptomatic relief of dysuria, urgency, nocturia, suprapubic pain, urinary frequency and incontinence.
Actions: Counteracts smooth muscle spasm of the urinary tract.
Dosage: 100–200 mg PO TID–QID.
Supplied: Tablets 100 mg.
Notes: May cause drowsiness, blurred vision, and dry mouth.

■ Fluconazole (Diflucan)
Indications: Oropharyngeal and esophageal candidiasis, cryptococcal meningitis, *Candida* infections of the lungs, peritoneum, and urinary tract; prevention of candidiasis in bone marrow transplant patients on chemotherapy or radiation; *Candida* vaginitis.
Actions: Antifungal; inhibits fungal cytochrome P-450 sterol demethylation.
Dosage: 100–400 mg PO or IV Q day.
       Vaginitis: 150 mg PO as single dose.
Supplied: Tablets 50 mg, 100 mg, 150 mg, 200 mg; injection 2 mg/mL.

Notes: Adjust dose in renal insufficiency; oral dosing produces the same blood levels as intravenously, therefore the oral route should be used whenever possible. For *Candida* vaginitis, give 150 mg PO as a single dose.

■ Flucytosine (Ancobon)

Indications: Serious infections caused by susceptible strains of *Candida* or *Cryptococcus*.

Actions: Antifungal.

Dosage: 50–150 mg/kg/day divided Q 6 hr.

Supplied: Capsules 250 mg, 500 mg.

Notes: May cause nausea, vomiting, and diarrhea. Instruct patient to take capsules a few at a time over 15 min.

■ Fludarabine Phosphate (Fludara)

Indications: Treatment of leukemia.

Actions: Antimetabolite, antineoplastic.

Dosage: 25 mg/m^2 IV for 5 consecutive days. Give every 28 days (counting from Day 1 of series).

Supplied: Powder for injection.

Notes: May cause severe bone marrow suppression and neurologic toxicity.

■ Fludrocortisone Acetate (Florinef)

Indications: Partial treatment for adrenocortical insufficiency.

Actions: Mineralocorticoid replacement.

Dosage: 0.05–0.1 mg PO Q day.

Supplied: Tablets 0.1 mg.

Notes: For adrenal insufficiency, must be used in conjunction with a glucocorticoid supplement; dosage changes based on plasma renin activity.

■ Flumazenil (Romazicon)

Indications: For complete or partial reversal of the sedative effects of benzodiazepines.

Actions: Benzodiazepine receptor antagonist.

Dosage: 0.2 mg IV over 15 sec, dose may be repeated if the desired level of consciousness is not obtained to a maximum dose of 1 mg.

Supplied: Injection 0.1 mg/mL.

■ Flunisolide (AeroBid)

Indications: Control of bronchial asthma in patients requiring chronic corticosteroid therapy.

Actions: Topical steroid.

Dosage: 2–4 inhalations BID.

Supplied: Metered-dose aerosol 250 μg.

Notes: May cause oral candidiasis. Not to be used for acute asthma attacks.

■ Fluorouracil (Adrucil)

Indications: Management of carcinoma of the colon, rectum, breast, stomach, and pancreas.

Actions: Antimetabolite, antineoplastic.

Dosage: Varies with individual protocol.

Supplied: Injection 50 mg/mL.

■ Fluoxetine (Prozac)

Indications: Treatment of depression and obsessive-compulsive disorders.

Actions: Selective serotonin reuptake inhibitor.

Dosage: 20 mg PO Q day initially; titrate to maximum dose of 80 mg/ 24 hr.

Supplied: Capsules 10 mg, 20 mg; solution 20 mg/5 mL.

Notes: May cause nausea, nervousness, and weight loss. Avoid concurrent use with astemizole and terfenadine.

■ Fluphenazine (Prolixin, Permitil)

Indications: Psychotic disorders.

Actions: Phenothiazine antipsychotic.

Dosage: 0.5–10 mg/day in divided doses PO Q 6–8 hr; average maintenance 5.0 mg/day or 1.25 mg IM initially; then 2.5–10 mg/day in divided doses Q 6–8 hr PRN.

Supplied: Tablets 1 mg, 2.5 mg, 5 mg, 10 mg; concentrate 5 mg/mL; elixir 2.5 mg/5 mL; injection 2.5 mg/mL.

Notes: Reduce dose in elderly; monitor liver functions; may cause drowsiness. Do not administer concentrate with caffeine, tannic acid, or products containing pectin.

■ Flurazepam (Dalmane) [C]

Indications: Insomnia.

Actions: Benzodiazepine.

Dosage: 15–30 mg PO Q HS PRN.

Supplied: Capsules 15 mg, 30 mg.

Notes: Reduce dose in the elderly.

■ Flurbiprofen (Ansaid) [See Table 7–10, p 532]

■ Flutamide (Eulexin)

Indications: Prostate cancer with hormone ablation.

Actions: Hormone.

Dosage: 3 capsules PO Q 8 hr.
Supplied: Capsules 125 mg.

■ Fluvastatin (Lescol)
Indications: Adjunct to diet in the treatment of elevated total cholesterol.
Actions: HMG-CoA reductase inhibitor.
Dosage: 20–40 mg PO Q HS.
Supplied: Capsules 20 mg, 40 mg.
Notes: Avoid concurrent use with gemfibrozil.

■ Folic Acid
Indications: Macrocytic anemia.
Actions: Dietary supplementation.
Dosage: *Supplement:* 0.4 mg PO Q day.
   Pregnancy: 0.8 mg PO Q day.
   Folate deficiency: 1.0 mg PO Q day–TID.
Supplied: Tablets 0.1 mg, 0.4 mg, 0.8 mg, 1.0 mg; injection 5 mg/mL; 10 mg/mL.
Notes: Recommended for all women of child-bearing years; routine administration would decrease neural-tube defects by 50%.

■ Foscarnet (Foscavir)
Indications: Treatment of cytomegalovirus retinitis in patients with AIDS and acyclovir-resistant herpes infections.
Actions: Inhibits viral DNA polymerase and reverse transcriptase.
Dosage: *Induction:* 60 mg/kg IV Q 8 hr.
   Maintenance: 90-120 mg/kg IV Q day (Mon-Fri).
Supplied: Injection 24 mg/mL.
Notes: Dosage *must* be adjusted for renal function; nephrotoxic; monitor ionized calcium closely (causes electrolyte abnormalities); administer through a central line.

■ Fosinopril (Monopril) [See Table 7–3, p 527]

■ Furosemide (Lasix)
Indications: Edema, hypertension, congestive heart failure.
Actions: Loop diuretic.
Dosage: 20–80 mg PO or IV Q day or BID.
Supplied: Tablets 20 mg, 40 mg, 80 mg; solution 10 mg/mL; injection 10 mg/mL.
Notes: Monitor for hypokalemia; use with caution in hepatic disease; high IV doses may cause ototoxicity.

■ Gabapentin (Neurontin)
Indications: Adjunctive therapy in the treatment of partial seizures.
Actions: Anticonvulsant.
Dosage: 900–1800 mg/day PO in three divided doses.
Supplied: Capsules 100 mg, 300 mg, 400 mg.
Notes: It is not necessary to monitor serum gabapentin levels.

■ Gallium nitrate (Ganite)
Indications: Treatment of hypercalcemia of malignancy.
Actions: Inhibits resorption of calcium from bone.
Dosage: 100–200 mg/m^2/day for 5 days.
Supplied: Injection 25 mg/mL.
Notes: Can cause renal insufficiency; < 1% of patients develop acute optic neuritis.

■ Ganciclovir (Cytovene)
Indications: Treatment of CMV retinitis and prevention of CMV disease in transplant recipients.
Actions: Inhibits viral DNA synthesis.
Dosage: *IV:* 5 mg/kg IV Q 12 hr for 14–21 days; then maintenance of 5 mg/kg IV Q day for 7 days/week, or 6 mg/kg IV Q day for 5 days/week.
     Oral: Following induction, 1000 mg PO Q 8 hr.
Supplied: Capsules 250 mg; injection 500 mg.
Notes: Ganciclovir is not a cure for CMV; granulocytopenia and thrombocytopenia are the major toxicities; injection should be handled with cytotoxic precautions. Instruct patient to take capsules with food.

■ Gemfibrozil (Lopid)
Indications: Hypertriglyceridemia (Types IV and V hyperlipoproteinemia).
Actions: Lipid regulating agent.
Dosage: 1200 mg/day PO in two divided doses 30 min before the morning and evening meals.
Supplied: Capsules 300 mg; tablets 600 mg.
Notes: Monitor AST, ALT, LDH, Alk Phos and serum lipids during therapy. Cholelithiasis may occur secondary to treatment; drug may enhance the effect of warfarin. Avoid concurrent use with HMG-CoA reductase inhibitors (fluvastatin, lovastatin, pravastatin, and simvastatin).

■ Gentamicin (Garamycin)
Indications: Serious infections caused by susceptible *Pseudomonas, Proteus, E coli, Klebsiella, Enterobacter,* and *Serratia;* and for initial treatment of gram-negative sepsis.

Actions: Bactericidal; inhibits protein synthesis.

Dosage: Loading dose of 1.5–2.0 mg per kg; then 2–5 mg/kg/24 hr IV divided Q 8–24 hr based on renal function. Refer to aminoglycoside dosing in Table 7–15, p 537. **OR:** give 7 mg per kg per 24 hr as a single dose (3 mg per kg if creatinine clearance < 40 mg per min per 1.73 m².)

Supplied: Injection 2 mg/mL, 10 mg/mL, 40 mg/mL.

Notes: Nephrotoxic and ototoxic; decrease dose with renal insufficiency; monitor serum creatinine and serum concentration of gentamicin for dosage adjustments. See Drug Levels, Table 7–14, p 536.

■ Gentamicin, Ophthalmic (Garamycin Ophthalmic) [See Table 7–11, pp 533 & 534]

■ Glipizide (Glucotrol) [See Table 7–12, p 535]

■ Glucagon

Indications: Treatment of severe hypoglycemic reactions in diabetic patients with sufficient liver glycogen stores or beta-blocker overdose.

Actions: Accelerates liver gluconeogenesis.

Dosage: Severe hypoglycemia: 0.5–1.0 mg SC, IM, or IV, repeated after 20 min as needed.

   Beta-blocker overdose: 3–10 mg IV, repeat in 10 min as needed, may be given as a continuous infusion.

Supplied: Powder for injection 1 mg, 10 mg.

Notes: Administration of glucose IV is necessary; glucagon is ineffective in states of starvation, adrenal insufficiency, or chronic hypoglycemia.

■ Glyburide (DiaBeta, Micronase) [See Table 7–12, p 535]

■ Glycerin

Indications: Constipation.

Actions: Hyperosmolar laxative.

Dosage: 1 suppository or enema, PR, PRN.

Supplied: Suppositories adult, infant.

■ Gonadorelin (Lutrepulse)

Indications: Primary hypothalamic amenorrhea.

Actions: Stimulates the pituitary to release the gonadotropins LH and FSH.

Dosage: 5–20 µg IV Q 90 min for 21 days, using a reservoir and pump.

Supplied: Injection 800 µg, 3.2 mg.
Notes: Risk of multiple pregnancies.

■ Goserelin (Zoladex)
Indications: Treatment of prostate cancer and endometriosis.
Actions: Gonadotropin-releasing hormone analogue.
Dosage: 3.6 mg SC once Q 28 days into the abdominal wall.
Supplied: Implant 3.6 mg.

■ Granisetron (Kytril)
Indications: Prevention of nausea and vomiting associated with emetogenic cancer therapy.
Actions: Serotonin receptor antagonist.
Dosage: 10 µg/kg IV 30 min prior to initiation of chemotherapy; OR 1 mg PO 1 hr before chemotherapy, then 12 hr after.
Supplied: Tablets 1 mg; injection 1 mg/mL.

■ Guaifenesin (Robitussin, Others)
Indications: Symptomatic relief of dry nonproductive cough.
Actions: Expectorant.
Dosage: 200–400 mg (10–20 mL) PO Q 4 hr.
Supplied: Tablets 100 mg, 200 mg; SR tablets 600 mg; capsules 200 mg; SR capsules 300 mg; syrup 67 mg/5 mL, 100 mg/5 mL, 200 mg/5 mL.

■ Guanabenz (Wytensin)
Indications: Hypertension.
Actions: Central alpha-adrenergic agonist.
Dosage: Initial dosage 4 mg PO BID; increase by 4 mg/day increments at 1–2 week intervals, up to 32 mg BID.
Supplied: Tablets 4 mg, 8 mg.
Notes: Sedation, dry mouth, dizziness, and headache are common side effects.

■ Guanadrel (Hylorel)
Indications: Hypertension.
Actions: Inhibits norepinephrine release from peripheral storage sites.
Dosage: 5 mg PO BID initially; increase up to 10 mg/day increments at 1 week intervals up to 75 mg PO BID.
Supplied: Tablets 10 mg, 25 mg.
Notes: Interactions with tricyclic antidepressants may reduce hypotensive effects of guanadrel. Drug has lower incidence of orthostatic changes and impotence than guanethidine.

■ Guanethidine (Ismelin)

Indications: Treatment of moderate to severe hypertension or renal hypertension.

Actions: Inhibits release of norepinephrine from peripheral storage sites.

Dosage: Initial dose 10–25 mg PO Q day; increase dose based on response.

Supplied: Tablets 10 mg, 25 mg.

Notes: May produce profound orthostatic hypotension especially with diuretic use. May potentiate effects of vasopressor agents; may increase frequency of bowel movements or produce explosive diarrhea. Interaction with tricyclic antidepressants reduces the effectiveness of guanethidine.

■ Guanfacine (Tenex)

Indications: Hypertension.

Actions: Centrally acting alpha-adrenergic agonist.

Dosage: 1 mg Q HS initially; increase by 1 mg/24 hr increments to maximum dose of 3 mg/24 hr; split dose BID if BP increases at end of dosing interval.

Supplied: Tablets 1 mg, 2 mg.

Notes: Use with thiazide diuretic is recommended; sedation, drowsiness common; rebound hypertension may occur with abrupt cessation of therapy.

■ Haloperidol (Haldol)

Indications: Management of psychotic disorders; agitation; Tourette's syndrome.

Actions: Antipsychotic, neuroleptic.

Dosage: *Moderate symptoms:* 0.5–2.0 mg PO BID–TID.

Severe symptoms or agitation: 3–5 mg PO BID–TID; OR 1–5 mg IM Q 4 hr PRN (maximum 100 mg/day).

Supplied: Tablets 0.5 mg, 1 mg, 2 mg, 5 mg, 10 mg, 20 mg; concentrate liquid 2 mg/mL; injection 5 mg/mL; deconate injection 50 mg/mL.

Notes: Can cause extrapyramidal symptoms, hypotension; reduce dose in the elderly.

■ Heparin Sodium

Indications: Treatment and prevention of venous thrombosis and pulmonary emboli, atrial fibrillation with emboli formation, acute arterial occlusion including a myocardial infarction.

Actions: Acts with antithrombin III to inactivate thrombin and to inhibit thromboplastin formation.

Dosage: *Prophylaxis:* 3000–5000 U SC Q 8–12 hr.

Treatment of thrombosis: Loading dose of 50–75 U/kg IV; then 10–20 U/kg IV Q hr (adjust dosage according to PTT).

Supplied: Injection 10 U/mL, 100 U/mL, 1000 U/mL, 5000 U/mL, 10,000 U/mL, 20,000 U/mL, 40,000 U/mL.

Notes: Follow PTT, TT, or activated clotting time to assess effectiveness; heparin has little effect on the prothrombin time (PT); with proper dosing PT should be 1½–2 times control for most indications. Heparin can cause thrombocytopenia 5% of the time; follow platelet counts.

■ Hepatitis A Vaccine (Havrix)

Indications: Prevention of hepatitis A in high-risk subpopulations, such as travelers in countries with poor sanitation, government employees and medical professionals in such areas, or persons engaged in high-risk behavior.

Actions: Provides active immunity against hepatitis A.

Dosage: 1440 EL.U. as a single IM dose.

Supplied: Injection 360 EL.U./0.5 mL, 1440 EL.U./1 mL.

Notes: Booster is recommended at 6–12 months after primary vaccination.

■ Hepatitis B Immune Globulin (HyperHep, H-BIG, Hep-B-Gammagee)

Indications: Exposure to HBsAg-positive materials such as blood, plasma, or serum (accidental needle-stick, mucous membrane contact, oral ingestion).

Actions: Supplies passive immunization.

Dosage: 0.06 mL/kg IM to maximum of 5 mL; within 24 hr of needle-stick or percutaneous exposure; within 14 days of sexual contact.

Supplied: Injection in 1 mL, 4 mL, and 5 mL vials.

Notes: Administered in gluteal or deltoid muscle; if exposure continues, patient should receive hepatitis B vaccine.

■ Hepatitis B Vaccine (Engerix-B, Recombivax HB)

Indications: Prevention of hepatitis B.

Actions: Active immunization.

Dosage: Three IM doses of 1 mL each, the first two given 1 month apart, the third 6 months after the first. Should be given in the deltoid muscle.

Supplied: Engerix-B: Injection 20 µg/mL; pediatric injection 10 µg/0.5 mL.

Recombivax HB: Injection 10 µg/mL, 40 µg/mL; pediatric injection 2.5 µg/0.5 mL, 5 µg/0.5 mL.

Notes: In adults, IM injections may cause fever or injection site soreness; derived from recombinant DNA technology.

■ Hetastarch (Hespan)

Indications: Plasma volume expansion as an adjunct in treatment of shock due to hemorrhage, surgery, burns, and other trauma.

Actions: Synthetic colloid with actions similar to albumin.

Dosage: 500–1000 mL (not to exceed 1500 mL/day) IV at a rate not to exceed 20 mL/kg/hr.

Supplied: Injection 30 gm/500 mL in 0.9% sodium chloride.

Notes and Caution: Hetastarch is *not* a substitute for blood or plasma; contraindicated in patients with severe bleeding disorders, severe CHF, or renal failure with oliguria or anuria.

■ Hydralazine (Apresoline)

Indications: Moderate to severe hypertension; congestive heart failure with concurrent use of nitrates.

Actions: Peripheral arterial vasodilator.

Dosage: Initial dose 10 mg PO QID, then increase to 25 mg QID to a maximum of 300 mg/day.

Supplied: Tablets 10 mg, 25 mg, 50 mg, 100 mg.

Notes and Caution: Use cautiously with impaired hepatic function or coronary artery disease. Compensatory sinus tachycardia can be eliminated with the addition of a beta-blocker. Chronically high doses of hydralazine can cause SLE-like syndrome. SVT can occur following IM administration.

■ Hydrochlorothiazide (HydroDiuril, Esidrix, Others)

Indications: Edema, hypertension, CHF.

Actions: Thiazide diuretic.

Dosage: 25–100 mg PO Q day in single or divided doses.

Supplied: Tablets 25 mg, 50 mg, 100 mg; oral solution 50 mg/5mL, 100 mg/mL.

Notes: Hypokalemia is frequent; hyperglycemia, hyperuricemia, hypomagnesemia, hyperlipidemia, and hyponatremia can also occur.

■ Hydrochlorothiazide and Amiloride (Moduretic)

Indications: Hypertension; adjunctive therapy for congestive heart failure.

Actions: Combined effects of a thiazide diuretic and a potassium-sparing diuretic.

Dosage: 1–2 tablets PO Q day.

Supplied: Tablets 5 mg amiloride/50 mg hydrochlorothiazide.

Notes: Compound should not be given to diabetics or patients with renal failure.

■ Hydrochlorothiazide and Spironolactone (Aldactazide)

Indications: Edema (CHF, cirrhosis); hypertension.

Actions: Combined effects of a thiazide diuretic and a potassium-sparing diuretic.

Dosage: 25–200 mg of each component Q day in divided doses.

Supplied: Tablets (hydrochlorothiazide/spironolactone) 25 mg/25 mg, 50 mg/50 mg.

■ Hydrochlorothiazide and Triamterene (Dyazide, Maxzide)

Indications: Edema, hypertension.

Actions: Combined effects of a thiazide diuretic and a potassium-sparing diuretic.

Dosage: Dyazide: 1–2 capsules PO Q day–BID.

Maxzide: ½–1 tablet PO Q day.

Supplied: Dyazide capsule: 50 mg triamterene/25 mg HCTZ.

Maxzide: 25 mg tablet: 37.5 mg triamterene/25 mg HCTZ.

Maxzide tablet: 50 mg tablet: 75 mg triamterene/50 mg HCTZ.

Notes: Hydrochlorothiazide component in Maxzide is more bioavailable than in Dyazide. Drug can cause hyperkalemia as well as hypokalemia; follow serum potassium.

■ Hydrocortisone (Cortef) [See Table 7–2, p 526]

■ Hydromorphone (Dilaudid) [C]

Indications: Moderate to severe pain.

Actions: Narcotic analgesic.

Dosage: 1–4 mg PO, IM, IV, or PR, Q 4–6 hr PRN.

Supplied: Tablets 1 mg, 2 mg, 3 mg, 4 mg; injection 1 mg/mL, 2 mg/mL, 3 mg/mL, 4 mg/mL, 10 mg/mL; suppositories 3 mg.

Notes: 1.5 mg IM equivalent to 10 mg morphine IM.

■ Hydroxyurea (Hydrea)

Indications: Treatment of cervical and ovarian cancer, melanoma, and leukemia.

Actions: Unknown; has some antimetabolite activity.

Dosage: Continuous therapy: 20–30 mg/kg PO Q day.

Intermittent therapy: 80 mg/kg Q 3 days.

Supplied: Capsules 500 mg.

■ Hydroxyzine (Atarax, Vistaril)

Indications: Anxiety, tension, sedation, itching.

Actions: Antihistamine, anxiolytic.

Dosage: Anxiety or need for sedation: 50–100 mg PO or IM QID or PRN (maximum of 600 mg Q day).

Itching: 25–50 mg PO or IM TID–QID.

Supplied: Tablets 10 mg, 25 mg, 50 mg, 100 mg; capsules 25 mg, 50 mg, 100 mg; syrup 10 mg/5mL; injection 25 mg/mL, 50 mg/mL.

Notes and Caution: Useful in potentiating the effects of narcotics. Do *not* give drug through IV. Drowsiness and anticholinergic effects are common.

■ Ibuprofen (Motrin, Advil, Others) [See Table 7–10, p 532]

■ Idarubicin (Idamycin)
Indications: Treatment of leukemia.
Actions: Anthracycline antineoplastic.
Dosage: 12 mg/m^2 Q day for 3 days.
Supplied: Injection 5 mg, 10 mg.
Notes: Do not administer if bilirubin is > 5 mg/dL.

■ Ifosfamide (Ifex)
Indications: Treatment of testicular, breast, and ovarian cancer.
Actions: Alkylating agent.
Dosage: 1.2 gm/m^2/day for 5 consecutive days. Repeat course every 3 weeks.
Supplied: Injection 1 gm, 3 gm.
Notes and Caution: May cause hemorrhagic cystitis; hydrate patient well before giving ifosfamide. Administer ifosfamide with mesna to prevent/lessen hemorrhagic cystitis.

■ Imipenem/Cilastatin (Primaxin)
Indications: Treatment of serious infections caused by a wide variety of susceptible bacteria; inactive against *S aureus,* group A and B streptococci, and others.
Actions: Bactericidal, interferes with cell wall synthesis.
Dosage: 250–500 mg (imipenem) IV Q 6 hr.
Supplied: Injection (imipenem/cilastatin) 250 mg/250 mg, 500 mg/500 mg.
Notes: Seizures may occur if drug accumulates; adjust dosage if calculated creatinine clearance is < 70 mL/min to avoid drug accumulation. Would avoid use in patients allergic to penicillin.

■ Imipramine (Tofranil)
Indications: Depression.
Actions: Tricyclic antidepressant.
Dosage: *Hospitalized patient:* Initial dose 100 mg/24 hr PO or IV in divided doses; may be increased over several weeks to 250–300 mg/24 hr.

Outpatient: Maintenance dose of 50–150 mg PO Q HS, not to exceed 200 mg/24 hr.

Supplied: Tablets 10 mg, 25 mg, 50 mg; Capsules 75 mg, 100 mg, 125 mg, 150 mg; injection 12.5 mg/mL.

Notes: Do not use with MAO inhibitors; less sedation than amitriptyline.

■ Immune Globulin Intravenous (Gamimune N, Sandoglobulin, Gammar IV)

Indications: IgG antibody deficiency diseases such as congenital agammaglobulinemia, common variable hypogammaglobulinemia; idiopathic thrombocytopenic purpura (ITP).

Actions: IgG supplementation.

Dosage: *Immunodeficiency:* 100–200 mg/kg IV monthly at rate of 0.01–0.04 mL/kg/minute up to maximum of 400 mg/kg/dose.

ITP: 400 mg/kg/dose IV Q day × 5 days.

Supplied: Injection 50 mg/mL; powder for injection 0.5 gm, 1 gm, 2.5 gm, 3 gm, 5 gm, 6 gm, 10 gm vials.

Notes: Adverse effects associated mostly with rate of infusion.

■ Indapamide (Lozol)

Indications: Hypertension, congestive heart failure.

Actions: Thiazide diuretic.

Dosage: 2.5–5.0 mg PO Q day.

Supplied: Tablets 2.5 mg.

Notes: Doses > 5 mg do not have additional effects on lowering BP.

■ Indomethacin (Indocin) [See Table 7–10, p 532]

■ Insulin

Indications: Diabetes mellitus that cannot be controlled by diet or oral hypoglycemic agents.

Actions: Insulin supplementation.

Dosage: Based on serum glucose levels; usually given SC, regular may also be given IV or IM to decrease glucose quickly. Maximal effect with intravenous insulin is within 1 hour.

Supplied: See Table 7–1, p 526.

Notes: The highly purified insulins provide an increase in free insulin; monitor patients closely for several weeks when changing doses.

■ Interferon Alfa (Roferon-A, Intron A)

Indications: Hairy cell leukemia.

Actions: Direct antiproliferative action against tumor cells and modulation of the host immune response.

Dosage: *Alfa-2A:* 3 million IU daily for 16–24 weeks SC or IM.
     Alfa-2B: 2 million IU/m^2 IM or SC 3 × week for 2–6 months.
Supplied: Injection.
Notes: Drug is being used in many investigational protocols for chronic Hepatitis B and C as well as many cancers and hematologic malignancies; flu-like symptoms are a common reaction.

■ Interferon Beta-1b (Betaseron)

Indications: Management of multiple sclerosis.
Actions: Biologic response modifier.
Dosage: 0.25 mg SC every other day.
Supplied: Powder for injection 0.3 mg.
Notes: May cause flu-like syndrome.

■ Interferon Gamma-1b (Actimmune)

Indications: Management of chronic granulomatous disease.
Actions: Biologic response modifier.
Dosage: 50 µg/m^2 SC 3 × weekly.
Supplied: Injection 100 µg.
Notes: 100 µg = 3 million U; may cause flu-like syndrome.

■ Ipecac Syrup

Indications: Treatment of drug overdoses and certain types of poisoning.
Actions: Irritation of GI mucosa and stimulation of chemoreceptor trigger zone.
Dosage: 15–30 mL PO followed by 200–300 mL water; if no emesis occurs in 20 min, may repeat × 1.
Supplied: Syrup 15 mL, 30 mL.
Notes and Caution: Do not use for ingestion of petroleum distillates, strong acid bases, or other corrosive or caustic agents. Do not use in comatose or unconscious patients; caution in CNS depressant overdose.

■ Ipratropium Bromide Inhalant (Atrovent)

Indications: Bronchospasm associated with COPD.
Actions: Synthetic anticholinergic agent similar to atropine.
Dosage: 2–4 inhalations QID.
Supplied: Metered dose inhaler (MDI), 18 µg/dose.
Notes: *Not* for initial treatment of acute episodes of bronchospasm.

■ Iron Dextran (Imferon)

Indications: In patients with iron deficiency when oral supplementation is unsatisfactory or impossible.

Actions: Parenteral iron supplementation.
Dosage: Based on estimate of iron deficiency (consult package insert).
Supplied: Injection 50 mg Fe per mL.
Notes: Test dose must be administered since anaphylaxis is a common reaction. Iron dextran may be given deep IM using "Z-track" technique, although IV administration is preferable.

■ Isoniazid (INH)
Indications: Treatment of *Mycobacterium* spp. infections.
Actions: Bactericidal, interferes with lipid and nucleic acid biosynthesis.
Dosage: Active TB: 5 mg/kg/24 hr PO or IM Q day (usually 300 mg/day).
    Prophylaxis: 300 mg PO Q day for 6–12 months.
Supplied: Tablets 50 mg, 100 mg, 300 mg; syrup 50 mg/5mL; injection 100 mg/mL.
Notes: Can cause severe hepatitis; incidence of hepatitis increases wtih age; given with other antituberculous drugs for active tuberculosis. IM route is rarely used. To prevent peripheral neuropathy (high-risk subpopulations for neuropathy: alcoholics and elderly), give pyridoxine 50–100 mg/day.

■ Isoproterenol (Isuprel)
Indications: Shock, cardiac arrest, AV nodal block.
Actions: Beta$_1$- and beta$_2$-receptor stimulant.
Dosage: Emergency cardiac care: 2–20 µg/min IV infusion, titrated to effect.
    Shock: 1–4 µg/min IV infusion, titrated to effect.
    AV nodal block: 20–60 µg IV push; dose may be repeated Q 3–5 min; 1–5 µg/min IV infusion maintenance.
Supplied: Injection 200 µg/mL.
Notes: Contraindications include tachycardia; pulse > 130 BPM may induce ventricular arrhythmias.

■ Isosorbide Dinitrate (Isordil)
Indications: Angina pectoris.
Actions: Relaxation of vascular smooth muscle.
Dosage: Acute angina: 2.5–10.0 mg PO (chewable tablet) or SL PRN Q 5–10 min. Should only be used to abort acute anginal attacks in patients intolerant of or unresponsive to sublingual NTG to provide more rapid relief of chest pain; > 3 doses should not be given in less than a 15–30 min period.
    Angina prophylaxis: 5–60 mg PO TID.
Supplied: Tablets 5 mg, 10 mg, 20 mg, 30 mg, 40 mg; SR tablets 40 mg; SL tablets 2.5 mg, 5 mg, 10 mg; chewable tablets 5 mg, 10 mg; capsules 40 mg; SR capsules 40 mg.

Notes: Nitrates should not be given on a chronic Q 6 hr or QID basis due to development of tolerance. Tolerance can be avoided by administering on a TID basis, (not Q8 hours). Last dose should not be given after 7 pm. It takes 1–2 weeks to develop tolerance. Isosorbide can cause headaches. Oral doses usually need to be higher than sublingual doses to achieve same results as with sublingual forms.

■ Isosorbide Monohydrate (ISMO, IMDUR)

Indications: Prevention of angina pectoris.
Actions: Causes relaxation of the vascular smooth muscle.
Dosage: 20 mg PO BID, with the 2 doses given 7 hours apart; OR extended-release 30–120 mg PO Q day.
Supplied: Tablets 10 mg, 20 mg; extended-release tablets 60 mg.

■ Isradipine (DynaCirc)

Indication: Hypertension.
Action: Calcium channel blocking agent.
Dosage: 2.5–5.0 mg PO BID.
Supplied: Capsules 2.5 mg, 5 mg.

■ Itraconazole (Sporanox)

Indications: Treatment of systemic fungal infections caused by *Aspergillus, Blastomycosis,* and *Histoplasma.* Treatment of onychomycosis with 200 mg Q day × 3 months.
Actions: Inhibits synthesis of ergosterol.
Dosage: Usual dose 200 mg PO Q day–BID. For onychomycosis 200 mg every day for 3 months.
Supplied: Capsules 100 mg
Notes: Avoid concurrent use with any agent increasing gastric pH (H_2 antagonists, omeprazole, antacids), and terfenadine, or astemizole.

■ Kaolin-Pectin (Kapectolin, Kao-spen)

Indications: Treatment of diarrhea.
Actions: Adsorbent demulcent.
Dosage: 60–120 mL PO after each loose stool; or Q 3–4 hr PRN.
Supplied: Oral suspension.

■ Ketoconazole (Nizoral)

Indications: Treatment of systemic fungal infections; topical cream for localized fungal infections due to dermatophytes and yeast.
Actions: Inhibits fungal cell wall synthesis.
Dosage: *Oral:* 200 mg PO Q day; increase to 400 mg PO Q day for very serious infections.
 Topical: Apply to affected area once daily.

Supplied: Tablets 200 mg; suspension 100 mg/5mL; topical cream 2%.
Notes and Caution: Ketoconazole is associated with severe hepato-toxicity; monitor LFTs closely throughout course of therapy. Avoid concurrent use with any drug increasing gastric pH (preventing absorption of ketoconazole); also avoid concurrent use with astemizole and terfenadine. Ketoconazole may enhance activity of oral anticoagulants; may react with alcohol to produce disulfiram-like reaction.

■ Ketoprofen (Orudis) [See Table 7–10, p 532]

■ Ketorolac (Toradol) [See Table 7–10, p 532]

■ Ketorolac (Acular)
Indications: Relief of ocular itching due to seasonal allergic conjunctivitis.
Actions: Nonsteroidal anti-inflammatory agent.
Dosage: 1 drop 4 × day.
Supplied: Solution 0.5%.

■ Labetalol (Trandate, Normodyne) [See Table 7–6, p 529]
Indications: Hypertension, hypertensive emergencies.
Actions: Alpha- and beta-adrenergic blocking agent.
Dosage: *Hypertension* 100 mg PO BID initially; then 200–400 mg PO BID.

Hypertensive emergency: 20–80 mg IV bolus; then 2 mg/min IV infusion titrated to effect.
Supplied: Tablets 100 mg, 200 mg, 300 mg; injection 5 mg/mL.

■ *Lactobacillus* (Lactinex Granules)
Indications: Control of diarrhea, especially after antibiotic therapy.
Actions: Replaces normal intestinal flora.
Dosage: 1 packet, 2 capsules, or 4 tablets with meals or liquids TID.
Supplied: Tablets; capsules; enteric-coated capsules; powder in 1-gm packets.

■ Lactulose (Chronulac, Cephulac)
Indications: Hepatic encephalopathy; post-barium studies of the gastrointestinal tract or chronic constipation.
Actions: Hyperosmotic laxative; acidifies the colon, allowing ammonia to diffuse into the colon.

Dosage: *Acute hepatic encephalopathy:* 30–45 mL PO Q 1 hr until soft stools are observed. Titrate to 2–3 stools per day (usually TID–QID).

Chronic laxative therapy: 30–45 mL PO TID–QID; adjust dosage Q 1–2 days to produce 2–3 soft stools Q day.

Supplied: Syrup 10 gm/15 mL.

Note and Caution: Drug can cause severe diarrhea which may result in life-threatening hypernatremia.

■ Lamotrigine (Lamictal)

Indications: Treatment of partial seizures.

Actions: Phenyltriazine antiepileptic.

Dosage: Initial dose 50 mg PO once daily, followed by 50 mg PO BID for 2 weeks, then maintenance dose of 300–500 mg/day in two divided doses.

Supplied: Tablets 25 mg, 100 mg, 150 mg, 200 mg.

Notes: May cause rash and photosensitity; the value of therapeutic monitoring has not been established.

■ Lansoprazole (Prevacid)

Indications: Treatment of duodenal ulcers, erosive esophagitis, and hypersecretory conditions.

Actions: Proton pump inhibitor.

Dosage: 15–30 mg PO once Q day.

Supplied: Capsules 15 mg, 30 mg.

■ Leucovorin Calcium (Wellcovorin)

Indications: Overdoses of folic acid antagonists (eg, methotrexate).

Actions: Antianemic agent; circumvents the action of folate reductase inhibitors.

Dosage: *Methotrexate rescue:* 10–100 mg/m^2/dose IV or PO Q 3–6 hr.

Adjunct to antimicrobials: 5–10 mg PO Q day.

Supplied: Tablets 5 mg, 25 mg; solution 1 mg/mL; injection 5 mg/mL, 10 mg/mL.

Notes: Many different dosing schedules exist for leucovorin rescue following methotrexate therapy.

■ Leuprolide (Lupron)

Indications: Treatment of prostate cancer, endometriosis, and central precocious puberty.

Actions: LH-RH agonist.

Dosage: *Prostate:* 1 mg SC Q day or 7.5 mg IM monthly of depot preparation.

Endometriosis: (depot only) 3.75 mg IM as a single monthly dose.

Supplied: Injection 5 mg/mL; depot preparation 3.75 mg, 7.5 mg; Depot-Ped 7.5 mg, 11.25 mg, 15 mg.

■ Levobunolol (Betagan) [See Table 7–11, pp 533 & 534]

■ Levonorgestrel Implants (Norplant)
Indications: Prevention of pregnancy.
Dosage: Implantation of six capsules in the mid-forearm.
Supplied: Kits containing 6 implantable capsules, each containing 36 mg.
Notes: Prevents pregnancy for up to 5 years; capsules may be removed if pregnancy is desired. Implantation and removal require local anesthesia.

■ Levorphanol (Levo-Dromoran) [C]
Indications: Moderate to severe pain.
Actions: Narcotic analgesic; antipyretic.
Dosage: 2 mg PO or SC PRN.
Supplied: Tablets 2 mg; injection 2 mg/mL.

■ Levothyroxine (Synthroid)
Indications: Hypothyroidism.
Actions: Supplementation of L-thyroxine (T_4).
Dosage: 25–50 µg/day PO or IV initially; increase by 25–50 µg/day orally Q week to Q month; usual dose 75–200 µg/day.
Supplied: Tablets 0.025 mg, 0.05 mg, 0.075 mg, 0.1 mg, 0.125 mg, 0.15 mg, 0.175 mg, 0.2 mg, 0.3 mg; injection 0.2 mg, 0.5 mg.
Notes: Titrate dosage based on clinical response and thyroid function tests; dosage can be increased more rapidly in young to middle-aged patients versus elderly patients.

■ Lidocaine (Xylocaine)
Indications: Need for local anesthesia; treatment of cardiac arrhythmias.
Actions: Anesthetic; Class Ib antiarrhythmic.
Dosage: Arrhythmias: 1 mg/kg (50–100 mg) IV bolus; then 2–4 mg/min IV infusion; repeat bolus after 5 min.
　　　　Local anesthesia: Infiltrate a few mLs of a 0.5–1.0% solution.
Supplied: Injection 0.5%, 1%, 2%, 4%, 10%, 20%.
Notes and Cautions: Epinephrine may be added for local anesthesia to prolong effect and help decrease bleeding. *Do not* use epinephrine with lidocaine on digits, ears, nose, etc. because vasoconstriction can cause necrosis. For IV forms, dosage reduction is required with liver disease and

CHF. Dizziness, paresthesias, and convulsions are associated with toxicity. See Drug Levels, Table 7–13, p 536.

■ Lindane (Kwell)
Indications: Infestation by head lice, crab lice, scabies.
Actions: An ectoparasiticide and ovicide.
Dosage: *Cream or lotion:* Apply thin layer after bathing and leave in place for 8–12 hrs; pour on laundry.
       Shampoo: Apply 30 mL and develop lather with warm water for 4 min; comb out nits.
Supplied: Cream 1%, lotion 1%, shampoo 1%.
Notes: Caution patient about overuse; drug may be absorbed into blood. Avoid applying to face, mucous membranes, open cuts or abrasions.

■ Liothyronine (Cytomel)
Indications: Hypothyroidism.
Actions: T_3 replacement.
Dosage: Initial dose of 25 µg/24 hr, then titration Q 1–2 weeks according to clinical response and thyroid function tests, to maintenance dose of 25–75 µg PO Q day.
Supplied: Tablets 5 µg, 25 µg, 50 µg.
Notes: Reduce dose in elderly; monitor thyroid function test. Shorter half-life than levothyroxine.

■ Lisinopril (Prinivil, Zestril) [See Table 7–3, p 527]

■ Lithium Carbonate (Eskalith, Others)
Indications: Manic episodes of manic-depressive illness; maintenance therapy in recurrent disease.
Actions: Effects a shift toward intraneuronal metabolism of catecholamines.
Dosage: *Acute mania:* 600 mg PO TID or 900 mg SR BID.
       Maintenance: 300 mg PO TID–QID.
Supplied: Capsules 150 mg, 300 mg, 600 mg; tablets 300 mg; sustained-release tablets 300 mg, 450 mg; syrup 300 mg/5 mL.
Notes: Dosage must be titrated; follow serum levels. See Drug Levels, Table 7–13, p 536. Common side effects are polyuria, tremor; contraindicated in patients with severe renal impairment. Sodium retention or diuretic use may potentiate toxicity.

■ Lomefloxacin (Maxaquin)
Indications: Treatment of UTI and lower respiratory tract infections caused by gram-negative bacteria; prophylaxis in transurethral procedures.

Actions: Quinolone antibiotic.
Dosage: 400 mg PO Q day.
Supplied: Tablets 400 mg.
Notes: May cause severe photosensitivity.

■ Loperamide (Imodium)
Indications: Diarrhea.
Actions: Slows intestinal motility.
Dosage: 4 mg PO initially; then 2 mg after each loose stool, up to 16 mg/day.
Supplied: Capsules 2 mg; liquid 1 mg/5 mL.
Notes: Do not use in acute diarrhea caused by *Salmonella, Shigella,* or *C difficile*; can cause toxic megacolon.

■ Loracarbef (Lorabid) [See Table 7–8, p 530]

■ Loratadine (Claritin)
Indications: Treatment of allergic rhinitis.
Actions: Non-sedating antihistamine.
Dosage: 10 mg PO once Q day.
Supplied: Tablets 10 mg.
Notes: Instruct patient to take dose on an empty stomach.

■ Lorazepam (Ativan, Alzapam) [C]
Indications: Anxiety and anxiety mixed with depression; pre-op sedation; control of status epilepticus, alcohol withdrawal.
Actions: Benzodiazepine; anxiolytic.
Dosage: *Anxiety:* 0.5–1.0 mg PO BID–TID.
Pre-op sedation: 0.05 mg/kg up to maximum of 4 mg IM 2 hr prior to surgery.
Insomnia: 2–4 mg PO Q HS.
Status epilepticus: 2.5–10 mg/dose IV, repeated at 15–20 min interval × 2 PRN.
Alcohol withdrawal: See Section I, Chapter 16, Delirium Tremens (DTs): Major Alcohol Withdrawal, V.B.7. p 91.
Supplied: Tablets 0.5 mg, 1 mg, 2 mg; injection 2 mg/mL, 4 mg/mL.
Notes: Decrease dosage in elderly. Effects of drug may not be apparent for as long as 10 min when given IV.

■ Losartan (Cozaar)
Indications: Treatment of hypertension.
Actions: Angiotensin II receptor antagonist; first drug in a new class.
Dosage: 25–50 mg PO Q day–BID.
Supplied: Tablets 25 mg, 50 mg.
Notes and Caution: Contraindicated during pregnancy. Symptomatic hypotension may occur in patients taking diuretics.

■ Lovastatin (Mevacor)

Indications: Dietary adjunct for the reduction of elevated total and LDL cholesterol in patients with primary hypercholesterolemia (Types IIa and IIb).

Actions: HMG-CoA reductase inhibitor.

Dosage: 20 mg PO Q day with the evening meal; may be increased at 4-week intervals to maximum of 80 mg/day, taken with meals.

Supplied: Tablets 10 mg, 20 mg, 40 mg.

Notes: Patient should be maintained on standard cholesterol-lowering diet throughout treatment. Headache and GI intolerance are common side effects. Avoid concurrent use of gemfibrozil. Monitor LFTs every 6 weeks during first 3 months of therapy, then Q 6–12 weeks for 12 months; then every 6 months thereafter.

■ Magaldrate (Riopan, Lowsium)

Indications: Hyperacidity associated with peptic ulcer; gastritis, and hiatal hernia.

Actions: Low-sodium antacid.

Dosage: 1–2 tablets PO, or 5–10 mL PO between meals and HS.

Supplied: Tablets; suspension.

Notes: Contains < 0.3 mg sodium per tablet or teaspoon. Do *not* use in renal insufficiency.

■ Magnesium Citrate

Indications: Vigorous bowel prep; constipation.

Actions: Saline cathartic.

Dosage: 120–240 mL PO PRN.

Supplied: Effervescent solution.

Note: Do not use in renal insufficiency or intestinal obstruction.

■ Magnesium Hydroxide (Milk of Magnesia)

Indications: Constipation, short-term relief of hyperacidity.

Actions: Saline laxative; antacid.

Dosage: 15–30 mL; or one or two tablets, PO PRN.

Supplied: Aqueous suspension 8%; tablets 325 mg.

Notes: Do not use in renal insufficiency or intestinal obstruction. For antacid use, give before meals and mix suspension with water.

■ Magnesium Oxide (Uro-Mag, Mag-Ox 400, Maox)

Indications: Replacement for low plasma levels of magnesium.

Actions: Magnesium supplementation; antacid.

Dosage: 400–800 mg/day divided Q day–QID.

Supplied: Capsules 140 mg; tablets 400 mg, 420 mg.

Notes: May cause diarrhea.

■ Magnesium Sulfate

Indications: Replacement for low plasma magnesium levels; refractory hypokalemia and hypocalcemia; pre-eclampsia and premature labor.

Actions: Magnesium supplement; saline cathartic; anticonvulsant.

Dosage: *Supplement:* 1–2 gm IM or IV; repeat dosing based on response and continued hypomagnesemia.

Pre-eclampsia, premature labor: 1–4 gm/hr IV infusion.

Supplied: Injection 100 mg/mL, 125 mg/mL, 250 mg/mL, 500 mg/mL.

Notes: Reduce dose with low urine output or renal insufficiency.

■ Mannitol

Indications: Conditions requiring osmotic diuresis (eg, cerebral edema, oliguria, anuria, myoglobinuria).

Actions: Osmotic diuretic.

Dosage: *Oliguria, anuria, myoglobinuria:* 0.2 gm/kg/dose IV over 3–5 min; if no diuresis within 2 hr, discontinue.

Cerebral edema: 0.25 gm/kg/dose IV push repeated at 5 min intervals PRN; increase incrementally to 1 gm/kg/dose PRN for intracranial hypertension.

Supplied: Injection 5%, 10%, 15%, 20%, 25%.

Notes: Use cautiously with CHF or volume overload.

■ Maprotiline (Ludiomil)

Indications: Depressive neurosis; manic-depressive illness; major depressive disorder; anxiety associated with depression.

Actions: Tetracyclic antidepressant.

Dosage: 75–150 mg/day Q HS, maximum dose 300 mg/day.

Supplied: Tablets 25 mg, 50 mg, 75 mg.

Notes: Contraindicated with history of seizures or concurrent use of MAO inhibitors. For patients > 60 years of age, give only 50–75 mg/day. Drug has anticholinergic side effects.

■ Meclizine (Antivert)

Indications: Motion sickness, vertigo associated with diseases of the vestibular system.

Actions: Antiemetic, anticholinergic, and antihistaminic properties.

Dosage: 25 mg PO TID–QID PRN.

Supplied: Tablets 12.5 mg, 25 mg; chewable tablets 25 mg; capsules 25 mg.

Notes: Drowsiness, dry mouth, blurred vision are common side effects.

■ Medroxyprogesterone (Provera)

Indications: Secondary amenorrhea; dysfunctional uterine bleeding due to hormonal imbalance; endometrial cancer; to decrease the risk of endometrial cancer use medroxyprogesterone concurrently with estrogen for hormonal replacement if the uterus has not been surgically removed.

Actions: Progestin supplement; antineoplastic.
Dosage:

- *Secondary amenorrhea:* 5–10 mg PO Q day for 5–10 days.
- *Abnormal uterine bleeding:* 5–10 mg PO Q day for 5–10 days beginning on day 16 or day 21 of menstrual cycle.
- *Cancer:* 400–1000 mg IM Q week.
- *Hormonal replacement:* (with estrogen) 5–10 mg PO on day 13 or day 16 through day 25; OR 2.5 mg Q day.

Supplied: Tablets 2.5 mg, 5 mg, 10 mg; Depo-injection 100 mg/mL, 400 mg/mL.
Note: Contraindicated in patients with histories of thromboembolic disorders or hepatic disease.

■ Megestrol Acetate (Megace)
Indications: Treatment of breast and endometrial cancer; appetite stimulant in HIV-related cachexia.
Actions: Hormone; antineoplastic.
Dosage: *Cancer:* 40–320 mg/day PO in divided doses.
      Appetite regulation: 800 mg PO Q day.
Supplied: Tablets 20 mg, 40 mg; solution 40mg/mL.

■ Melphalan (Alkeran)
Indications: Treatment of breast and ovarian cancer, and multiple myeloma.
Actions: Alkylating agent.
Dosage: 6 mg/day PO as single dose; or 16 mg/m^2 IV Q 2 weeks for 4 doses.
Supplied: Tablets 2 mg; Injection 50 mg.
Notes: Monitor blood counts closely.

■ Meperidine (Demerol) [C]
Indications: Relief of moderate to severe pain.
Actions: Narcotic analgesic.
Dosage: 50–100 mg PO or IM Q 3–4 hr PRN.
Supplied: Tablets 50 mg, 100 mg; syrup 50 mg/mL; injection 10 mg/mL, 25 mg/mL, 50 mg/mL, 75 mg/mL, 100 mg/mL.
Notes and Caution: 75 mg IM equivalent to 10 mg morphine IM. Watch for signs of respiratory depression; instruct patient to avoid alcohol and other CNS depressants.

■ Mercaptopurine (Purinethol)
Indications: Treatment of leukemia.
Actions: Antimetabolite; antineoplastic.

Dosage: 2.5 mg/kg/day PO.
Supplied: Tablets 50 mg.

■ Mesalamine (Rowasa)
Indications: Treatment of mild to moderate distal ulcerative colitis, proctosigmoiditis, or proctitis.
Actions: Unknown; may topically inhibit prostaglandins.
Dosage: Retention enema Q HS.
Supplied: Rectal suspension 4 gm/60 mL.

■ Mesna (Mesnex)
Indications: Reduction of the incidence of ifosfamide-induced hemorrhagic cystitis.
Actions: Antidote; detoxifying agent.
Dosage: 20% of the ifosfamide dose (w/w) IV at the time of ifosfamide infusion; and 4 and 8 hr after, for a total dose = 60% of the ifosfamide dose.
Supplied: Injection 100 mg/mL.

■ Mesoridazine (Serentil)
Indications: Schizophrenia; acute and chronic alcoholism; chronic brain syndrome.
Actions: Phenothiazine antipsychotic.
Dosage: 25–50 mg PO or IV TID initially; titrate to maximum of 300–400 mg/day.
Supplied: Tablets 10 mg, 25 mg, 50 mg, 100 mg; oral concentrate 25 mg/mL; injection 25 mg/mL.
Note: Drug has low incidence of extrapyramidal side effects.

■ Metaproterenol (Alupent, Metaprel)
Indications: Bronchodilator for asthma and reversible bronchospasm.
Actions: Sympathomimetic bronchodilator.
Dosage: Inhalation: 1–3 inhalations Q 3–4 hr to a maximum of 12–16 inhalations Q 24 hrs; allow at least 2 min between inhalations.
  Oral: 20 mg Q 6–8 hr.
Supplied: Metered-dose inhaler 650 µg/dose; solution for inhalation 0.5%, 0.6%; tablets 10 mg, 20 mg; syrup 10 mg/5 mL.
Notes: Metaproterenol has fewer beta-1 effects than isoproterenol and is longer-acting.

■ Metformin (Glucophage)
Indications: Treatment of NIDDM (Non-insulin-dependent diabetes mellitus).
Actions: Decreases hepatic glucose production and intestinal absorption of glucose, and improves insulin sensitivity.

Dosage: Initial dose of 500 mg PO BID; dose may be increased to a maximum daily dose of 2500 mg.

Supplied: Tablets 500 mg, 850 mg.

Notes and Caution: Administer with morning and evening meals. May cause lactic acidosis. *Do not use metformin* if serum creatinine is > 1.4 mg/dL in female patients or > 1.5 mg/dL in males.

■ Methadone (Dolophine) [C]

Indications: Severe pain; detoxification and maintenance of narcotic addiction.

Actions: Narcotic analgesic.

Dosage: 2.5–10 mg IM Q 8 hr; OR 5–15 mg PO Q 8 hr (titrate as needed).

Supplied: Tablets 5 mg, 10 mg; oral solution 5 mg/5 mL, 10 mg/5 mL; injection 10 mg/mL.

Notes: Equianalgesic with parenteral morphine; has long half-life. Increase dose slowly to avoid respiratory depression.

■ Methimazole (Tapazole)

Indications: Hyperthyroidism; preparation for thyroid surgery or radiation.

Actions: Blocks the formation of T_3 and T_4.

Dosage: Initial dosage 15–60 mg/day PO divided TID; maintenance dosage of 5–15 mg PO Q day.

Supplied: Tablets 5 mg, 10 mg.

Notes: Follow patient clinically; monitor thyroid function tests carefully.

■ Methocarbamol (Robaxin)

Indications: Relief of discomfort associated with painful musculo-skeletal conditions.

Actions: Centrally acting skeletal muscle relaxant.

Dosage: 1.5 gm PO QID for 2–3 days; then 1.5 gm PO TID or 1 gm QID maintenance therapy; IV form rarely indicated.

Supplied: Tablets 500 mg, 750 mg; injection 100 mg/mL.

Notes: Methocarbamol may discolor urine; may cause drowsiness or GI upset. Contraindicated in patients with myasthenia gravis.

■ Methotrexate (Folex)

Indications: Treatment of gestational trophoblastic disease; breast, ovarian, lung, head, or neck cancer; leukemia; psoriasis; rheumatoid arthritis.

Actions: Antimetabolite antineoplastic.

Dosage: *Cancer:* Dosage varies with type of cancer and individual protocol.

Rheumatoid arthritis: 7.5 mg/week PO as a single dose each week; OR 2.5 mg Q 12 hr PO for 3 doses each week.

Supplied: Tablets 2.5 mg; injection 2.5 mg/mL, 25 mg/mL; preservative free injection 25 mg/mL.

Notes and Caution: Utilize leucovorin rescue with high doses of methotrexate. Monitor blood counts and methotrexate levels carefully.

■ Methyldopa (Aldomet)

Indications: Essential hypertension.

Actions: Central-acting antihypertensive.

Dosage: 250–500 mg PO BID–TID (maximum 2–3 gm/day); or 250 mg–1 gm IV Q 4–8 hr.

Supplied: Tablets 125 mg, 250 mg, 500 mg; oral suspension 250 mg/5 mL; injection 250 mg/5 mL.

Notes: Do not use methyldopa in presence of liver disease. May discolor urine. Initial transient sedation or drowsiness are frequent side effects.

■ Methylprednisolone (Solu-Medrol, Medrol) [See Table 7–2, p 526]

■ Metipranolol (Optipranolol) [See Table 7–11, pp 533 & 534]

■ Metoclopramide (Reglan, Clopra, Others)

Indications: Relief of diabetic gastroparesis; symptomatic gastro-esophageal reflux; relief of cancer chemotherapy-induced nausea and vomiting.

Actions: Stimulates motility of the upper GI tract.

Dosage:

- *Diabetic gastroparesis:* 10 mg PO 30 min AC and HS for 2–8 weeks PRN; OR same dose given IV for 10 days, then switch to PO.
- *Reflux:* 10–15 mg PO 30 min AC and HS.
- *Antiemetic:* 1–3 mg/kg/dose IV 30 min prior to antineoplastic agent; then Q 2 hr for two doses; then Q 3 hr for three doses.

Supplied: Tablets 5 mg, 10 mg; syrup 5 mg/5 mL; injection 5 mg/mL.

Notes: Dystonic reactions common with high doses, can be treated with IV diphenhydramine. Metoclopramide can also be used to facilitate small bowel intubation and radiological evaluation of the upper GI tract.

■ Metolazone (Diulo, Zaroxolyn)

Indications: Mild to moderate essential hypertension; edema of renal disease or cardiac failure.

Actions: Thiazide-like diuretic.

Dosage: Hypertension: 2.5–5 mg PO Q day.
　　　Edema: 5–20 mg PO Q day.
Supplied: Tablets 2.5 mg, 5 mg, 10 mg.
Notes: Monitor patient's fluid and electrolyte status during treatment.

■ Metoprolol (Lopressor, Toprol XL) [See Table 7–6, p 529]

■ Metronidazole (Flagyl)
Indications: Amebiasis, trichomoniasis, bacterial vaginosis, infections caused by *C difficile*, and anaerobic infections.
Actions: Interferes with DNA synthesis.
Dosage:

- *Anaerobic infections:* 500 mg IV Q 6–8 hr.
- *Amebic dysentery:* 750 mg PO Q day for 5–10 days.
- *Trichomoniasis:* 250 mg PO TID for 7 days; Or 2 gm PO in 1 dose.
- *C difficile:* 500 mg PO every 8 hours for 7–10 days.
- *Bacterial vaginosis:* 500 mg PO BID for 7 days.

Supplied: Tablets 250 mg, 500 mg; injection 500 mg.
Notes: For *Trichomonas* infections, treat patient's partner also. Reduce dose in hepatic failure. Metronidazole has no activity against aerobic bacteria; use in combination in serious mixed infections. Drug may cause disulfiram-like reaction.

■ Metyrapone (Metopirone)
Indications: Diagnostic test for hypothalamic-pituitary ACTH function.
Actions: Inhibits adrenocortical synthesis by blocking 11-beta hydroxylase.
Dosage: Metapyrone test:

- *Day 1:* Control period: collect 24-hr urine to measure 17-hydroxycorticosteroids (17-OHCS) or 17-ketogenic steroids (17-KSG).
- *Day 2:* ACTH test: 50 U ACTH infused over 8 hr; measure 24-hour urinary steroids.
- *Days 3-4:* Rest period.
- *Day 5:* Administer metyrapone 750 mg PO Q 4 hr for six doses; give with milk or snack.
- *Day 6:* Determine 24-hr urinary steroids.

Supplied: Tablets 250 mg.
Notes: Normal 24-hr urine 17-OHCS is 3–12 mg; following ACTH, it increases to 15–45 mg/24 hours. Normal response to metyrapone is a twofold to fourfold increase in 17-OHCS excretion. Drug interactions with phenytoin, cyproheptadine, and estrogens may lead to subnormal response.

■ Mexiletine (Mexitil)

Indications: Suppression of symptomatic ventricular arrhythmias.
Actions: Class Ib antiarrhythmic.
Dosage: Administer with food or antacids; 200–300 mg PO Q 8 hr; do not exceed 1200 mg/day.
Supplied: Capsules 150 mg, 200 mg, 250 mg.
Notes and Cautions: Not to be used in cardiogenic shock, second- or third-degree AV block if no pacemaker is present. Drug may worsen severe arrhythmias. Monitor liver function during therapy; drug interactions with hepatic enzyme inducers and suppressors requiring dosage changes.

■ Mezlocillin (Mezlin) [See Table 7–5, p 528]

■ Miconazole (Monistat)

Indications: Severe systemic fungal infections including coccidioidomycosis, candidiasis, cryptococcal infections, and others; various tinea forms; cutaneous candidiasis; vulvovaginal candidiasis; tinea versicolor.
Actions: Antibiotic; fungicidal, alters permeability of the fungal cell membrane.
Dosage: Systemic: Dosage range from 200–3600 mg/24 hr IV based on diagnosis and divided into three doses.
　　　　Topical: Apply to affected area twice daily for 2–4 weeks.
　　　　Intravaginal: Insert one full applicator or suppository at bedtime for 7 days.
Supplied: Injection 10 mg/mL; topical cream 2%, lotion 2%, powder 2%, spray 2%, vaginal suppositories 200 mg; vaginal cream 2%.
Notes: Miconazole is antagonistic to amphotericin-B in vivo. Rapid IV infusion may cause tachycardia or arrhythmias. Miconazole may also potentiate warfarin drug activity.

■ Midazolam (Versed) [C]

Indications: Preoperative sedation; conscious sedation for short procedures; induction of general anesthesia.
Actions: Short-acting benzodiazepine.
Dosage: 1–5 mg IV or IM; titrate dose to effect.
Supplied: Injection 1 mg/mL, 5 mg/mL.
Notes and Caution: Monitor patient for respiratory depression. Midazolam may produce hypotension in conscious sedation.

■ Milrinone (Primacor)

Indications: Treatment of congestive heart failure.
Actions: Positive inotrope and vasodilator, with little chronotropic activity.

Dosage: Loading dose of 50 µg/kg, followed by a continuous infusion of 0.375–0.75 µg/kg/min.
Supplied: Injection 1 mg/mL.
Notes: Carefully monitor fluid and electrolyte status.

■ Mineral Oil
Indications: Constipation.
Actions: Emollient laxative.
Dosage: 15–45 mL PO PRN.
Supplied: Liquid.
Notes: Most patients find mineral oil less objectionable when taken with orange juice.

■ Minoxidil (Loniten)
Indications: Severe hypertension; treatment of male and female pattern baldness.
Actions: Peripheral vasodilator; stimulates vertex hair growth.
Dosage: *Oral:* 2.5–10 mg PO BID–QID.
            Topical: Apply twice daily to affected area.
Supplied: Tablets 2.5 mg, 10 mg; topical solution 2%.
Notes: Pericardial effusion and volume overload may occur; hypertrichosis after chronic use.

■ Misoprostol (Cytotec)
Indications: Prevention of NSAID-induced gastric ulcers.
Actions: Synthetic prostaglandin with both antisecretory and mucosal protective properties.
Dosage: 200 µg PO QID.
Supplied: Tablets 200 µg.
Notes and Caution: Contraindicated during pregnancy; misoprostol can cause miscarriage with potentially dangerous bleeding. GI side effects are also common.

■ Mitomycin (Mutamycin)
Indications: Treatment of breast, cervical, and ovarian cancer; and adenocarcinoma.
Actions: Antibiotic, antineoplastic agent.
Dosage: 20 mg/m^{2}IV as a single dose Q 6–8 weeks.
Supplied: Injection 5 mg, 20 mg, 40 mg.
Notes: May cause cumulative myelosuppression.

■ Mitoxantrone (Novantrone)
Indications: Treatment of leukemia, lymphoma, and breast cancer.

Actions: Antibiotic, antineoplastic.
Dosage: 12 mg/m²/day IV infusion for 2–3 days of each chemotherapy cycle.
Supplied: Injection 2 mg/mL.
Notes: Causes severe myelosuppression.

■ Moexipril (Univasc) [See Table 7–3, p 527]

■ Morphine Sulfate [C]
Indications: Relief of severe pain.
Actions: Narcotic analgesic.
Dosage: *Oral:* 10–30 mg Q 4 hr PRN; sustained-release tablets 30-60 mg Q 8–12 hr.
       IV/IM: 2.5–15 mg Q 4 hr PRN.
Supplied: Tablets 10 mg, 15 mg, 30 mg; SR tablets 15 mg, 30 mg, 60 mg; solution 10 mg/5 mL, 20 mg/5 mL, 100 mg/5 mL; suppositories 5 mg, 10 mg, 20 mg; injection 2 mg/mL, 4 mg/mL, 5 mg/mL, 8 mg/mL, 10 mg/mL, 15 mg/mL; preservative-free injection 0.5 mg/mL, 1 mg/mL.
Notes: Morphine has a large number of narcotic side effects; may require scheduled dosing to relieve severe chronic pain.

■ Muromonab-CD3 (Orthoclone OKT3)
Indications: Treatment of acute rejection following organ transplantation.
Actions: Immunosuppressant; blocks T-cell function.
Dosage: 5 mg IV Q day for 10–14 days.
Supplied: Injection 5 mg/5 mL.
Notes: Muromonab is a murine antibody; may cause significant fever and chills after the first dose.

■ Mycophenolate Mofetil (CellCept)
Indications: Prevention of organ rejection following transplantation.
Actions: Inhibits immunologically mediated inflammatory responses.
Dosage: 1 gm PO BID.
Supplied: Capsules 250 mg.
Notes: Used in conjunction with corticosteroids and cyclosporin.

■ Nabumetone (Relafen) [See Table 7–10, p 532]

■ Nadolol (Corgard) [See Table 7–6, p 529]

■ Nafcillin [See Table 7–4, p 527]

■ Nalbuphine (Nubain)
Indications: Moderate to severe pain.
Actions: Narcotic agonist-antagonist.
Dosage: 10–20 mg IM, IV, SC Q 4–6 hr PRN.
Supplied: Injection 10 mg/mL, 20 mg/mL.
Notes and Caution: Nalbuphine causes CNS depression and drowsiness. Use with caution in patients receiving opiate drugs.

■ Naloxone (Narcan)
Indications: Reversal of narcotic effect.
Actions: Competitive narcotic antagonist.
Dosage: 0.4–2.0 mg IV, IM or SC Q 5 min; maximum total dose of 10 mg.
Supplied: Injection 0.4 mg/mL, 1.0 mg/mL; neonatal injection 0.02 mg/mL.
Notes: May precipitate acute withdrawal in addicts; if no response after 10 mg, suspect a non-narcotic cause.

■ Naproxen (Naprosyn, Anaprox) [See Table 7–10, p 532]

■ Nedocromil (Tilade)
Indications: Management of patients with mild to moderate asthma.
Actions: Anti-inflammatory agent.
Dosage: Two inhalations 4 × day.
Supplied: Metered-dose inhaler.

■ Nefazodone (Serzone)
Indications: Treatment of depression.
Actions: Inhibits neuronal uptake of serotonin and norepinephrine.
Dosage: Initial dose 100 mg PO BID; usual effective range is 300–600 mg/day in two divided doses.
Supplied: Tablets 100 mg, 150 mg, 200 mg, 250 mg.
Notes: May cause postural hypotension and allergic reactions.

■ Neomycin Sulfate
Indications: Hepatic coma; pre-op bowel prep.
Actions: Aminoglycoside; suppresses GI bacterial flora.
Dosage: 3–12 gm/24 hr PO in 3–4 divided doses.
Supplied: Tablets 500 mg; oral solution 125 mg/5 mL.

■ Niacin (Nicolar)

Indications: Adjunctive therapy in patients with significant hyperlipidemia who do not respond adequately to diet and weight loss.

Actions: Inhibits lipolysis; decreases esterification of triglyceride; increases lipoprotein lipase activity.

Dosage: 500 mg–2 gm PO TID with meals; up to 6 gm Q day.

Supplied: 50 mg and 100 mg tablets; elixir 50 mg/5 mL.

Notes and Caution: Upper body and facial flushing or warmth following dose are common side effects. Flushing can be alleviated with aspirin 325 mg PO ½ hr before dose and taking niacin with meals. Drug may cause GI upset or precipitate gout. *Do not use* sustained-release products.

■ Nicardipine (Cardene)

Indications: Chronic stable angina, hypertension.

Actions: Calcium channel blocking agent.

Dosage: *Oral:* 20–40 mg PO TID; sustained-release, 30–60 mg PO BID.

   IV: 0.5–15 mg/hr continuous IV infusion; titrate to desired blood pressure.

Supplied: Capsules 20 mg, 30 mg; SR capsules 30 mg, 45 mg, 60 mg; injection 2.5 mg/mL.

Notes: Oral to IV conversion: 20 mg TID = 0.5 mg/hr; 30 mg TID = 1.2 mg/hr; 40 mg TID = 2.2 mg/hr.

■ Nifedipine (Procardia, Procardia XL, Adalat, Adalat CC)

Indications: Vasospastic or chronic stable angina; hypertension; accelerated hypertension.

Actions: Calcium channel blocking agent.

Dosage: *Hypertension:* SR tablets 30–90 mg Q day–BID.

   Hypertensive emergency: 10–20 mg PO as single dose.

Supplied: Capsules 10 mg, 20 mg; tablets SR 30 mg, 60 mg, 90 mg.

Notes and Caution: Headaches common during initial treatment; reflex tachycardia may occur with nonsustained release forms. Adalat CC and Procardia XL are *not* interchangeable dosage forms. An increase in mortality has been associated with short-acting nifedipine used to treat hypertension.

■ Nitrofurantoin (Macrodantin, Furadantin)

Indications: Urinary tract infections.

Actions: Bacteriostatic; interferes with carbohydrate metabolism.

Dosage: *Suppression:* 50–100 mg PO Q day.

   Treatment: 50–100 mg PO QID; macrocrystal/monohydrate 100 mg Q 12 hr.

Supplied: Capsules and tablets 50 mg, 100 mg; macrocrystal/mono-hydrate 25 mg, 50 mg, 100 mg; suspension 25 mg/5 mL.

Notes: GI side effects common; drug should be taken with food, milk, or antacid. Macrocrystals (Macrodantin) cause less nausea than other forms of drug.

■ Nitroglycerin (Nitrostat, Nitrolingual, Nitro-Bid Ointment, Nitro-Bid IV, Nitrodisc, Transderm-Nitro, Others)

Indications: Angina pectoris; acute and prophylactic therapy; conges-tive heart failure, blood pressure control.

Actions: Relaxation of vascular smooth muscle.

Dosage:

- *Sublingual:* 1 tablet SL Q 5 min PRN up to three doses.
- *Translingual:* 1–2 metered doses sprayed onto oral mucosa.
- *Oral:* 2.5–9 mg TID.
- *Intravenous:* 5–20 µg/min titrated to effect.
- *Topical:* 1/2–2 inches of ointment to chest wall Q 6 hr, then wipe off at night.
- *Transdermal:* 5–20 cm patch Q day, remove at night.

Supplied: Sublingual tablets 0.15 mg, 0.3 mg, 0.4 mg, 0.6 mg; translin-gual spray 0.4 mg/dose; SR capsules 2.5 mg, 6.5 mg, 9 mg; tablets SR 2.6 mg, 6.5 mg, 9.0 mg; injection 0.5 mg/mL, 0.8 mg/mL, 5 mg/mL, 10 mg/mL; ointment 2%; transdermal patches delivering 2.5, 5, 7.5, 10 or 15 mg/24 hr.

Notes: Tolerance to nitrates will develop with chronic use after 1–2 weeks; this can be avoided by providing a nitrate-free period each day. Shorter-acting nitrates should be used on a TID basis; longer-acting patches and ointment should be removed before bedtime in order to pre-vent development of tolerance.

■ Nitroprusside (Nipride, Nitropress)

Indications: Hypertensive emergency, aortic dissection, pulmonary edema.

Actions: Reduces systemic vascular resistance.

Dosage: 0.5–10 µg/kg/min IV infusion titrated to desired effect.

Supplied: Injection 50 mg.

Notes and Caution: Thiocyanate, the metabolite, is excreted by the kidney. Thiocyanate toxicity occurs at plasma levels of 5–10 mg/dL. If nitroprusside is used to treat aortic dissection, a beta-blocker must be used concomitantly.

■ Nizatidine (Axid)

Indications: Treatment of duodenal ulcers; gastroesophageal reflux disease (GERD).

Actions: H_2 receptor antagonist.

Dosage: *Active ulcer:* 150 mg PO BID; OR 300 mg PO Q HS; maintenance dose 150 mg PO Q HS.

GERD: 150 mg PO BID; maintenance dose 75 mg PO before bed or BID.

Supplied: Capsules 150 mg, 300 mg.

■ Norepinephrine (Levophed)

Indications: Acute hypotensive states.

Actions: Peripheral vasoconstrictor acting on both the arterial and venous beds.

Dosage: 8–12 µg/min IV titrated to desired effect.

Supplied: Injection 1 mg/mL.

Notes and Caution: Correct blood volume depletion as much as possible prior to initiation of vasopressor therapy. Drug may interact with tricyclic antidepressants to produce severe prolonged hypertension. Infuse into large vein to avoid extravasation; phentolamine 5–10 mg/10 mL NSS may be injected locally as antidote to extravasation.

■ Norfloxacin (Noroxin)

Indications: Treatment of complicated and uncomplicated urinary tract infections due to a wide variety of gram-negative bacteria, and prostatitis. Also used to prevent spontaneous bacterial peritonitis in patients with cirrhosis.

Actions: Inhibits DNA gyrase.

Dosage: UTI and prostatitis 400 mg PO BID; SBP prophylaxis 400 mg per day.

Supplied: Tablets 400 mg.

Notes and Caution: *Not* for use in pregnancy; drug interactions with antacids, theophylline, and caffeine. Good drug levels in the kidney and urine, poor drug levels in the blood. *Do not use* in urosepsis.

■ Nortriptyline (Aventyl, Pamelor)

Indications: Endogenous depression.

Actions: Tricyclic antidepressant.

Dosage: 25 mg PO TID–QID. Doses > 100 mg/day are not recommended.

Supplied: Capsules 10 mg, 25 mg, 50 mg, 75 mg; solution 10 mg/5 mL.

Notes: Drug has many anticholinergic side effects including blurred vision, urinary retention, dry mouth.

■ Nystatin (Mycostatin, Nilstat)

Indications: Treatment of mucocutaneous *Candida* infections (thrush, vaginitis).

Actions: Alters membrane permeability.
Dosage: *Oral:* 400,000–600,000 U PO "swish and swallow" QID.
           Intravaginal: 1 tablet Q HS.
           Topical: Apply 2–3 times Q day to affected area.
Supplied: Oral suspension 100,000 U/mL; oral tablets 500,000 U; troches 200,000 U; vaginal tablets 100,000 U; topical cream and ointment 100,000 U/gm.
Notes: Nystatin is not absorbed orally, therefore is not effective for systemic infections.

■ Octreotide Acetate (Sandostatin)

Indications: Suppresses or inhibits severe diarrhea associated with carcinoid and vasoactive intestinal tumors; treatment of variceal hemorrhage.
Actions: Long-acting peptide that mimics the natural hormone somatostatin.
Dosage: *Diarrhea:* 100–600 µg/day SC in 2–4 divided doses.
           Variceal hemorrhage: 25–50 µg/hr for 48 hr.
Supplied: Injection 0.05 mg/mL, 0.1 mg/mL, 0.5 mg/mL.
Notes: May cause nausea, vomiting, and abdominal discomfort.

■ Ofloxacin (Floxin)

Indications: Treatment of infections of the lower respiratory tract, skin and skin structure, and urinary tract; prostatitis; uncomplicated gonorrhea; and *Chlamydia* infections.
Actions: Bactericidal, inhibits DNA gyrase.
Dosage: 200–400 mg PO BID or IV Q 12 hr.
Supplied: Tablets 200 mg, 300 mg, 400 mg; injection 20 mg/mL, 40 mg/mL.
Notes: Drug may cause nausea, vomiting, diarrhea, insomnia and headache; may increase theophylline levels. Ofloxacin interacts with antacids, sucralfate, and iron and zinc containing products which decrease its absorption.

■ Olsalazine (Dipentum)

Indications: Maintenance of remission of ulcerative colitis.
Actions: Anti-inflammatory activity.
Dosage: 500 mg PO BID.
Supplied: Capsules 250 mg.
Notes: Instruct patient to take drug with food. May cause diarrhea.

■ Omeprazole (Prilosec)

Indications: Treatment of duodenal ulcers, Zollinger-Ellison syndrome, and gastroesophageal reflux (GERD).
Actions: Proton-pump inhibitor.

Dosage: 20–40 mg Q day.
Supplied: Capsules 20 mg.

■ Ondansetron (Zofran)
Indications: Prevention of nausea and vomiting associated with cancer chemotherapy; prevention of post-operative nausea and vomiting.
Actions: Serotonin receptor antagonist.
Dosage: *Chemotherapy:* 0.15 mg/kg/dose IV prior to chemotherapy; then repeated 4 and 8 hr after the first dose; OR 4–8 mg PO TID, administer first dose 30–60 min prior to chemotherapy.
　　　Post-op: 4 mg IV immediately before induction or post-op.
Supplied: Tablets 4 mg, 8 mg; injection 2 mg/mL.
Notes: Drug may cause diarrhea and headache.

■ Oxacillin (Bactocill, Prostaphlin) [See Table 7–4, p 527]

■ Oxaprozin (Daypro) [See Table 7–10, p 532]

■ Oxazepam (Serax) [C]
Indications: Anxiety; acute alcohol withdrawal; anxiety with depressive symptoms.
Actions: Benzodiazepine anxiolytic.
Dosage: 10–15 mg PO TID–QID. Severe anxiety and alcohol withdrawal may require up to 30 mg QID.
Supplied: Capsules 10 mg, 15 mg, 30 mg; tablets 15 mg.
Notes: Oxazepam is one of the metabolites of diazepam (Valium).

■ Oxybutynin (Ditropan)
Indications: Symptomatic relief of urgency, nocturia, and incontinence associated with neurogenic or reflex neurogenic bladder.
Actions: Antispasmodic.
Dosage: 5 mg PO BID–QID.
Supplied: Tablets 5 mg; syrup 5 mg/5 mL.
Note: Anticholinergic side effects.

■ Oxycodone (Percocet, Percodan, Tylox) [C]
Indications: Moderate to severe pain.
Actions: Narcotic analgesic.
Dosage: 1–2 tablets/capsules PO Q 4–6 hr PRN.
Supplied: Percocet tablets: 5 mg oxycodone, 325 mg acetaminophen.
　　　　　Percodan tablet: 4.5 mg oxycodone, 325 mg aspirin.
　　　　　Tylox capsule: 5 mg oxycodone, 500 mg acetaminophen.

Notes: Evaluate patient's ongoing need for oxycodone preparations; drug has high potential for tolerance and dependence.

■ Oxytocin (Pitocin, Syntocinon)

Indications: Induction of labor; control of postpartum hemorrhage.
Actions: Stimulates uterine contractions.
Dosage: 0.001–0.002 U/min, IV infusion; titrate to desired effect, to a maximum of 0.02 U/min.
Supplied: Injection 10 U/mL.
Notes and Caution: Oxytocin can cause uterine rupture and fetal death; monitor patient's vital signs closely.

■ Paclitaxel (Taxol)

Indications: Treatment of ovarian cancer.
Actions: Antimicrotubule antineoplastic agent.
Dosage: 135 mg/m^{2}IV Q 3 weeks.
Supplied: Injection 30 mg/5 mL.
Notes: Drug may cause severe neutropenia.

■ Pamidronate (Aredia)

Indications: Treatment of hypercalcemia of malignancy and Paget's disease.
Actions: Inhibition of normal and abnormal bone resorption.
Dosage: *Hypercalcemia:* 60 mg IV over 4 hr or 90 mg IV over 24 hr. Lower doses (15–45 mg/day) can be repeated daily up to 6 days. For higher doses (60–90 mg), a period of 7 days should elapse before starting a 2nd course.
　　　　Paget's disease: 30 mg IV Q day for 3 days.
Supplied: Powder for injection 30 mg, 60 mg, 90 mg.
Notes: Drug may cause hypokalemia, hypomagnesemia and hypophosphatemia.

■ Pancreatin, Pancrelipase (Pancrease, Cotazyme)

Indications: For patients deficient in exocrine pancreatic secretions (cystic fibrosis, chronic pancreatitis, other causes of pancreatic insufficiency), and for steatorrhea of malabsorption syndrome.
Actions: Pancreatic enzyme supplementation.
Dosage: 1–3 capsules or tablets with meals and snacks; dosage may be increased up to 32,000 U or more if necessary with each meal and snack.
Supplied: Capsules; tablets. Various amounts of lipase, amylase and protease; recommendations of dosage based on amount of lipase.
Notes: Instruct patient to avoid antacids, and not to crush or chew enteric-coated products. Drug may cause nausea, abdominal cramps, or diarrhea.

■ Pancuronium (Pavulon)

Indications: Assistance in the management of patients on mechanical ventilators.

Actions: Nondepolarizing neuromuscular blocker.

Dosage: 2–4 mg IV Q 2–4 hr PRN; OR 0.02–0.10 mg/kg/dose Q 2–4 hr PRN.

Supplied: Injection 1 mg/mL, 2 mg/mL.

Notes: Patient must be intubated and on controlled ventilation; use adequate amount of sedation or analgesia.

■ Paroxetine (Paxil)

Indications: Treatment of depression.

Actions: Serotonin reuptake inhibitor.

Dosage: 20–50 mg PO as a single daily dose.

Supplied: Tablets 20 mg, 30 mg.

Notes: Avoid concurrent use with astemizole and terfenadine.

■ Penbutolol (Levatol) [See Table 7–6, p 529]

■ Penicillin G Aqueous (Potassium or Sodium) (Pfizerpen, Pentids)

Indications: Most gram-positive infectious agents (except penicillin-resistant staphylococci), including streptococci, *N meningitidis, T pallidum,* clostridia, corynebacteria, and some coliforms.

Actions: Bactericidal, inhibits cell wall synthesis.

Dosage: 400,000–800,000 U PO QID; IV doses vary greatly depending on indications, range from 1.2–24 million U/day.

Supplied: Tablets 200,000 U, 250,000 U, 400,000 U, 800,000 U; suspension 200,000 U/5 mL, 400,000 U/5 mL; powder for injection.

Notes and Caution: 400,000 U = 250 mg. Monitor patient for hypersensitivity reactions. Penicillin G is drug of choice for group A streptococcal infections and syphilis. High doses can cause seizures, especially in the presence of renal insufficiency.

■ Penicillin G Benzathine (Bicillin)

Indications: Useful as a single-dose treatment regimen for streptococcal pharyngitis, rheumatic fever and glomerulonephritis prophylaxis, as well as syphilis.

Actions: Bactericidal; inhibits cell wall synthesis.

Dosage: 1.2–2.4 million U, deep IM injection Q 2–4 weeks.

Supplied: Injection 300,000 U/mL, 600,000 U/mL.

Notes: Has sustained action with detectable levels up to 4 weeks; considered drug of choice for treatment of noncongenital syphilis. Bicillin L-A contains the benzathine salt only; Bicillin C-R contains a combination of benzathine and procaine salts and is used for most acute strep infections

(300,000 U procaine with 300,000 U benzathine/mL, or 900,000 U benzathine with 300,000 U procaine/2 mL). Intramuscularly administered penicillin more likely to cause anaphylactic reaction than oral penicillin.

■ Penicillin G Procaine (Wycillin, Others)

Indications: Moderately severe infections caused by penicillin G-sensitive organisms that respond to low persistent serum levels of penicillin (syphilis and uncomplicated pneumococcal pneumonia).

Actions: Bactericidal; inhibits cell wall synthesis.

Dosage: 300,000–1.2 million U/day IM, divided Q day–BID.

Supplied: Injection 300,000 units/mL, 500,000 units/mL, 600,000 units/mL.

Notes: A long-acting parenteral penicillin; provides measurable blood levels up to 15 hr. Give probenecid at least 30 min prior to administration of penicillin to prolong action. Intramuscularly administered pencillin more likely to cause anaphylactic reaction than oral pencillin.

■ Penicillin V (Pen-Vee K, Veetids, Others)

Indications: Most gram-positive infectious agents (except penicillin-resistant staphylococci), including streptococci, *N meningitidis, T pallidum,* clostridia, corynebacteria, and some coliforms.

Actions: Bactericidal; inhibits cell wall synthesis.

Dosage: 250–500 mg PO Q 6 hr.

Supplied: Tablets 125 mg, 250 mg, 500 mg; suspension 125 mg/5 mL, 250 mg/5 mL.

Notes: A well-tolerated oral penicillin; 250 mg = 400,000 U Pen G.

■ Pentamidine Isoethionate (Pentam 300, Nebupent)

Indications: Treatment and prevention of *Pneumocystis carinii* pneumonia.

Actions: Inhibits DNA, RNA, phospholipids and protein synthesis.

Dosage: IV treatment: 4 mg/kg/24 hr IV Q day for 14–21 days.

    Prevention: 300 mg once Q 4 weeks, administered via Respirgard II nebulizer.

Supplied: Injection 300 mg/vial; aerosol 300 mg.

Notes and Caution: Monitor patient for severe hypotension following IV administration. Drug is associated with pancreatic islet cell necrosis leading to hypoglycemia or hyperglycemia. Monitor for leukopenia and thrombocytopenia.

■ Pentazocine (Talwin) [C]

Indications: Moderate to severe pain.

Actions: Partial narcotic agonist-antagonist.

Dosage: 30 mg IM or IV; 50–100 mg PO Q 3–4 hr PRN.

Supplied: Tablets 50 mg (with naloxone 0.5 mg); injection 30 mg/mL.

Notes: 30–60 mg IM equianalgesic to 10 mg morphine IM. Drug is associated with considerable dysphoria.

■ Pentobarbital (Nembutal, Others) [C]
Indications: Insomnia, convulsions, induced coma following severe head injury.
Actions: Barbiturate; anxiolytic.
Dosage: *Sedative:* 20–40 mg PO or PR Q 6–12 hr.
      Hypnotic: 100–200 mg PO or PR Q HS PRN.
      Induced coma: Loading dose 3–5 mg/kg IV × 1; then maintenance 2–3.5 mg/kg/dose IV Q 1 hr PRN to keep level between 25–40 µg/mL.
Supplied: Capsules 50 mg, 100 mg; elixir 20 mg/5 mL; suppositories 30 mg, 60 mg, 120 mg, 200 mg; injection 50 mg/mL.
Notes and Caution: Drug can cause respiratory depression. May produce profound hypotension when given aggressively intravenously for cerebral edema. Tolerance to sedative-hypnotic effect acquired within 1–2 weeks.

■ Pentoxifylline (Trental)
Indications: Intermittent claudication.
Actions: Lowers blood cell viscosity by restoring erythrocyte flexibility.
Dosage: 400 mg PO TID with meals.
Supplied: Tablets 400 mg.
Note: Treat for at least 8 weeks to see full effect.

■ Pergolide (Permax)
Indications: Parkinson's disease.
Actions: Dopamine receptor agonist.
Dosage: Initial dose 0.05 mg PO TID, titrated Q 2–3 days to desired effect.
Supplied: Tablets 0.05 mg, 0.25 mg, 1.0 mg.
Notes: May cause hypotension during initiation of therapy.

■ Permethrin (Nix)
Indications: Infestation by lice.
Actions: Pediculicide.
Dosage: Saturate hair and scalp; allow to remain in hair for 10 min before rinsing.
Supplied: Liquid 1%.
Notes: Instruct patient to shampoo, rinse, and dry hair prior to treatment with permethrin; drug is not a shampoo.

■ Perphenazine (Trilafon)
Indications: Psychotic disorders, intractable hiccups, severe nausea.

Actions: Phenothiazine antipsychotic; antiemetic.

Dosage: *Antipsychotic:* 4–8 mg PO TID, maximum 64 mg/day.

Hiccups: 5 mg IM Q 6 hr PRN; OR 1 mg IV at not less than 1–2 mg/min intervals up to 5 mg.

Antiemetic: 5 mg IM Q 6 hr PRN. Do not exceed 15 mg in ambulatory or 30 mg in hospitalized patients.

Supplied: Tablets 2 mg, 4 mg, 6 mg, 16 mg; repetabs 8 mg; oral concentrate 16 mg/5 mL; injection 5 mg/mL.

■ Phenazopyridine (Pyridium, Others)

Indications: Symptomatic relief of discomfort from lower urinary tract irritation/infection.

Actions: Local anesthetic on urinary tract mucosa.

Dosage: 200 mg PO TID.

Supplied: Tablets 100 mg, 200 mg.

Notes: Side effects include GI disturbances. Drug discolors urine red–orange, which may stain clothing, bed linens, contacts, et al.

■ Phenobarbital [C]

Indications: Seizure disorders, insomnia, anxiety.

Actions: Barbiturate.

Dosage: *Sedative-hypnotic:* 30–120 mg PO or IM Q day PRN.

Anticonvulsant: Loading dose of 10–12 mg/kg in three divided doses; then 1–3 mg/kg/24 hr PO, IM, or IV.

Supplied: Tablets 8 mg, 15 mg, 30 mg, 60 mg, 100 mg; elixir 15 mg/5 mL, 20 mg/5 mL; injection 30 mg/mL, 60 mg/mL, 65 mg/mL, 130 mg/mL.

Notes: Tolerance develops to sedation. Paradoxical hyperactivity may be seen in pediatric patients. Long half-life allows single daily dosing. For drug levels, consult Table 7–13, p 536.

■ Phenylephrine (Neo-Synephrine)

Indications: Treatment of vascular failure in shock, hypersensitivity, or drug-induced hypotension; nasal congestion; mydriatic.

Actions: Alpha-adrenergic agonist.

Dosage: *Mild to moderate hypotension:* 2–5 mg IM or SC elevates BP for 2 hr; 0.1–0.5 mg IV elevates BP for 15 min.

Severe hypotension or shock: Initiate continuous infusion at 100–180 µg/min; after BP stabilized, maintenance rate of 40–60 µg/min.

Nasal congestion: 1–2 sprays into each nostril PRN.

Supplied: Injection 10 mg/mL; nasal solution 0.125%, 0.16%, 0.2%, 0.25%, 0.5%, 1%; ophthalmic solution 0.12%, 2.5%, 10%.

Notes and Caution: Promptly restore blood volume if volume loss has occurred. Use with extreme caution in patients with hyperthyroidism, bradycardia, partial heart block, myocardial disease, or severe arteriosclerosis. Use large veins for infusion to avoid extravasation; phentolamine 10 mg in 10–15 mL NSS may be injected locally as antidote for extravasation. Activity of drug is potentiated by oxytocin, MAOIs, and tricyclic antidepressants.

■ Phenytoin (Dilantin)

Indications: Tonic-clonic and partial seizures.

Actions: Inhibits seizure spread in motor cortex.

Dosage: Loading dose: 15–20 mg/Kg, IV infusion rate is usually 10–25 mg/min up to a maximum rate of 50 mg/min. Blood pressure should be checked Q 5 min three times then every 15 min till end of the infusion; OR PO in 400 mg doses Q 4 hr.

    Maintenance: 200 mg PO or IV BID; OR 100 mg TID (5–7 mg/kg/day) initially,then once seizure control is established with divided doses, once-a-day dosage of 300 mg Q HS can be considered. Then follow serum concentrations. Therapeutic range: 10–20 µg/mL.

Supplied: Capsules 30 mg, 100 mg; chewable tablets 50 mg; oral suspension 30 mg/5mL, 125 mg/5mL; injection 50 mg/mL.

Notes and Caution: Be alert for cardiac depressant side effects, especially with IV administration; follow levels as needed (Drug Levels, Table 7–13, p 536). Nystagmus and ataxia are early signs of toxicity; gum hyperplasia occurs with long-term use. Avoid use of oral suspension if possible because of erratic absorption. Dilantin is contraindicated in pregnancy. Phenytoin sodium contains 92% phenytoin.

■ Physostigmine (Antilirium)

Indications: Antidote for atropine and scopolamine overdose.

Actions: Reversible cholinesterase inhibitor.

Dosage: 2 mg IV/IM Q 15 min.

Supplied: Injection 1 mg/mL.

Notes: Rapid IV administration associated with convulsions. Drug has cholinergic side effects; may cause asystole.

■ Phytonadione [Vitamin K] (AquaMEPHYTON, Others)

Indications: Coagulation disorders caused by faulty formation of Factors II, VII, IX, and X; hyperalimentation.

Actions: Supplementation needed for the production of Factors II, VII, IX, and X.

Dosage: Anticoagulant-induced prothrombin deficiency: 1.0–10.0 mg PO; OR 0.5–10.0 mg IM, SC, or IV slowly.

    Hyperalimentation: 10 mg IM or IV Q week.

Supplied: Tablets 5 mg; injection 2 mg/mL, 10 mg/mL.

Notes: With parenteral treatment, prothrombin time will usually improve within 12–24 hr. Anaphylaxis can result from IV dosage; drug should therefore be administered *slowly* when this route is used.

■ **Pindolol (Visken) [See Table 7–6, p 529]**

■ **Piperacillin (Pipracil) [See Table 7–5, p 528]**

■ **Piperacillin/Tazobactam (Zosyn) [See Table 7–5, p 528]**

■ **Pirbuterol (Maxair)**
Indications: Prevention and reversal of bronchospasm.
Actions: Sympathomimetic.
Dosage: Two inhalations Q 4–6 hr, maximum of 12 inhalations/day.
Supplied: Aerosol 0.2 mg/actuation.

■ **Piroxicam (Feldene) [See Table 7–10, p 532]**

■ **Plasma Protein Fraction (Plasmanate, Others)**
Indications: Shock and hypotension.
Actions: Plasma volume expansion.
Dosage: Initial dose 250–500 mL IV (not > 10 mL/min); subsequent infusions should depend upon clinical response.
Supplied: Injection 5%.
Notes and Caution: Hypotension associated with rapid infusion. Preparation contains 130–160 mEq sodium per liter. Do *not* use as a substitute for red cells.

■ **Plicamycin (Mithracin)**
Indications: Treatment of hypercalcemia of malignancy.
Actions: Antibiotic; antineoplastic.
Dosage: 25 µg/kg/day IV for 3–4 days.
Supplied: Injection 2500 µg.

■ **Pneumococcal Vaccine, Polyvalent (Pneumovax-23)**
Indications: Immunization against pneumococcal infections in patients predisposed to or at high risk of acquiring these infections.
Actions: Active immunization.
Dosage: 0.5 mL IM.
Supplied: Injection, 25 µg each of polysaccharide isolates per 0.5 mL dose.
Notes: Do not vaccinate during immunosuppressive therapy; re-vaccinate every 6 years if high risk for loss of immunity (nephrotic syndrome, renal failure, status-post transplant) or highest risk for fatal pneumococcal infection (asplenia).

■ Polyethylene Glycol-Electrolyte Solution (GoLYTELY, CoLyte)
Indications: Bowel cleansing prior to examination or surgery.
Actions: Osmotic cathartic.
Dosage: Have patient fast for 3–4 hr; then administer PO 240 mL of solution Q 10 min until patient has consumed 4 L.
Supplied: Powder for reconstitution to 4 L in container.
Notes: First bowel movement should occur in ~1 hr; solution may cause some cramping or nausea.

■ Potassium Supplements
Indications: Prevention or treatment of hypokalemia.
Actions: Supplementation of potassium.
Dosage: 8–30 mEq PO Q day–BID.
Supplied:
Potassium chloride:

- Liquid: 20 mEq/15 mL, 30 mEq/15 mL, 40 mEq/15 mL.
- Powder packets: 15 mEq, 20 mEq, 25 mEq.
- Tablets CR: 6.7 mEq, 8 mEq, 10 mEq, 20 mEq.
- Capsules CR: 8 mEq, 10 mEq.

Potassium bicarbonate: Effervescent tablets: 20 mEq, 25 mEq, 50 mEq.
Notes and Caution: Potassium supplements can cause GI irritation. Powder and liquids must be mixed with beverage (unsalted tomato juice very palatable). Use cautiously in renal insufficiency, and along with NSAIDs and ACE inhibitors.

■ Pravastatin (Pravachol)
Indications: Reduction of elevated cholesterol levels.
Actions: HMG-CoA reductase inhibitor.
Dosage: 10–40 mg PO Q HS.
Supplied: Tablets 10 mg, 20 mg, 40 mg.
Notes: Avoid concurrent use with gemfibrozil.

■ Prazosin (Minipress)
Indications: Hypertension.
Actions: Peripherally acting alpha-adrenergic blocker.
Dosage: 1 mg PO TID; may be increased to a total daily dose of 5 mg QID.
Supplied: Capsules 1 mg, 2 mg, 5 mg.
Notes: Prazosin may cause orthostatic hypotension; therefore, patient should take first dose at bedtime; tolerance develops to this effect; tachyphylaxis may result.

■ Prednisolone (Delta-Cortef) [See Table 7–2, p 526]

■ Prednisone (Deltasone) [See Table 7–2, p 526]

■ Probenecid (Benemid, Others)
Indications: Gout; maintenance of serum levels of penicillins or cephalosporins.
Actions: Renal tubular blocking agent.
Dosage: Gout: 0.25 gm BID for 1 week; then 0.5 gm PO BID.
    Enhance antibiotic effect: 1–2 gm PO 30 min prior to dose of antibiotic.
Supplied: Tablets 500 mg.

■ Procainamide (Pronestyl, Procan)
Indications: Treatment of supraventricular and ventricular arrhythmias.
Actions: Class 1a antiarrhythmic.
Dosage: Emergency cardiac care: 100–200 mg/dose IV Q 5 min until dysrhythmia resolves, hypotension ensues, or dose totals 1 gm; then maintenance dose of 1–4 mg/min IV infusion.
    Chronic dosing: 50 mg/kg/day PO in divided doses Q 4–6 hr.
Supplied: Tablets and capsules 250 mg, 375 mg, 500 mg; SR tablets 250 mg, 500 mg, 750 mg, 1000 mg; injection 100 mg/mL, 500 mg/mL.
Notes: Drug can cause hypotension and an SLE-like syndrome. Dosage must be adjusted with renal impairment; see Drug Levels, Table 7–13, p 536.

■ Prochlorperazine (Compazine)
Indications: Nausea, vomiting, agitation, psychotic disorders.
Actions: Phenothiazine antiemetic and antipsychotic.
Dosage: Antiemetic: 5–10 mg PO TID–QID; OR 25 mg PR BID; OR 5–10 mg deep IM Q 4–6 hr.
    Antipsychotic: 10–20 mg IM in acute situations; OR 5–10 mg PO TID–QID for maintenance.
Supplied: Tablets 5 mg, 10 mg, 25 mg; SR capsules 10 mg, 15 mg, 30 mg; syrup 5 mg/5mL; suppositories 2.5 mg, 5 mg, 25 mg; injection 5 mg/mL.
Notes: Much larger dose may be required for antipsychotic effect. Extrapyramidal side effects are common. Treat acute extrapyramidal reactions with diphenhydramine.

■ Promethazine (Phenergan)
Indications: Nausea, vomiting, motion sickness.
Actions: Phenothiazine antihistamine, antiemetic.
Dosage: 12.5–50 mg PO, PR, or IM BID–QID PRN.
Supplied: Tablets 12.5 mg, 25 mg, 50 mg; syrup 6.25 mg/mL, 25 mg/mL; suppositories 12.5 mg, 25 mg, 50 mg; injection 25 mg/mL, 50 mg/mL.
Notes: Drug has high incidence of drowsiness.

■ Propafenone (Rythmol)
Indications: Treatment of life-threatening ventricular arrhythmias; treatment of atrial fibrillation.

Actions: Class Ic antiarrhythmic.

Dosage: 150–300 mg PO Q 8 hr.

Supplied: Tablets 150 mg, 300 mg.

Notes and Caution: Drug may cause dizziness, taste alterations, and first-degree heart block. May also cause prolongation of QRS and QT intervals.

■ Propantheline (Pro-Banthine)
Indications: Symptomatic treatment of small intestine hypermotility, spastic colon, ureteral spasm, bladder spasm, pylorospasm.

Actions: Antimuscarinic agent.

Dosage: 15 mg PO before meals and 30 mg PO HS.

Supplied: Tablets 7.5 mg, 15 mg.

Notes: Anticholinergic side effects such as dry mouth, blurred vision, etc., are common.

■ Propofol (Diprivan)
Indications: Induction or maintenance of anesthesia; continuous sedation in intubated patients.

Actions: Sedative-hypnotic.

Dosage: *Anesthesia:* 20–40 mg Q 10 min until onset of induction; then 50–200 µg/kg/min continuous infusion.

ICU sedation: 5–50 µg/kg/min continuous infusion.

Supplied: Injection 10 mg/mL.

Notes: 1 mL of propofol contains 0.1 gm fat; preparation may increase serum triglycerides when administered for extended periods of time.

■ Propoxyphene (Darvon, Darvocet) [C]
Indications: Mild to moderate pain.

Actions: Narcotic analgesic.

Dosage: 32–65 mg PO Q 4 hr PRN.

Supplied:

- Darvon (Propoxyphene HCl) 32 mg, 65 mg;
- Darvon-N (Propoxyphene Napsylate) 100 mg (= 65 mg of Propoxyphene HCl);
- Darvocet-N: Propoxyphene Napsylate/acetaminophen
- Darvon Compound: Propoxyphene HCl/aspirin/caffeine

Notes and Caution: Intentional overdose can be lethal. Drug interacts with alcohol and other CNS depressants.

■ Propranolol (Inderal) [See Table 7–6, p 529]

■ Propylthiouracil (PTU)

Indications: Hyperthyroidism.

Actions: Inhibits production of T_3 and T_4, and conversion of T_4 to T_3.

Dosage: Begin at 100 mg PO Q 8 hr (may need up to 1200 mg/day for control); after patient is euthyroid (6–8 weeks), taper dose by $1/3$ Q 4–6 weeks to a maintenance dose of 50–150 mg/24 hr. Treatment may usually be discontinued within 2–3 years.

Supplied: Tablets 50 mg.

Notes: Follow patient clinically; monitor thyroid function tests.

■ Protamine Sulfate

Indications: Reversal of heparin effect.

Actions: Antidote; neutralizes heparin.

Dosage: Based on amount of heparin reversal desired; given slow IV, 1 mg will reverse approximately 100 units of heparin given in the preceding 3–4 hr, to max dose of 50 mg.

Supplied: Injection 10 mg/mL.

Notes: Follow coagulation studies. Drug may have anticoagulant effect if given without heparin.

■ Pseudoephedrine (Sudafed, Novafed, Afrinol, Others)

Indications: Decongestant.

Actions: Sympathomimetic.

Dosage: 30–60 mg PO Q 6–8 hr; SR capsules 120 mg PO Q 12 hr.

Supplied: Tablets 30 mg, 60 mg; SR capsules 120 mg; liquid 15 mg/5mL; syrup 30 mg/5mL.

Notes: Contraindicated in patients with poorly controlled hypertension or coronary artery disease, and patients taking MAO inhibitors concurrently. Pseudoephedrine is an ingredient in many cough and cold preparations; may interact with OTC medications.

■ Psyllium (Metamucil, Serutan, Effer-Syllium)

Indications: Constipation, diverticular disease of the colon.

Actions: Bulk laxative.

Dosage: 1 tsp (7 gm) in a glass of water Q day–TID.

Supplied: Granules 4 gm/tsp, 25 gm/tsp; powder 3.5 gm/packet.

Notes and Caution: Psyllium is one of the safest laxatives. Do not, however, use if bowel obstruction is suspected. The effervescent (Effer-Syllium) form usually contains potassium and should be used with caution in patients with renal failure, or in patients taking potassium-sparing diuretics (spironolactone, triamterene) or angiotensin-converting enzyme inhibitors (ACE inhibitors) (captopril, enalapril, see Table 7–3, p 527).

■ Pyrazinamide
Indications: Treatment of active tuberculosis.
Actions: Bacteriostatic; precise mechanism is unknown.
Dosage: 20–35 mg/kg/24 hr PO, divided TID–QID; maximum dose is 3 gm/day.
Supplied: Tablets 500 mg.
Notes: May cause hepatotoxicity; use in combination with other antituberculosis drugs.

■ Pyridoxine (Vitamin B_6)
Indications: Treatment and prevention of vitamin B_6 deficiency.
Actions: Supplementation of vitamin B_6.
Dosage: *Deficiency:* 2.5–10.0 mg PO Q day.
  Drug-induced neuritis: 50 mg PO Q day.
Supplied: Tablets 10 mg, 25 mg, 50 mg, 100 mg, 200 mg, 250 mg, 500 mg; injection 100 mg/mL.

■ Quinapril (Accupril) [See Table 7–3, p 527]

■ Quinidine (Quinidex, Quinaglute)
Indications: Treatment of tachyarrhythmias.
Actions: Class 1a antiarrhythmic.
Dosage: *Premature atrial and ventricular contractions:* 200–300 mg PO TID–QID.

  Conversion of atrial fibrillation or flutter: use after digitalization, 200 mg Q 2–3 hr for eight doses; then increase daily dose to maximum of 3–4 gm or until normal rhythm is restored.
Supplied: *Sulfate:* Tablets 100 mg, 200 mg, 300 mg; capsules 200 mg, 300 mg; SR tablets 300 mg; injection 200 mg/mL.
  Gluconate: SR Tablets 324 mg, 330 mg; injection 80 mg/mL.
Notes and Caution: Contraindicated in digitalis toxicity or AV block; follow serum levels if available (Drug Levels, Table 7–13, p 536). Associated with a number of drug interactions. Extreme hypotension may occur with IV administration. Sulfate salt contains 83% quinidine; gluconate salt contains 62% quinidine. Quinidine increases conduction through the AV node; should therefore be used with a drug that slows conduction through the AV node such as digoxin, verapamil, diltiazem, or a beta-blocker. If used with digoxin, the digoxin dose may need to be reduced by as musch as 50% when quinidine is initiated because of quinidine's effect on digoxin metabolism.

■ Ramipril (Altace) [See Table 7–3, p 527]

■ Ranitidine (Zantac)
Indications: Duodenal ulcer, active benign ulcers, hypersecretory conditions, gastroesophageal reflux disease (GERD).

Actions: H_2 receptor antagonist
Dosage: *Ulcer:* 150 mg PO BID, 300 mg PO Q HS, or 50 mg IV Q 6–8 hr; OR 400 mg IV/day continuous infusion. Maintenance dose 150 mg PO Q HS.

> *Hypersecretion:* 150 mg PO BID.
> *GERD:* Initial dose 300 mg PO BID; maintenance 300 mg PO Q HS.

Supplied: Tablets 150 mg, 300 mg; syrup 15 mg/mL; injection 25 mg/mL.
Notes: Reduce dose with renal failure. Note that oral and parenteral doses different.

■ Rifabutin (Mycobutin)

Indications: Prevention of *Mycobacterium avium* complex (MAC) infection in late-stage HIV patients with a CD4 count <100.
Actions: Inhibits DNA-dependent RNA polymerase activity.
Dosage: 300 mg PO Q day.
Supplied: Capsules 150 mg.
Notes: Has adverse effects and drug interactions similar to those of rifampin.

■ Rifampin (Rifadin)

Indications: Tuberculosis; treatment and prophylaxis of *N meningitidis, H influenzae,* or *S aureus* carriers.
Actions: Inhibits DNA-dependent RNA polymerase activity.
Dosage: Exposure to *N meningitidis or H influenzae:* 600 mg PO Q day × 4 days.

> *Tuberculosis:* 600 mg PO or IV Q day; OR twice weekly. Use in combination with other antituberculosis drugs.

Supplied: Capsules 150 mg, 300 mg; injection 600 mg.
Notes: Drug has multiple side effects. Causes orange–red discoloration of bodily secretions, including tears. Rifampin should never be used as a single agent to treat active tuberculosis infections.

■ Rimantidine (Flumadine)

Indications: Prophylaxis and treatment of influenza A virus infections.
Actions: Antiviral agent.
Dosage: 100 mg PO BID.
Supplied: Tablets 100 mg; syrup 50 mg/5 mL.

■ Risperidone (Risperdal)

Indications: Management of psychotic disorders.
Actions: Benzisoxasole antipsychotic agent.
Dosage: 1–8 mg PO BID.
Supplied: Tablets 1 mg, 2 mg, 3 mg, 4 mg.

■ Salmeterol (Serevent)
Indications: Treatment of asthma and exercise-induced bronchospasm.
Actions: Sympathomimetic bronchodilator.
Dosage: Two inhalations BID.
Supplied: Metered-dose inhaler.
Notes and Caution: *Do not use* for acute bronchospasm.

■ Sargramostim [GM-CSF] (Prokine, Leukine)
Indications: Treatment of myeloid recovery following bone marrow transplantation.
Actions: Activates mature granulocytes and macrophages.
Dosage: 250 mg/m^2/day IV for 21 days.
Supplied: Injection 500 mg.
Notes: May cause bone pain.

■ Secobarbital (Seconal) [C]
Indications: Insomnia.
Actions: Rapid-acting barbiturate.
Dosage: 100 mg PO, or IM Q HS PRN.
Supplied: Capsules 50 mg, 100 mg; tablets 100 mg; injection 50 mg/mL.
Notes: Monitor patient for respiratory depression. Tolerance acquired within 1–2 weeks.

■ Selegiline (Eldepryl)
Indications: Parkinson's disease.
Actions: Inhibits monoamine oxidase activity.
Dosage: 5 mg PO BID.
Supplied: Tablets 5 mg.
Notes: May cause nausea and dizziness.

■ Sertraline (Zoloft)
Indications: Treatment of depression.
Actions: Inhibits neuronal uptake of serotonin.
Dosage: 50–200 mg PO Q day.
Supplied: Tablets 50 mg, 100 mg.
Notes and Caution: Sertraline can activate manic/hypomanic states. Has caused weight loss in clinical trials. Avoid concurrent use with astemizole and terfenadine.

■ Silver Sulfadiazine (Silvadene)
Indications: Prevention of sepsis in second- and third-degree burns.

Actions: Bactericidal.
Dosage: Aseptically cover affected area with 1/16-inch coating BID.
Supplied: Cream 1%.
Notes: Drug may be systemically absorbed from application site with extensive application.

■ Simethicone (Mylicon)
Indications: Symptomatic treatment of flatulence.
Actions: Defoaming action.
Dosage: 40–125 mg PO after meals and HS PRN.
Supplied: Tablets 40 mg, 80 mg, 125 mg; capsules 125 mg; drops 40 mg/0.6 mL.

■ Simvastatin (Zocor)
Indications: Reduction of elevated cholesterol levels.
Actions: HMG-CoA reductase inhibitor.
Dosage: 5–40 mg PO Q HS.
Supplied: Tablets 5 mg, 10 mg, 20 mg, 40 mg.
Notes: Avoid concurrent use with gemfibrozil.

■ Sodium Bicarbonate
Indications: Alkalinization of urine, treatment of metabolic acidosis. For severe metabolic acidosis (pH < 7.10), correct to a pH of bicarbonate of 10–15 mmol/L.
Dosage: Titrate to effect based on blood gases or urine pH.
Supplied: Injection 0.5 mEq/mL, 1 mEq/mL; tablets 325 mg, 650 mg.
Notes: 1 gr neutralizes 12 mEq of acid. A normal osmolar bicarbonate drip can be made by adding three ampoules of sodium bicarbonate (50 meq of HCO_3 in 50 ml) to 1 liter of D5W.

■ Sodium Polystyrene Sulfonate (Kayexalate)
Indications: Treatment of hyperkalemia.
Actions: Sodium and potassium ion exchange resin.
Dosage: 15–60 gm PO; OR 30–60 gm PR Q 6 hr based on serum K^+.
Supplied: Powder; suspension 15 gm/60 mL sorbitol.
Notes: Preparation can cause hypernatremia. Given with laxative such as sorbitol to promote movement through bowel.

■ Sorbitol
Indications: Constipation.
Actions: Laxative.
Dosage: 30–60 mL of a 20–70% solution PRN.
Supplied: Liquid 70%.

■ Sotalol (Betapace)

Indications: Treatment of ventricular arrhythmias.
Actions: Beta-adrenergic blocking agent.
Dosage: 80 mg PO BID; may be increased to 240–320 mg Q day.
Supplied: Tablets 80 mg, 160 mg, 240 mg.
Notes: Dosage should be adjusted for renal insufficiency.

■ Spironolactone (Aldactone)

Indications: Treatment of hyperaldosteronism, essential hypertension, edematous states (CHF, cirrhosis).
Actions: Aldosterone antagonist, potassium-sparing diuretic.
Dosage: 25–100 mg PO QID.
Supplied: Tablets 25 mg, 50 mg, 100 mg.
Notes: Drug can cause hyperkalemia and gynecomastia. Avoid prolonged use. Diuretic of choice for edema and ascites associated with cirrhosis.

■ SSKI

Indications: As an expectorant to help thin tenacious mucus in various pulmonary conditions; treatment of thyroid storm.
Actions: Enhances secretion of respiratory fluids, thus decreasing viscosity of mucus; blocks release of preformed thyroid hormone, to be given after medication to block synthesis (propylthiouracil or methimazole).
Dosage: 0.3–0.6 mL (300–600 mg) TID–QID diluted in water. Maximum dosage is 6 mL (6 g) Q day.
Thyroid storm: 5 drops Q 6 hr.
Supplied: Solution 1000 mg/mL.
Notes and Caution: Not for use during pregnancy as it may lead to fetal goiter. Drug interacts with lithium and antithyroid drugs to enhance hypothyroid effects. Thyroid function tests may be altered. Monitor patient for chronic iodine poisoning.

■ Stavudine (Zerit)

Indications: Treatment of adults with advanced HIV disease.
Actions: Reverse transcriptase inhibitor.
Dosage: Persons > 60 kg, 40 mg BID; persons < 60 kg, 30 mg BID.
Supplied: Capsules 15 mg, 20 mg, 30 mg, 40 mg.
Notes: Drug may cause peripheral neuropathy. Not a cure for HIV.

■ Steroids:

The following information relates only to the commonly used systemic glucocorticoids:
Indications:

- Endocrine disorders (adrenal insufficiency)
- Rheumatoid disorders

- Collagen-vascular diseases
- Atopic dermatitis and other skin eruptions
- Allergic states
- Edematous states (cerebral, nephrotic syndrome)
- Immunosuppression for transplantation
- Hypercalcemia
- Malignant neoplasms (breast, lymphomas)
- Preoperatively (in any patient who has been on steroids in the previous year, known hypoadrenalism, pre-op for adrenalectomy).

Dosage: Varies with indications and institutional protocols. Some commonly used dosages are listed here:

- *Acute adrenal insufficiency (Addisonian crisis):* Hydrocortisone 100 mg IV Q 8 hr.
- *Chronic adrenal insufficiency:* Hydrocortisone 20 mg PO Q AM, 10 mg PO Q PM; may need mineralocorticoid supplementation with Florinef (fludrocortisone acetate) or similar agent.
- *Perioperative steroid coverage:* Variable dosing; two typical regimens are as follows:
  1. Hydrocortisone 100 mg IV night prior to surgery, 1 hr pre-op, intraoperatively, and 4, 8, and 12 hr postoperatively; POD#1 100 mg IV Q 6 hr; POD#2 100 mg IV Q 8 hr; POD#3 100 mg IV Q 12 hr; POD#4 50 mg IV Q 12 hr; POD#5 25 mg IV Q 12 hr. Then resume prior oral dosing if steroids have been used chronically; discontinue if only perioperative coverage is required.
  2. Hydrocortisone 100 mg 1 hr pre-op, then 100 mg Q 6 hr for four doses, then 50 mg Q 6 hr for four doses, then 25 mg Q 6 hr for four doses, then 25 mg Q 8 hr for three doses, then 25 mg Q 12 hr for two doses. Then resume prior oral dosing if chronic dosing or discontinue if only perioperative coverage.
- *Cerebral edema:* Dexamethasone 10 mg IV; then 4 mg IV Q 4–6 hr.

Notes and Caution: See Table 7–2, p 526. All steroids may cause hyperglycemia and adrenal suppression. *Never* stop steroid treatment abruptly, especially if patient has been receiving chronic treatment; taper dose. Steroids may also cause hypokalemia, hypernatremia, hyperglycemia, hypertension, and osteoporosis.

■ Streptokinase (Streptase, Kabikinase)

Indications: Coronary artery thrombosis; acute massive pulmonary embolism; deep vein thrombosis; some occluded vascular grafts.

Actions: Activates plasminogen to plasmin that degrades fibrin.

Dosage: *Pulmonary embolus:* Loading dose of 250,000 IU IV through a peripheral vein over 30 min; then 100,000 U/hr IV for 24–72 hr.

    Coronary artery thrombosis: 1,500,000 U IV over 60 min.

    Deep vein thrombosis or arterial embolism: Load as with pulmonary embolus; then 100,000 U/hr for 72 hours.

Supplied: Powder for injection 250,000 U, 600,000 U, 750,000 U.

Notes: If maintenance infusion is not adequate to maintain thrombin clotting time 2–5 × control, refer to package insert, PDR, or Hospital Formulary Service for adjustments.

■ Streptomycin

Indications: Tuberculosis; bacterial endocarditis.

Actions: Aminoglycoside antibiotic; interferes with protein synthesis.

Dosage: 1-4 gm/day IM in 2–4 divided doses.

Supplied: Injection 400 mg/mL; powder for injection 1 g, 5 g.

Notes and Caution: Drug is nephrotoxic and ototoxic. Decrease dose in renal insufficiency. Availability may be limited. For tuberculosis always use in combination with other drugs.

■ Succimer (Chemet)

Indications: Treatment of lead poisoning.

Actions: Heavy metal chelating agent.

Dosage: Dosage is determined by the patient's weight:

- 8–15 kg 100 mg PO.
- 16–23 kg 200 mg PO.
- 24–34 kg 300 mg PO.
- 35–44 kg 400 mg PO.
- 45 kg 500 mg PO.

Give the above dose Q 8 hr for 5 days, then Q 12 hr for 14 days.

Supplied: Capsules 100 mg.

Notes: Preparation may cause rash. Instruct patient to increase fluid intake.

■ Succinylcholine (Anectine, Quelicin, Sucostrin)

Indications: Adjunct to general anesthesia to facilitate endotracheal intubation and to induce skeletal muscle relaxation during surgery or mechanically supported ventilation.

Actions: Depolarizing neuromuscular blocking agent.

Dosage: 0.6 mg/kg IV over 10–30 sec, followed by 0.04–0.07 mg/kg as needed to maintain muscle relaxation.

Supplied: Injection 20 mg/mL, 50 mg/mL, 100 mg/mL; powder for injection 100 mg, 500 mg, 1 gm per vial.

Notes and Caution: Drug may precipitate malignant hyperthermia; respiratory depression or prolonged apnea may also occur. Succinylcholine has many drug interactions potentiating its activity; monitor patient for cardiovascular effects. Use only freshly prepared solutions.

■ Sucralfate (Carafate)

Indications: Treatment of duodenal and gastric ulcers.

Actions: Forms ulcer-adherent complex that protects mucosa against stomach acid, pepsin, and bile.

Dosage: 1 gm PO QID, 1 hr before meals and HS.

Supplied: Tablets 1 gm; suspension 1 mg/10 mL.

Notes: Treatment should be continued for 4–8 weeks unless healing demonstrated by x-ray or endoscopy. Constipation is the most frequent side effect.

■ Sulfacetamide (Sodium Sulamyd, Bleph-10 Ophthalmic, Blephamide Ophthalmic) [See Table 7–11, pp 533 & 534]

■ Sulfasalazine (Azulfidine)
Indications: Ulcerative colitis.

Actions: Sulfonamide; precise antiinfective actions not clear.

Dosage: Initial dose 1–2 gm PO; increase to maximum of 8 gm/day in 3–4 divided doses; maintenance dose 500 mg PO QID.

Supplied: Tablets 500 mg; enteric-coated tablets 500 mg; oral suspension 250 mg/5 mL.

Notes: Drug can cause severe GI upset; discolors urine orange–yellow.

■ Sulfinpyrazone (Anturane)
Indications: Acute and chronic gout.

Actions: Inhibits renal tubular absorption of uric acid.

Dosage: 100–200 mg PO BID for 1 week; then increase as needed to maintenance of 200–400 mg BID.

Supplied: Tablets 100 mg; capsules 200 mg.

■ Sulindac (Clinoril) [See Table 7–10, p 532]

■ Sumatriptan (Imitrex)
Indications: Treatment of acute migraine attacks.

Actions: Vascular serotonin receptor agonist.

Dosage: 6 mg SC as a single dose; may be repeated in 1 hr, for a maximum dose of 12 mg per 24-hr period. Tablets: 25 mg–100 mg PO x 1, additional doses may be taken at 2 hr intervals up to a maximum daily dose of 300 mg.

Supplied: Injection 12 mg/mL; tablets 25 mg, 50 mg.

Notes: Drug may cause pain and bruising at injection site. Should not be used in patients with ischemic heart disease, uncontrolled hypertension, or patients receiving ergotamine preperations because of its potential to cause coronary vasospasm.

■ Tacrine (Cognex)
Indications: Treatment of mild to moderate dementia in Alzheimer's disease.
Actions: Cholinerase inhibitor.
Dosage: 10–40 mg PO QID.
Supplied: Capsules 10 mg, 20 mg, 30 mg, 40 mg.
Notes: May cause elevations in transaminase levels; LFTs should be monitored regularly. Drug may also cause GI distress.

■ Tacrolimus (Prograf) [FK-506]
Indications: Prophylaxis of organ rejection.
Actions: Macrolide immunosuppressant.
Dosage: IV: 0.05–0.1 mg/kg/day as continuous infusion.
  PO: 0.15–0.3 mg/kg/day divided into two doses.
Supplied: Capsules 1 mg, 5 mg; injection 5 mg/mL.
Notes: Drug may cause neurotoxicity and nephrotoxicity.

■ Tamoxifen (Nolvadex)
Indications: Treatment of breast cancer.
Actions: Antiestrogen antineoplastic.
Dosage: 10–20 mg PO BID.
Supplied: Tablets 10 mg, 20 mg.
Notes: Tamoxifen may increase the risk of secondary uterine cancer.

■ Temazepam (Restoril) [C]
Indications: Insomnia.
Actions: Benzodiazepine anxiolytic; sedative-hypnotic.
Dosage: 15–30 mg PO Q HS PRN.
Supplied: Capsules 15 mg, 30 mg.
Notes: Reduce dose in elderly. Instruct patient to avoid use of alcohol and other CNS depressants.

■ Teniposide (Vumon)
Indications: Treatment of leukemia.
Actions: Mitotic inhibitor.
Dosage: 165 mg/m^2 IV 2 $\times$ week for 8–9 doses.
Supplied: Injection 50 mg.

■ Terazosin (Hytrin)
Indications: Treatment of hypertension and benign prostatic hyperplasia.
Actions: Alpha$_1$-blocker.
Dosage: Initial dose 1 mg PO HS; titrate up to maximum of 20 mg PO Q HS.

Supplied: Tablets and capsules 1 mg, 2 mg, 5 mg, 10 mg.

Notes: Patient may experience hypotension and syncope following first dose; dizziness, weakness, nasal congestion, peripheral edema are common side effects.

■ Terbutaline (Brethine, Bricanyl)

Indications: Reversible bronchospasm (asthma, COPD); inhibition of labor.

Actions: Sympathomimetic; brochodilator.

Dosage: *Brochodilator:* 2.5–5 mg PO QID or 0.25 mg SC; may repeat in 15 min (maximum 0.5 mg in 4 hr). Two inhalations Q 4–6 hr via metered-dose inhaler.

Premature labor: 10–80 µg/min IV infusion for 4 hr; then 2.5 mg PO Q 4–6 hr until term.

Supplied: Tablets 2.5 mg, 5 mg; injection 1 mg/mL; metered-dose inhaler 200 mg/dose.

Notes: Use cautiously with diabetes, hypertension, hyperthyroidism; high doses may precipitate beta-1 adrenergic effects. Tolerance may develop with long-term use.

■ Terconazole (Terazol 7)

Indications: Vaginal fungal infections.

Actions: Topical antifungal.

Dosage: One applicatorful intravaginally Q HS for 7 days.

Supplied: Vaginal cream 0.4%.

■ Terfenadine (Seldane)

Indications: Seasonal allergic rhinitis.

Actions: Non-sedating antihistamine.

Dosage: 60 mg PO BID; children 3–5 yrs: 15 mg PO BID.

Supplied: Tablets 60 mg.

Notes and Caution: Life-threatening arrhythmias have been reported. Do *not* use concurrently with ketoconazole, itraconazole, the macrolide antibiotics or the selective serotonin reuptake inhibitor antidepressants (fluoxetine, paroxetine, and sertraline).

■ Tetanus Immune Globulin

Indications: Passive immunization against tetanus for any person with a suspected contaminated wound and unknown immunization status.

Actions: Passive immunization.

Dosage: 250–500 U IM (higher doses if initiation of therapy is delayed).

Supplied: Injection, 250-U vial or syringe.

Notes: Clinician may begin active immunization series at different injection site if required.

■ Tetanus Toxoid
Indications: Protection against tetanus.
Actions: Active immunization.
Dosage: 0.5 mL IM of tetanus-diphtheria toxoid.
Supplied: Injection: Tetanus toxoid, fluid 4–5 Lf U/0.5 mL; tetanus toxoid, adsorbed 5 Lf U/0.5 mL, 10 Lf U/0.5 mL.

■ Tetracycline (Achromycin V, Sumycin)
Indication: Broad-spectrum antibiotic, active against staphylococci, streptococci, chlamydiae, rickettsiae, and mycoplasma.
Actions: Interferes with protein synthesis.
Supplied: Capsules 100 mg, 250 mg, 500 mg; tablets 250 mg, 500 mg; oral suspension 250 mg per 5 mL.
Notes and Cautions: Do not use in pregnancy. *Do not use* in patients with impaired renal function; doxycycline (which can be taken with food) is preferred in most instances. Dairy products, antacids, laxatives or iron-containing products will impair absorption. Tetracycline may cause photosensitivity rash.

■ Theophylline (Theolair, Theo-Dur, Somophyllin, Others)
Indications: Asthma, bronchospasm.
Actions: Relaxes smooth muscle of the bronchi and pulmonary blood vessels.
Dosage: 12–20 mg/kg/day (typically do not exceed 900 mg/day). PO divided Q 6 hr; SR products may be divided Q 8–12 hr.
Supplied: Elixir 80 mg/15 mL, 150 mg/15 mL; liquid 80 mg/15 mL, 160 mg/15 mL; capsules 100 mg, 200 mg, 250 mg; tablets 100 mg, 125 mg, 200 mg, 225 mg, 250 mg, 300 mg; SR capsules 50 mg, 75 mg, 100 mg, 125 mg, 200 mg, 250 mg, 260 mg, 300 mg; SR tablets 100 mg, 200 mg, 250 mg, 300 mg, 400 mg, 450 mg, 500 mg.
Notes: See Drug Levels, Table 7–13, p 536. Theophylline has many drug interactions; side effects include nausea, vomiting, tremor, tachycardia, and seizures.

■ Thiamine (Vitamin B₁)
Indications: Thiamine deficiency (beriberi); alcoholic neuritis; Wernicke's encephalopathy.
Actions: Dietary supplementation.
Dosage: Deficiency: 100 mg IM Q day for 2 weeks; then 5–10 mg PO Q day for 1 month.
          Wernicke's encephalopathy: 100 mg IV × 1 dose, then 100 mg IM Q day for 2 weeks.
Supplied: Tablets 5 mg, 10 mg, 25 mg, 50 mg, 100 mg, 500 mg; injection 100 mg/mL, 200 mg/mL.

Notes: IV thiamine administration may be associated with anaphylactic reaction. Drug must be given slowly IV.

■ Thiethylperazine (Torecan)
Indications: Nausea and vomiting.
Actions: Antidopaminergic antiemetic.
Dosage: 10 mg PO, PR or IM Q day–TID.
Supplied: Tablets 10 mg; suppositories 10 mg; injection 5 mg/mL.
Notes: Extrapyramidal reactions may occur.

■ Thioridazine (Mellaril)
Indications: Psychotic disorders; short-term treatment of depression, agitation, organic brain syndrome.
Actions: Phenothiazine antipsychotic.
Dosage: Initial dose 50–100 mg PO TID; maintenance dose 200–800 mg/24 hr PO in 2–4 divided doses.
Supplied: Tablets 10 mg, 15 mg, 25 mg, 50 mg, 100 mg, 150 mg, 200 mg; oral concentrate 30 mg/mL, 100 mg/mL; oral suspension 25 mg/5 mL, 100 mg/5 mL.
Notes: Low incidence of extrapyramidal effects. Instruct patient to avoid use of alcohol.

■ Thiotepa (TSPA)
Indications: Treatment of breast and ovarian cancer.
Actions: Alkylating agent.
Dosage: 0.3–0.4 mg/kg IV at 1–4 week intervals.
Supplied: Injection 15 mg.

■ Thiothixene (Navane)
Indications: Psychotic disorders.
Actions: Phenothiazine antipsychotic.
Dosage: *Mild to moderate psychosis:* 2 mg PO TID.
     Severe psychosis: 5 mg PO BID; increase to maximum dose of 60 mg/24 hr PRN.
     IM administration: 16–20 mg/24 hr divided BID–QID; maximum 30 mg/day.
Supplied: Capsules 1 mg, 2 mg, 5 mg, 10 mg, 20 mg; oral concentrate 5 mg/mL; injection 2 mg/mL, 5 mg/mL.
Notes and Caution: Drowsiness and extrapyramidal side effects most common. Warn patient to avoid concurrent use of alcohol and other CNS depressants.

■ Ticarcillin (Ticar) [See Table 7–5, p 528]

■ Ticarcillin/Potassium Clavulanate (Timentin) [See Table 7–5, p 528]

■ Ticlopidine (Ticlid)
Indications: Reduction of risk of thrombotic stroke.
Actions: Platelet aggregation inhibitor.
Dosage: 250 mg PO BID.
Supplied: Tablets 250 mg.
Notes: Instruct patient to take with food. Ticlopidine may cause severe neutropenia. Regular monitoring of CBC and white cell differential essential during first 3 months of therapy.

■ Timolol (Blocadren) [See Table 7–6, p 529]

■ Timolol (Timoptic) [See Table 7–11, pp 533 & 534]

■ Tioconazole (Vagistat)
Indications: Vaginal fungal infections.
Actions: Topical antifungal agent.
Dosage: One applicatorful intravaginally Q HS (single dose).
Supplied: Vaginal ointment 6.5%.

■ Tobramycin (Nebcin)
Indications: Serious gram-negative infections, especially *Pseudomonas*.
Actions: Aminoglycoside antibiotic; inhibits protein synthesis.
Dosage: Loading dose of 1.5–2.0 mg per kg; then 2–5 mg per kg per 24 hr IV, divided Q 8–24 hr based on renal function. Refer to Aminoglycoside Dosing, Table 7–15, p 537. **OR:** give 7 mg per kg per 24 hr as a single dose (3 mg per kg if creatinine clearance < 40 mg/min per 1.73 m^2).
Supplied: Injection 10 mg/mL, 40 mg/mL.
Notes: Drug is nephrotoxic and ototoxic. Decrease dose with renal insufficiency; monitor creatinine clearance and serum concentrations for dosage adjustments. See Drug Levels, Table 7–14, p 536.

■ Tocainide (Tonocard)
Indications: Suppression of ventricular arrhythmias including premature ventricular contractions and ventricular tachycardia.
Actions: Class 1b antiarrhythmic.
Dosage: 400–600 mg PO Q 8 hr.
Supplied: Tablets 400 mg, 600 mg.
Notes: Has properties similar to lidocaine; reduce dose in renal failure. CNS and GI side effects common.

■ Tolazamide (Tolinase) [See Table 7–12, p 535]

■ Tolbutamide (Orinase) [See Table 7–12, p 535]

■ Tolmetin (Tolectin) [See Table 7–10, p 532]

■ Torsemide (Demadex)
Indications: Edema, hypertension, congestive heart failure, and hepatic cirrhosis.
Actions: Loop diuretic.
Dosage: 5–20 mg PO or IV once Q day.
Supplied: Tablets 5 mg, 10 mg, 20 mg, 100 mg; injection 10 mg/mL.

■ Tramadol (Ultram)
Indications: Management of moderate to severe pain.
Actions: Centrally acting analgesic.
Dosage: 50–100 mg PO Q 4–6 hr PRN, not to exceed 400 mg/day.
Supplied: Tablets 50 mg.

■ Trazodone (Desyrel)
Indications: Major depression.
Actions: Antidepressant.
Dosage: 50–150 mg PO Q day–QID; maximum 600 mg/day.
Supplied: Tablets 50 mg, 100 mg, 150 mg.
Notes: Symptomatic improvement may take 1–2 weeks. Drug has anticholinergic side effects. Drug should be discontinued prior to elective surgery.

■ Triazolam (Halcion) [C]
Indications: Insomnia.
Actions: Benzodiazepine anxiolytic; sedative-hypnotic.
Dosage: 0.125–0.5 mg PO Q HS PRN.
Supplied: Tablets 0.125 mg, 0.25 mg, 0.5 mg.
Notes: Additive CNS depression with alcohol and other CNS depressants. Patients may develop tolerance with long-term use.

■ Trifluoperazine (Stelazine)
Indications: Psychotic disorders.
Actions: Phenothiazine antipsychotic.
Dosage: 2–10 mg PO BID.
Supplied: Tablets 1 mg, 2 mg, 5 mg, 10 mg; oral concentrate 10 mg/mL; injection 2 mg/mL.
Notes: Decrease dosage in elderly and debilitated patients. Oral concentrate must be diluted to 60 mL or more prior to administration.

■ Trihexyphenidyl (Artane)
Indications: Parkinsonism.
Actions: Anticholinergic; antispasmodic.
Dosage: 2–5 mg PO Q day–QID.
Supplied: Tablets 2 mg, 5 mg; SR capsules 5 mg; elixir 2 mg/5 mL.
Notes: Contraindicated in narrow-angle glaucoma. Dry mouth is common side effect.

■ Trimethobenzamide (Tigan)
Indications: Nausea and vomiting.
Actions: Antihistamine antiemetic.
Dosage: 250 mg PO or 200 mg PR or IM TID–QID PRN.
Supplied: Capsules 100 mg, 250 mg; suppositories 100 mg, 200 mg; injection 100 mg/mL.
Notes: Drug may contribute to Reye's syndrome in the presence of viral infections. May also cause parkinson-like syndrome.

■ Trimethoprim (Trimpex, Proloprim)
Indications: Urinary tract infections caused by susceptible gram-positive and gram-negative bacteria. Often used for suppression.
Actions: Inhibits dihydrofolate reductase.
Dosage: 100 mg PO BID; OR 200 mg PO Q day.
Supplied: Tablets 100 mg, 200 mg.
Notes: Reduce dose in renal failure. If creatinine clearance 15–30 mL per min, give ½ dose. Drug has not been well studied with creatinine clearance < 15 mL per min.

■ Trimethoprim-Sulfamethoxazole (Co-Trimoxazole, Bactrim, Septra)
Indications: Urinary tract infections, otitis media, sinusitis, bronchitis; infections caused by *Shigella, Pneumocystis carinii, Nocardia* .
Actions: Dual effect of sulfamethoxazole-inhibiting synthesis of dihydrofolic acid and trimethoprim-inhibiting dihydrofolate reductase to cause impaired protein synthesis.
Usual Dosage: One double-strength (DS) tablet PO BID; OR 5–10 mg/kg/24 hr (based on trimethoprim component) IV in 3–4 divided doses.
  Pneumocystis carinii: 15–20 mg/kg/day IV or PO (trimethoprim component) in four divided doses.
  Nocardia: 10–15 mg per kg IV or PO in four divided doses.
Supplied: Tablets: Regular 80 mg TMP and 400 mg SMX, DS 160 mg TMP and 800 mg SMX; oral suspension 40 mg TMP and 200 mg SMX per 5 mL; injection 80 mg TMP and 400 mg SMX per 5 mL.
Notes: Synergistic combination; reduce dosage in renal failure.

■ Trimetrexate (Neutrexin)
Indications: Treatment of moderate to severe *Pneumocystis carinii* pneumonia.

Actions: Inhibits dihydrofolate reductase.
Dosage: 45 mg/m^2 IV Q 24 hr for 21 days.
Supplied: Injection: lyphilized powder 25 mg.
Notes: Trimetrexate *must* be administered with leucovorin 20 mg/m^2 IV Q 6 hr for 24 days; use cytotoxic precautions.

■ Trimipramine (Surmontil)
Indications: Treatment of depression.
Actions: Tricyclic antidepressant.
Dosage: 75–300 mg PO Q HS.
Supplied: Capsules 25 mg, 50 mg, 100 mg.
Notes: Orthostatic hypotension and dry mouth are common side effects.

■ Urokinase (Abbokinase)
Indications: Pulmonary embolism, deep venous thrombosis, restoration of patency to IV catheters.
Actions: Converts plasminogen to plasmin that causes clot lysis.
Dosage: Systemic effect: 4400 U/kg IV over 10 min, followed by 4400 U/kg/hr for 12 hr.
     Catheter patency: Inject 5000 U into catheter and aspirate gently.
Supplied: Powder for injection 5000 U/mL, 250,000 U/5 mL vial.
Notes: Do not use systemically within 10 days of surgery, delivery, or organ biopsy.

■ Valacyclovir (Valtrex)
Indications: Treatment of herpes zoster.
Actions: Prodrug of acyclovir; inhibits viral DNA replication.
Dosage: 1 gm PO TID.
Supplied: Caplets 500 mg.

■ Valproic Acid and Divalproex (Depakene and Depakote)
Indications: Absence seizures; in combination for tonic/clonic seizures.
Actions: Anticonvulsant; precise mechanism unknown.
Dosage: 30–60 mg/kg/24 hr PO divided TID.
Supplied: Valproic acid: Capsules 250 mg; syrup 250 mg/5 mL. *Divalproex:* Enteric-coated tablets 125 mg, 250 mg, 500 mg.
Notes: Monitor liver functions and follow serum levels (see Drug Levels, Table 7–13, p 536). Concurrent use of phenobarbital and phenytoin may alter serum levels of these agents.

■ Vancomycin (Vancocin, Vancoled)
Indications: Serious infections due to methicillin-resistant staphylococci, enterococcal endocarditis in combination with aminoglycosides and

serious gram-positive infections in penicillin-allergic patients; oral treatment of *C difficile* pseudomembranous colitis.

Actions: Inhibits cell wall synthesis.

Dosage: 1 gm IV Q 12 hr with normal renal function, for pseudomembranous colitis 250–500 mg PO Q 6 hr.

Supplied: Capsules 125 mg, 250 mg; powder for oral solution; powder for injection 500 mg, 1000 mg, 10 gm per vial.

Notes: Drug is nephrotoxic, ototoxicity has been reported, reversible neutropenia can occur; not absorbed orally, provides local effect in gut only. IV dose must be given slowly over 1 hr to prevent "red-man syndrome." Adjust dose in renal failure. See Drug Levels, Table 7–14, p 536.

■ Varicella Virus Vaccine (Varivax)

Indications: Prevention of varicella infection.

Actions: Active immunization.

Dosage: 0.5 mL SC, repeated in 4–8 weeks.

Supplied: Powder for injection.

Notes and Caution: Vaccine contains live virus; **do not** administer to immunocompromised patients. May cause mild varicella infection.

■ Vasopressin (Antidiuretic hormone) (Pitressin)

Indications: Treatment of diabetes insipidus; relief of gaseous GI tract distention; severe GI bleeding.

Actions: Posterior pituitary hormone, potent GI vasoconstrictor.

Dosage: *Diabetes insipidus:* 2.5–10 U SC or IM TID–QID; OR 1.5–5.0 U IM Q 1–3 days of vasopressin tannate.

GI hemorrhage: 20 U in 50–100 cc D5W or NS given IV over 15–30 min.

Supplied: Injection 20 U/mL.

Notes: Use with caution with any vascular disease. Do not administer vasopressin tannate IV. Tannate is preferred for chronic therapy.

■ Vecuronium (Norcuron)

Indications: Skeletal muscle relaxation during surgery or mechanical ventilation.

Actions: Nondepolarizing neuromuscular blocker.

Dosage: 0.08–0.1 mg/kg IV bolus; maintenance dose of 0.010–0.015 mg/kg after 25–40 min, followed with additional doses Q 12–15 min.

Supplied: Powder for injection 10 mg.

Notes: Drug interactions leading to increased effect of vecuronium include aminoglycosides, tetracycline, and succinylcholine. Drug has fewer cardiac effects then pancuronium.

■ Venlafaxine (Effexor)

Indications: Treatment of depression.

Actions: Potentiation of CNS neurotransmitter activity.

Dosage: 75–225 mg/day divided into 2–3 equal doses.
Supplied: Tablets 25 mg, 37.5 mg, 50 mg, 75 mg, 100 mg.

■ Verapamil (Calan, Isoptin)
Indications: Treatment of angina, essential hypertension, and arrhythmias.
Actions: Calcium channel blocker.
Dosage: Arrhythmias: 5–10 mg IV over 2 min (may repeat in 30 min); 240–480 mg/day PO in 3–4 divided doses.
     Angina: 80–120 mg PO TID.
     Hypertension: SR tablet 120–240 mg PO Q day to 240 mg BID.
Supplied: Tablets 40 mg, 80 mg, 120 mg; SR tablets 120 mg, 180 mg, 240 mg; capsules 120 mg; capsules SR 240 mg; injection 5 mg/2 mL.
Notes and Caution: Use with caution with elderly patients. Reduce dose in renal failure. Constipation is a common side effect.

■ Vinblastine (Velban)
Indications: Treatment of Hodgkin's disease; lymphoma; testicular and ovarian cancer.
Actions: Mitotic inhibitor.
Dosage: Varies with individual protocol.
Supplied: Injection 1 mg/mL.
Notes: May cause severe leukopenia and mucositis. Extravasation causes tissue necrosis.

■ Vincristine (Oncovin)
Indications: Treatment of cervical and ovarian cancer, sarcoma, leukemia, and Hodgkin's disease.
Actions: Mitotic inhibitor.
Dosage: 1.4–2 mg/m^2 IV once Q week.
Supplied: Injection 1 mg/mL.
Notes and Caution: May cause severe neurotoxicity. *Never administer vincristine intrathecally. Extravasation causes tissue necrosis.*

■ Vitamin B$_1$: See *Thiamine*

■ Vitamin B$_6$: See **Pyridoxine**

■ Vitamin B$_{12}$: See **Cyanocobalamin**

■ Vitamin K: See **Phytonadione**

■ Warfarin Sodium (Coumadin)
Indications: Prophylaxis and treatment of pulmonary embolism and venous thrombosis, atrial fibrillation with embolization, cerebral thrombosis and embolization, prevention of thrombosis of artificial heart valves.

Actions: Inhibits vitamin K-dependent production of clotting factors in the order: VII–IX–X–II.

Dosage: Dosage should be individualized to keep international normalized ratio (INR) 2.0–3.0 for most indications; for mechanical heart valves desired INR is 2.5–3.5. INR is the preferred laboratory test rather than the ratio of the patients prothrombin time (PT) to control. See Section 2, Laboratory and Diagnosis, p 320. Initial dose is 5–10 mg PO, or IV Q day for 1–2 days; then maintenance dose of 2–10 mg PO, or IV Q day (range may extend from 0.5 mg every other day to 15–20 mg Q day); follow daily PT/INR during initial phase to guide dosage.

Supplied: Tablets 2 mg, 2.5 mg, 5 mg, 7.5 mg, 10 mg; powder for injection 50 mg/vial.

Notes and Cautions: PT must be checked periodically while on maintenance dose; monitor patient for bleeding caused by over-anticoagulation (PT > 3 × control or INR > 5.0–6.0). Caution patient on effects of taking Coumadin with other medications, especially aspirin. To correct over-coumadinization rapidly, use intravenous vitamin K (10 mg) or fresh frozen plasma or both. Coumadin is highly teratogenic; do not use in pregnancy.

■ Zalcitabine (Hivid)

Indications: Management of patients with HIV infection who are intolerant of zidovudine and didanosine.

Actions: Antiretroviral agent.

Dosage: 0.75 mg PO TID.

Supplied: Tablets 0.375 mg, 0.75 mg.

Notes: May be used in combination with zidovudine. May cause peripheral neuropathy.

■ Zidovudine (Retrovir)

Indications: Management of patients with HIV infection.

Actions: Inhibits reverse transcriptase.

Dosage: 100 mg PO 5 times Q day; or 200 mg PO TID; or 1–2 mg/kg/dose IV Q 4 hr.

Pregnancy: 100 mg PO 5 times Q day until the start of labor; then during labor 2 mg/kg IV over 1 hr followed by 1 mg/kg/hr until clamping of the umbilical cord.

Supplied: Capsules 100 mg; syrup 50 mg/5 mL; injection 10 mg/mL.

Note: Not a cure for HIV infection.

■ Zolpidem (Ambien) [C]

Indications: Short-term treatment of insomnia.

Actions: Hypnotic agent.

Dosage: 5–10 mg PO Q HS PRN.

Supplied: Tablets 5 mg, 10 mg.

Notes: Should not be administered for more than 7–10 days. Instruct patient to avoid use of alcohol.

TABLE 7–1. INSULINS.

Type of insulin	Onset (h)	Peak (h)	Duration (h)	Compatible to Mix With
■ Rapid-acting				
Regular Iletin II	0.5–1	5–10	6–8	All
Humulin R	0.5–1	5–10	6–8	All
Novolin R	0.5–1	5–10	6–8	All
■ Intermediate-acting				
NPH Iletin II	1–1.5	4–6	24	Regular
Humulin N	1–1.5	4–6	24	Regular
Novolin N	1–1.5	4–6	24	Regular
Lente Iletin II	1–2.5	7.5	24	Regular, Semilente
■ Long-acting				
Humulin U	4–8	10–30	36	Regular
Ultralente	4–8	10–30	36	Regular
■ Combinations				
Humulin 70/30	0.5	4–8	24	
Novolin 70/30	0.5	4–8	24	

TABLE 7–2. COMPARISON OF GLUCOCORTICOIDS.

Drug (Trade)	Equivalent Dose (mg)	Anti-inflammatory Potency	Mineralocorticoid Potency
■ Short-acting			
Cortisone (Cortone)	25	0.8	2
Hydrocortisone (Cortef)	20	1	2
■ Intermediate-acting			
Methylprednisoline (Medrol)	4	5	0
Prednisone (Deltasone)	5	4	1
Prednisolone (Delta-Cortef)	5	4	1
■ Long-acting			
Betamethasone (Celestone)	0.6–0.75	20–30	0
Dexamethasone (Decadron)	0.75	20–30	0

TABLE 7–3. ANGIOTENSIN-CONVERTING ENZYME INHIBITORS.[1]

Drug (Trade)	Hypertension	Heart Failure	Left Ventricular Dysfunction
Benazepril (Lotensin)	10–40 mg/day divided qd-bid		
Captopril (Capoten)	25–50 mg bid-tid	6.25–25 mg tid	Titrate to 50 mg tid
Enalapril (Vasotec)	5–40 mg/day divided qd-bid	2.5–10 mg bid	Titrate to 10 mg bid
Fosinopril (Monopril)	10–40 mg qd	10–40 mg qd	
Lisinopril (Prinivil, Zestril)	10–40 mg qd	5–20 mg qd	
Moexipril (Univasc)	7.5–30 mg/day divided qd-bid		
Quinapril (Accupril)	10–80 mg qd	5–20 mg bid	
Ramipril (Altace)	2.5–20 mg/day divided qd-bid	1.25–5 mg bid	

[1] **Notes:**
1. Pro-drugs (metabolized to active agent): Benazepril, Enalapril, Fosinopril, Moexipril, Quinapril, Ramipril.
2. Persistent, nonproductive cough has occurred with the use of *all* ACE inhibitors. Cough typically resolves within one to four days after therapy is discontinued. Angiotensin-II receptor inhibitor (Losarten) does not have cough as a potential side-effect.
3. Co-administration of ACE inhibitors with potassium preparations may result in elevated serum potassium concentrations.
4. Strictly contraindicated in pregnancy. Women of child-bearing age should be warned regarding risk of teratogenicity and use of ACE inhibitors.

TABLE 7–4. ANTISTAPHYLOCOCCAL PENICILLINS.[1, 2]

Drug (Brand)	Dosage	Dosing Interval	Supplied	Notes
Oxacillin (Bactocill)	1–2 gm	4–6 hr	Injection	
Nafcillin (Nafcil, Unipen)	1–2 gm	4–6 hr	Injection	No dosage adjustments for renal function
Cloxacillin (Cloxapen, Tegopen)	250–500 mg	6 hr	Oral	Administer on an empty stomach
Dicloxacillin (Dynapen, Dycill)	250–500 mg	6 hr	Oral	Administer on an empty stomach

[1] **Indications:** Treatment of infections caused by susceptible strains of *Staphylococcus* and *Streptococcus*.
[2] **Actions:** Bactericidal; inhibits cell wall synthesis.

TABLE 7–5. EXTENDED-SPECTRUM PENICILLINS.[1, 2, 3]

Drug (Brand)	Dose	Dosing Interval	mEq Na$^+$ Per Gram	Notes
Ticarcillin (Ticar)	3 gm	4–6 hr	5.2	May cause hypokalemia/ sodium overload, acquired platelet dysfunction with the potential for bleeding to occur
Ticarcillin-clavulanate (Timentin)	3.1 gm	4–6 hr	4.75	Clavulanate is a beta-lactamase inhibitor
Mezlocillin (Mezlin)	3 gm	4–6 hr	1.85	Activity against Enterobacteriacae
Piperacillin (Pipracil)	3 gm	4–6 hr	1.85	Best activity against *Pseudomonas*
Piperacillin-tazobactam (Zosyn)	3.375 gm	6 hr		Tazobactam is a beta-lactamase inhibitor (Does not improve activity against *Pseudomonas* when compared to piperacillin without tazobactam)

[1] *Indications:* Treatment of infections caused by susceptible gram-negative bacteria (including *Klebsiella, Proteus, E. coli, Enterobacter, P. aeruginosa, Serratia*) involving the skin, bone and joints, respiratory tract, urinary tract, abdomen and vascular system.

[2] *Actions:* Bactericidal, inhibits cell wall synthesis.

[3] *Notes:* These agents are often used in combination with an aminoglycoside to treat *P. aeroginosa* and in neutropenic patients with a fever. Dosage adjustment necessary in renal impairment.

TABLE 7–6. BETA-ADRENERGIC BLOCKING AGENTS.

Drug (Trade)	Receptor	Angina	Hypertension	Myocardial infarction
Acebutolol (Sectral)	B₁, ISA		200–400 mg BID	
Atenolol (Tenormin)	B₁	50–100 mg QD	50–100 mg QD	5 mg IV X 2 doses, then 50 mg PO BID
Betaxolol (Kerlone)	B₁		10–20 mg QD	
Bisoprolol (Zebeta)	B₁		5–10 mg QD	
Carteolol (Cartrol)	B₁, B₂, ISA		2.5–5 mg QD	
Carvedilol (Coreg)	B₁,, B₂, α		6.25–25 mg BID	
Labetalol (Trandate, Normodyne)	B₁, B₂, α₁		100–400 mg BID	
Metoprolol (Lopressor, Toprol XL)	B₁	50–100 mg BID	100–450 mg QD	5 mg IV X 3 doses, then 50 mg PO q6h X 48 hr, then 100 mg PO BID
Nadolol (Corgard)	B₁, B₂	40–80 mg QD	40–80 mg QD	
Penbutolol (Levatol)	B₁, B₂		20–40 mg QD	
Pindolol (Visken)	B₁, B₂, ISA		5–10 mg BID	
Propranolol (Inderal)	B₁, B₂	160 mg SR QD	120–160 mg SR QD	60 mg TID-QID
Sotalol (Betapace)	See p 519			
Timolol (Blocadren)	B₁, B₂		10–20 mg BID	10 mg BID

Notes: ISA = intrinsic sympathomimetic activity

Other Uses:	Cardiac Arrythmias:	Various agents and doses
	Migraine Prophylaxis:	Atenolol 50–100 mg/d
		Nadolol 40–80 mg/d
		[1]Propranolol 80–240 mg/d
	Essential Tremor:	Propranolol 40 mg BID; maximal dose 320 mg/day
	Adjunctive Therapy:	Pheochromocytoma (after alpha-adrenergic drugs are added)
		Hyperthyroidism (propranolol)
		Rebleeding of esophageal varices in cirrhotic patients
		Alcohol withdrawal (atenolol)

[1] FDA-approved indication

Precautions:
1. Use with caution in diabetic patients. May blunt symptoms/signs of acute hypoglycemia; nonselective agents may potentiate insulin-induced hypoglycemia. Beta-blockade also reduces the release of insulin in response to hyperglycemia.
2. May increase serum lipid concentrations. May not be as pronounced with agents having intrinsic sympathomimetic activity.
3. Use with caution in patients with congestive heart failure (decreased myocardial contractility) and chronic obstructive pulmonary disease (potential blockade of B₂ receptors).
4. When discontinuing chronically administered beta-blockers, particularly in patients with ischemic heart disease, reduce dose gradually, especially with agents with a short half-life (propranolol, metoprolol).

TABLE 7–7. FIRST-GENERATION CEPHALOSPORINS.[1, 2, 3]

Drug (Brand)	Dose	Dosing Interval	Supplied	Notes
Cefadroxil (Duricef, Ultracef)	500 mg–1 gm	12–24 hr	Capsules, tablets	
Cefazolin (Ancef, Kefzol)	1–2 gm	8 hr	Injection	For surgical prophylaxis most widely used antibiotic
Cephalexin (Keflex)	250–500 mg	QID	Capsules, tablets	
Cephalothin (Keflin)	1–2 gm	6 hr	Injection	
Cephapirin (Cefadyl)	1–2 gm	6 hr	Injection	
Cephradine (Velosef)	250–500 mg	QID	Capsules	
	1 gm	6 hr	Injection	

[1] *Indications:* Treatment of infections caused by susceptible strains of *Streptococcus, Staphylococcus, E. coli, Proteus,* and *Klebsiella* involving the skin, bone and joints, upper and lower respiratory tract, and urinary tract.
[2] *Actions:* Bactericidal; inhibits cell wall synthesis.
[3] *Dosage adjustment* necessary in renal impairment.

TABLE 7–8. SECOND-GENERATION CEPHALOSPORINS.[1, 2, 3]

Drug (Brand)	Dose	Dosing Interval	Supplied	Notes
Cefaclor (Ceclor)	250–500 mg	8 hr	Capsules	Good activity against *H influenzae*
Cefamandole (Mandol)	1–2 gm	4–6 hr	Injection	
Cefmetazole (Zefazone)	1–2 gm	8 hr	Injection	Activity against anaerobes
Cefonicid (Monocid)	1–2 gm	24 hr	Injection	
Cefotetan (Cefotan)	1–2 gm	12 hr	Injection	Activity against anaerobes
Cefoxitin (Mefoxin)	1–2 gm	6 hr	Injection	Best activity against anaerobes
Cefprozil (Cefzil)	250–500 mg	QD–BID	Tablets	Use higher doses for otitis and pneumonia
Cefuroxime (Zinacef, Ceftin)	750 mg–1.5 gm	8 hr	Injection	Ceftin should be taken with food
	250–500 mg	BID	Tablets	
Loracarbef (Lorabid)	200–400 mg	BID	Capsules	Similar to cefaclor

[1] *Indications:* Treatment of infections caused by susceptible bacteria involving the upper and lower respiratory tract, skin, bone, urinary tract, abdomen, and female reproductive system.
[2] *Actions:* Bactericidal; inhibits cell wall synthesis.
[3] *Notes:* More active than 1st-generation agents against *H. influenzae, E. coli, Klebsiella* species and *P. mirabilis.* Risk of hypoprothrombinemia or bleeding has been associated with cephalosporins containing the N-methylthiotetrazole (NMTT) side chain. These agents include cefotetan, cefamandole and cefoperazone (3rd-generation). Administration of vitamin K will prevent clinical bleeding associated with these drugs. Dosage adjustment necessary in renal impairment.

TABLE 7–9. THIRD-GENERATION CEPHALOSPORINS.[1, 2, 3]

Drug (Brand)	Dose	Interval	Supplied	Notes
Cefixime (Suprax)	200–400 mg	12–24 hr	Tablets, suspension	Use suspension for otitis media
Cefoperazone (Cefobid)	1–2 gm	12 hr	Injection	Administer Vitamin K with cefoperazone
Cefotaxime (Claforan)	1–2 gm	4–8 hr	Injection	Crosses the blood-brain barrier
Cefpodoxime (Vantin)	200–400 mg	12 hr	Tablets	Drug interactions with agents increasing the gastric pH
Ceftazidime (Fortax, Ceptaz) (Tazidine, Tazicef)	1–2 gm	8 hr	Injection	Best activity against *Pseudomonas.* Crosses the blood-brain barrier
Ceftizoxime (Cefizox)	1–2 gm	8–12 hr	Injection	
Ceftriaxone (Rocephin)	1–2 gm	12–24 hr	Injection	Treatment of choice for gonorrhea. Crosses the blood-brain barrier.

[1] *Indications:* Treatment of infections caused by susceptible bacteria involving the respiratory tract, skin, bone and joints, urinary tract; treatment of meningitis, febrile neutropenia and septicemia.

[2] *Actions:* Bactericidal; inhibits cell wall synthesis.

[3] *Notes:* Less active against gram-positive cocci than 1st- and 2nd-generation agents. Increased activity against gram-negative aerobes (Enterobacteriaceae including *Enterobacter* and *Serratia*) due to increased stability to beta-lactamases. May be used in combination with an aminoglycoside. Dosage adjustment necessary in renal impairment.

TABLE 7–10. NONSTEROIDAL ANTI-INFLAMMATORY DRUGS.

Drug (Trade)	Arthritis	Analgesia	Dysmenorrhea	Maximum Daily Dose (mg)
■ Acetic acids				
Diclofenas (Cataflam, Voltaren)	50–75 mg bid-tid	50 mg tid	50 mg tid	200
Etodolac (Lodine)	200–400 mg bid-tid	200–400 mg q6–8h		1200
Indomethacin (Indocin)	25–50 mg bid-tid			200 SR: 150
Ketorolac (Toradol)		IV/IM 15–30 mg q6h PO: 10 mg q6h		IV:120; PO 40 Max 5 days therapy
Nabumetone (Relafen)	1000–2000 mg/day divided qd–bid			2000
Sulindac (Clinoril)	150–200 mg bid			400
Tolmetin (Tolectin)	200–600 mg tid			2000
■ Oxicams				
Piroxicam (Feldene)	10–20 mg qd			20
■ Propionic acids				
Fenoprofen (Nalfon)	300–600 mg tid-qid	200 mg q4–6h		3200
Flurbiprofen (Ansaid)	50–100 mg bid-qid			300
Ibuprofen (Advil, Motrin)	400–800 mg tid-qid	400 mg q4–6h	400 mg q4h	3200
Ketoprofen (Orudis)	50–75 mg tid-qid	25–50 mg q6–8h		300
Naproxen (Naprosyn)	250–500 mg bid	250 mg q6–8h	250 mg q6–8h	1500
Naproxen sodium (Aleve, Anaprox)	275–550 mg bid	275 mg q6–8h	275 mg q6–8h	1375
Oxaprozin (Daypro)	600–1200 mg qd			

TABLE 7–11. OPHTHALMIC AGENTS.

Drug (Trade)	Strength (%)	Dosing Schedule
■ **Agents for glaucoma**		
Sympathomimetics		
Apraclonidine (Iopidine)	1.0	1 gtt in operative eye 1 hr prior to surgery
Dipivefrin (Propine)	0.1	1 gtt q 12 hr
Beta-Blockers		
Betaxolol (Betoptic-S, Betoptic)	0.25, 05	1 gtt bid
Levobunolol (Betagan Liquifilm)	0.25, 0.5	1 gtt qd-bid
Metipranolol (OptiPranolol)	0.3	1 gtt bid
Timolol (Timoptic)	0.25, 0.5	1 gtt qd-bid
Miotics, Direct-Acting		
Acetylcholine (Miochol)	1.0	Used only for miosis during surgery
Carbachol (Isopto Carbachol)	0.75–3	1–2 gtts tid
Pilocarpine (Isopto Carpine, Pilocar)	0.25–10	1–2 gtts up to 6 × per day
(Pilopine HS gel)	4.0	0.5 inch HS
Miotics, Cholinesterase Inhibitors		
Physostigmine (Isopto Eserine)	0.25, 0.5	2 gtts up to qid
Demecarium (Humorsol)	0.125, 0.25	1–2 gtts twice weekly, up to 1–2 gtts bid

(continued)

TABLE 7–11. *(Continued)*

Drug (Trade)	Strength (%)	Dosing Schedule
■ Antibiotics		
Chloramphenicol (AK-Chlor)	oint/sol	1–2 gtts or 0.5 inch q 3–4 hr
Ciprofloxacin (Ciloxin)	solution	1–2 gtts 4–6 × per day
Erythromycin (AK-Mycin, Ilotycin)	ointment	0.5 inch 2–8 × per day
Gentamicin (Garamycin)	oint/sol	1–2 gtts or 0.5 inch 2–3 × per day, up to q 3–4 hr
Neomycin, Polymyxin B, Hydrocortisone 1% (Cortisporin)	sus	1–2 gtts q 3–4 hr
Sulfacetamide Sodium (Sodium Sulamyd, Bleph 10)	10–30% oint/sol	1–2 gtts q 1–3 hr or 0.5 inch qd-qid
Tobramycin (Tobrex)	oint/sol	1–2 gtts or 0.5 inch 2–3 × per day, up to q 3–4 hr
■ Anti-inflammatory		
NSAIDS		
Diclofenac (Voltaren)	0.1%	1 gtt qid (Tx of post-op inflammation following cataract surgery)
Ketorolac (Acular)	0.5%	1 gtt qid (Relief of ocular itching due to season allergic conjunctivitis)
Corticosteroids		
Prednisolone (AK-Pred, Pred Forte)	0.12%, 0.125%, 1.0%	1–2 gtt q 1 hr during day & q 2 hr at night till favorable response, than 1 gtt q 4 hr

TABLE 7–12. SULFONYLUREAS.[1, 2]

Drug (Trade)	Duration of Activity (hr)	Equivalent Dose (mg)	Dosing Schedule
■ First-generation			
Acetohexamide (Dymelor)	24	500	250–1500 mg qd
Chlorpropamide (Diabinese)	≥60	250	100–500 mg qd
Tolazamide (Tolinase)	12–24	250	100–500 mg qd
Tolbutamide (Orinase)	6–12	1000	500–1000 mg bid
■ Second-generation			
Glipizide[3] (Glucotrol, Glucotrol-XL)	10–16	10	5–15 mg qd-bid
Glyburide non-micronized[4] (DiaBeta, Micronase)	24	5	1.25–10 mg qd-bid
Glyburide micronized[4] (Glynase)	24	3	1.5–6 mg qd-bid

[1] *Indications:* Management of non-insulin-dependent diabetes mellitus (NIDDM).

[2] *Actions:* Stimulates the release of insulin from the pancreas; increases insulin sensitivity at peripheral sites; reduces glucose output from the liver.

[3] *Glipizide:* Give approximately 30 minutes before a meal. Divide total daily doses when doses exceed 15 mg. Maximum daily recommended daily dose is 40 mg.

[4] *Glyburide:* Administer with first main meal. Maximum recommended daily dose: non-micronized, 20 mg; micronized, 12 mg.

TABLE 7–13. DRUG LEVELS.[1]

Drug	Therapeutic Level	Toxic Level
Carbamazepine	8.0–12.0 µg/mL	>15.0 µg/mL
Digoxin	0.8–2.0 ng/mL	>2.4 ng/mL
Ethanol		>100 mg/100 mL (legally intoxicated in most states)
		100–200 mg/100 mL labile
		150–300 mg/100 mL (confusion)
		250–400 mg/100 mL (stupor)
		350–500 mg/100 mL (coma)
		>450 mg/100 mL (death)
Ethosuximide	40–100 µg/mL	>150 µg/mL
Lidocaine	1.5–6.5 µg/mL	>6.0–8.0 µg/mL
Lithium	0.6–1.2 mmol/L	>2.0 mmol/L
Phenobarbital	15.0–40.0 µg/mL	>45.0 µg/mL
Phenytoin	10.0–20.0 µg/mL	>25.0 µg/mL
Procainamide N-acetylprocainamide (NAPA-active metabolite of procainamide)	4.0–10.0 µg/mL	>16.0 µg/mL
Quinidine	3.0–5.0 µg/mL	>7 µg/mL
Salicylate	20–30 µg/mL	40–50 µg/dL
Theophylline	10.0–20.0 µg/mL	>20.0 µg/mL
Valproic acid	50–100 µg/mL	>150 µg/mL

Note: Each lab may have its own set values that vary slightly from those given.
[1] Modified and reproduced with permission from Gomella LG, ed: *Clinician's Pocket Reference.* 7th ed.: Appleton & Lange; 1993.

TABLE 7–14. DRUG LEVELS: ANTIBIOTICS.[1]

Antibiotic	Trough (µg/mL) (Maintain Below Upper Limit)	Peak (µg/mL)
Amikacin	5.0–7.5	25–35
Gentamicin	1.0–2.0	5–8
Gentamicin (24-hour dosing with normal renal function)	1.0–2.0	>10
Tobramycin	1.0–2.0	5–8
Tobramycin (24-hour dosing with normal renal function)	1.0–2.0	>10
Vancomycin	5.0–10.0	20–40

[1] Modified and reproduced with permission from Gomella LG, ed: *Clinician's Pocket Reference.* 7th ed.: Appleton & Lange; 1993.

TABLE 7–15. FOR 8- OR 12-HOUR AMINOGLYCOSIDE DOSING IN ADULTS[1] (FOR Q DAY DOSING OF GENTAMICIN AND TOBRAMYCIN SEE PAGES 466 AND 428 RESPECTIVELY).

1. Select the loading dose:
   Gentamicin 1.5–2.0 mg/kg
   Tobramycin 1.5–2.0 mg/kg
   Amikacin   5.0–7.5 mg/kg

2. Calculate the estimated creatinine clearance (CrCl) based on serum creatinine (SCr), age, and weight (kg); OR order a formal creatinine clearance, if time permits.

$$\text{CrCl for male} = \frac{(140 - \text{age}) \times (\text{weight in kg})}{(\text{ScCr}) \times (72)} \times 100.$$

   CrCl for female = $0.85 \times$ (CrCl male)

3. By using Table 7–16 you can now select the maintenance dose (as a percentage of the chosen loading dose) most appropriate for the patient's renal function based on CrCl and dosing interval. Shaded areas are the percentages and intervals suggested for any given creatinine clearance. For patients over 60 years old, it is recommended to give the dose no more frequently than every 12 hours.

4. Empiric dosing, as above, is used to begin therapy. Serum levels (see Table 7–14, p 536) should be monitored and adjustments made in the dosing based on the drug levels for optimal therapy.

Note: See Table 7–14, p 536, for the trough and peak levels of the aminoglycosides gentamicin, tobramycin, and amikacin. Peak levels should be drawn 30 minutes after the dose is completely infused; trough levels should be drawn 30 minutes prior to the dose. As a general rule, draw the peak and trough around the fourth maintenance dose. Therapy can be initiated with the recommended guidelines. **These calculations are not valid for netilmicin.**

[1] Modified and reproduced with permission from Gomella LG, ed: *Clinician's Pocket Reference.* 7th ed.: Appleton & Lange; 1993.

TABLE 7–16. PERCENTAGE OF LOADING DOSE REQUIRED FOR DOSAGE INTERVAL SELECTED.[1]

Creatinine Clearance (mL/min)	Dosing Interval (hr)		
	8	12	24
90	90%	—	—
80	88	—	—
70	84	—	—
60	79	91%	—
50	74	87	—
40	66	80	—
30	57	72	92%
25	51	66	88
20	45	59	83
15	37	50	75
10	29	40	64
7	24	33	55
5	20	28	48
2	14	20	35
0	9	13	25

Note: Shaded areas indicate suggested dosage intervals.
[1] Reproduced with permission from Hull JH, Sarubbi FA: Gentamicin serum concentrations: Pharmacokinetic predictions. *Ann Inter Med* 1976; 85:183–189.

Appendix

Contents

TABLE A–1. TEMPERATURE CONVERSION.[1]

°F	°C	°C	°F
95.0	35.0	35.0	95.0
96.0	35.5	35.5	95.9
97.0	36.1	36.0	96.8
98.0	36.6	36.5	97.7
98.6	37.0	37.0	98.6
99.0	37.2	37.5	99.5
100.0	37.7	38.0	100.4
101.0	38.3	38.5	101.3
102.0	38.8	39.0	102.2
103.0	39.4	39.5	103.1
104.0	40.0	40.0	104.0
105.0	40.5	40.5	104.9
106.0	41.1	41.0	105.8
$°C = (°F - 32) \times 5/9$		$°F = (°C \times 9/5) + 32$	

[1] Modified and reproduced with permission from Gomella LG, ed: *Clinician's Pocket Reference.* 7th ed.: Appleton & Lange; 1993.

TABLE A–2. POUNDS AND KILOGRAMS WEIGHT CONVERSION.[1]

lb	kg	kg	lb
1	0.5	1	2.2
2	0.9	2	4.4
4	1.8	3	6.6
6	2.7	4	8.8
8	3.6	5	11.0
10	4.5	6	13.2
20	9.1	8	17.6
30	13.6	10	22.0
40	18.2	20	44.0
50	22.7	30	66.0
60	27.3	40	88.0
70	31.8	50	110.0
80	36.4	60	132.0
90	40.9	70	154.0
100	45.4	80	176.0
150	68.2	90	198.0
200	90.8	100	220.0
$kg = lb \times 0.454$		$lb = kg \times 2.2$	

[1] Reproduced with permission from Gomella LG, ed: *Clinician's Pocket Reference.* 7th ed.: Appleton & Lange; 1993.

TABLE A–3. GLASGOW COMA SCALE.[1]

Parameter	Response		Score
Eyes	Open	Spontaneously	4
		To verbal command	3
		To pain	2
		No response	1
Best motor response	To verbal command	Obeys	6
	To painful stimulus	Localizes pain	5
		Flexion-withdrawal	4
		Decorticate (flex)	3
		Decerebrate (extend)	2
		No response	1
Best verbal response		Oriented, converses	5
		Disoriented, converses	4
		Inappropriate responses	3
		Incomprehensible sounds	2
		No response	1

Note: The Glasgow Coma Scale (EMV Scale) is a fairly reliable, objective way to monitor changes in levels of consciousness. It is based on eye opening, motor responses, and verbal responses (EMV). A person's EMV score is based on the total of the three different responses. The score ranges from 3 (lowest) to 15 (highest).

[1] Modified and reproduced with permission from Gomella LG, ed: *Clinician's Pocket Reference.* 7th ed.: Appleton & Lange; 1993.

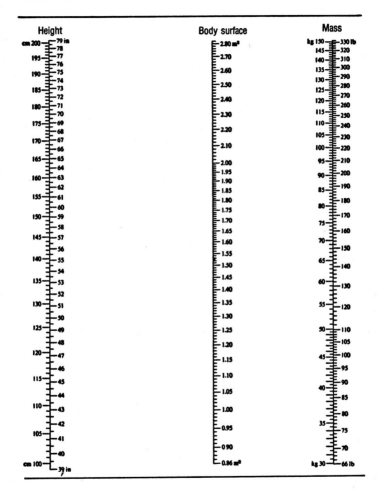

Figure A–1. Body surface area. To determine the body surface of an adult, use a straight-edge to connect height and mass. The point of intersection in the body surface line gives the body surface area in meters squared (m²). (From Lentner C. ed. *Gelgy Scientific Tables*. 8th ed. Basel: CIBA Glegy; 1981:vol 1. p 227.)

TABLE A–4. ENDOCARDITIS PROPHYLAXIS.[1]

	Dosage for Adults
■ **Dental and upper respiratory procedures[2]**	
Oral[3]	
Amoxicillin[4]	3 g 1 h before procedure and 1.5 g 6 h late
Penicillin allergy: Erythromycin	1 g 2 h before procedure and 500 mg 6 h later
Parenteral[3,5]	
Ampicillin	2 g IM or IV 30 min before procedure
plus	
Gentamicin	1.5 mg/kg IM or IV 30 min before procedure
Penicillin allergy: Vancomycin	1 g IV infused *slowly over 1 h* beginning 1 h before procedure
■ **Gastrointestinal and genitourinary procedures[2]**	
Oral[3]	
Amoxicillin[4]	3 g 1 h before procedure and 1.5 g 6 h later
Parenteral[3,5]	
Ampicillin	2 g IM or IV 30 min before procedure
plus	
Gentamicin	1.5 mg/kg IM or IV 30 min before procedure
Penicillin allergy: Vancomycin	1 g IV infused *slowly over 1 h* beginning 1 h before procedure
plus	
Gentamicin	1.5 mg/kg IM or IV 30 min before procedure

[1] For patients with previous endocarditis, valvular heart disease, prosthetic heart valves, most forms of congenital heart disease (but not uncomplicated secundum atrial septal defect), idiopathic hypertrophic subaortic stenosis, and mitral valve prolapse with regurgitation are the most common cause of endocarditis after dental or upper respiratory procedures; enterococci are the most common cause of endocarditis after gastrointestional or genitourinary procedures. Reproduced with permission from Med Lett 1989; 31:112.

[2] For a review of the risk of bacteremia and endocarditis with various procedures, see Durack DT, Prophylaxis of Infection Endocarditis. In: Mandell GL, Bennett JE, Dolin R, eds. *Principles and Practice of Infectious Disease.* 4th ed., New York: Churchill Livingstone; 1995: 793–799.

[3] Oral regimens are more convenient and safer. Parenteral regimens are more likely to be effective; they are recommended especially for patients with prosthetic heart valves, those who have had endocarditis previously, or those taking continuous oral penicillin for rheumatic fever prophylaxis.

[4] Amoxicillin is recommended because of its excellent bioavailability and good activity against streptococci and enterococci.

[5] A single dose of parenteral drugs is probably adequate, because bacteremia after most dental and diagnostic procedures is of short duration. An additional dose may be given 8 hours later in patients judged to be at higher risk.

TABLE A–5. SPECIMENS TUBES FOR VENIPUNCTURE.[1]

Tube Color	Additives	General Use
Red	None	Clot tube to collect serum for chemistry, cross-matching, serology
Red and black (hot pink)	Silicone gel for rapid clot	As above, but not for osmolality or blood bank work
Blue	Sodium citrate (binds calcium)	Coagulation studies (best kept on ice, not for fibrin split products)
Blue/yellow label		Fibrin split products
Royal blue		Heavy metals, arsenic
Purple	Disodium EDTA (binds calcium)	Hematology, not for lipid profiles
Green	Sodium heparin	Ammonia, cortisol, ionized calcium (best kept on ice)
Green/glass beads		LE prep
Gray	Sodium fluoride	Lactic acid
Yellow	Transport medium	Blood cultures

Note: Individual labs may vary slightly from these listings.

[1] Reproduced with permission from Gomella LG, Lefor AT: *Surgery On Call.* 2nd ed.: Appleton & Lange; 1996.

Index

NOTE: A *t* following a page number indicates tabular material and an *f* following a page number indicates a figure. Drugs are listed under their generic names. When a drug trade name is listed, the reader is referred to the generic name.